BIOMEDICAL IMAGING

BIOMEDICAL IMAGING

Principles and Applications

Edited by

REINER SALZER

WILEY

A JOHN WILEY & SONS, INC., PUBLICATION

Published by John Wiley & Sons, Inc., Hoboken, New Jersey
Published simultaneously in Canada

Library of Congress Cataloging-in-Publication Data:

Biomedical imaging : principles and applications / [edited by] Reiner Salzer.
p. ; cm.
ISBN 978-0-470-64847-6 (hardback)
I. Salzer, Reiner, 1942–
[DNLM: 1. Diagnostic Imaging. 2. Spectrum Analysis. WN 180]

616.07′54–dc23

2011042654

Printed in the United States of America
10 9 8 7 6 5 4 3 2 1

CONTENTS

PREFACE

Biomedical imaging is improving healthcare and helps selecting the most efficient therapy. Imaging technologies provide snapshots of biomarkers and diseases such as cancer. Imaging can take this information even a step further, showing the activity of these markers *in vivo* and how their location changes over time. Advances in experimental and clinical imaging are likely to enable doctors not only to locate and delineate the disease but also to assess the activity of the biological processes and to provide localized treatment. New imaging technologies are increasingly being used to understand the biological complexity, diversity, and the *in vivo* behaviour. Imaging is considered an important bridge between basic research and bed-side application.

A wide range of technologies is already available for *in vivo*, *ex vivo*, and *in vitro* imaging. The introduction of new imaging instrumentation requires the combination of know-how in medicine and biology, in data processing, in engineering, and in science. Biologists and MDs are interested in technical basics and methods of measurement. Engineers need detailed descriptions of the biomedical basis of the measured data. Scientists want more background information on instrumentation and measurement techniques. Different imaging modalities always have specific strengths and weaknesses. For each modality, the basics of how it works, important information parameters, and the state-of-the-art instrumentation are described in this book. Examples of imaging applications are presented.

X-rays, gamma rays, radiofrequency signals, and ultrasound waves are standard probes, but others such as visible and infrared light, microwaves, terahertz rays, and intrinsic and applied electric and magnetic fields are being explored. Some of the younger technologies, such as molecular imaging, may enhance existing imaging modalities; however, they also, in combination with nanotechnology, biotechnology, bioinformatics, and new forms of computational hardware and software, may well lead to novel approaches to clinical imaging. This review provides a brief overview of the current state of image-based diagnostic medicine and offers comments on the directions in which some of its subfields may be heading.

Visualization can augment our ability to reason about complex data, thereby increasing the efficiency of manual analyses. In some cases, the appropriate image makes the solution obvious. The first two chapters give an overview of existing methods and tools for visualization and highlight some of their limitations and challenges. The next chapters describe technology and applications of established imaging modalities such as X-ray imaging, CT (Computed Tomography), MRI (Magnetic Resonance Imaging), and tracer imaging. The final part deals with imaging technologies using light (fluorescence imaging, infrared and Raman imaging, CARS microscopy) or sound (biomedical sonography and acoustic microscopy).

Thanks go to all authors for their efforts and commitments to the publication of this volume. The support by the publisher WILEY in the final composition and edition of the book should be acknowledged as well. The greatest debt of gratitude goes to our families for their patience and encouragement.

CONTRIBUTORS

Jürgen Bereiter-Hahn, Institut für Zellbiologie und Neurowissenschaft, Johann-Wolfgang-Goethe-Universität, Frankfurt/M, Germany

Stefan Bernet, Department für Physiologie und Medizinische Physik, Medizinische Universität Innsbruck, Innsbruck, Austria

Christian Brackmann, Department of Chemical and Biological Engineering, Chalmers University of Technology, Göteborg, Sweden

Lutgarde M.C. Buydens, Radboud University Nijmegen, Institute for Molecules and Materials, Department of Analytical Chemistry/Chemometrics, Nijmegen, The Netherlands

Nikolaos C. Deliolanis, Institute for Biological and Medical Imaging (IBMI), Helmholtz Zentrum München and Technische Universität München, Munich, Germany

Annika Enejder, Department of Chemical and Biological Engineering, Chalmers University of Technology, Göteborg, Sweden

Thomas Flohr, Computed Tomography Department, Siemens Healthcare, Forchheim, Germany

Christoph Heinrich, Department für Physiologie und Medizinische Physik, Medizinische Universität Innsbruck, Innsbruck, Austria

Volker Hietschold, Department of Radiology, University Hospital, "Carl Gustav Carus," Dresden, Germany

Rainer Hinz, Wolfson Molecular Imaging Centre, University of Manchester, Manchester, UK

Karen A. Jansen, Department of Molecular Cell Biology, Leiden University Medical Center, Leiden, The Netherlands

Abraham J. Koster, Department of Molecular Cell Biology, Leiden University Medical Center, Leiden, The Netherlands

Patrick W.T. Krooshof, Radboud University Nijmegen, Institute for Molecules and Materials, Department of Analytical Chemistry/Chemometrics, Nijmegen, The Netherlands

Willem J. Melssen, Radboud University Nijmegen, Institute for Molecules and Materials, Department of Analytical Chemistry/Chemometrics, Nijmegen, The Netherlands

Vasilis Ntziachristos, Institute for Biological and Medical Imaging (IBMI), Helmholtz Zentrum München and Technische Universität München, Munich, Germany

Geert J. Postma, Radboud University Nijmegen, Institute for Molecules and Materials, Department of Analytical Chemistry/Chemometrics, Nijmegen, The Netherlands

Monika Ritsch-Marte, Department für Physiologie und Medizinische Physik, Medizinische Universität Innsbruck, Innsbruck, Austria

Reiner Salzer, Department of Chemistry and Food Chemistry, Technische Universität Dresden, Dresden, Germany

Georg Schmitz, Department for Electrical Engineering and Information Technology, Medical Engineering, Ruhr-University, Bochum, Germany

Christian P. Schultz, Siemens Medical and Center for Molecular Imaging Research, Massachusetts General Hospital, Charlestown, MA, USA

Jonathan C. Sharp, Institute for Biodiagnostics (West), National Research Council of Canada, Calgary, AB, Canada

Gerald Steiner, Clinical Sensoring and Monitoring, Medical Faculty Carl Gustav Carus, Dresden University of Technology, Dresden, Germany

Boguslaw Tomanek, Institute for Biodiagnostics (West), National Research Council of Canada, Calgary, AB, Canada

Stefan Ulzheimer, Computed Tomography Department, Siemens Healthcare, Forchheim, Germany

Jack A. Valentijn, Department of Molecular Cell Biology, Leiden University Medical Center, Leiden, The Netherlands

Karine M. Valentijn, Department of Molecular Cell Biology, Leiden University Medical Center, Leiden, The Netherlands

Jörg van den Hoff, Department of Positron Emission Tomography, Institute of Radiopharmacy, Helmholtz-Zentrum Dresden-Rossendorf, Dresden, Germany

Linda F. van Driel, Department of Molecular Cell Biology, Leiden University Medical Center, Leiden, The Netherlands

1

EVALUATION OF SPECTROSCOPIC IMAGES

PATRICK W.T. KROOSHOF, GEERT J. POSTMA, WILLEM J. MELSSEN, AND LUTGARDE M.C. BUYDENS

Radboud University Nijmegen, Institute for Molecules and Materials, Department of Analytical Chemistry/Chemometrics, Nijmegen, The Netherlands

1.1 INTRODUCTION

Many sophisticated techniques are currently used for an accurate recognition and diagnosis of different diseases. Advanced imaging techniques are useful in studying medical conditions in a noninvasive manner. Common imaging methodologies to visualize and study anatomical structures include Computed Tomography (CT, Chapter 4), Magnetic Resonance Imaging (MRI, Chapter 5), and Positron Emission Tomography (PET, Chapter 7). Recent developments are focused on understanding the molecular mechanisms of diseases and the response to therapy. Magnetic Resonance Spectroscopy (MRS) (Section 5.12), for example, provides chemical information about particular regions within an organism or sample. This technique has been used on patients with a wide range of neurological and psychiatric disorders, such as stroke, epilepsy, multiple sclerosis, dementia, and schizophrenia.

Examination of the images, obtained by any of the imaging techniques to visualize and study anatomical structures, is a straightforward task. In many situations, abnormalities are clearly visible in the acquired images and often the particular disease can also be identified by the clinician. However, in some cases, it is more difficult to make the diagnosis. The spectral data obtained from MRS can then assist, to a large extent, in the noninvasive diagnosis of diseases.

Biomedical Imaging: Principles and Applications, First Edition. Edited by Reiner Salzer.

However, the appearance of the spectral data is different compared to the image data (Fig. 1.5). Although spectra obtained from diseased tissues are different from spectra obtained from normal tissue, the complexity of the data limits the interpretability. Furthermore, the amount of spectral data can be overwhelming, which makes the data analysis even more difficult and time consuming. In order to use the information in MR spectra effectively, a (statistical) model is required, which reduces the complexity and provides an output that can easily be interpreted by clinicians. Preferably, the output of the model should be some kind of an image that can be compared to MRI images to obtain a better diagnosis.

In this chapter, the application of a chemometric approach to facilitate the analysis of image data is explained. This approach is based on a similarity measure between data obtained from a patient and reference data by searching for patterns in the data. In particular, when the amount of data is large, the use of such a mathematical approach has proved to be useful. The basics of pattern recognition methods are discussed in Section 1.2. A distinction is made between commonly used methods and several advantages and disadvantages are discussed. The application of a useful pattern recognition technique is presented in Section 1.3. The required data processing and quantitation steps are mentioned, and subsequently, data of different patients is classified. Finally, results are shown to illustrate the applicability of pattern recognition techniques.

1.2 DATA ANALYSIS

Chemometrics is a field in chemistry that helps improve the understanding of chemical data (1–3). With the use of mathematical and statistical methods, chemical data is studied to obtain maximum information and knowledge about the data. Chemometrics is typically used to explore patterns in data sets, that is, to discover relations between samples. In particular, when the data is complex and the amount of data is large, chemometrics can assist in data analysis. A technique that is frequently applied to compress the information into a more comprehensible form is Principal Component Analysis (PCA) (2, 4). Another application of chemometrics is to predict properties of a sample on the basis of the information in a set of known measurements. Such techniques are found very useful in process monitoring and process control to predict and make decisions about product quality (3, 5). Finally, chemometrics can be used to make classification models that divide samples into several distinct groups (6, 7).

This last mentioned application of chemometrics could be very helpful, for example, in the discrimination of the different and complex spectra acquired by MRS examinations. Patient diagnosis and treatment can be improved if chemometric techniques can automatically distinguish diseased tissue from normal tissue.

The aim of such pattern recognition techniques is to search for patterns in the data. Individual measurements are grouped into several categories on the basis of a similarity measure (7–9). If class membership is used in the grouping of objects, the classification is called *supervised pattern recognition* (6, 8). Pattern recognition can also be unsupervised, where no predefined classes are available. The grouping of objects is then obtained by the data itself. Unsupervised pattern recognition is also called *clustering* (7–9).

The resulting clusters obtained by pattern recognition contain objects, for example, MR spectra, which are more similar to each other compared to objects in the other clusters. If the spectra of a patient with brain tumor are considered, the data could be divided into two groups: one group contains normal spectra and the other group contains spectra acquired from the tumorous tissue. If the group that contains normal spectra and the group that contains tumorous spectra can be identified, this grouping can be used for classification. The tissue from a region of the brain can be classified as normal or tumorous by matching its spectra to the class that contains the most similar spectra.

1.2.1 Similarity Measures

Most essential in pattern recognition is the definition of the similarity measure. Usually, the (dis)similarity between a set of objects is calculated using a distance measure, of which the Euclidean distance is most popular (6–8, 10). The dissimilarity between two objects $\mathbf{x}_i$ and $\mathbf{x}_j$ is calculated as in Equation 1.1.

$$d^2_{\mathrm{euc}}(\mathbf{x}_\mathrm{i}, \mathbf{x}_\mathrm{j}) = \sum_{l=1}^{P} (x_{il} - x_{jl})^2 \tag{1.1}$$

where $\mathbf{x}_i = \{\mathbf{x}_{i1}, \ldots, \mathbf{x}_{iP}\}$, in which P denotes the number of measured variables. In vector notation, this can be written as

$$d^2_{\mathrm{euc}}(\mathbf{x}_i, \mathbf{x}_j) = (\mathbf{x}_i - \mathbf{x}_j)^T(\mathbf{x}_i - \mathbf{x}_j) \tag{1.2}$$

Another widely used distance measure is the Mahalanobis distance, which incorporates the correlations between variables in the calculations (6, 7, 11). To calculate the distance between an object $\mathbf{x}_i$ and the centroid (mean) of a group of objects, $\mu_\mathbf{k}$, it takes the covariance matrix $\mathbf{C}_k$ of the cluster into account, that is, the size and shape of the cluster. The squared Mahalanobis distance is given by

$$d^2_{\mathrm{mah}}(\mathbf{x}_i, \mu_k) = (\mathbf{x}_i - \mu_k)^T \mathbf{C}_k^{-1}(\mathbf{x}_i - \mu_k) \tag{1.3}$$

Several variants of these distance measures exist, such as the Manhattan or Bhattacharyya distance (3, 6–8), but are not commonly used in practice.

Instead of clustering the data using distances as a similarity measure, the data can also be modeled by several distributions such as the normal distribution. In that case, the likelihood, which is discussed in Section 1.2.2.1, is used as a criterion function (12, 13).

1.2.2 Unsupervised Pattern Recognition

A large variety of clustering methods have been developed for different kinds of problems (6–8, 14). A distinction between these different approaches can be made on the basis of their definition of a cluster. The techniques can be categorized into three main types: partitional (15, 16), hierarchical (17, 18), and density based (19).

1.2.2.1 Partitional Clustering. The type of clustering techniques that are most widely applied obtain a single partition of the data. These partitional clustering methods try to divide the data into a predefined number of clusters. Usually, the techniques divide the data into several clusters by optimizing a criterion or cost function. In the popular K-means algorithm (15, 16, 20), for example, the sum of squares of within-cluster distances is minimized (Equation 1.4). This is obtained by iteratively transferring objects between clusters, until the data is partitioned into well-separated and compact clusters. Because compact clusters contain objects with a relatively small distance to the mean of the cluster, these clusters result in a small value for the criterion function.

$$E = \sum_{k=1}^{K} \sum_{i \in k} d^2(\mathbf{x}_i, \mu_k) \tag{1.4}$$

The K-means algorithm starts with a random selection of K cluster centers. In the next step, each object of the data set is assigned to the closest cluster. To determine the closest cluster, the distances of a particular object to the cluster centers, $d(\mathbf{x}_i, \mu_k)$, are calculated using one of the similarity measures. Subsequently, the cluster centers are updated, and this process is repeated until a stop criterion is met, such as a threshold for the criterion function. In the end, each object is assigned to one cluster.

This clustering algorithm requires short computation time and is therefore suitable to handle large data sets. A major disadvantage, however, is the sensitivity to the cluster centers chosen initially, which makes the clustering results hard to reproduce. Another drawback is that the number of clusters has to be defined in advance (6, 7).

It is also possible to associate each object to every cluster using a membership function. Membership reflects the probability that the object belongs to the particular cluster. The K-means variant, which results in a fuzzy clustering by including cluster memberships, is fuzzy c-means (16, 21). The membership function u_{ik}, which is used in fuzzy c-means, is given in Equation 1.5 and represents the probability of object $\mathbf{x}_i$ belonging to cluster k. This membership is dependent on the distance of the object to the cluster center. If the distance to a cluster center is small, the membership for this cluster becomes relatively large (22).

$$u_{ik} = \frac{1}{\sum_{j=1}^{K} \left(\frac{d(\mathbf{x}_i, \mu_k)}{d(\mathbf{x}_i, \mu_j)} \right)^{\frac{1}{\gamma - 1}}} \tag{1.5}$$

In addition to the distances, the membership also depends on the fuzziness index γ, which is 2 in most situations. By taking smaller values for the index, the membership for clusters close to object $\mathbf{x}_i$ is increased. If two clusters overlap in variable space, the membership of an object will be low for both clusters because the uncertainty of belonging to a particular cluster is high. This is an attractive property of fuzzy methods. Because the problem with overlapping clusters is common in cluster analysis, fuzzy clustering algorithms are frequently applied.

The partitional methods that have been described earlier are based on a distance measure to calculate cluster similarities. Another variant to determine clusters in a data set is based on a statistical approach and is called *model-based clustering* or *mixture modeling* (7, 13, 23). It describes the data by mixtures of multivariate distributions. The density of objects in a particular cluster can, for example, be described by a P-dimensional Gaussian distribution. The formula of the distribution is given in Equation 1.6, where μ_k and $\mathbf{C}_k$ are the mean and covariance matrix of the data in cluster k, respectively.

$$\mathbf{F}_{ki} = (2\pi)^{-P/2} \cdot \mathbf{C}_k^{-1/2} \cdot e^{\left(-\frac{1}{2}(\mathbf{x}_i - \boldsymbol{\mu}_\mathbf{k})^\mathbf{T} \mathbf{C}_\mathbf{k}^{-1} (\mathbf{x}_i - \boldsymbol{\mu}_\mathbf{k})\right)} \tag{1.6}$$

If the sum of the Gaussians, which describe the density of objects in the individual clusters, exactly fits the original data, the entire data set is perfectly described. Each Gaussian can then be considered as one cluster. For the one-dimensional data set presented in Figure 1.1a three Gaussian distributions (dashed lines) are required to obtain a proper fit of the density of objects in the original data (solid line) (24).

With the use of multidimensional Gaussian distributions, more complicated data sets can be modeled. The density of objects in a data set consisting of two variables can be modeled by two-dimensional distributions, as illustrated in Figure 1.1b. In this situation also, three clusters are present, and therefore,

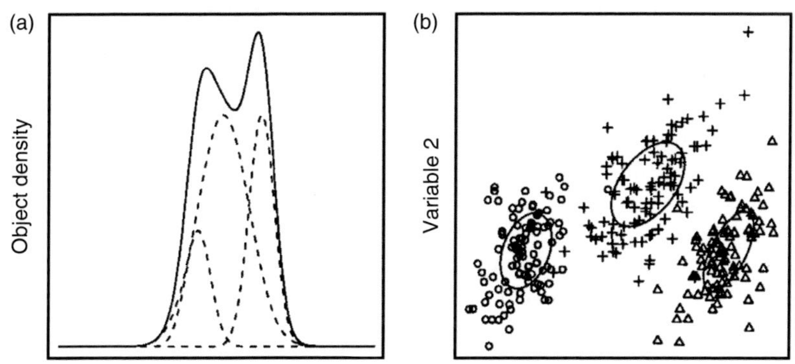

Figure 1.1. Example of modeling the density of objects by three Gaussian distributions for (a) one-dimensional and (b) two-dimensional data sets (25).

three distributions are required to obtain a good fit of the object density in the entire data.

The goodness of fit is evaluated by the log-likelihood criterion function, which is given in Equation 1.7 (13). The distributions are weighted by the mixture proportion τ_k, which corresponds to the fraction of objects in the particular cluster. The log-likelihood depends also on the cluster memberships of each of the N objects. In Equation 1.7, this is expressed as u_{ik}, which represents the probability that object $\mathbf{x}_i$ belongs to cluster k, similar to the membership function given in Equation 1.5. The data set is optimally described by the distributions when the criterion function is maximized (13).

$$\log L = \sum_{k=1}^{K} \sum_{i=1}^{N} u_{ik} \cdot \log(\tau_k \cdot \mathbf{F}_{ki}) \tag{1.7}$$

The optimal partitioning of the data is usually obtained by the Expectation-Maximization (EM) algorithm (4, 7, 26). In the first step of EM, the probabilities u_{ik} are estimated by an initial guess of some statistical parameters of each cluster. These parameters are the means, covariances, and mixture proportions of the cluster. Subsequently, the statistical parameters are recalculated using these estimated probabilities (4). This process is iterated until convergence of the log-likelihood criterion. The data is eventually clustered according to the calculated probabilities of each object to belong to the particular clusters. It is an advantage that model-based clustering yields cluster memberships instead of assigning each object to one particular cluster. However, because of the random initialization of the parameters, the results of mixture modeling are not robust. Furthermore, the number of distributions to describe the data has to be defined ahead of the clustering procedure (7, 24).

1.2.2.2 Hierarchical Clustering. Another approach to clustering is to obtain a clustering structure instead of a single partitioning of the data. Such a hierarchical clustering can be agglomerative or divisive. The agglomerative strategy starts with assigning each object to an individual cluster (16, 17, 27). Subsequently, the two most similar clusters are iteratively merged, until the data is grouped in one single cluster. Once an object is merged to a cluster, it cannot join another cluster. Divisive hierarchical clustering is similar to the agglomerative strategy, but starts with one cluster that is divided into two clusters that have least similarity. This process is repeated until all clusters contain only one object. Repeated application of hierarchical clustering will result in identical merging or splitting sequences, and thus the results are reproducible (12).

Agglomerative methods are more commonly used. On the basis of the definition of the similarity measure, several variants exist: single, complete, average, and centroid linkage (28, 29). In single linkage, the (updated) distance between the objects of a particular cluster (e.g. c_1 and c_2) and an object x_i is the minimum distance ($d_{\min}$) between x_i and the objects of the cluster. The maximum ($d_{\max}$) and average (d_{avg}) of the distances between the particular object x_i and

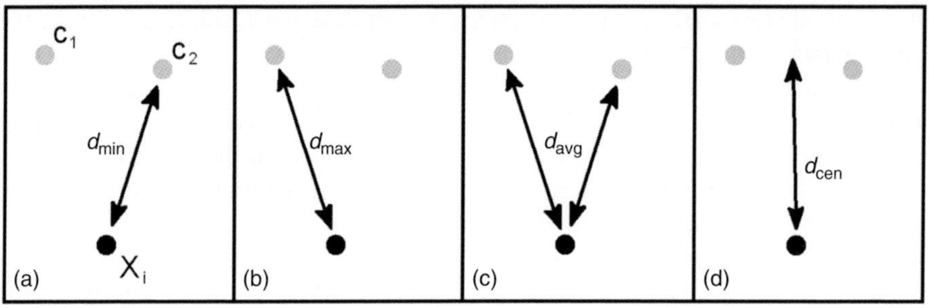

Figure 1.2. Distances between clusters used in hierarchical clustering. (a) Single linkage. (b) Complete linkage. (c) Average linkage. (d) Centroid linkage.

the objects of the cluster is used in complete and average linkage, respectively. In centroid linkage, the distance between an object and the centroid of the cluster (d_{cen}) is used. This is schematically represented in Figure 1.2.

Analogous to the methods based on distance measures, hierarchical clustering can also be performed by model-based clustering. The hierarchical approach is an adaptation from the partitional approach of model-based clustering (12, 23). Model-based agglomerative clustering also starts with individual objects, but merges the pair of objects that lead to the largest increase in the log-likelihood criterion (see Eq. 1.7). This process then continues until all objects are grouped into one cluster (23).

The sequence of merging or splitting can be visualized in a dendrogram, representing, in a treelike manner, the similarity levels at which clusters are merged. The dendrogram can be cut at a particular level to obtain a clustering with a desired number of clusters. The results with different number of clusters can then be easily compared. The dendrogram obtained by average linkage, applied to MR spectra of a patient, is given in Figure 1.3. If, for example, the data should be clustered into four groups, the dendrogram should be cut at a distance of 11,700. This threshold is indicated by the red line in Figure 1.3.

Hierarchical clustering methods are not sensitive to outliers because outliers will be assigned to distinct clusters (6). A possible drawback is the computation time. Hierarchical clustering of large data sets will require the merging of many objects: at each merging step, the similarities between pairs of objects need to be recalculated (6, 12, 23, 30).

1.2.2.3 Density-Based Clustering. The third type of clustering methods is based on the density of objects in variable space (7, 19, 31). Clusters are formed by high density areas, and the boundaries of the clusters are given by less dense regions. These densities are determined by a threshold. Another parameter that has to be defined is the size of the volume for which the density is estimated. Objects are then assigned to a cluster when the density within this volume exceeds the predefined threshold. The number of areas with high density indicates the number of clusters in the clustering result. Objects that are not assigned to a cluster are considered as noise or outliers.

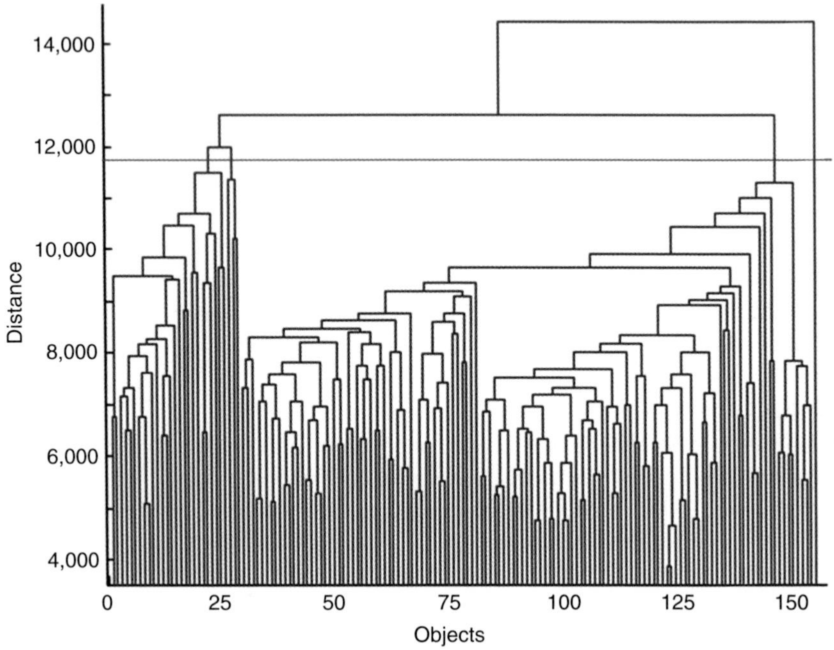

Figure 1.3. Dendrogram showing the sequence of merging MR spectral data by hierarchical clustering. The red line indicates the threshold to obtain four clusters.

DBSCAN is a well-known method to cluster data into regions using high density constraints (19, 22). The algorithm scans an area within a certain radius from a particular object and determines the number of other objects within this neighborhood. The size of the area and the minimum number of objects in the neighborhood have to be defined in advance. If the neighborhood contains more objects than the threshold, then every object in the neighborhood is assigned to one cluster. Subsequently, the neighborhood of another object in the particular cluster is scanned to expand the cluster. When the cluster does not grow anymore, the neighborhood of another object, not belonging to this cluster, is considered. If this object is also located in a dense region, a second cluster is found, and the whole procedure is repeated. With fewer objects in the neighborhood than the threshold, an object is assigned to a group of noisy objects.

Originally, density-based clustering was developed to detect clusters in a data set with exceptional shapes and to exclude noise and outliers. However, the method fails to simultaneously detect clusters with different densities (22). Clusters with a relatively low density will then be considered as noise. Another limitation is the computation time for calculating the density estimation for each object. Moreover, it can be difficult to determine proper settings for the size of the neighborhood and the threshold for the number of objects.

1.2.3 Supervised Pattern Recognition

Pattern recognition can also be supervised, by including class information in the grouping of objects (6, 8). Predefined classes are used by this type of pattern recognition for the classification of unknown objects. For example, the distance of an unidentified object to all the objects in the reference data set can be calculated by a particular distance measure, to determine the most similar (closest) object. The unknown object can then be assigned to the class to which this nearest neighbor belongs. This is the basic principle of the k-nearest neighbor (kNN) method (3, 6, 7). A little more sophisticated approach is to extend the number of neighbors. In that case, there is a problem if the nearest neighbors are from different classes. Usually, a majority rule is applied to assign the object to the class to which the majority of the nearest neighbors belong. If the majority rule cannot be applied because there is a tie, that is, the number of nearest neighbors of several classes is equal, another approach is required. The unknown object can, for example, randomly be assigned to a predefined class. Another method is to assign the object, in this situation, to the class to which its nearest neighbor belongs (7).

Another type of supervised pattern recognition is discriminant analysis (3, 7, 32). These methods are designed to find boundaries between classes. One of the best-known methods is Linear Discriminant Analysis (LDA). With the assumption that the classes have a common covariance matrix, it describes the boundaries by straight lines. More generally, an unknown object is assigned to the class for which the Mahalanobis distance (Eq. 1.3) is minimal. Because the covariance matrices of the classes are assumed to be equal, the pooled covariance matrix is used to calculate the Mahalanobis distances:

$$\mathbf{C} = \frac{1}{n-K}\sum_{k=1}^{K} n_k \mathbf{C}_k \tag{1.8}$$

where $\mathbf{C}_k$ and n_k are the covariance matrix and the number of objects in cluster k, K is the number of predefined classes, and n is the total number of objects in the data set.

In Quadratic Discriminant Analysis (QDA), the covariance matrices of the classes are not assumed to be equal. Each class is described by its own covariance matrix (3, 7, 32). Similar to LDA, QDA calculates the Mahalanobis distances of unknown objects to the predefined classes and assigns the objects to the closest class. Other more sophisticated techniques also exist, such as support vector machines (33) or neural networks (34), but these approaches are beyond the scope of this chapter.

1.2.3.1 Probability of Class Membership. To reflect the reliability of the classification, the probabilities of class membership could be calculated. This is especially useful to detect overlapping classes. An object will then have a relatively high probability to belong to two or more classes. Furthermore, the probabilities can be used to find new classes, which are not present in the reference data set. If the class membership is low for the predefined classes, the unknown object probably belongs to a totally different class.

The probabilities of class membership can be estimated on the basis of the distribution of the objects in the classes (6, 7). The density of objects at a particular distance from a class centroid is a direct estimator of the probability that an object at this distance belongs to the class. If it is assumed that the data follows a normal distribution, the density of objects can be expressed as in Equation 1.6. If the distance of a new object to a class centroid is known, the density and thus the probability of class membership can be calculated on the basis of Equation 1.6 (3, 7, 32).

A more straightforward approach is based on the actual distribution of the objects, without the assumption that the data can be described by a theoretical distribution (35). In this method, the Mahalanobis distances of the objects in a particular class, say class A, with respect to the centroid of this class are calculated. Also, the Mahalanobis distances of the other objects (not belonging to class A) with respect to the centroid of class A are calculated. This procedure is repeated for every class present in the data set. Eventually, the distances are used to determine the number of objects within certain distances from the centroid of each class. These distributions of objects can be visualized in a plot as presented in Figure 1.4 (36). The solid line represents the percentage of objects from class A within certain Mahalanobis distances (d) from the centroid of class A. Every object of class A is within a distance of $6d$ from the particular centroid. The dotted line represents the percentage of other objects (not from class A) within certain distances from the centroid of class A. In this example, there is little overlap between objects from class A and the other objects, indicating that class A is well separated from the other classes.

The percentage of objects within a particular distance from a class centroid reflects the object density of the class at this distance. Therefore, these percentages

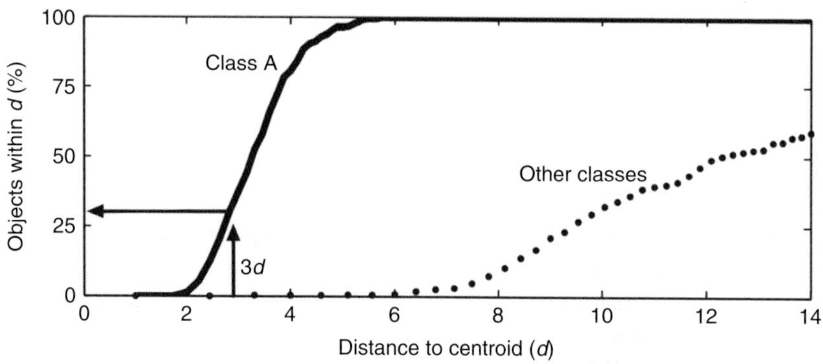

Figure 1.4. Distribution of objects belonging to class A (solid line) and objects belonging to other classes (dotted line) with respect to the centroid of class A (36).

can be used to estimate the probabilities of class membership for the classes that are present in the data set. At a distance $3d$ from the centroid of class A, for example, about 30% of the objects belonging to class A are within this distance. This is illustrated in Figure 1.4. If the Mahalanobis distance of an unknown object with respect to the centroid of class A is $3d$, the estimated probability is then 70%. By comparing the probabilities of class membership for each class, the unknown objects can be classified and conclusions can be drawn about the reliability of classification (35).

1.3 APPLICATIONS

Pattern recognition techniques can be applied to magnetic resonance data to improve the noninvasive diagnosis of brain tumors (37–41). Because the spectra obtained by MRS are complex, statistical models can facilitate data analysis. The application of pattern recognition techniques to MR spectra and MRI image data is illustrated using research performed on a widely studied data set (24, 35). This data set was constructed during a project called INTERPRET, which was funded by the European Commission to develop new methodologies for automatic tumor type recognition in the human brain (42).

1.3.1 Brain Tumor Diagnosis

Uncontrolled growth of cells is a major issue in medicine, as it results in a malignant or benign tumor. If the tumor spreads to vital organs, such as the brain, tumor growth can even be life threatening (43). Brain tumors are the leading cause of cancer death in children and third leading cause of cancer death in young adults. Only one-third of people diagnosed with a brain tumor survive more than 5 years from the moment of diagnosis (44).

Two commonly used techniques to diagnose brain tumors are magnetic resonance imaging (MRI, Chapter 5) and magnetic resonance spectroscopy (MRS, Section 5.12). MRI provides detailed pictures of organs and soft tissues within the human body (45, 46). This technique merely shows the differences in the water content and composition of various tissues. Because tumorous tissues have a composition (and water content) different from that of normal tissues, MRI can be used to detect tumors, as shown in Figure 1.5a. Even different types of tissue within the same organ, such as white and gray matter in the brain, can easily be distinguished (46).

Magnetic resonance spectroscopy (MRS) is another technique that can be used for diagnosing brain tumors (47–49). It allows the qualitative and quantitative assessment of the biochemical composition in specific brain regions (50). A disadvantage of the technique is that interpretation of the resulting spectra representing the compounds present in the human tissue is difficult and time consuming. Several spectra acquired from a tumorous region in the brain are presented in Figure 1.5b to illustrate the complexity of the data. To compare

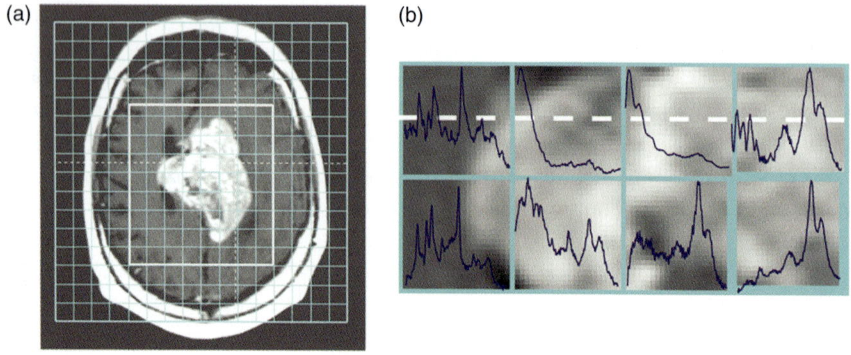

Figure 1.5. Example of the data obtained by MRI and MRS. (a) An MRI image of the brain that clearly shows the presence of abnormal tissue. The grid on the MRI image indicates the resolution of the spectroscopic data. (b) Part of the spectroscopic data, showing the spectra obtained by MRS from several regions of the brain.

the differences in resolution, the MR spectra are visualized on top of the corresponding region of the MRI image. Another limitation of MRS is that the size of the investigated region, for example, of the brain, might be larger than the suspected lesion. The heterogeneity of the tissue under examination will then disturb the spectra, making characterization of the region more difficult (51).

1.3.2 MRS Data Processing

Before chemometrics can be applied to the complex spectra obtained by MRS, these spectra require some processing. Owing to time constraints, the quality of the acquired MR spectra is often very poor. The spectra frequently contain relatively small signals and a large amount of noise: the so-called signal-to-noise ratio is low. Furthermore, several artifacts are introduced by the properties of the MR system. For example, magnetic field inhomogeneities result in distortion of the spectra. Also, patient movement during the MR examinations will introduce artifacts. Another characteristic of the spectra is the appearance of broad background signals from macromolecules and the presence of a large water peak.

1.3.2.1 Removing MRS Artifacts. In order to remove the previously mentioned artifacts, several processing steps need to be performed (26). Different software packages are commercially available to process and analyze MR spectra (43, 52, 53) and, in general, they apply some commonly used correction methods. These methods include eddy current correction (54), residual water filtering (55), phase and frequency shift correction (56), and a baseline correction method (26).

Eddy current correction is performed to correct for magnetic field inhomogeneities, induced in the magnetic system during data acquisition (54, 57). One method to correct for these distortions is to measure the field variation as a function of time. This can be achieved by measuring the phase of the much stronger signal of water. The actual signal can then be divided by this phase factor in order to remove the effect of field variation (57).

Residual water filtering is required to remove the intense water peak that is still present in the spectra after correction for eddy current distortions. A useful filtering method is based on Hankel-Lanczos Singular Value Decomposition (HLSVD) (58). Resonances between 4.1 and 5.1 ppm, as determined by the HLSVD algorithm, are subtracted from the spectra. Water resonates at approximately 4.7 ppm, and therefore, the water peak and its large tails are removed from the spectra without affecting the peak areas of other compounds (55, 58).

Several small phase differences between the peaks in a spectrum may still be present after eddy current correction. In addition, frequency shifts between spectra of different regions, for example, of the brain, may also be present. These peak shifts may be induced by patient movement. A correction method based on PCA can be applied to eliminate the phase and frequency shift variations of a single resonance peak across a series of spectra. PCA methodology is used to model the effects of phase and frequency shifts, and this information can then be used to remove the variations (56, 59).

Broad resonances of large molecules or influences from the large water peak may contribute to baseline distortions, which make the quantification of the resonances of small compounds more difficult. The removal of these broad resonances improves the accuracy of quantification and appearance of the spectrum. Usually, the correction is performed by estimating the baseline using polynomial functions, followed by subtraction from the original signal (26).

1.3.2.2 MRS Data Quantitation. After processing the spectra obtained by MRS, the data can be interpreted. As the spectra contain information from important brain metabolites, deviation in the spectra, and thus in metabolite concentrations, might be indicative of the presence of abnormal tissue. Two different MR spectra are shown in Figure 1.6. The spectrum in Figure 1.6a is acquired from a normal region of the brain and the spectrum in Figure 1.6b originates from a malignant region. The differences between these spectra are obvious and MRS could therefore be used to detect abnormal tissues. Several metabolites are particularly useful for tumor diagnosis, and some of these are creatine (resonates at 3.95 and 3.02 ppm), glutamate (3.75 and 2.20 ppm), glutamine (3.75 and 2.20 ppm), myoinositol (3.56 ppm), choline (3.20 ppm), *N*-acetyl aspartate (NAA, 2.02 ppm), lactate (1.33 ppm), and fatty acids (1.3 and 0.90 ppm) (25, 60, 61).

To use the metabolic information in the MR spectra for diagnosis of brain tumors, the intensity of the signals in the spectra requires quantitation (62). A simple approach is to integrate several spectral regions, assuming that each region contains information from one single metabolite. Because some metabolites show overlap in the spectra, for example, glutamate and glutamine, more sophisticated methods could be applied. More accurate methods fit the spectrum by a specific lineshape function, using a reference set of model spectra. A method that has been introduced for the analysis of MR spectra is the LCModel (52, 62, 63). This method analyzes a spectrum as linear combinations of a set of model

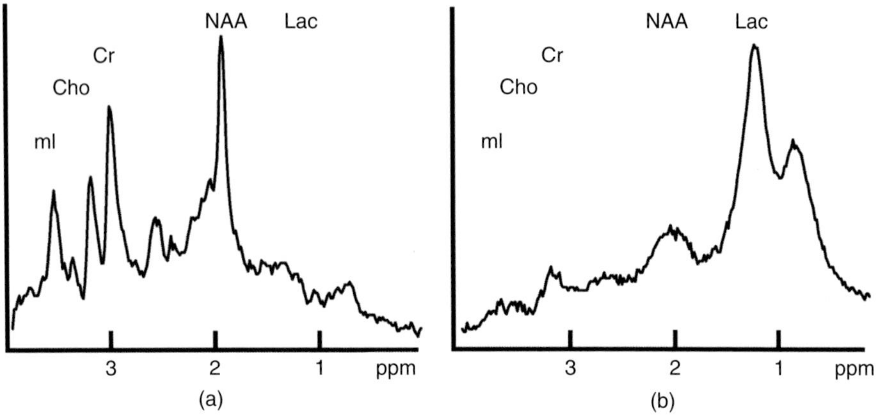

Figure 1.6. Two MR spectra, illustrating the difference between spectra obtained from a normal region (a) and a malignant region (b) of the brain. The signals of some metabolites are indicated in the figure: myoinositol (mI) at 3.56 ppm, choline (Cho) at 3.20 ppm, creatine (Cr) at 3.02 ppm, NAA at 2.02 ppm, and lactate (Lac) at 1.33 ppm.

spectra from individual metabolites in solution. Another powerful tool for processing and quantitation of MR spectra is MRUI (64, 65). This program has a graphical user interface and is able to analyze the MR spectra and present the results in an accessible manner.

Differences in the quantitated metabolite levels are often used to diagnose the malignancy of a tumor. But even when only the peak intensities of the previously mentioned metabolites are quantitated and interpreted, the amount of data is still large. Especially if MRS is applied to a large region of the brain, to obtain multiple spectra, many metabolite concentrations have to be compared. To facilitate the data analysis, the relative metabolite concentrations within different regions (or actually volumes) could be presented in an image. These regions are referred to as *voxels*. The resulting metabolic maps visualize the spatial distribution of the concentration of several metabolic compounds, and this can be used to localize or diagnose brain tumors. This is shown in Figure 1.7, in which the relative metabolite concentrations of choline, creatine, and NAA are presented. As shown, an increased concentration of choline is detected in the tumorous region, and reduced concentrations of creatine and NAA are found. Another application of such metabolic maps is to study tumor heterogeneity since this is important for an accurate diagnosis (66–68).

1.3.3 MRI Data Processing

As mentioned in Section 5.7, the echo time (TE) and the repetition time (TR) are acquisition parameters that determine the T_1- and T_2-sensitivity of the acquired images. By using different settings for these parameters, different MRI images are obtained (45, 46). Examples of these images are given in Figure 1.8. In the

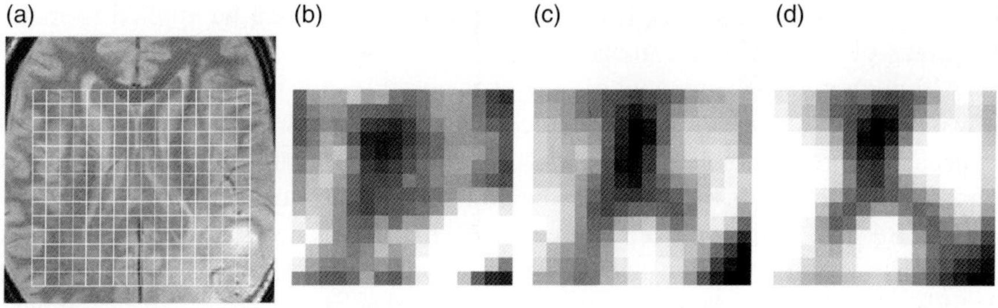

Figure 1.7. Metabolic maps constructed from MRS data. (a) The MRI image shows the presence of a tumor in the lower right corner of the image. The differences in metabolic concentration are illustrated for (b) choline, (c) creatine, and (d) NAA. Bright pixels represent a high concentration of the particular metabolite.

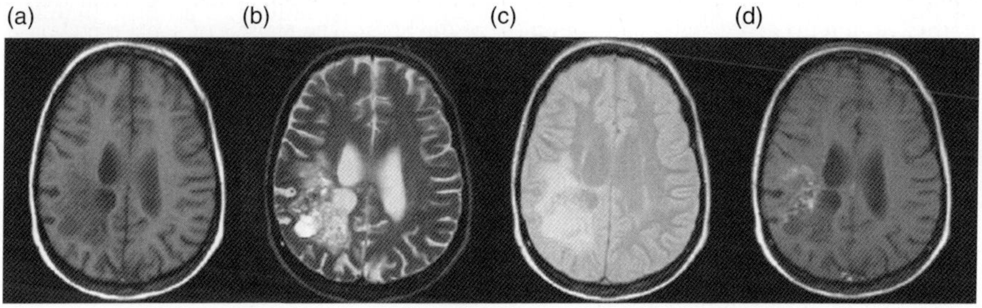

Figure 1.8. MRI images obtained by different acquisition parameters. (a) T_1-weighted image. (b) T_2-weighted image. (c) Proton density image. (d) T_1-weighted image after administration of a gadolinium tracer.

T_1- and T_2-weighted images (Fig. 1.8a and b), the differences in contrast reveal the ventricles while this is less visible in the PD-weighted image (Fig. 1.8c).

T_1-, T_2-, and PD-weighted images are commonly acquired with different combinations of TR and TE to be able to discriminate between different tissues. For tumor diagnosis, a contrast medium can be used to improve the tissue differentiation. Usually, gadolinium (Gd) is used as a contrast agent to enhance lesions where the blood–brain barrier is defective. An example of a T_1-weighted image enhanced by gadolinium is presented in Figure 1.8d (69).

When the different images need to be compared, they should be aligned with respect to each other. This is necessary because when patients move during the acquisition of the different MRI images, artifacts may be introduced, which complicates the data analysis.

1.3.3.1 Image Registration. Image registration is the alignment of the different images obtained by MRI examinations. This alignment compensates for differences in the position or orientation of the brain in the images due to patient movement. If the images are taken from a series of MRI examinations to study tumor growth or shrinkage after radiation treatment, differences in image size or resolution may be obtained. Image registration should then be applied to match the areas of interest in the images (36).

Although manual alignment of images is possible, it is time consuming and not always reproducible. Automated procedures are therefore preferred. Numerous approaches are available for medical images (69, 70), and in general, they are based on a similarity measure between an image and a corresponding reference image. Because patient movement results in small shifts between different images, a simple cross-correlation method can be used to correct for this artifact (71). However, sensitivity to large intensity differences in different contrast images limits the use of cross-correlation methods. To perform the alignment by matching specific features in the images, which are insensitive to changes in tissue or acquisition, the registration can be improved. These features are, for example, edges and corners in normal brain tissue regions. The chemometric technique Procrustes analysis can then be applied to match the specific features by means of translation, rotation, and uniform scaling transformations. The best match is found when the least-squares solution is obtained by minimizing the distance between all pairs of points in the two images (3, 72).

1.3.4 Combining MRI and MRS Data

If the magnetic resonance data is properly processed, tumorous tissue may be distinguished from normal or other abnormal nonmalignant tissue types, such as necrosis, edema, or scar tissue, by examining the data. However, from the standard acquired MRI images, it is often difficult to properly discriminate tissues within the tumorous region. This can be improved by the contrast-enhanced image, which reveals the lesion where the blood–brain barrier is defective. But because this barrier may variably be affected, the size of the tumor may be under- or overestimated. This has been observed in some brain tumor studies, where the contrast-enhanced lesion was found to be much smaller than the region of abnormal metabolism (73). In addition, MRS examinations have shown that metabolite levels are highly variable for particular tissue types. Also, overlap of metabolite levels between different tumor grades has been observed (73). These findings indicate that MRI and MRS are two complementary techniques for brain tumor diagnosis. MRS provides metabolic information on a low spatial resolution, and MRI provides morphological information on a high spatial resolution. Therefore, the analysis of MRI images and metabolic maps should be performed simultaneously. One of the possibilities is to display a specific metabolic map over an MRI image. Examination of these overlay images facilitates the differentiation between tissue types. For example, the delineation of a viable tumor can be detected more accurately. This is important for studying the effect of chemotherapy or radiation treatment. The combination of MRI and MRS data will improve patient diagnosis and treatment or will facilitate the sampling of biopsies to regions of tumorous tissue.

1.3.4.1 Reference Data Set. For pattern recognition, the data from several patients with a brain tumor and several volunteers was selected from the

INTERPRET database (42). After reaching consensus about the histopathology, three tumor types were identified according to the World Health Organization classification system. These three classes contained glial tumors with different grades, indicating the level of malignancy. If a tumor could be assigned to more than one grade, the highest malignancy level determined the grade for the entire tumor, even if most of the tumor is of a lower grade (74). The brain tumors of six patients were diagnosed as grade II, of four patients as grade III, and of five patients as grade IV glial tumors. In addition, classes of normal tissue and Cerebrospinal Fluid (CSF) were created from the patient and volunteer data.

For each predefined class, a selection of voxels from different patients was made. Only voxels from regions that clearly consisted of tissue belonging to the particular class were selected. The data for the normal class was selected from the volunteers or from the contralateral brain region of the patients. The CSF class contained only data from CSF regions that were not in close contact with the tumor region (35).

From the MR spectra of these selected voxels, only the regions where important metabolites appear were selected, as these regions contain most information for the discrimination between brain tumors. The remaining regions contain mainly spectral noise. Besides excluding noise, this also results in a significant reduction in the amount of data.

The estimated metabolite levels should be subsequently combined with the MRI data to improve data analysis (75–77). However, the spatial resolution of MRI images is much higher than the resolution of MRS data. Therefore, to combine MRI with MRS data, the resolution of the MRI images was lowered to the resolution of the MRS data by averaging the pixel intensities within each spectroscopic voxel. To equally weigh the influence from both data modalities in the classification process, the averaged intensities were scaled to the range of the spectral data.

Different (statistical) methods are available to classify the processed data (see Section 1.2). Application of these methods to the data will result in a classification for each individual voxel. It is also possible to calculate an accuracy measure to indicate the reliability of the classification outcome. An example of a classification method with a statistical basis and the possibility of determining the reliability are discussed in the following sections.

1.3.5 Probability of Class Memberships

After processing the data of the reference set, the distribution of objects in each class can be investigated. By determining the percentage of objects within certain distances from the class centroids, as explained in Section 1.2.3.1, separated and overlapping classes can be found. To investigate which classes are overlapping, the Mahalanobis distance of the objects in each surrounding tissue class with respect to a class centroid was calculated. The surrounding of an isolated class will contain no objects from other classes, whereas the neighborhood of overlapping classes will contain objects belonging to multiple classes. The distributions of the classes in the reference data set are presented in Figure 1.9 (35). Within a distance of about 6*d* from the centroid of the normal class, every object belonging to this class and some objects from the cerebrospinal fluid class are found. The CSF class shows some overlap with the normal class, but is well separated from the other classes, as depicted in Figure 1.9b. This indicates that the normal and CSF classes are isolated from the tumor classes, and thus, a classification method should discriminate well between normal tissue and malignant tumors.

More overlap exists between grade II and III classes. Although at a distance of 5.5*d* from the centroid of grade II class, almost every object from this class is found; also, about 25% of the objects from grade III class appear within this distance. Less overlap is found with grade IV class. Therefore, discrimination between grade II and grade IV is possible, but grade II class is difficult to be separated from grade III class. The same can be concluded from the distribution of grade III class (Fig. 1.9d). Because grade IV class is isolated from the other classes, this type of tumor can probably be classified with a high reliability (Fig. 1.9e).

1.3.6 Class Membership of Individual Voxels

The distribution of objects can be used to estimate probabilities of class membership for a new patient, as discussed in Section 1.2.3.1. Four patients (A–D) were analyzed; histopathological examination of the brain tissue resulted in the diagnosis of grade III (patient A and D), grade II (patient B), and grade IV (patient C) tumors. The probability maps calculated for the patients are presented in Figure 1.10. Dark voxels in the map represent a high probability that the underlying tissue belongs to the particular class. The probability maps need to be compared regionwise because the probabilities are relative, that is, the intensities are scaled to its maximum value. If a region in the map, for example, of grade II, is dark, while it is bright in the other maps, the estimated probability for grade II class is high (close to 100%). If the region is dark in several maps, the estimated probability of the class membership is lower, and a black pixel does not correspond with a probability of 100%. The probabilities may, therefore, also assist in the assessment of tumor heterogeneity. If the probability is high exclusively for one class, then the tissue will be homogeneous. If the probability is high for two tissue classes, the region might be a mixture of these tissues and might therefore be heterogeneous. However, if a mixture of these two tissues is not possible from a clinical point of view, the high probabilities for both classes indicate a low classification reliability.

The probability maps for the four patients show that large regions have a high probability to belong to the normal class while these regions have a low probability to belong to another class. The CSF and grade IV regions of the patients show a similar behavior. The voxels with a high probability for the CSF or grade IV class have low probabilities to belong to the other classes. This indicates that these classes are well separated from other classes and that the reliability of classification is high.

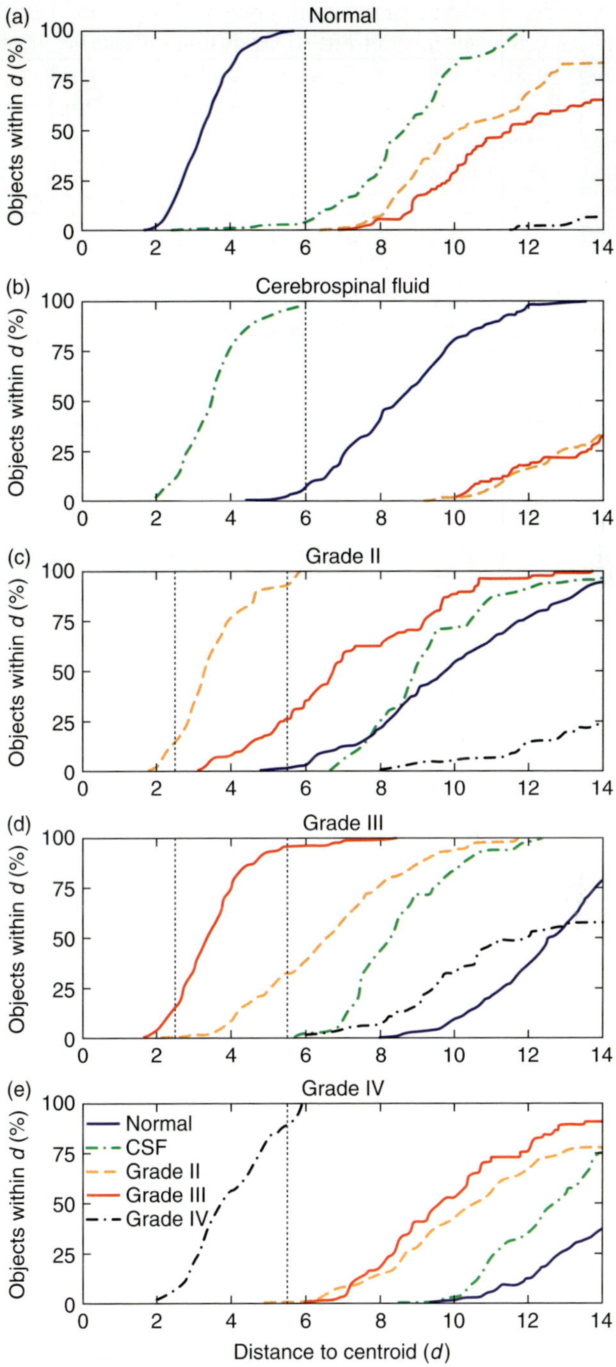

Figure 1.9. Distribution of the objects in different classes with respect to the centroid of the (a) normal, (b) CSF, (c) grade II, (d) grade III, and (e) grade IV class. The vertical dotted lines indicate thresholds that are used in the classification.

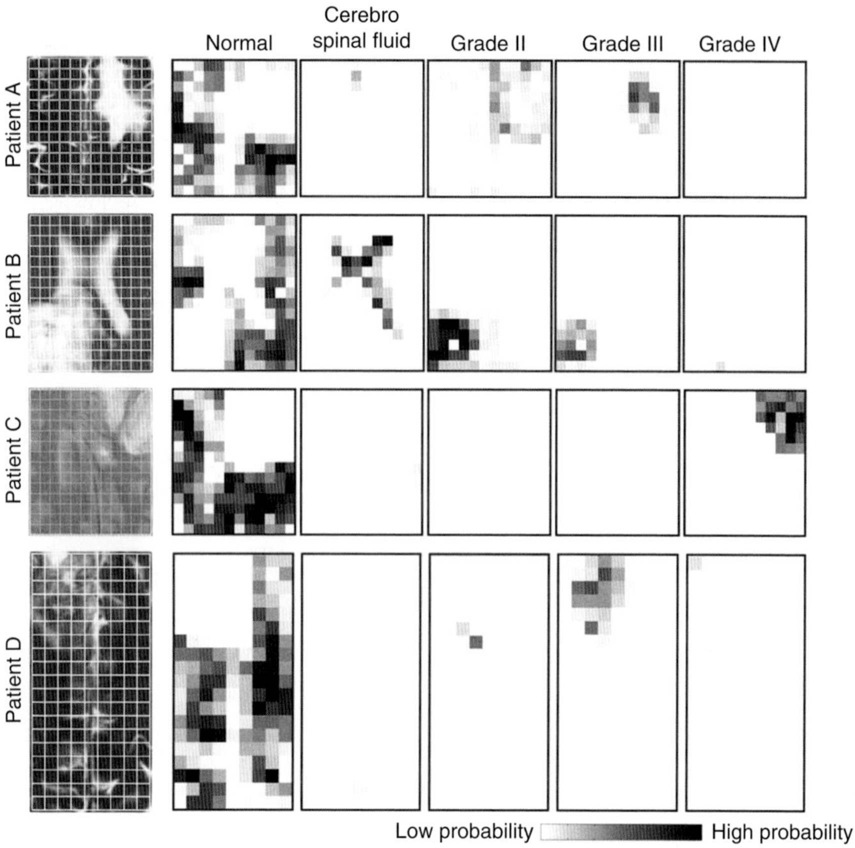

Figure 1.10. Probability maps of four patients (A–D). For comparison, an MRI image of each patient is shown on the left. The probability of each voxel to belong to the normal, CSF, grade II, grade III, and grade IV class are shown. Patients A and D are diagnosed with a grade III tumor, patient B with a grade II tumor, and patient C with a grade IV tumor.

Different results are obtained for grade II and grade III classes. The regions where the estimated probability is high for belonging to grade II class also have a high probability to belong to grade III class. In particular, patients A and B show clearly the overlapping problem of these two tissue classes. This could indicate the presence of heterogeneous tumor tissue in these regions and that the reliability of the classification is low.

1.3.7 Classification of Individual Voxels

The estimated probabilities of class membership can be used for classification by assigning each voxel to the class for which it has the highest probability. To define specific classification accuracies, thresholds are set for each class. For a correct classification of 99% of the normal objects, and thus an α-error of 1%, the threshold was set at the position shown in Figure 1.9a. However, with the threshold set at $6d$, about 3% of the objects will be classified incorrectly (β-error) as normal. Similar to the normal class, the threshold for the CSF objects was also set at $6d$ to obtain a low α-error. To minimize the chance that normal or CSF objects are classified as grade IV, the specific threshold for grade IV class was set at $5.5d$ even though the α-error is then relatively large. Because of the overlap between grade II and III classes, additional thresholds were defined. To obtain a low β-error, an object is directly assigned to grade II when the distance to the particular centroid is very small. With larger distances to grade II class (between $2.5d$ and $5.5d$), the object is assigned to this class only if the distance to grade III class is 1.3 times larger than to grade II class. Otherwise, the object is located in the area of overlap between both classes and the object is assigned to an "undecided" class. The value of 1.3 is obtained after optimization. Identical thresholds are used when the object is closest to grade III class (Fig. 1.9d). If the distance of an object exceeds the specific thresholds for each individual class, the object probably does not belong to any of the classes in the reference data set, and the object is therefore assigned to an "unknown" class.

By applying these thresholds to the classification of the four patients A–D, good results are obtained, as shown in Figure 1.11. The results of pattern recognition are projected over different MRI images to compare the results with morphological information. Patient A was diagnosed with a grade III tumor, and the classification result shows the presence of regions of grade II and grade III tumors. But because a tumor is diagnosed by the most malignant tissue present, the result of the statistical method is in agreement with histopathology. From the maps in Figure 1.10, it was clear that some voxels in the tumorous region have equal probability of belonging to grade II and grade III classes. This indicates

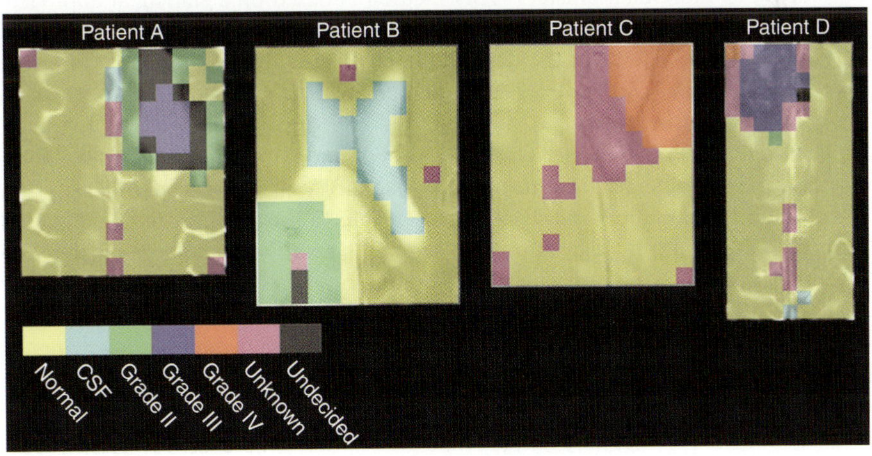

Figure 1.11. Classification results of patients A–D. Classification was performed by applying specific thresholds to define classification accuracies.

the presence of a heterogeneous tumor. Therefore, the voxels in the overlapping region of grade II and III tumors are assigned to the undecided class. The voxels in the center of the tumor have the highest probability of belonging to grade III class and are therefore assigned to this class. The tumors of patients B and C are classified as grade II and grade IV tumor in correspondence with the histopathology. Although the tumorous voxels of patient B also have a relatively high probability to belong to grade III class, the estimated probability for grade II class is much higher, and the voxels are classified as grade II. One region of patient C is classified as unknown. This is probably because the particular class is not represented in the reference data set. One voxel of patient D has been misclassified as a grade IV tumor while the patient was diagnosed with a grade III tumor. The reason for this could be that the voxel is a corner voxel, where the MRS signal is low because of the characteristics of the MRS data acquisition.

1.3.8 Clustering into Segments

More robust classification results can be obtained by grouping similar voxels in advance of the classification. The voxels that are grouped in one cluster will then be assigned to the same class. The voxels within a region covering a brain tumor, for example, will be grouped in one cluster, and this cluster will subsequently be classified as tumorous tissue. Because a tumor is often larger than the size of a voxel, it could be advantageous to combine the voxels within the tumorous region for classification purposes. However, when the information of the voxels within the tumor is averaged, it is not possible to discover any spatial heterogeneity of the tumor. Therefore, a clustering method that groups only similar voxels instead of grouping neighboring voxels should be applied. One of the methods that could be used to cluster similar voxels is mixture modeling (see Section 1.2.2.1), which describes the spread of the data by a set of distributions. Similar objects will be described by the same distribution and the resulting distributions can be considered as individual clusters. This method is based on a statistical approach, which makes it possible to calculate the probability of an object to belong to a particular cluster. The fit of the data can be evaluated by the likelihood criterion given in Equation 1.7. However, the number of distributions, and thus clusters, has to be defined in advance.

The voxels of a patient are clustered to obtain a partitioning with three, four, five, and six segments. The results for patient A are given in Figure 1.12a (78). The different colors in the clustering results are used only for visualization purpose. Clustering the data into three segments results in one large cluster representing normal tissue and one cluster of tumorous tissue, with a third cluster scattered over the recorded image. If the data is partitioned into more clusters, the voxels covering the tumorous region are divided into multiple segments as illustrated in Figure 1.12a. For example, by clustering the data of patient A into five segments, the tumorous region is covered by three clusters, which could indicate tumor heterogeneity.

The optimal number of segments can be obtained by comparing the estimated probabilities of class membership. Similar to the calculation for individual voxels,

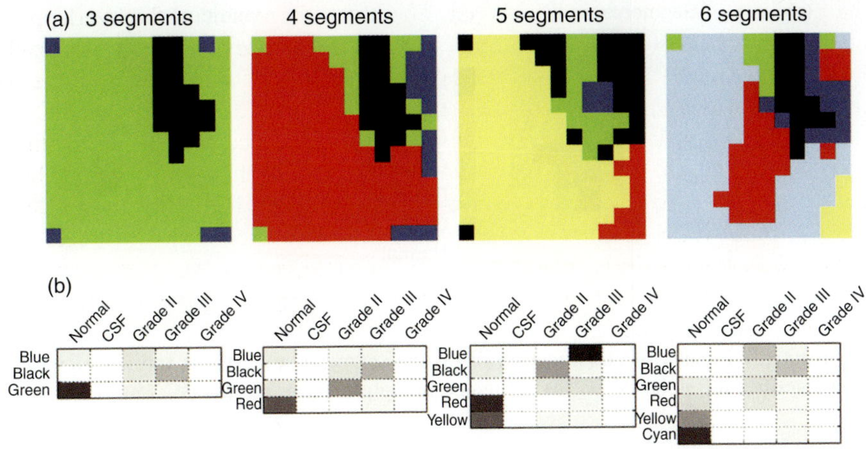

Figure 1.12. (a) Results of clustering patient A into three, four, five, and six segments. Clustering was performed by mixture modeling. (b) Estimated probabilities of each segment for each of the five classes. Dark areas correspond to a high probability.

the estimated probabilities can be determined for each segment. This is performed by averaging the MRI and MRS information in each segment. Subsequently, the Mahalanobis distances to the classes in a reference data set are calculated. The estimated probabilities of each segment in the clustering results of patient A are given in the bottom of Figure 1.12b. Each row shows, for a specific segment, the probability of membership for all investigated classes. Dark areas represent high probabilities.

In the three segments solution, the first row represents the probabilities for the blue segment. The probabilities are relatively low, and this could indicate that the blue segment does not belong to any of the classes in the reference data set. The black segment has the highest probability for grade III class, and also some for grade II. The green segment probably contains voxels of the normal class.

In the five cluster solution, more segments are obtained with a high probability for a particular class. Therefore, clustering the patient in five segments is preferred. The blue segment most probably belongs to grade III and the black segment to grade II class. The green segment has a high probability for grade II and III class. The red and yellow segments have a high probability to contain normal tissue.

1.3.9 Classification of Segments

The calculated probabilities can be used to assign each segment to a particular class. With the specific thresholds used in the classification, the result presented in Figure 1.13a is obtained. Each class is color coded according to the legend shown in Figure 1.13. The blue segment of the five cluster solution is classified as grade III and the black segment as grade II (Fig. 1.12). The green segment has

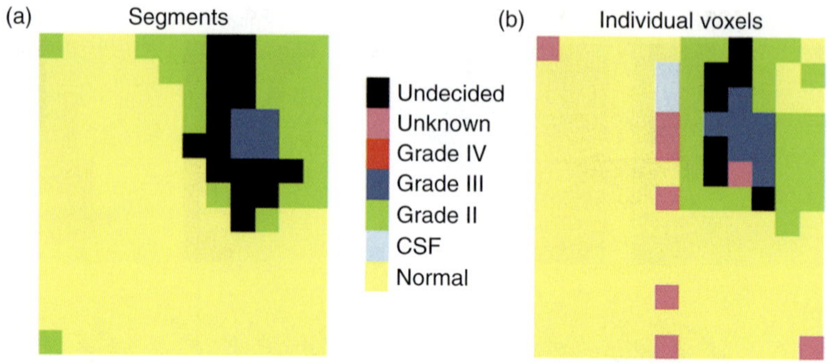

Figure 1.13. Results of classification of (a) the segments and (b) the individual voxels. The classification is based on the estimated probabilities for each class.

equal probabilities to belong to grade II and grade III and is therefore classified as undecided. The red and yellow segments have the highest probability to belong to the normal class, and therefore both segments are classified as normal. Because the probabilities of four segments are high for only one class, the classification of these segments is reliable. The reliability of the green segment is low, or the high probability for more classes could indicate that the underlying tissue is heterogeneous. Overall, the classification indicates that the most malignant tumor of this patient is of grade III, and this is in agreement with the pathology.

For comparison, the result of the classification of individual voxels is shown in Figure 1.13b. Although the classes after classification of the individual voxels are more scattered and the clustered result seems more robust, both results indicate the presence of a grade III tumor. Because the estimated probability of classification of some segments is higher than any of the probabilities of the individual voxels, it could be advantageous to cluster the data first.

Presented as images, the results of classification could facilitate the diagnosis of brain tumors. The probabilities of class membership are also important as they give an indication about the reliability of classification and/or the heterogeneity of the tissue.

1.3.10 Future Directions

In the procedures described, the data of each voxel was classified without including the spatial relation between voxels. By including the neighborhood information in the classification, the results can be improved (79). In one paper, Canonical Correlation Analysis (CCA) was used to study the effect of including spatial information in the classification of MRS data (80). This technique is based on the correlation between variables (3), for example, MR spectra of a patient and several model (reference) spectra. The problem with heterogeneous tissues is addressed by incorporating mixed spectra of normal and tumorous tissues in the set of model spectra. The application of this approach to the data of patient

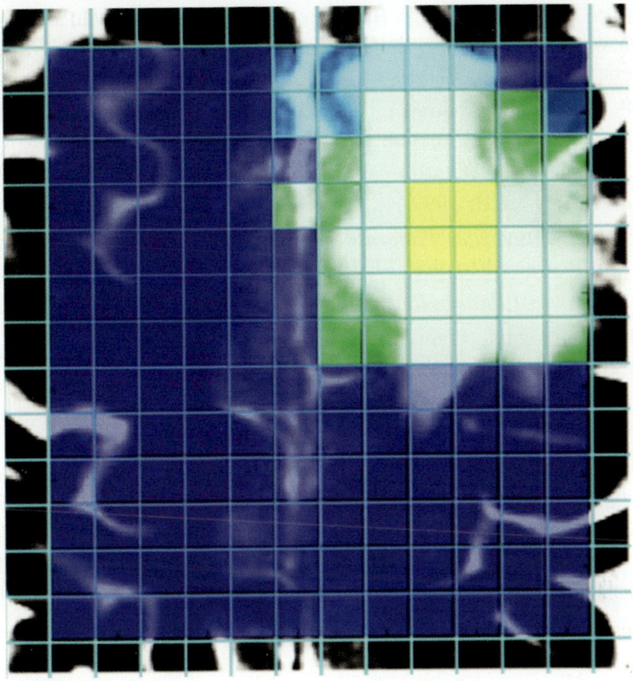

Figure 1.14. Classification result of canonical correlation analysis after the inclusion of neighborhood information, applied on the data of patient A. *Source*: Adapted from Reference (80).

A results in the classification presented in Figure 1.14, in which distinct regions are obtained. Further details are given in De Vos et al. (80).

The improvement of the classification accuracy by taking the neighboring voxels into account can be extended further by considering three-dimensional data. This kind of data becomes more widely available with recent developments in the instrumentation. As more neighboring voxels are available in three-dimensional data, more information is used to obtain more robust classification results.

Another future direction could be to combine MRS data with the data obtained from other imaging techniques, such as CT and PET. As other data modalities may contain different information, the fusion of these images may contribute to an improved tumor diagnosis.

REFERENCES

1. Beebe KR, Pell RJ, Seasholtz MB. *Chemometrics: A Practical Guide*. New York: John Wiley and Sons, Inc.; 1998.
2. Massart DL, Vandeginste BGM, Buydens LMC, de Jong S, Lewi PJ, Smeyers-Verbeke J. *Handbook of Chemometrics and Qualimetrics: Part A*. Amsterdam: Elsevier Science Publishers; 1998.

3. Vandeginste BGM, Massart DL, Buydens LMC, de Jong S, Lewi PJ, Smeyers-Verbeke J. *Handbook of Chemometrics and Qualimetrics: Part B*. Amsterdam: Elsevier Science Publishers; 1998.
4. Geladi P, Isaksson H, Lindqvis L, Wold S, Esbensen K. Principal component analysis of multivariate images. Chemom Intell Lab Syst 1989;5:209–220.
5. Otto M. *Chemometrics, Statistics and Computer Applications in Analytical Chemistry*. Weinheim: Wiley-VCH; 1999.
6. Brereton RG. *Multivariate Pattern Recognition in Chemometrics, Illustrated by Case Studies*. Amsterdam: Elsevier; 1992.
7. Webb A. *Statistical Pattern Recognition*. Malvern: John Wiley and Sons; 2002.
8. Jain AK, Murty MN, Flynn PJ. Data clustering: a review. ACM Comput Surv 1991;31:264.
9. Fukunaga K. *Introduction to Statistical Pattern Recognition*. 2nd ed. London: Academic Press; 1990.
10. Richards JA, Jia X. *Remote Sensing Digital Image Analysis*. Berlin: Springer; 1999.
11. Mao J, Jain AK. A self-organizing network for hyperellipsoidal clustering. IEEE Trans Neural Networks 1996;7:16–29.
12. Fraley C. Algorithms for model-based Gaussian hierarchical clustering. SIAM J Sci Comput 1998;20:270–281.
13. McLachlan G, Peel D. *Finite Mixture Models*. New York: John Wiley and Sons; 2000.
14. Halkidi M, Batistakis Y, Vazirgiannis M. On clustering validation techniques. J Intell Inf Syst 2001;17:107–145.
15. Noordam JC, van den Broek WHAM. Multivariate image segmentation based on geometrically guided fuzzy C-means clustering. J Chemom 2002;16:1–11.
16. Teppola P, Mujunen SP, Minkkinen P. Adaptive fuzzy C-means clustering in process monitoring. Chemom Intell Lab Syst 1999;45:23–38.
17. Smolinski A, Walczak B, Einax JW. Hierarchical clustering extended with visual complements of environmental data set. Chemom Intell Lab Syst 2002;64:45–54.
18. Liang J, Kachalo S. Computational analysis of microarray gene expression profiles: clustering, classification, and beyond. Chemom Intell Lab Syst 2002;62:199–216.
19. Daszykowski M, Walczak B, Massart DL. Looking for natural patterns in data Part 1. Density-based approach. Chemom Intell Lab Syst 2001;56:83–92.
20. Anderberg MR. *Cluster Analysis for Applications*. New York: Academic Press; 1973.
21. Bezdek JC. *Pattern Recognition with Fuzzy Objective Function Algorithms*. New York: Plenum; 1981.
22. Tran TN, Wehrens R, Buydens LMC. Clustering multispectral images: a tutorial. Chemom Intell Lab Syst 2005;77:3–17.
23. Fraley C, Raftery AE. Model-based clustering, discriminant analysis, and density estimation. J Am Stat Assoc 2002;97(458): 611–631.
24. Wehrens R, Simonetti AW, Buydens LMC. Mixture modeling of medical magnetic resonance data. J Chemom 2002;16:274–282.
25. Rijpkema M, Schuuring J, van der Meulen Y, van der Graaf M, Bernsen H, Boerman R, van der Kogel A, Heerschap A. Characterization of oligodendrogliomas using short echo time 1H MR spectroscopic imaging. NMR Biomed 2003;16:12–18.

26. Zandt HJA, van der Graaf M, Heerschap A. Common processing of in vivo MR spectra. NMR Biomed 2001;14:224–232.
27. Pham DL. Spatial models for fuzzy clustering. Comput Vis Image Underst 2001;84:285–297.
28. Li SZ. *Markov Random Field Modeling in Image Analysis*. Tokyo: Springer-Verlag; 2001.
29. Besag J. On the statistical analysis of dirty pictures. J R Stat Soc Series B-Methodol 1986;48:259.
30. Sneath PHA, Sokal RR. *Numerical Taxonomy*. London: Freeman; 1973.
31. Yizong C. Mean shift, mode seeking, and clustering. IEEE Trans Pattern Anal Mach Intell 1995;17:790–799.
32. Hastie T, Tibshirani R, Friedman J. *The Elements of Statistical Learning, Data Mining, Inference, and Prediction*. New York: Springer; 2001.
33. Lukas L, Devos A, Suykens JAK, Vanhamme L, Howe FA, Majos C, Moreno-Torres A, van der Graaf M, Tate AR, Arus C, van Huffel S. Brain tumor classification based on long echo proton MRS signals. Artif Intell Med 2004;31:73–89.
34. Melssen W, Wehrens R, Buydens L. Supervised Kohonen networks for classification problems. Chemom Intell Lab Syst 2006;83:99–113.
35. Simonetti AW, Melssen WJ, van der Graaf M, Postma GJ, Heerschap A, Buydens LMC. A chemometric approach for brain tumor classification using magnetic resonance imaging and spectroscopy. Anal Chem 2003;75:5352–5361.
36. Hutton BF, Braun M, Thurfjell L, Lau DYH. Image registration: an essential tool for nuclear medicine. Eur J Nucl Med 2002;29:559–577.
37. Howells SL, Maxwell RJ, Griffiths JR. Classification of tumour 1H NMR spectra by pattern recognition. NMR Biomed 1992;5:59–64.
38. Preul MC, Caramanos Z, Leblanc R, Villemure JG, Arnold DL. Using pattern analysis of in vivo proton MRSI data to improve the diagnosis and surgical management of patients with brain tumors. NMR Biomed 1998;11:192–200.
39. Tate AR, Majos C, Moreno A, Howe FA, Griffiths JR, Arus C. Automated classification of short echo time in vivo 1H brain tumor spectra: a multicenter study. Magn Reson Med 2003;49:26–36.
40. Szabo de Edelenyi F, Rubin C, Esteve F, Grand S, Decorps M, Lefournier V, Le Bas J, Remy C. A new approach for analyzing proton magnetic resonance spectroscopic images of brain tumors: nosologic images. Nat Med 2000;6:1287–1289.
41. Herminghaus S, Dierks T, Pilatus U, Moller-Hartmann W, Wittsack J, Marquardt G, Labisch C, Lenfermann H, Schlote W, Zanella FE. Determination of histopathological tumor grade in neuroepithelial brain tumors by using spectral pattern analysis of in vivo spectroscopic data. J Neurosurg 2003;98:74–81.
42. INTERPRET. Website by Universitat Autonoma de Barcelona. Last accessed: February 6th, 2012. Available at http://azizu.uab.es/INTERPRET/index.html.
43. Feinberg AP, Ohlsson R, Henikoff S. The epigenetic progenitor origin of human cancer. Nat Rev Genet 2006;7:21–33.
44. National Brain Tumor Society. Website by National Brain Tumor Society. Last accessed: February 6th, 2012. Available at http://www.braintumor.org.
45. Gadian DG. *NMR and its Applications to Living Systems*. 2nd ed. Oxford: Oxford Science Publications; 1995.

46. Schild HH. *MRI Made Easy (... well almost)*. Berlin: Schering AG; 1990.
47. Andrews C, Simmons A, Williams S. Magnetic resonance imaging and spectroscopy. Phys Educ 1996;31:80–85.
48. Barker PB, Lin DDM. In vivo proton MR spectroscopy of the human brain. Prog Nucl Magn Reson Spectrosc 2006;49:99–128.
49. Gujar SK, Maheshwari S, Bjorkman-Burtscher I, Sundgren PC. Magnetic resonance spectroscopy. J Neuro-Ophthalmol 2005;25(3): 217–226.
50. Stanley JA. In vivo magnetic resonance spectroscopy and its application to neuropsychiatric disorders. Can J Psychiatry 2002;47:315–326.
51. Sibtain NA, Howe FA, Saunders DE. The clinical value of proton magnetic resonance spectroscopy in adult brain tumours. Clin Radiol 2007;62:109–119.
52. Provencher SW. Estimation of metabolite concentrations from localized in vivo proton NMR spectra. Magn Reson Med 1993;30:672–679.
53. van den Boogaart A. *MRUI Manual v96.3 A User's Guide to the Magnetic Resonance User Interface Software Package*. Delft: Delft Technical University Press; 1997.
54. Klose U. In vivo proton spectroscopy in presence of eddy currents. Magn Reson Med 1990;14:26–30.
55. Vanhamme L, Fierro RD, van Huffel S, de Beer R. Fast removal of residual water in proton spectra. J Magn Reson 1998;132:197–203.
56. Brown TR, Stoyanova R. NMR spectral quantitation by principal-component analysis. II. Determination of frequency and phase shifts. J Magn Reson 1996;112:32–43.
57. Ordidge RJ, Cresshull ID. The correction of transient Bo field shifts following the application of pulsed gradients by phase correction in the time domain. J Magn Reson 1986;69:151–155.
58. Pijnappel WWF, van den Boogaart A, de Beer R, van Ormondt D. SVD-based quantification of magnetic resonance signals. J Magn Reson 1992;97:122–134.
59. Witjes H, Melssen WJ, Zandt HJA, van der Graaf M, Heerschap A, Buydens LMC. Automatic correction for phase shifts, frequency shifts, and lineshape distortions across a series of single resonance lines in large spectral data sets. J Magn Reson 2000;144:35–44.
60. Govindaraju V, Young K, Maudsley AA. Proton NMR chemical shifts and coupling constants for brain metabolites. NMR Biomed 2000;13:129–153.
61. Castillo M, Smith JK, Kwock L. Correlation of myo-inositol levels and grading of cerebral astrocytomas. Am J Neuroradiol 2000;21:1645–1649.
62. Mierisova S, Ala-Korpela M. MR spectroscopy quantitation: a review of frequency domain methods. NMR Biomed 2001;14:247–259.
63. Provencher SW. Automatic quantitation of localized in vivo 1H spectra with LCModel. NMR Biomed 2001;14:260–264.
64. van den Boogaart A. *MRUI Manual v.96.3. A User's Guide to the Magnetic Resonance User Interface Software Package*. Delft: Delft Technical University Press; 2000.
65. Naressi A, Couturier C, Castang I, de Beer R, Graveron-Demilly D. Java-based graphical user-interface for MRUI, a software package for quantitation of in vivo/medical magnetic resonance spectroscopy signals. Comput Biol Med 2001;31:269–286.
66. Fulhan MJ, Bizzi A, Dietz MJ, Shih HHL, Raman R, Sobering GS, Frank JA, Dwyer AJ, Alger JR, Di Chiro G. Mapping of brain tumor metabolites with proton MR spectroscopic imaging: clinical relevance. Radiology 1992;185:675–686.

67. Furuya S, Naruse S, Ide M, Morishita H, Kizu O, Ueda S, Maeda T. Evaluation of metabolic heterogeneity in brain tumors using 1H-chemical shift imaging method. NMR Biomed 1997;10:25–30.

68. Segebarth C, Balériaux D, Luyten PR, den Hollander JA. Detection of metabolic heterogeneity of human intracranial tumors in vivo by 1H NMR spectroscopic imaging. Magn Reson Med 1990;13:62–76.

69. Weinmann HJ, Ebert W, Misselwitz B, Schmitt-Willich H. Tissue-specific MR contrast agents. Eur J Radiol 2003;46:33–44.

70. Maintz JBA, Viergever MA. A survey of medical image registration. Med Image Anal 1998;2:1–36.

71. Pratt WK. *Digital Image Processing*. New York: John Wiley & Sons; 1978. pp. 526–566.

72. Evans EC, Collins DL, Neelin P, MacDonald D, Kamber M, Marret TS. Three-dimensional correlative imaging: applications in human brain imaging. In: Thatcher RW, Hallett M, Zeffiro T, John ER, Huerta M, editors. *Functional Neuroimaging: Technical Foundations*. Orlando: Academic Press; 1994. pp. 145–161.

73. Nelson SJ, Vigneron DB, Dillon WP. Serial evaluation of patients with brain tumors using volume MRI and 3D 1H MRSI. NMR Biomed 1999;12:123–138.

74. American Joint Committee on Cancer. *AJCC Cancer Staging Manual*. 6th ed. New York: Springer; 2002.

75. Simonetti AW, Melssen WJ, Szabo de Edelenyi F, van Asten JA, Heerschap A, Buydens LMC. Combination of feature-reduced MR spectroscopic and MR imaging data for improved brain tumor classification. NMR Biomed 2005;18:34–43.

76. Devos A, Simonetti AW, van der Graaf M, Lukas L, Suykens JAK, Vanhamme L, Buydens LMC, Heerschap A, van Huffel S. The use of multivariate MR imaging intensities versus metabolic data from MR spectroscopic imaging for brain tumour classification. J Magn Reson 2005;173:218–228.

77. Galanaud D, Nicoli F, Chinot O, Confort-Gouny S, Figarella-Branger D, Roche P, Fuentes S, Le Fur Y, Ranjeva JP, Cozzone PJ. Noninvasive diagnostic assessment of brain tumors using combined in vivo MR imaging and spectroscopy. Magn Reson Med 2006;55:1236–1245.

78. Simonetti AW. Investigation of brain tumor classification and its reliability using chemometrics on MR spectroscopy and MR imaging data. [PhD thesis]. Radboud University Nijmegen, Nijmegen; 2004. pp. 115–137.

79. Krooshof PWT, Tran TN, Postma GJ, Melssen WJ, Buydens LMC. Effects of including spatial information in clustering multivariate image data. Trends Anal Chem 2006;25(11): 1067–1080.

80. de Vos M, Laudadio T, Simonetti AW, Heerschap A, van Huffel S. Fast nosologic imaging of the brain. J Magn Reson 2007;184:292–301.

2

EVALUATION OF TOMOGRAPHIC DATA

JÖRG VAN DEN HOFF
Department of Positron Emission Tomography, Institute of Radiopharmacy, Helmholtz-Zentrum Dresden-Rossendorf, Dresden, Germany

2.1 INTRODUCTION

Through the last decades tomographic techniques have gained an ever-increasing importance in biomedical imaging. The great benefit of these techniques is the ability to assess noninvasively (and nondestructively) the three-dimensional structure of the investigated objects.

With regards to biomedical applications, several, but not all, available tomographic techniques allow the investigation of dynamic processes (e.g., transport phenomena) and repeated measurements in a single organism. One thus can differentiate between these *in vivo* techniques and *in vitro* techniques, which are suitable, for example, for investigations of tissue samples. Electron tomography (Chapter 6) belongs to the latter group. X-ray Computed Tomography (CT, Chapter 4), Magnetic Resonance Imaging (MRI, Chapter 5), as well as Single Photon Emission Computed Tomography and Positron Emission Tomography (SPECT and PET, Chapter 7) are generally (SPECT and PET exclusively) used for the noninvasive 3D imaging of living organisms. The aforementioned techniques are well suited to generate three-dimensional tomographic image volumes even of complete organisms such as the human body.

This contrasts with more recent developments in the area of optical imaging such as Optical Coherence Tomography (OCT), which utilize light sources within or near the visible range. Owing to the usually high absorption and scattering

Biomedical Imaging: Principles and Applications, First Edition. Edited by Reiner Salzer.

of light in tissue, the application of optical tomographic methods is generally restricted to investigation of near-surface structures such as the skin or the eye.

This chapter provides a rather general outline of the principal problems that one faces when evaluating tomographic data, with focus on the analysis of the image data. The important but highly specialized field of tomographic image reconstruction will be discussed only very shortly. The four tomographic *in vivo* techniques that currently are of relevance not only in basic research but also in clinical routine are as follows.

X-ray Computed Tomography (CT): This is currently certainly the most widespread tomographic technique encountered in the clinical setting. CT uses an external X-ray source and images the tissue-dependent X-ray absorption.

Magnetic Resonance Imaging (MRI): MRI is based on the nuclear magnetic resonance effect. It utilizes static magnetic and Radio Frequency (rf) fields for the imaging process. Compared to CT the method provides superior soft tissue differentiation.

Single Photon Emission Computed Tomography (SPECT): This method detects γ-radiation emitted from molecules labeled with radioactive isotopes that are injected into the organism. The method is very sensitive and able to detect the injected tracers at very low concentrations (several orders of magnitude lower than those necessary in contrast agent enhanced CT or MRI).

Positron Emission Tomography (PET): Similar to SPECT, PET is a technique using radioactive tracers, but in PET the coincident annihilation radiation from positron-emitting isotopes is the image-generating signal. There are important differences between the two techniques, which result from the use of positron emitters. Apart from differences in the chemical and biological properties of the used tracers, the different detection mechanism of PET results in a much larger detection efficiency of PET (allowing measurements of tracer concentrations in the nano- to picomolar range) and superior spatial resolution (only exceeded by special low sensitivity pinhole SPECT systems). Last but not least, PET is the only one of the listed modalities that routinely allows truly quantitative measurements of the tracer concentrations, which is a prerequisite of all further quantitative evaluations.

As already indicated, the different methods probe different properties of the living organisms investigated:

CT: tissue dependent attenuation of X-ray radiation (essentially determined by the atomic electron density, which in turn is related to tissue density),

MRI: tissue dependent absorption from rf fields (essentially determined by hydrogen/proton density) and related effects such as spin–lattice and spin–spin relaxation times of the resonance absorption signal,

SPECT and PET: tissue dependent tracer concentration, which is related to the traced biochemical and (patho)physiological process (such as blood flow, glucose consumption, protein synthesis, etc.)

All tomographic techniques share, to a varying degree, the following characteristics:

1. Ability to acquire noninvasively tomographic, that is, overlap-free cross-sectional (2D) images of the interior parts of the investigated organism or sample.
2. Generation of 3D image data: the ability to image a certain target volume by closely spaced cross-sectional images.
3. Selective sensitivity of the imaging process to specific morphological properties and/or physiological and biochemical processes.
4. A need for mathematical algorithms to achieve optimal image reconstruction from the acquired raw data.
5. Necessity to manage potentially huge amounts of raw and image data.
6. A need for dedicated tools to handle, display, and analyze 3D image data.

Formally, evaluation of the tomographic data can be pursued along two different approaches.

On the one hand, tomographic data are, first and foremost, three-dimensional image data that provide information concerning the regional variation of the parameter producing the signal. Depending on the tomographic method used and on the experimental setting, it might not be possible (or necessary) to evaluate the data beyond visual inspection. This is, for instance, true if one is aiming solely at getting qualitative structural/anatomical information (e.g., investigating bone structures with X-ray CT).

In such a situation, methods for optimal image display, digital image processing, and especially tools for efficient 3D image data visualization such as volume rendering are of primary interest.

On the other hand, tomographic data frequently are valuable also in the sense that the image-generating signal is itself of interest as a quantitative measure. For example: while CT data are more often than not evaluated in a qualitative fashion, it is also possible to use the measured attenuation of the X-ray radiation to derive quantitative information concerning bone density. Some tomographic methods are more "quantitative" than others in the sense that they provide an image signal that is related in a better known way to the quantity of interest. Most desirable is the situation where the image signal is simply proportional to such a quantity, which allows, for example, direct interpretation of all image contrasts in terms of that quantity.

Probably the best example for this is the PET method. Here, the images represent quantitatively the number of radioactive decays of the applied tracer in the respective image pixel. Since this number in turn is directly proportional to the amount of tracer substance in the corresponding pixel volume, one obtains a direct measure of this quantity. PET images are therefore directly interpretable as quantitative tracer concentration maps.

For other modalities the situation usually is a bit more complicated. Taking MRI as an example, the images provide detailed information especially concerning the soft tissue anatomy, but it is rather difficult to derive reliable quantitative information such as concentrations of systemic substances. If contrast agents are applied, which is in a way the analogue of the tracers used in PET, although the applied amounts are larger by a factor of 10^6 or so in the case of MRI, one usually is not at all able to deduce the local contrast agent concentration quantitatively. This difficulty has its origin in the fact that the relationship between the concentration of the contrast agent and the contrast-agent-induced changes of the image signal is influenced by a number of factors whose precise effect cannot be quantified accurately. Therefore, the MRI image signal usually cannot be translated into truly quantitative measures of concentrations.

The discussion of the different quantitative capabilities of the above-mentioned different methods refers to the primary images that are delivered by the respective method. In doing so, one further important parameter that could be used has been ignored, namely, investigation of time-dependent processes by so-called dynamic investigations (in contrast to static "snapshot"-like studies).

Dynamic tomography requires the ability to perform the measurements for a single tomographic data set so fast that a sufficiently large number of such measurements can be performed over the interesting time window of the investigated process.

Depending on the method used, different factors limit the obtainable temporal resolution that typically goes down to the order of seconds in the case of CT, MRI, or PET.

2.2 IMAGE RECONSTRUCTION

The basic idea of most tomographic approaches is to acquire two-dimensional projection images from various directions around the object of interest. It is necessary that the radiation, which directly or indirectly generates each image (X-rays, electron rays, γ-radiation, rf fields, etc.), is penetrating in the sense that each two-dimensional image can be seen as a projection of the real three-dimensional object onto the image plane*. The most straightforward example might be X-ray CT, where each projection is the same as a standard X-ray image acquired under that orientation.

*This description is not really suitable for all techniques. For example, in the case of magnetic resonance imaging the raw data are not projection data but are rather directly acquired in Fourier space. Moreover, in this case, directional information does not stem from the applied rf field itself but from its combination with a suitable gradient of the magnetic field utilized in the measurement. The basic strategy of using a penetrating radiation applies nevertheless.

Having acquired the projection data for a sufficiently complete set of directions, usually covering an angular range of 360° or 180° around the patient, the next step is tomographic image reconstruction.

Various standard mathematical techniques exist to calculate from a sufficiently complete set of projections the complete three-dimensional structure of the investigated object.

The algorithms can be roughly divided into two groups: analytical and iterative procedures.

The analytical procedures utilize variants of the filtered backprojection approach. This approach is based on a mathematical theorem that goes back to 1911, namely, the Radon transformation, which in two dimensions defines the relationship between the complete set of all possible line integrals (the projections or Radon transform) through a two-dimensional function $f(x, y)$ and that function itself (which represents a cross-sectional slice through our object).

Iterative image reconstruction utilizes well-defined trial-and-error approaches whose background lies in mathematical statistics. Here, image reconstruction consists in providing the algorithm with an initial guess of the object that then is subjected to a simulated imaging process, thus generating artificial projection data that are compared with the actual measured data. From this comparison, correction factors are derived, which in turn are applied to each image pixel of the first image estimate, thus generating a new improved image estimate. This iterative loop of image estimation, simulated projection and image estimate improvement, is repeated until some convergence criterion is met.

Analytical image reconstruction is applied whenever the nature of the data allows it since the computational burden is much smaller than is the case for the iterative approaches. Analytical reconstruction is the default approach in CT as well as in MRI.

For SPECT and PET applicability of analytic procedures is limited. This is due to the fact that these tracer techniques operate at extremely high sensitivities (compared to CT and MRI) but suffer from influences of the statistical nature of the decay of the radioactive tracers, which translates into considerable statistical noise of the projection data. This in turn frequently leads to sizable artifacts during image reconstruction. In recent years, the ever-increasing computer speed allowed to move to iterative algorithms as the default reconstruction method in SPECT and PET.

2.3 IMAGE DATA REPRESENTATION: PIXEL SIZE AND IMAGE RESOLUTION

The early tomographs usually acquired only single cross-sectional slices of an appreciable slice thickness (that is, low spatial resolution perpendicular to the primary image plane). Nowadays, tomographic techniques are capable of producing not only single cross-sectional images but, rather, contiguous stacks of such images representing consecutive cross-sections through the investigated object. The spatial orientation of the cross sections (i.e., image plane orientation) is usually determined by the orientation of the object within the Field of View (FOV) of the tomograph: with the exception of MRI the major techniques generate cross sections whose orientation is collinear to the symmetry axis of the tomograph's gantry, that is, the image plane is parallel to the plane defined by the tomograph's gantry. This slice orientation is usually called transaxial.

Despite the fact that the transaxial image plane is usually the one that has been measured in the first place, it is now primarily a matter of taste, whether one prefers to view data organized as a stack of consecutive two-dimensional transaxial images or as representing a three-dimensional digital image volume, which then can be "sliced" via suitable software tools to yield cross sections of arbitrary orientation.

The latter approach (arbitrary slicing of 3D volumes) only works well if the spatial resolution is similar along each direction within the image volume. This is guaranteed in modern designs where spatial resolution is indeed approximately isotropic.

From a user point of view, a tomograph can be then seen as a kind of 3D digital camera. As is the case for any digital camera, one has to be careful not to confuse actual image resolution with the digital grid on which the data are displayed. This point is at the same time trivial and a source of recurring confusion and will, therefore, be now examined more closely.

It is common usage to specify the number of image pixels along both axes of the image matrix to characterize a digital camera. In the case of three-dimensional tomographic data, one has three such axes. Let the primary transaxial image plane be the x/y-plane, and let the z-axis point along the image stack. The number of resolution cells across each axis of the FOV is also called the sampling of the digital image volume†. A typical figure for clinical whole body spiral CT would be

$$n_x \times n_y \times n_z = 1024 \times 1024 \times 1000$$

and for a clinical PET tomograph

$$n_x \times n_y \times n_z = 256 \times 256 \times 250$$

Three-dimensional image pixels are more accurately called voxels. Each voxel represents a constant small volume within the FOV of the tomograph. The voxel size is simply equal to the ratio of the actual metric extension of the imaged volume along each axis divided by the number of resolution cells along the same

†We view sampling here as being contiguous across the data so that each pixel contains the average of the input signal over the pixel extension (histogramming). A slightly different, more common definition would be to represent the imaging process by equally spaced "point samples" from the continuous input signal. The difference between both definitions is small for densely sampled data but can be notable otherwise. For the tomographic techniques discussed here, the histogramming description is more adequate.

axis. The important point to realize is that the voxel size in general does not describe the spatial resolution of the image data. Using the example of a digital camera again, the achievable spatial resolution is controlled by the optical system (i.e., the lens) and the resulting image is then discretized into a finite number of pixels by the Charge-Coupled Device (CCD) detector chip located in the focal plane. In a reasonable design, the number of pixels has to be chosen in such a way that each pixel is significantly smaller than the smallest structure that can be resolved by the camera. Only if this requirement is not fulfilled, that is, if the pixel size is larger than the resolving power of the optical system, is the effective image resolution controlled by the image matrix size (i.e., the number of pixels along each axis). On the other hand, if the pixel size is decreased well below the resolution limit, no quality gain will be noticed in the digital image.

Exactly the same holds true for tomographic data; the image voxel size should be chosen in such a way that the voxels, which, contrary to usual digital photographies, need not be cubic, are significantly, but not excessively, smaller than the known spatial resolution limit of the respective tomograph. This is reflected in the typical figures given earlier. CT data are stored in much finer sampled digital image volumes than PET data simply because the spatial resolution typically is better by about a factor of 5. If, on the other hand, one would decide to store a given PET image volume using the much finer sampling (larger 3D image matrix) as used in CT this would obviously not result in improved spatial resolution of the PET data.

This qualitative statement can be made mathematically exact. This is the content of the Nyquist-Shannon sampling theorem; readers may refer (Nyquist, 1928; Shannon, 1949), or any good textbook on digital image processing, such as Gonzalez and Woods, 2007. A continuous signal can be restored from equally spaced discrete point samples if the sampling rate (in our context the number of samples per unit of length) is at least equal to twice the highest frequency occurring in the Fourier spectrum of the signal. (Signals conforming to the implied assumption that the Fourier spectrum has a finite upper limiting frequency are called band limited).

As discussed in more detail in the next section, the image of a point source is adequately represented by a Gaussian function with a standard deviation σ that depends on the spatial resolving power of the imaging device. The relationship between a Gaussian and its Fourier transform is given by

$$g(x) = \mathrm{e}^{-\frac{1}{2}\frac{x^2}{\sigma^2}} \Rightarrow G(f) = \sqrt{\frac{\pi}{2}}\mathrm{e}^{-\frac{1}{2}\sigma^2 \cdot f^2}$$

Thus, the Fourier spectrum is not really band limited in this case but at least it drops off very rapidly at high frequencies. The standard deviation of $G(f)$ is $1/\sigma$, and going up to twice this frequency already covers about 95% of the area under the curve. Thus, a crude (rather low) estimate of the effective frequency limit is given by

$$f_{\text{lim}} \approx \frac{1}{\sigma}$$

that is, the inverse of the standard deviation of the original Gaussian $g(x)$.

Leaving further mathematical details as well as considerations concerning the consequences of violating the assumptions (discrete point samples from a band-limited signal) aside, the sampling theorem implies that a reasonable estimate of the sampling rate required for approximately restoring the continuous Gaussian $g(x)$ from discrete samples is two times the above limiting frequency, that is, $2/\sigma$. This means, one would need approximately two samples over a length σ, which is about the same as four samples across the Full Width at Half Maximum (FWHM) of the Gaussian.

This number should not be taken literally, but only as a rough estimate of the sampling rate that will be necessary if one wants to "reconstruct" the continuous Gaussian from its discrete samples. Even if one is not interested in actually performing this task, it is obvious that the same sampling rate will suffice to map the relevant structural details of the continuous signal (otherwise the reconstruction of the continuous signal would not be possible) and thus to obtain a digital image whose quality is limited not by the discretization but by the intrinsic resolution of the imaging device.

The one-dimensional case will serve to illustrate the above a bit more. In Figure 2.1 an idealized object, indicated in gray, is shown, consisting of several rectangular structures of different sizes and signal intensities that are superimposed on a constant background that is assumed to extend well beyond the plot boundaries.

The black curve is the image of this object obtained at a given finite intrinsic spatial resolution of the imaging system. The implications of finite resolution with regards to quantitative measurements in the tomographic data are discussed in the next section. Here, we want to concentrate on the effects of final sampling, that is, of final pixel size. These effects can be appreciated when looking at the red curves in the figure. From Figure 2.1a–c, the number of pixels is increased consecutively by a factor of 4. When the pixel size decreases and falls sufficiently below the intrinsic spatial resolution (which is set to 4 mm in Fig. 2.1), the measured signal (the red curve) approximates the black curve with increasing accuracy. In Figure 2.1c the sampling is equal to the given estimate (four samples across the FWHM of the peaks). As explained earlier, this sampling density is more or less sufficient to restore the continuous signal (the black curves) from the discrete samples. At this sampling rate the discretized signal (the red curve) can itself serve as a reasonable approximation of the object (without the need to actually use the sampling theorem). Decreasing the pixel size (at the expense of increasing the total number of pixels) much further would not result in a better spatial resolution but only in an increase of image size and, thus, computer memory usage.

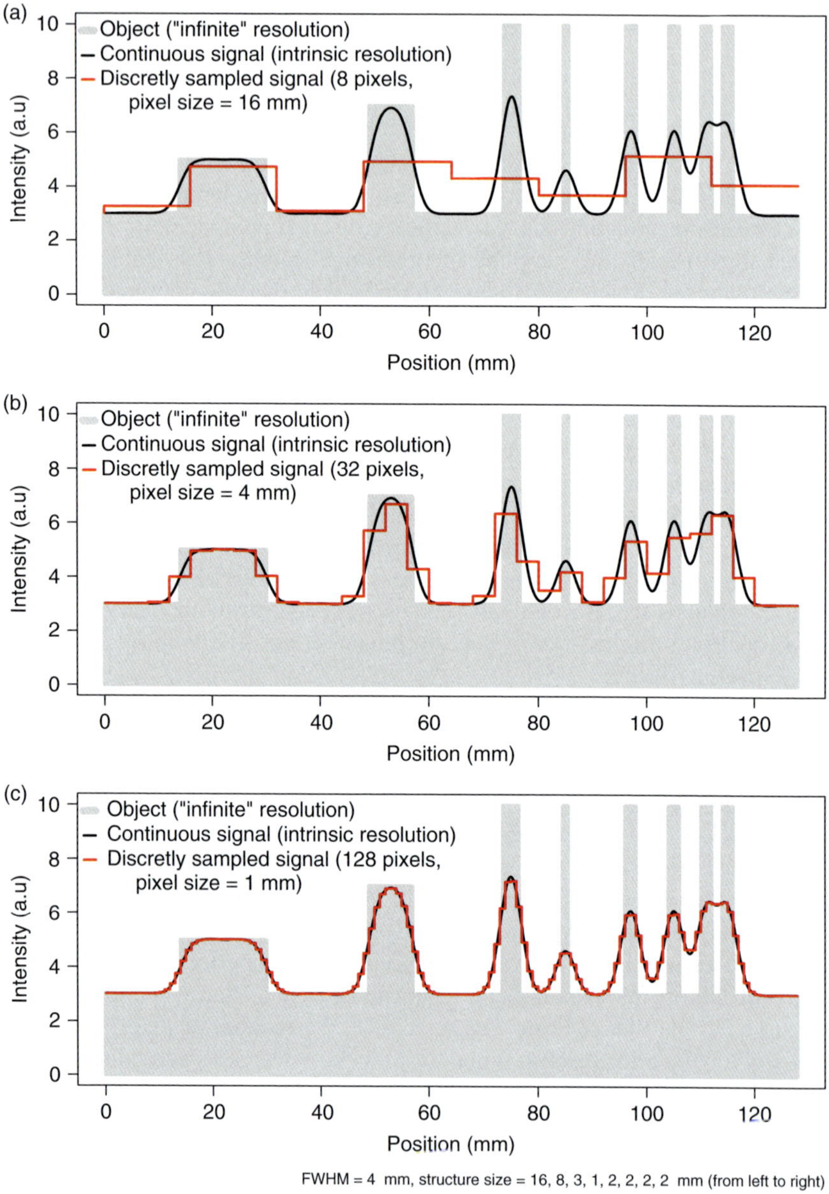

Figure 2.1. Effects of finite sampling on object delineation in the one-dimensional case. Shown in solid gray is the true object consisting of several rectangular peaks of varying sizes and signal intensities. The imaging device is assumed to have a spatial resolution of 4 mm FWHM. The black curve then represents the result of the imaging process in the continuous case. Using finite sampling, the object is actually imaged as shown in red for three different pixel sizes. When the pixel size approaches or exceeds the intrinsic spatial resolution, a significant quality loss is observed.

On the other hand (Fig. 2.1a and b), if the pixel size is larger than the intrinsic resolution of the imaging device, the effective resolution in the image is limited by this inadequate pixel size. This results in increasing loss of detail (different peaks no longer resolved) and discretization artifacts such as apparent shift of peak position and discontinuous jumps in image intensity. In our example, at the largest pixel size (Fig. 2.1a) the four separate peaks at the right hand side are no longer resolved.

In summary, one has to choose a pixel size that is adapted to the given resolution of the imaging device. As a rule of thumb, the pixel size should not exceed one half of the effective peak width (i.e., FWHM) in order to keep discretization errors tolerable, and reducing the pixel size by another factor of 2 (resulting in 4 pixels across the FWHM) is generally a good choice.

2.4 CONSEQUENCES OF LIMITED SPATIAL RESOLUTION

A major figure of merit for any tomographic technique is the achieved spatial resolution. Table 2.1 gives some typical numbers for the major approaches discussed here.

These values are valid for the primary image plane (which usually will be the transaxial plane). As has been indicated, modern tomographs are able to provide near-isotropic resolution in all three dimensions, that is, the resolution along the scanner axis is very nearly identical to that achieved in the transaxial plane.

Now, what exactly is meant by this kind of number, that is, what does it mean if spatial resolution is specified as being equal to 1 mm? Only the case of isotropic (direction independent) resolution will be discussed, but the adaption to the nonisotropic case should be straightforward.

Generally, spatial resolution is characterized by the Point Spread Function (PSF).

The PSF is the image of a point source (i.e., an infinitely small source; in practice this is a source whose linear dimensions are much smaller than the spatial

TABLE 2.1. Typical Spatial Resolution of Different Tomographic Techniques

Technique	Typical Spatial Resolution (mm)
Clinical CT	1
Clinical MRI	1
Clinical PET	5
Small animal CT	0.03
Small animal MRI	0.06
Small animal PET	1.5

resolution of the imaging device under consideration). The precise shape of the PSF depends on the imaging device, but usually a three-dimensional Gaussian

$$PSF(r) = \frac{1}{(\sqrt{2\pi}\sigma)^3} e^{-\frac{1}{2}\frac{r^2}{\sigma^2}}$$

is an adequate description. (This might be seen as a consequence of the central limit theorem of mathematical statistics: each superposition of sufficiently many random processes with a probability density function dropping sufficiently rapid to zero for large deviations from the mean yields a normal distribution. In the current context, this corresponds to the superposition of the large number of factors contributing to the spatial resolution of the finally resulting tomographic image data.) The standard deviation σ of this Gaussian describes the spatial resolution. Instead of using σ, it is more common to specify the FWHM of the PSF (simply because this figure is directly accessible in measurements). The FWHM is the distance of the two points left and right of the center where the PSF has dropped to 50% of its center (maximum) value. For the Gaussian, the relation with the standard deviation σ is given by

$$FWHM = 2\sqrt{2 \cdot \ln(2)}\sigma \approx 2.355 \cdot \sigma \approx 1.177 \cdot 2\sigma$$

that is, as a rule of thumb the FWHM is about twice the size of σ. The FWHM is not the strict limit for the minimal distance necessary to differentiate between two structures within the image. Rather, this figure is an approximate limit near which differentiation becomes increasingly difficult. This is illustrated in Figure 2.1. The two rightmost peaks have a distance equal to the FWHM of 4 mm and are barely discriminated in the measured signal. In the presence of image noise, differentiation of these two peaks would no longer be possible at all.

Loss of identifiability of adjacent peaks is only one aspect of finite spatial resolution. Another one is the mutual "cross talk" of neighboring structures. This phenomenon is usually referred to as the Partial Volume Effect (PVE) with regards to a loss of signal intensity from the Region of Interest (ROI) and called spillover when referring to a (undesired) gain of signal intensity from neighboring high intensity structures. The effect can be appreciated in Figure 2.1 in several respects by comparing the continuous signal with the true object. For one, all object boundaries exhibit an apparent smooth transit in signal intensity between target and background (loss of precise definition of the boundaries). Moreover, closely neighbored peaks acquire a slightly elevated signal intensity from the mutual cross talk of the signal intensities in comparison to a more distant peak of the same size (see the group of the four 2-mm peaks at the right hand side of the figure). At the same time, the target to background contrast is heavily reduced because of signal spillover into the background region between the peaks.

Another important aspect of limited spatial resolution is the limited recovery of the correct original signal intensity even for well isolated peaks. In order to assess the effect quantitatively, the Recovery Coefficient (RC) is used, which is defined as the ratio (after background subtraction) of the measured signal intensity maximum to the true intensity of the respective structure. As shown in Figure 2.1, the measured peaks only reach the original signal intensity if the size of the imaged structure is significantly larger than the spatial resolution limit as described by the FWHM.

Recovery limitation massively limits structure identification simply by decreasing the signal to background ratio and frequently leads to underestimates of signal intensity. For the smallest structure in Figure 2.1 (with a structure width of 1 mm, that is, 1/4 of the FWHM), the RC is less than 25% of the true signal intensity.

Limited recovery is an even more serious problem in the two- and three-dimensional case in comparison to the one-dimensional example of Figure 2.1. Figure 2.2 shows RC for homogeneous objects of three simple shapes for varying object size. By "slab" we designate an object whose spatial extent in two of its dimensions is much larger than the spatial resolution of the tomograph. The spatial extent in these dimensions can then be considered as "infinite" and does have no influence on the imaging process of cross sections through the slab. Therefore, the slab curve corresponds to the one-dimensional situation already shown in Figure 2.1. As a practical example, imaging of the myocardial wall corresponds approximately to this case, since the curvature of the myocardium is small compared to the spatial resolution (as well as compared to the wall thickness) and can therefore be neglected when estimating the recovery effects. Similarly, a (circular) "rod" is an object whose extent along one dimension can be considered as infinite and does not influence the cross-sectional imaging. This is thus the analog of simple two-dimensional imaging. As a practical example, consider imaging of the aorta or some other vessel. The third shape (sphere) approximates the imaging of localized structures whose extent in all three dimensions is comparable (as might be the case, e.g., for metastases of a tumor disease).

For these simple object shapes (or any combination of them in order to describe more complex structures), simulation of the imaging process is rather straightforward (analytic convolution of the object with the PSF of the imaging device) and yields formulas that describe the spatial variation of the measured signal for any given spatial resolution (e.g., the continuous signal curve in Fig. 2.1 has been determined in this way).

The resulting formulas especially provide the intensity value at the center of the imaged structure. By dividing these values through the true intensity (i.e., by normalizing to unit intensity) one obtains the RC s as defined by the following expressions:

$$RC_{\text{slab}} = erf(Z)$$

$$RC_{\text{rod}} = 1 - \mathrm{e}^{-Z^2}$$

$$RC_{\text{sphere}} = erf(Z) - \frac{2}{\sqrt{\pi}} Z\, \mathrm{e}^{-Z^2}$$

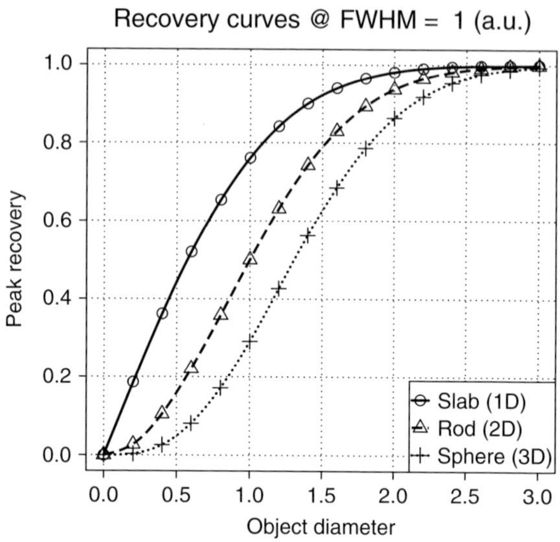

Figure 2.2. Recovery curves for three simple object shapes. The object diameter is specified in multiples of the FWHM of the PSF. If the object diameter drops below about two times the FWHM, recovery is rapidly decreasing, especially for rods and spheres.

where

$$erf(Z) = \frac{2}{\sqrt{\pi}} \int_0^Z e^{-x^2} dx$$

is the so-called error function and

$$Z = \frac{1}{\sqrt{2}} \frac{R}{\sigma} = 2\sqrt{\ln(2)} \frac{D}{FWHM} \approx 1.67 \frac{D}{FWHM}.$$

For a more detailed discussion of recovery-related effects see (Kessler et al., 1984) (note that these authors use a different, and unusual, definition of the error function that might be a potential source of error when applying their formulas).

The RCs are not dependent on the absolute object size, but rather on the size of the object relative to the spatial resolution of the imaging device. Reducing at the same time object size and the width of the PSF by the same factor leaves the recovery unaltered. The curves in Figure 2.2 show the (peak) RCs as explained earlier, that is, the ratio of the measured peak intensity (in the center of the object) to the true intensity (which is assumed to be constant across the object). The recovery values approach a value of one only for object diameters of about three times the FWHM. For smaller objects, recovery decreases, most rapidly in the 3D case. The differences between the curves become very large for objects smaller than the FWHM. Already at a diameter of one-half of the FWHM, the peak recovery for a sphere is below 5% and about a factor of 10 smaller than for a slab of the same diameter. In the presence of finite image noise and background, such a small sphere will most probably not even be detectable, let alone assessable in any quantitative fashion.

These cumulative adverse consequences of limited spatial resolution and image noise are demonstrated in Figure 2.3, which uses the same sampling as in Figure 2.1c and superimposes noise on the measured signal.

As can be seen by comparison with Figure 2.1c, objects near the resolution limit can no longer be correctly identified even at rather low noise levels. Both discrimination of adjacent peaks as well as identification of isolated small structures are compromised.

Up to now the consequences of limited spatial resolution with regard to measured signal intensity and detectability have been discussed.

Another point of interest is how accurately object boundaries can be localized. Since all sharp edges present in the image are smeared out by the finite resolution, one has to decide where on the slope the true boundary is located. For arbitrary shapes, this question cannot easily be answered since this would require a reversal of the imaging process (deconvolution), which can at best be carried out approximately. It is useful, nevertheless, to investigate the situation encountered with the simple object shapes discussed earlier.

It turns out that for the one-dimensional case ("slab"), the object boundaries are usually located at a threshold of 50% of the peak intensity (after subtraction of potential background) except for very thin slabs near or below the resolution limit. Here the correct threshold becomes extremely size dependent and a reliable determination of object size is no longer possible.

In the two- and three-dimensional cases, it turns out that the threshold is generally size dependent and the threshold approaches the value of 50% only very slowly with increasing object size. This is illustrated in Figure 2.4 for the case of spheres.

Figure 2.5 shows the resulting dependence of the "edge detecting" threshold for our three simple geometries as a function of object size. The object size dependence persists (for rods and spheres) well beyond the range where recovery limitations play a role. In contrast, the increase of the threshold at very small object sizes is simply a consequence of the rapidly decreasing RC in this range.

The situation described earlier imposes certain restrictions on the ability to delineate object boundaries in the image data correctly. If one resorts to interactive visual delineation of the object boundary in the image data, the uncertainties can be of the order of the FWHM, or even more, since the visual impression is very sensitive to details of the chosen color table and thresholding of the display. Depending on the relative size D/FWHM of the target structure and the question to be answered, this uncertainty might be irrelevant in one case and intolerable in the other. For example, for PET-based radiotherapy planning, unambiguous and accurate definition of boundaries is of paramount importance even for larger target structures.

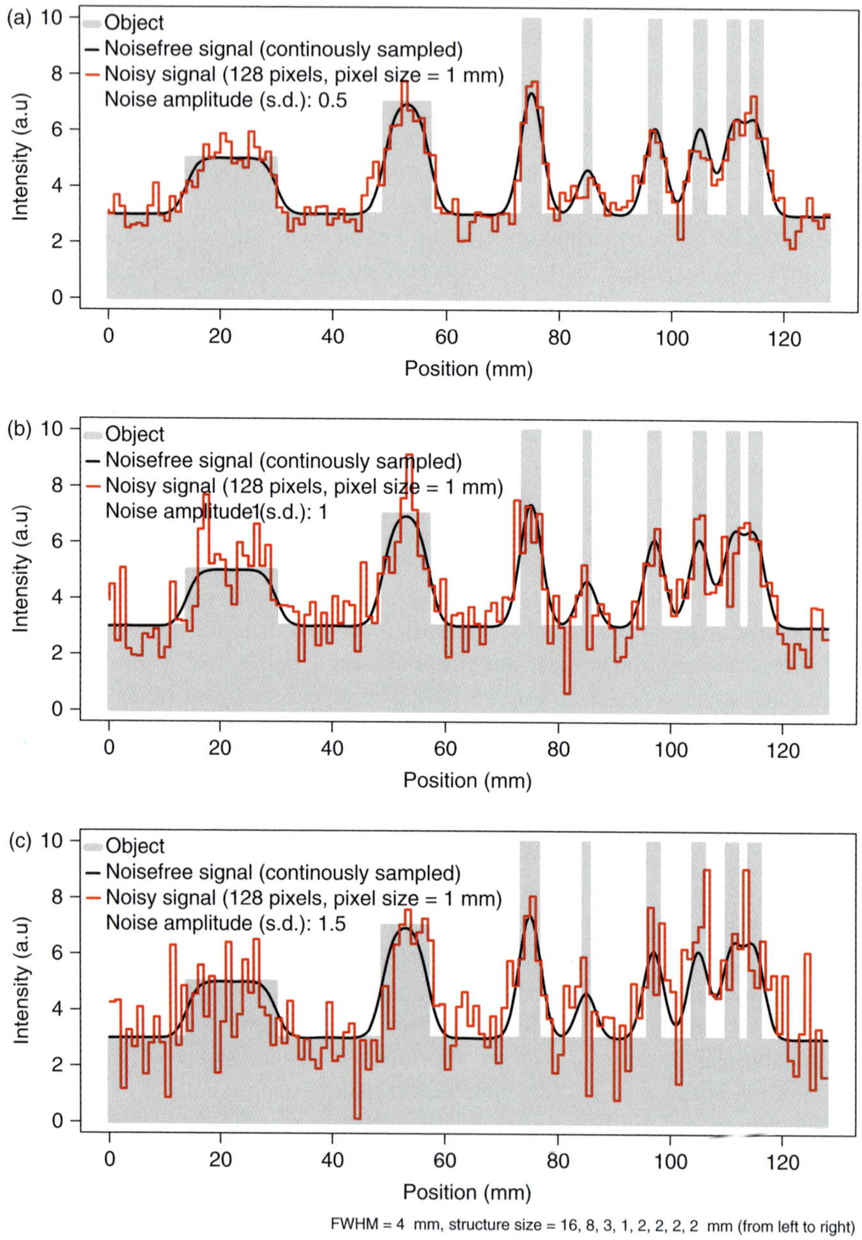

Figure 2.3. Influence of image noise and finite spatial resolution (using the same configuration as in Fig. 2.1). For a given signal level, image noise most seriously affects structures near the resolution limit.

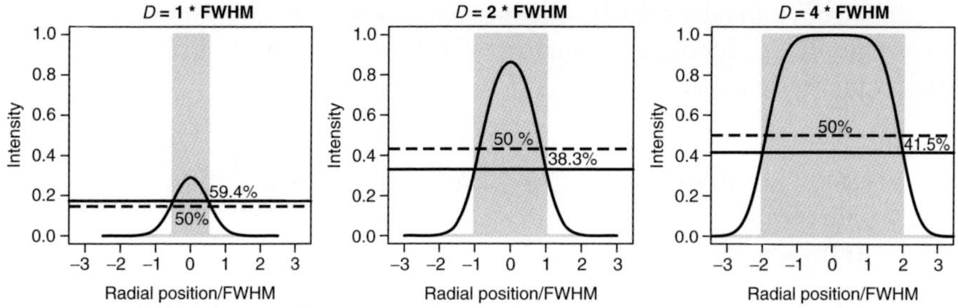

Figure 2.4. Profile through the center of a sphere for three different sphere diameters. The solid horizontal line represents the threshold intersecting the profiles at the true object boundary. The threshold generally is size dependent and usually smaller than 50% except for very small sphere diameters.

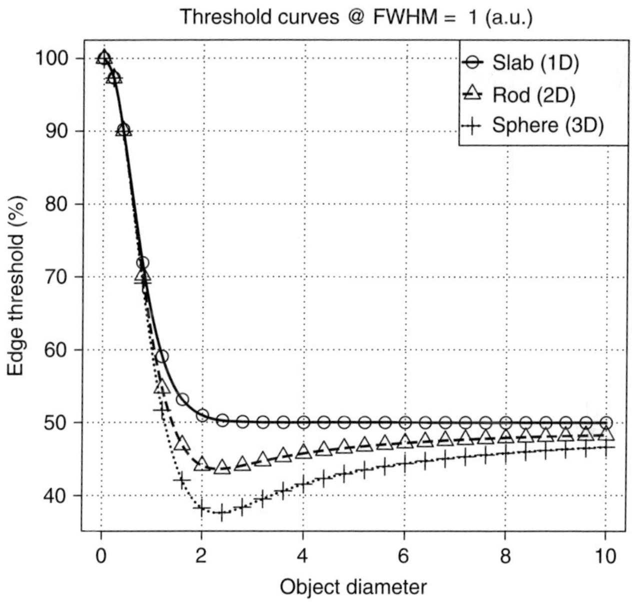

Figure 2.5. Object size dependence of the threshold intersecting the object boundary for three simple object shapes. The threshold is specified as a percentage of the measured (background corrected) signal maximum in the center of the object.

It is therefore necessary to use algorithmic approaches that are able to account for effects such as those discussed above. Moreover, the presented results are valid in this form only under idealized circumstances (with respect to object shape, assumption of noise-free data, and Gaussian PSF and the assumption of an otherwise perfect imaging process). The lesson is that, for any given tomograph, it is necessary to investigate via phantom studies the exact behavior of the respective device under realistic circumstances and to use this information to optimize algorithmic approaches, which are able to perform the desired quantitatively correct object delineation.

2.5 TOMOGRAPHIC DATA EVALUATION: TASKS

2.5.1 Software Tools

Evaluation of tomographic data has two aspects: qualitative visual assessment of the images and extraction of quantitative data.

Any commercial tomograph will come together with a set of (possibly insufficient) evaluation tools. These will at least encompass 2D visualization facilities and functionality for defining two-dimensional ROIs. ROIs are finite size regions in the images for which the user desires to get quantitative measures (e.g., diameter, area, mean/minimum/maximum signal intensity). For ROI definition, the user can select between different options, including prescribed shapes (rectangles, circles, ellipses), irregular polygons, and threshold-based approaches.

Once the ROI is defined, the numerical data for the ROI are computed and usually saved to a text file for further processing.

If one looks at the visualization and data evaluation software accompanying the tomographs, usually some problems become apparent:

1. The standard software is often rather basic and does not always address the special needs of experimental work.
2. Quality differences between products of different vendors are frequently more severe in the software area than concerning the hardware.
3. Costs for additional vendor-provided visualization/evaluation workstations are far from negligible and can, in a multiuser setting, constitute a sizable fraction of the overall installation costs.
4. Customizability/extensibility of the software is usually restricted or not possible.

From these observations it follows that restricting oneself to the possibilities provided by the standard software tools coming with the tomograph is not reasonable. Instead, one should define the evaluation tasks and then look for the best tools available or, if this is an option, develop (part of) the necessary tools in-house.

Medical imaging is a highly technical field that requires dedicated tools. One consequence of this is that commercially provided tools are usually quite expensive. Nevertheless, prices for products providing similar functionality can vary extensively. It is always a good idea to check the availability of third-party products that sometimes are reasonable (or superior) alternatives to vendor-provided additional data evaluation workstations or "extension packages."

Last, one should check out the tools that are provided as open Source or are otherwise are freely available in the public domain. As is true for other areas as well, there is a substantial amount of high quality software to be found here, which might suit the user's needs.

It would not make sense to give a comprehensive overview of the existing commercial and open source tools; such an overview would be outdated very rapidly, but two freely available and very valuable multipurpose tools should be mentioned: octave and R. Both can be used as interactive data exploration and visualization environments and include high level programming languages and numerical libraries, allowing the automation of complex data evaluation tasks without the need for low level programming in compiled languages (Eaton, 2011; R, 2011). A number of data processing tasks that are frequently relevant irrespective of which tomographic technique is used are discussed next.

2.5.2 Data Access

If one concludes that the available (or affordable) vendor-provided software tools are insufficient, the only remedy is to look for third-party software or implement the missing functionality in-house.

A necessary requirement is that the tomographic data are available in an accessible file format. A couple of years ago a multitude of proprietary file formats was still in use. Proprietary formats always pose the problem that interfacing the image data has to be solved for each vendor/modality separately.

The problem persists to a certain extent for the experimental devices used in small-animal imaging, but at least for the tomographic techniques that have found their way into clinical application one can safely expect that they provide the image data in a form compliant with the DICOM standard (DICOM Standards Committee, 2011).

Principally, adhering to a standard format is a good thing. With respect to DICOM, however, the standard is complex and allows for many vendor-specific entries (private tags) in the metadata part of the files. Interoperability between different vendors cannot always be taken for granted.

If one plans to process the images with third-party software or own tools, access to DICOM files is a must. Luckily, some noncommercial solutions exist, for instance, the DCMTK DICOM toolkit (OFFIS e.V., 2011), which provides a C library on top of which one's own applications can be built.

2.5.3 Image Processing

Once the access to the tomographic data is solved, the next requirement is to be able to perform standard image processing operations on the data. For slice-oriented (two-dimensional) processing of the tomographic data, one can resort to many different general purpose tools, but if the same tasks are to be performed on 3D image volumes, it is necessary to resort to programs specially designed for this. Generally, it is desirable to save the processed image data finally in the original source file format in order to make use of the available viewing software.

There are a number of recurring image processing tasks that one will encounter during evaluation of tomographic images.

2.5.3.1 ***Slice Averaging.*** This is the easiest way of achieving reduction of image noise and might especially be desirable if one deals with dynamic data where the statistical quality of each image volume is usually reduced because of shorter acquisition times. Averaging (or simply summing) slice ranges is nothing more than increasing the effective slice thickness of the tomographic images.

2.5.3.2 ***Image Smoothing.*** Image smoothing is one of the important tasks for which efficient tools should be available. The degree of smoothing defines the effective spatial resolution of the final images. For many tomographic methods it is not always wise to require that the full spatial resolution of the tomograph is used. Doing so necessarily increases the noise component in the images. If it turns out that the noise becomes so large that it masks relevant signals, using adequate smoothing is usually the only sensible strategy. From a formal point of view, smoothing is a special kind of filtering the data (namely low pass filtering). The mathematical framework for this is digital signal processing. There are a multitude of possible filter shapes possessing different properties. Depending on the precise characteristics of the input data, one can optimize the filter shape with respect to some desirable criteria. From a more pragmatic point of view, most filters that progressively suppress high frequency components (going sufficiently rapid to zero at high frequencies) perform well.

With respect to smoothing of 3D tomographic data, one should always use 3D filtering and avoid a slice-by-slice approach. It is thus possible to achieve a much better noise reduction for any given spatial resolution.

Smoothing can be described as operating in the frequency domain (the Fourier transform of the original data). This offers theoretical advantages and can be computationally more efficient for certain types of filters (e.g., bandpath filters). But usually it is more intuitive to describe smoothing as a weighted moving average operating directly on the discrete image data. The filter is defined by the filter kernel, which is the discretized equivalent of the intrinsic PSF of the imaging device; the filter kernel can be interpreted as the result one obtains when smoothing an image containing a single nonzero pixel. A two-dimensional example is given in Figure 2.6.

The smoothing process is achieved by centering the filter kernel in turn on each image pixel, computing the average of the covered pixels weighted with the corresponding values of the filter kernel and assigning the resulting value to the current center pixel. A reasonable smoothing filter should be symmetric around its center and include weights that decrease monotonically toward the filter edges.

Formally, one can view smoothing (or arbitrary filtering) as modifying the intrinsic PSF of the imaging device. In the case of smoothing, the PSF will become broader, that is, the spatial resolution decreases. In the 3D case, the filter kernel becomes a cube instead of a square, but the averaging process is the same. If the procedure described earlier is implemented literally, the computation time increases with the third power of the filter width. If filtering a given image volume with a kernel size of $3 \times 3 \times 3$ would take 2 s, increasing

(a)

0	0	0	0	0	0	0
0	0	0	0	0	0	0
0	0	16	16	16	0	0
0	0	16	16	16	0	0
0	0	16	16	16	0	0
0	0	0	0	0	0	0
0	0	0	0	0	0	0

(b)

0	0	0	0	0	0	0
0	1	3	4	3	1	0
0	3	9	12	9	3	0
0	4	12	16	12	4	0
0	3	9	12	9	3	0
0	1	3	4	3	1	0
0	0	0	0	0	0	0

Figure 2.6. Example of image smoothing by using a two-dimensional moving average. (a) Original image matrix. (b) Smoothed image matrix obtained with the filter kernel $\frac{1}{16} \cdot \begin{pmatrix} 1 & 2 & 1 \\ 2 & 4 & 2 \\ 1 & 2 & 1 \end{pmatrix}$.

the kernel size to $9 \times 9 \times 9$ pixels would increase computation time by a factor of 27, that is, to about 1 min, making the approach unsuitable for large kernel sizes. One solution to the problem is to note that many filters, such as the one used in Figure 2.6, can be constructed from one-dimensional filters (in the above example from the single one-dimensional filter (1 2 1)) by multiplying the components of the one-dimensional filters that correspond to the coordinates in the multidimensional filters. For such separable filters it is much more efficient to perform three successive one-dimensional filterings along the three coordinates of the image volume. This yields exactly the same result as direct 3D filtering. The gain is especially dramatic for larger kernel sizes, since the computation time only increases linearly with the filter kernel size with this approach.

Reasonable 3D smoothing of the tomographic data can substantially improve the visual quality of the data; as discussed already, the data should be acquired with a pixel size that is smaller than the FWHM of the PSF of the tomograph. In this case, sizable intensity fluctuations between neighboring pixels will not correspond to actual signal variations in the imaged object, but will rather represent pure noise, that is, statistical fluctuations (Fig. 2.3). Filtering such data with a smoothing filter whose own effective FWHM is of the same order of magnitude than the intrinsic spatial resolution will deteriorate the final spatial resolution only to a limited extent but will reduce the noise amplitude massively.

Generally, the user should be aware that there always is a trade-off between maintaining maximal image resolution and minimizing noise. (This also holds true for the diametrical approach, namely trying to increase image resolution by deconvolving the PSF "out of" the measured data).

As an example, Figure 2.7 shows three orthogonal intersecting slices from a PET investigation of the human brain with the glucose analogue [^{18}F]-2-fluoro-2-deoxy-D-glucose (FDG). The leftmost column shows the original data. The degree of three-dimensional smoothing increases through the columns from left

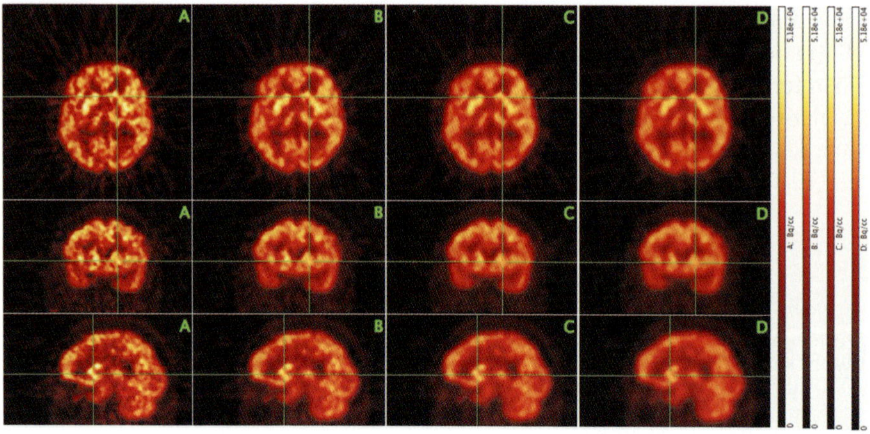

Figure 2.7. Effect of three-dimensional image smoothing on spatial resolution and noise level. Three orthogonal slices through the image volume from a PET investigation of the human brain with the glucose analogue FDG are shown (top row, transaxial; middle row, coronal; bottom row, sagittal). The leftmost column (A) shows the original image data that exhibit notable image noise. Columns B–D show the same slices after three-dimensional smoothing of the image volume with a cubic binomial filter kernel of width $N = 3, 5, 7$ pixels, respectively.

to right. In the second column, the smoothing leads to a significant noise reduction while leaving the spatial resolution essentially unaltered. Only in the third and fourth columns a loss of resolution becomes obvious.

A cubic binomial filter kernel of width $N = 3, 5, 7$ was used in this example. The filter weights are defined by products of binomial coefficients[‡]

$$w_{ijk} = w_i \cdot w_j \cdot w_k = \binom{N-1}{i-1} \cdot \binom{N-1}{j-1} \cdot \binom{N-1}{k-1}$$

where

$$\binom{N-1}{k-1} \equiv \frac{(N-1)!}{(k-1)!(N-k)!}, \quad k = 1, \ldots, N$$

For example, for $N = 5$, one gets $w = (1, 4, 6, 4, 1)$. This type of filter is similar in effect to Gaussian shaped filters and offers the advantage that the kernel width alone defines the filter characteristic (for a Gaussian filter, the filter width should be matched to the standard deviation in order to yield sensible results).

[‡]To simplify the formulas, we omit the necessary normalization to a value of one for the sum over all weights in the 3D filter kernel. Of course, this normalization should actually be included.

In Figure 2.7, the spatial resolution corresponds to a FWHM of 3–4 pixels (in accord with our previous considerations concerning adequate sampling). Therefore, the $3 \times 3 \times 3$–point binomial smoothing used in column B affects the resolution only marginally, but reduces the image noise notably. Increasing the filter kernel size does cause a slight reduction of the image resolution but might still be found acceptable, depending on circumstances.

2.5.3.3 Coregistration and Resampling. Another frequently necessary operation is resampling of the image data, that is, modification of the voxel size. If one wants to maintain the originally covered image volume, this implies change of the 3D image matrix size as well. The need for this transformation regularly occurs if tomographic data from different modalities are to be compared side by side in a parallel display.

In order to evaluate spatially corresponding areas easily and reliably, it is necessary to ensure first that both data sets are displayed with respect to a common frame of reference. In principle, it would suffice to know the spatial transformation that connects the two native reference frames of both data sets (at least a coupled 3D rotation/translation is required). If this transformation is known, a display program could theoretically handle the parallel display (taking additionally into account the differing pixel sizes).

Practically, such an approach is not suitable for reasons of additional complications in data management as well as recurring computational overhead during visualization. Therefore, the usual procedure consists in transforming both data sets to a common voxel and image matrix size (resampling) and spatially transforming one of the image volumes to match the other (coregistration).

Coregistration is a well-investigated field, and there are several methods available. Automatic algorithms use variants of multidimensional optimization strategies to minimize some goodness of fit criterion, for example, the correlation coefficient between the intensities of corresponding pixels from both image volumes. The algorithms usually perform best for coregistration of image data from the same modality. Difficulties increase if there is a need for plastic transformations, as is generally the case for intersubject coregistration but possible also for intrasubject coregistration, for example, in the thorax.

Both operations (resampling and coregistration) imply interpolation within the image data. For reasons of increased numerical accuracy, it is therefore advantageous to combine both steps and to reduce the number of interpolations to one.

Interpolation becomes necessary because the image data are known only for the given discrete voxels. A reduction of the voxel size and/or spatial transformation of the imaged object then always requires to determine new values "in between" the given data. For practical matters, it usually suffices to use trilinear interpolation in the given data instead of using the full mathematical apparatus of the sampling theorem. A nearest neighbor approach, on the other hand, is usually inadequate.

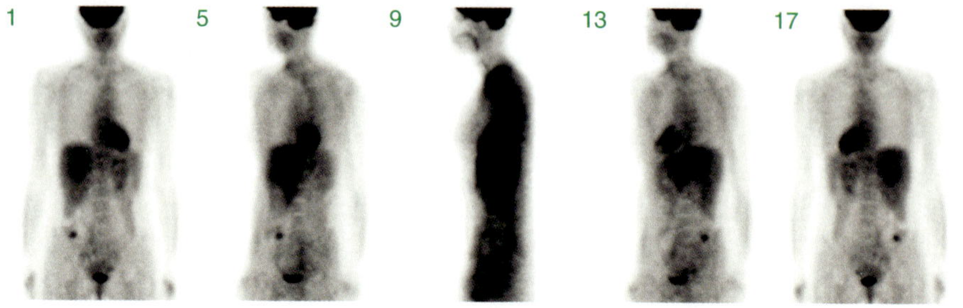

Figure 2.8. Sum projections along different directions. Shown are projections in angular steps of 45°, starting with a frontal view in projection 1. These data are part of the complete set of projection data from which the 3D tomographic volume is reconstructed.

2.5.4 Visualization

Tomographic data sets comprise large amounts of information. A single image volume can easily consist of several hundreds of slices. Therefore, efficient visualization tools are needed to analyze such data.

One useful technique is to navigate interactively through the image volumes with orthogonal viewers that allow the user to view simultaneously three orthogonal intersecting slices and to choose the slice positions interactively. Such viewers do exist as stand-alone applications or are integrated in dedicated data evaluation environments that offer additional functionality.

2.5.4.1 Maximum Intensity Projection (MIP). The large number of tomographic images in a typical investigation makes it desirable to utilize efficient visualization techniques to augment (or sometimes even replace) the tedious slice-by-slice inspection of the primary tomographic data.

Initially, most tomographic techniques measure projection data. Each measured tomographic projection corresponds to a summation through the imaged volume along the given projection direction. The complete set of projections along sufficiently many directions is the basis for the tomographic image reconstruction, that is, the projection set already contains the complete information concerning the interior structure of the imaged object. Each single projection, on the other hand, contains only a small fraction of this information. The cumulative contribution from overlapping structures along the projection direction especially complicates identification (let alone localization) of smaller structures. This is illustrated in Figure 2.8, which shows projections along selected directions (in steps of 45°).

The visual quality is low. Only prominent structures such as the heart, the bladder, or the liver are identifiable. After image reconstruction (based on the complete set of all projections, not only the few shown in the figure), a detailed assessment of interior structures is possible, as demonstrated in Figure 2.9, where coronal slices from the resulting tomographic image volume are shown.

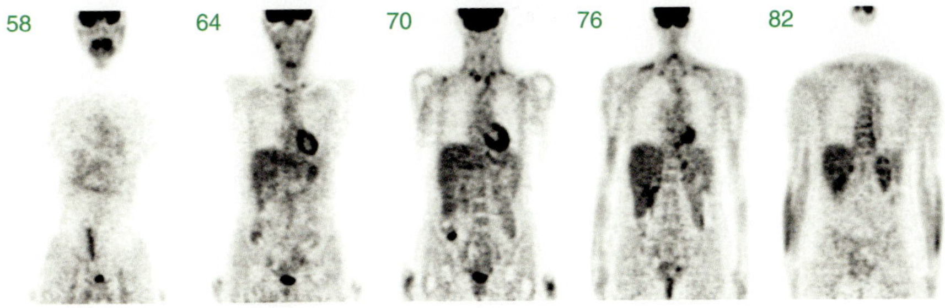

Figure 2.9. Selected coronal slices through the reconstructed tomographic image volume resulting from the complete set of projection data underlying Figure 2.8.

A comparison of the last two figures clearly demonstrates that the sum projections are usually not useful to get an alternative visualization of the tomographic data.

The idea of the Maximum Intensity Projection (MIP) consists in calculating projections through the tomographic image volume, but contrary to the initially measured sum projection data, one now looks for the maximum intensity pixel along each projection ray and uses its value in the projection image.

MIP is a very helpful method to get a quick overview of high signal intensity structures within an image volume. The approach works best for image data with high image contrast between target structures and the surrounding tissue.

In comparison to more sophisticated volume rendering algorithms, MIPs require only moderate computation time and might even be usable interactively in real-time if OpenGL support is available.

Usually the projection is performed within the transaxial image plane. Then, for each projection direction (from different angles around the edge of the transaxial slice), each transaxial slice contributes one row to the maximum projection image. Figure 2.10 illustrates this schematically.

Each resulting maximum projection is completely overlap-free. The single pixel of maximum intensity (along the given projection direction) determines the intensity value in the projection image. However, each projection does not contain any depth information, since the maximum projection will look the same whether the maximum pixel in the tomographic data set was "at the front" or "at the back" of the data set. But if the maximum projection is repeated along multiple viewing directions, any high intensity structure in the image volume will be visible in many or all of the projections and the spatial location can be assessed. MIPs are especially suitable for generation of animations for which maximum projections are acquired at tightly spaced angles and then displayed as a cyclic movie, yielding the impression of a rotating semitransparent object, providing a view of the high intensity structures from different angles. However, this type of visualization is no substitute for a thorough assessment of the tomographic data themselves; MIPs will, for any given projection angle, display the maximum intensities along each projection ray, that is, hide everything else. If some

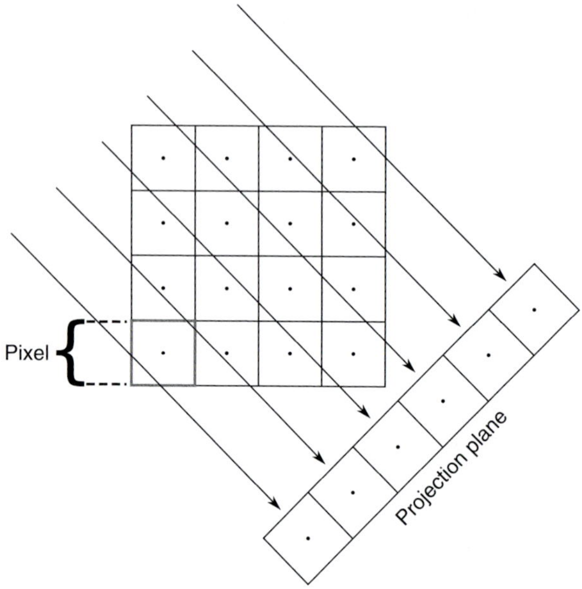

Figure 2.10. Illustration of MIP. Along all projection rays through the tomographic image, the maxima that generate one row in the projection plane are determined. Repeating this procedure for the whole stack of transaxial tomographic images generates the maximum intensity image corresponding to this projection angle.

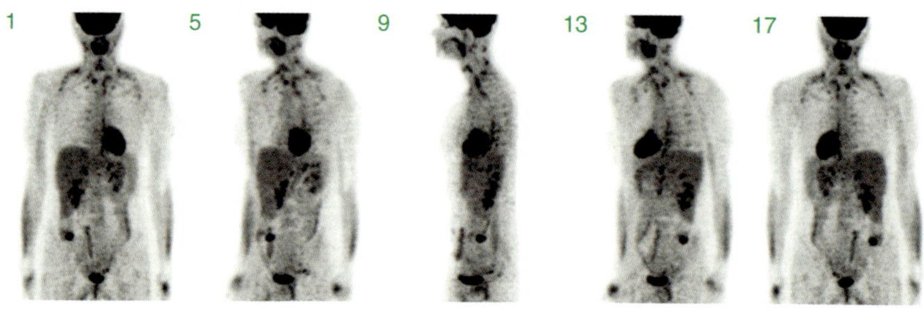

Figure 2.11. Example of volume rendering with maximum intensity projections (MIPs). Shown are projections in angular steps of 45°, starting with a frontal view in projection 1.

structure is lying inside a high intensity "shell," it will be completely invisible in a maximum projection. A central necrosis within a tumor, for instance, is not detectable at all in a MIP of a FDG-PET investigation, since the necrosis exhibits a much lower FDG uptake than the tumor rim, which "masks" the interior in the MIPs (in Fig. 2.11, this masking occurs for the cavity of the heart).

2.5.4.2 Volume Rendering and Segmentation. The maximum projection method is a simple and very useful visualization method in all situations where one is

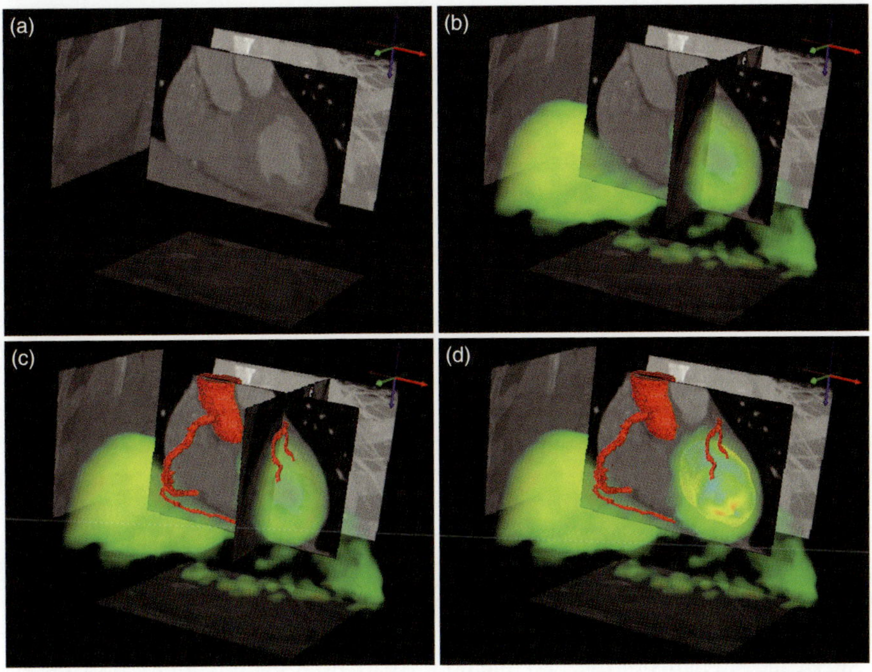

Figure 2.12. Example of the combination of different 3D visualization techniques. Two tomographic data sets (CT and PET) of a human heart are shown. The CT data are displayed in gray via selected tomographic slices as well as maximum projections onto three orthogonal planes. In addition, the blood vessel geometry as derived by segmentation of the CT data is shown in red. The PET data are displayed semitransparently by volume rendering in green together with the segmented myocardial wall. The color used for the PET data display represents variations in myocardial blood flow that can be compared with the CT-derived information concerning blood vessel integrity. Courtesy of Prof. W. Burchert, Department of Radiology, Nuclear Medicine and Molecular Imaging, Heart and Diabetes Center, NRW, Germany.

interested in well-defined (localized, high intensity) structures. The MIPs algorithm can be seen as the simplest example of a class of visualization techniques called volume rendering techniques.

Volume rendering is closely related to the problem of partitioning the image volume into different subvolumes (called segmentation) whose surfaces can then be displayed in different ways. One example of this is demonstrated in Figure 2.12.

This example shows CT and PET data of a human heart and combines several techniques of visualizing the data: tomographic slices, maximum projections, semitransparent volume rendering, and segmentation. This example combines the detailed anatomical structure of the coronary arteries (derived from the CT data set) with the metabolic information present in the PET data.

2.5.5 Dynamic Tomographic Data

If one acquires a whole series of time "frames" (image volumes) in order to investigate dynamic processes, one ends up with a fourth data dimension (besides the three spatial coordinates), identifying a single voxel in a single time frame. Such measurements are sometimes called 4D data sets (as in "4D CT"), but we prefer calling them simply dynamic data.

A related possibility is the acquisition of gated data sets that use a stroboscopic method to visualize the cyclic motion of the heart and the lung: external triggers (ECG or a breathing trigger) are used to monitor and subdivide the motion cycle into several "gates," which are mapped into separate image volumes. Each volume takes up a certain phase of the cyclic motion averaged over the duration of the data acquisition. One benefit of gating is the ability to correct for motion artifacts related to cyclic organ movement during the breathing cycle.

Dynamic measurements open up several possibilities not offered by static measurements since they allow the monitoring of *in vivo* physiological transport and metabolic processes. It is then possible to derive quantitative information for parameters such as blood flow, oxygen consumption, and blood volume for one or several ROIs or even each individual pixel within the tomographic image volume.

This ability to noninvasively quantify regional blood flow and metabolism is one of the strengths of the PET method. Apart from the possibility of using the biologically relevant molecules as tracers by labeling them with a suitable isotope, PET is superior to other tomographic methods because of the very good quantitative nature of the measurement process, which yields the regional tracer concentrations in absolute numbers, and its strict adherence to the tracer principle (introducing negligible amounts of the substance into the organism), which ensures that the measurement does not influence the investigated biological process.

Consequently, the kinetics of PET tracers can be treated as strictly linear, which allows the straightforward use of compartment modeling for the derivation of relevant parameters.

In principle, mathematical techniques similar to those used in PET can also be used to analyze contrast agent kinetics in CT or MRI. On closer inspection, however, the data evaluation is complicated by several factors. One of these factors concerns deviation from linearity because of the use of sizable amounts of contrast agent. This leads to deviations from linear kinetics (doubling the administered amount no longer doubles the response) as well as pharmacological effects that influence the outcome. For instance, one CT-based technique for the assessment of cerebral blood flow is based on administering stable xenon in sizable amounts that diffuse easily into brain tissue. The blood-flow-driven washout of xenon is then used to derive quantitative values for the local cerebral blood flow, in much the same mathematical way as when using PET with a freely diffusible tracer (such as ^{15}O-labeled water). But since xenon is an anesthetic and has to be administered in sizable amounts, this leads to pharmacological effects (drowsiness). It cannot be taken for granted that cerebral blood flow is unaffected by this circumstance.

More recently, perfusion CT, which analyzes the single pass kinetics of common intravasal contrast agents using very high time resolution, has become a very active field. The potential of this technique is obvious, but there remain open questions with regard to systematic accuracy and validity of the mathematical techniques applied (Ng et al., 2006; Stewart et al., 2006; St Lawrence et al., 1998; van den Hoff, 2007a; van den Hoff, 2007b).

2.5.5.1 Parametric Imaging. If quantitation of dynamic data is performed on a per-pixel basis, the results define a new tomographic image volume where the pixel values no longer represent the primary signal (e.g., tracer concentration, Hounsfield units) but yield directly the relevant biological information. This can be evaluated visually or quantitatively via suitable ROIs.

Such parametric images are a valuable way of maximizing the information accessible to the user. Since the parameters displayed in the images have a direct biological interpretation (blood flow, glucose consumption, etc.), the visible image contrast is directly interpretable in terms of these parameters. Usually this is not the case when looking at the underlying dynamic data itself. Only under favorable circumstances is it possible to select time frames from the series around a certain time point in such a way that the image content is approximately proportional to the actual quantity of interest.

2.5.5.2 Compartment Modeling of Tomographic Data. Only a basic account of this technique is given, and the reader is otherwise referred to the literature, for example, Carson, 2003; Lassen and Perl, 1979; van den Hoff, 2005; Willemsen et al., 2002.

Compartment models describe the kinetics of tracers or contrast agents as bidirectional transport between several "well-stirred" pools, that is, spaces that do not exhibit any internal concentration gradients. This description seems a priori inadequate. For instance, the bolus passage of a tracer (or contrast agent) through the so-called Krogh cylinder is shown in Figure 2.13, as derived from a detailed mathematical convection/diffusion simulation. The "compartment assumption" of homogeneous distribution is fulfilled neither for the capillary nor for the surrounding tissue.

Nevertheless, compartment models are frequently able to describe the measured data well and rarely lead to sizable bias in the derived parameters. Only at time scales shorter than the capillary transit time (requiring a corresponding time resolution of the experimental data), the compartment model description is no longer suitable.

For dynamic tomographic data, however, compartment models are usually adequate. Figure 2.14 shows the first step of translating the situation in Figure 2.13 to a workable compartment model.

In this model, the longitudinal concentration gradients are accounted for by subdividing the capillary and surrounding tissue into sufficiently short sections for which all internal gradients are negligible. In mathematical terms, going from Figure 2.13 to Figure 2.14 is equivalent to replacing a partial differential equation with a system of ordinary differential equations that is much easier to solve.

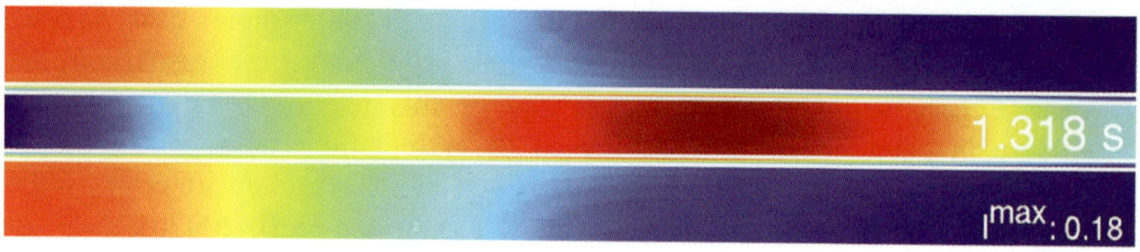

Figure 2.13. Numerical simulation of the capillary transit of a very short bolus of a permeable contrast agent or tracer through the Krogh cylinder. A longitudinal cross section through the capillary and surrounding tissue is shown. The capillary wall is indicated by the pair of white lines; the color indicates the concentration (blue, low; red, high) of the injected substance. The tracer is entering from the left at $t = 0.I_{\max}$ is the maximum concentration (specified as a fraction of the initial bolus amplitude at $t = 0$) in the system at the given time point $t = 1.3$ s.

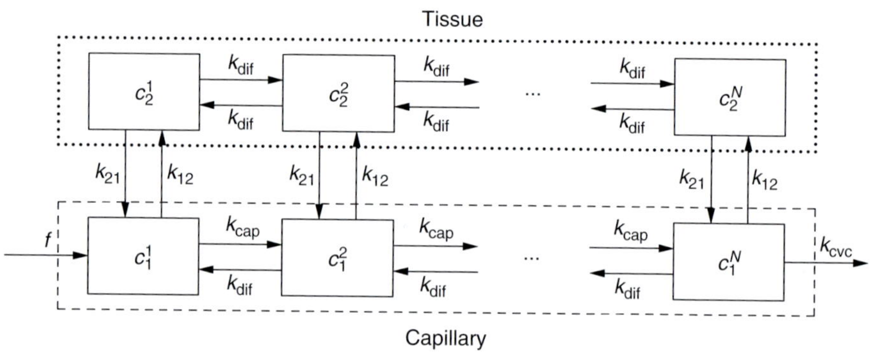

Figure 2.14. Linear chains of compartments describe the longitudinal concentration variations visible in Figure 2.13, where f specifies the perfusion, that is, the blood flow in units of (ml blood/min)/(ml tissue), c is tracer concentration, and k are rate constants (units min^{-1}). Referring, as usual in compartment modeling, all concentrations to the common total volume of the system have consequences for the interpretation of the model parameters (e.g., the apparent asymmetry of k vs k and f vs k).

Depending on the nature of the investigated system and/or the actual time resolution of the experimental data, this model configuration might be simplified further. In this example, at the usual time resolution of dynamic tomographic data, it is usually not possible to resolve details of thc bolus passage. In Figure 2.15, all concentration gradients inside the capillary and the tissue are ignored (the behavior of the system can be described sufficiently using the average concentrations in these spaces, which is a weaker assumption, as it only assumes that potential concentration gradients are stationary). This configuration represents a two-compartment model, modeling the capillary space as one of the compartments. Such a description might be adequate when modeling the transit of a CT-contrast agent bolus imaged with high time resolution.

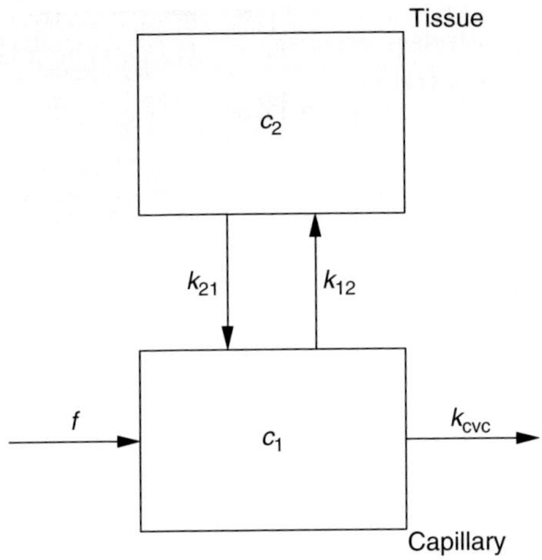

Figure 2.15. After the end of the capillary transit, the chain shown in Figure 2.14 can be collapsed into a single segment, which suffices to describe the "visible" tracer kinetics. For finite bolus duration (longer than the capillary transit time), this approach might also be adequate to describe the capillary transit itself.

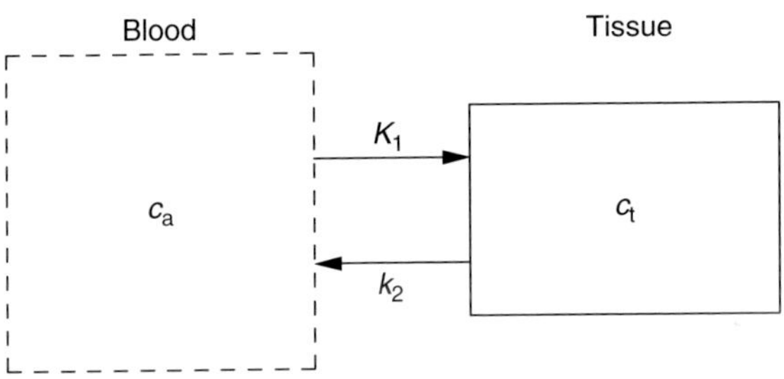

Figure 2.16. A further simplification, regularly applicable in PET (and generally for a time resolution not better than about 1 s), assumes that the time course of tracer concentration in the capillary blood space is identical to that in the arterial blood vessels.

It is possible to simplify the description even further, as depicted in Figure 2.16. This configuration represents a one-compartment model, assuming that the capillary promptly follows every concentration change in the arterial input. This description is adequate for description of diffusible (reversibly transported) tracers in PET.

The differences between the configurations in Figures 2.15 and 2.16 can be subtle, as demonstrated in Figure 2.17.

Both models fit the data well. Thus, selection of the correct model, which influences interpretation of the derived model parameters, must be done beforehand using available a priori information.

The above example is a special simple case. If the tracer kinetics is more complicated (e.g., if the tracer is trapped in the tissue or undergoes further metabolic

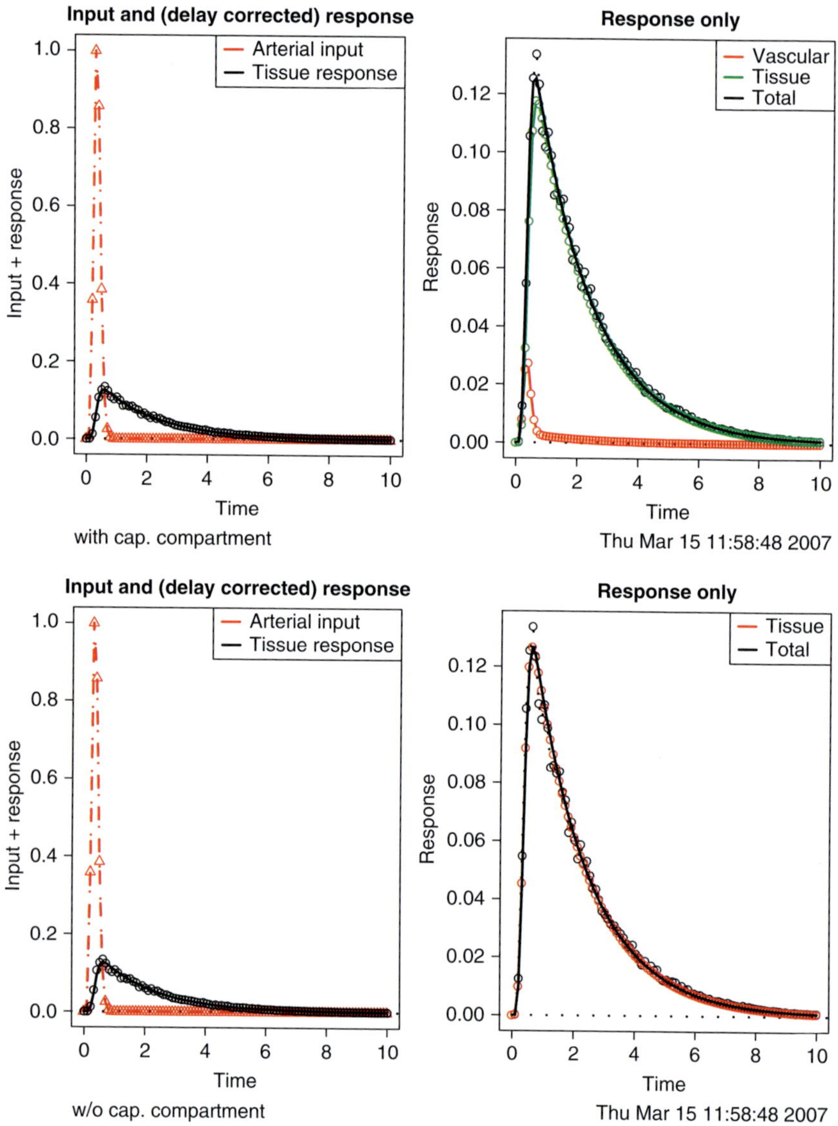

Figure 2.17. Simulated capillary passage of an idealized short bolus (red triangles) for a semipermeable contrast agent or tracer (time scale given in seconds). (a) The model from Figure 2.15 is used to generate a noisy artificial response curve (black circles) to which the model is fitted, yielding the decomposition in contributions from the capillary and from the tissue compartment. (b) The model from Figure 2.16 is used to fit the same artificial response curve. The capillary contribution is not modeled separately. Even in this idealized case, the data do not allow decision between the models.

steps), the compartment model has to account for this by adding further tissue compartments. In any case, the resulting model describes the measured data using standard optimization techniques to derive the model parameter values that yield the best fit of the model to the data. Performing this analysis on a per-pixel basis enables the generation of parametric images as explained in Section 2.5.5.1.

2.6 SUMMARY

Evaluation of tomographic data combines techniques from digital signal processing, image processing, multidimensional data visualization, and numerical mathematical methods related to modeling and fitting the experimental data. It also includes the tomographic image reconstruction itself.

Depending on the tomographic technique and the special question investigated, emphasis might lie on qualitative evaluation and, thus, on image processing and visualization or on derivation of quantitative measures by developing adequate models and utilizing them for data description.

Generally, all aspects play an equally important role. Adequate integration of all steps in the data evaluation ensures that the wealth of detailed information present in tomographic data is used in an optimal way.

REFERENCES

Carson RE. Tracer kinetic modeling in PET. In: Valk PE, Bailey DL, Townsend DW, Maisey MN, editors. *Positron Emission Tomography*. London: Springer; 2003. pp. 147–179, ISBN 1852334851.

DICOM Standards Committee. Digital Imaging and Communications in Medicine. 2011. Available at http://medical.nema.org.

Eaton JW. GNU Octave; 2011. Available at http://www.octave.org.

Gonzalez RC, Woods RE. *Digital Image Processing* (Prentice Hall International); 2007. pp. 976 ISBN 013168728X.

Kessler RM, Ellis JR Jr, Eden M. Analysis of emission tomographic scan data: limitations imposed by resolution and background. J Comput Assist Tomogr 1984;8(3):514–522.

Lassen N, Perl W. *Tracer Kinetic Methods in Medical Physiology*. New York: Raven Press; 1979, ISBN 0-89004-114-8.

Ng QS, Goh V, Fichte H, Klotz E, Fernie P, Saunders MI, Hoskin PJ, Padhani AR. Lung cancer perfusion at multi-detector row CT: reproducibility of whole tumor quantitative measurements. Radiology 2006;239(2):547–553.

Nyquist H. Certain topics in telegraph transmission theory. Trans AIEE 1928;47: 617–644.

OFFIS e.V. DCMTK - DICOM Toolkit. 2011. Available at http://www.dcmtk.org.

R Development Core Team. *R: A Language and Environment for Statistical Computing*. Vienna, Austria: R Foundation for Statistical Computing; 2011. ISBN 3-900051-07-0. Available at http://www.R-project.org.

Shannon CE. Communication in the presence of noise. Proc Inst Radio Eng 1949;37(1):10–21.

Stewart EE, Chen X, Hadway J, Lee TY. Correlation between hepatic tumor blood flow and glucose utilization in a rabbit liver tumor model. Radiology 2006;239(3):740–750.

St Lawrence KS, Lee TY. An adiabatic approximation to the tissue homogeneity model for water exchange in the brain: I. Theoretical derivation. J Cereb Blood Flow Metab 1998;18(12):1365–1377.

van den Hoff J. Principles of quantitative positron emission tomography. Amino Acids 2005;29(4):341–353.

van den Hoff J. Assessment of lung cancer perfusion using patlak analysis: what do we measure? Radiology 2007a;243(3):907–908.

van den Hoff J. Blood flow quantification with permeable contrast agents: a valid technique? Radiology 2007b;243(3):909–910.

Willemsen ATM, van den Hoff J, Quantitative PET. Fundamentals of data analysis. Curr Pharm Des 2002;8(16):1513–1526.

3

X-RAY IMAGING

VOLKER HIETSCHOLD
Department of Radiology, University Hospital, "Carl Gustav Carus", Dresden, Germany

3.1 BASICS

3.1.1 History

Wilhelm Conrad Röntgen was born in Lennep (nowadays a part of Remscheid/Germany) in 1845 and grew up in Apeldoorn (Holland). From 1865 to 1868 he studied mechanical engineering in Zürich, and in 1870 moved to Würzburg. After employment in Straßburg, Hohenheim, and Gießen, he was offered a professorship in Würzburg in 1888, and in 1893 he was elected as the rector of the University of Würzburg. His primary experiments were with cathode rays, which he had studied since 1894. On November 8, 1895, late in the evening, he happened to notice that a barium-platine-cyanuere coated screen fluoresced each time he switched on the cathode ray tube (a Hittorf-Crooke tube). This fortunate observation allowed him to reach the conclusion that the radiation responsible for the fluorescence must be able to penetrate opaque materials. About six weeks later, on December 22, he took the famous X-ray of his wife Bertha's hand (Leicht, 1994; Schedel, 1995). Röntgen termed this "unknown radiation" he had discovered "X-Strahlen" (X-rays). Although this terminology was kept unchanged by the English-speaking world, the radiation is called "Röntgenstrahlen" in German and "рентгеновское излучение" (rentgenovskoe izlučenie) in Russian, to honor its discoverer.

Biomedical Imaging: Principles and Applications, First Edition. Edited by Reiner Salzer.

3.1.2 Basic Physics

X-rays are part of the electromagnetic spectrum. By definition, X-rays are photon radiation generated either by the rapid acceleration (or deceleration) of charged particles ("Bremsstrahlung," from the German bremsen = to brake and Strahlung = radiation) or as a result of high energy transitions between the electron shells of atoms or molecules.

For diagnostic applications, X-rays usually are produced in X-ray tubes, in which electrons, accelerated to a certain kinetic energy using a high voltage, are shot onto a metallic target. They are decelerated mainly by the Coulomb interaction with the electron shell of the target material, and the difference in kinetic energy is emitted as electromagnetic radiation (bremsstrahlung). The intensity of bremsstrahlung is continuously distributed with a linear decrease down to the initial kinetic energy of the electrons. If the kinetic energy is sufficient to strip an electron from the inner shell of the target, an electron from the target's outer energy level may transition to this unoccupied energy level. The energy difference between the initial and final energy levels of the transitioning electron is emitted from the target's electron shell in the form of a photon. This emitted photon will have an energy characteristic of the electron shell of the target material. The contribution of this process to the energy distribution obtained from an X-ray tube (Fig. 3.1) is called the "characteristic spectrum."

When X-rays interact with matter, one part of the rays will simply penetrate it (transmission); another part will be deflected from their original direction, which can be accompanied by a change in their energy (scattering); and a third portion will be blocked by the matter and "become stuck" (absorption). In the range of photon energies that is relevant for imaging applications, the underlying processes are photoelectric effect, coherent (Rayleigh) scattering, and incoherent (Compton) scattering. All three processes contribute to the attenuation within

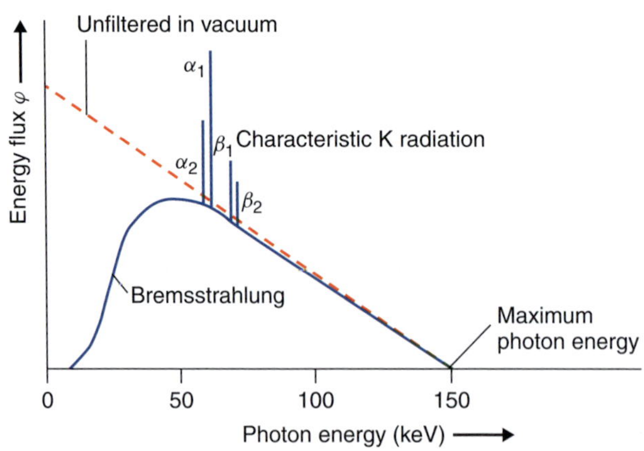

Figure 3.1. Schematic representation of a spectrum of an X-ray tube with tungsten anode operated at a high voltage of 150 kV (according to Morneburg, 1995).

an X-ray penetrating material. Their probabilities (which can be described with the cross sections $\sigma_{PE}, \sigma_{coherent}$, and $\sigma_{Compton}$, respectively) increase with the atomic number and decrease with the photon energy, as shown in Eq. (3.1)–(3.3).

In the photoelectric effect, the energy of one X-ray photon is completely transferred to an electron within the shell of an atom in the absorbing material. If the energy of the X-ray photon exceeds the binding energy of the electron in the absorbing material, the latter leaves the atom with a kinetic energy equal to the difference between the energy of the photon and the electron's binding energy. The dependence between the cross section (which expresses the likelihood of interaction between the photon and the electron sheath), the material (represented by its density ρ and its mean atomic number Z), and the photon energy E_γ can be approximately described by Eq. (3.1)–(3.3):

$$\sigma_{PE} \sim \rho \frac{Z^4}{E_\gamma^{3,5}} \tag{3.1}$$

$$\sigma_{coherent} \sim \rho \frac{Z^2}{E_\gamma^2} \tag{3.2}$$

$$\sigma_{Compton} \sim \rho \frac{Z}{E_\gamma} \tag{3.3}$$

The photoelectric effect, as well as Rayleigh and Compton scattering, contribute to the attenuation of X-rays. This attenuation can be described as a reduction of the intensity in the original direction of the beam by a certain percentage per amount of material through which it passes. In the simplest case, this amount of material can be described as the length or thickness d, but descriptions containing the density, the density per area, and so on, are used as well (for instance, in osteodensitometry). This attenuation law that relates the current intensity to the length (or thickness) of a zone of material and the initial intensity can be written as follows:

$$I = I_0 \exp(-\mu d) \tag{3.4}$$

where I_0 is the initial intensity and I is the intensity after passing a zone of material with an attenuation coefficient μ and thickness d. Similar to the cross sections σ (Eqs (3.1)–(3.3)), μ decreases with the photon energy E and increases with the mean atomic number Z (and in our notation, with the density ρ).

The high energy part of the spectrum emitted by the tube (the "harder radiation") will be less attenuated compared to its low energy part ("the softer radiation"), thus the term "the spectrum will be hardened". In other words, the low energy part (the soft radiation) will contribute to the X-ray image to a lesser degree compared to the high energy part. But the softer part of the spectrum will strongly contribute to the radiation exposure of the patient, since a higher percentage of its energy will be deposited in the patient compared to harder X radiation.

3.2 INSTRUMENTATION

X-ray imaging systems consist of the following components:

- high voltage generator
- X-ray tube
- beam filter for manipulation of the X-ray spectrum
- apertures for defining of the geometrical shape of the X-ray beam
- (often) a collimation unit for preventing scattered radiation from reaching the image detector
- image detector

Depending on the field of application, these components can form devices ranging from transportable units for static or dynamic imaging, including Bucky and fluoroscopic devices, to computed tomographs (which are dealt with in Chapter 4).

3.2.1 Components

3.2.1.1 Beam Generation. As mentioned earlier, for diagnostic applications X-rays are generated by an X-ray tube, in which the electrons are accelerated in an electric field of several tens up to about 150 kV. This high voltage is provided by the high voltage generator. High frequency (up to 20 kHz) converter generators allow for high power with comparatively small transformer size and negligible ripple, an advantage with respect to minimizing the radiation exposure of patients.

The basic structure of a conventional tube can be described briefly as follows: a vacuum tube contains a filament that is heated in order to thermally emit electrons. The heating current regulates the number of released electrons, which will be proportional to the X-ray dose. Electrons travel between the cathode and the anode via the applied high voltage electric field, which ranges in energy from several tens up to about 150 kV. In this electric field, electrons are accelerated and give rise to the bremsstrahlung and the characteristic spectrum formed during their interaction with the anode material.

One important parameter that determines maximum output power, as well as spatial resolution, is the focus size on the anode. The focus size describes the area of the anode on which the X-rays are generated. Since only about 1% of the electrical power is converted to X-rays, heating of the anode is a problem that limits the amount of irradiation achievable per focus area. In medical diagnostics, most of the heat is distributed over a larger amount of anode material by the application of rotating anodes. However, in the case of exposure to a series of images (or with fluoroscopy), the important parameters are the heat capacity of the anode and the tube assembly, as well as anode cooling. They are described in heat units (HU) (Eq. 3.5)

$$HU = U\,I\,t \tag{3.5}$$

where the voltage U is given in kilovolt peak (kVp), the mean tube current in milliamperes, and the exposure time in seconds. 1 HU is equivalent to 1 J. Equation (3.5) is valid for two-pulse generators, where the peak current is about 1.4 times the mean current. For lower ripple (three-pulse generators and better), where the peak current is nearly equal to the mean current, Eq. (3.5) has to be multiplied by a factor of 1.35.

X-rays generated at a certain depth in the anode leave its surface at different angles, and have to cover different distances within the anode material. This results in different attenuations, as well as hardening, of the beam. The resulting inhomogeneity in the intensity and mean energy is described as Heel effect.

As described earlier, photons from the low energy side of the spectrum contribute less effectively to the X-ray image than those from the high energy side. In terms of the radiation exposure of the patient, this means that low energy photons give less signal per unit of incident X-ray dose. An optimal relationship between contrast and patient dose could be achieved with monoenergetic radiation. However, the spectrum of the beam reaching the patient can be improved to a certain degree by application of appropriate beam filtering between the anode and the patient with aluminum, copper, or, in the case of mammography, even molybdenum or rhodium.

The radiation exposure the patient experiences must be limited to the region of clinical interest. For collimating the primary beam, opaque and semiopaque apertures can be positioned within the tube housing. Finally, the X-ray tube with the anode drive, part of the cooling system (often oil based), collimator, and light collimating system are enclosed in a tube shield or housing that prevents much of the radiation leakage.

3.2.1.2 Reduction of Scattered Radiation. The dominating mechanisms of interaction between diagnostic X-rays and matter are absorption via the photoelectric effect and Compton scattering. Scattering in the body of the patient results in rays that do not propagate in a direction originating at the tube focus, thus leading to blurred images. In imaging methods based on monochromatic radiation, Compton scattered photons can be recognized by their reduced energy compared to the unscattered photons. However, since the X-ray tube emits a spectral distribution, this criterion is not useful in radiological diagnostics. Here, three different approaches—all based on the different origins of scattered photons compared to the unscattered ones—can be applied (Fig. 3.2).

The most commonly applied method is the insertion of an antiscatter grid, which consists of absorbing lamellas, mostly arranged in parallel (occasionally

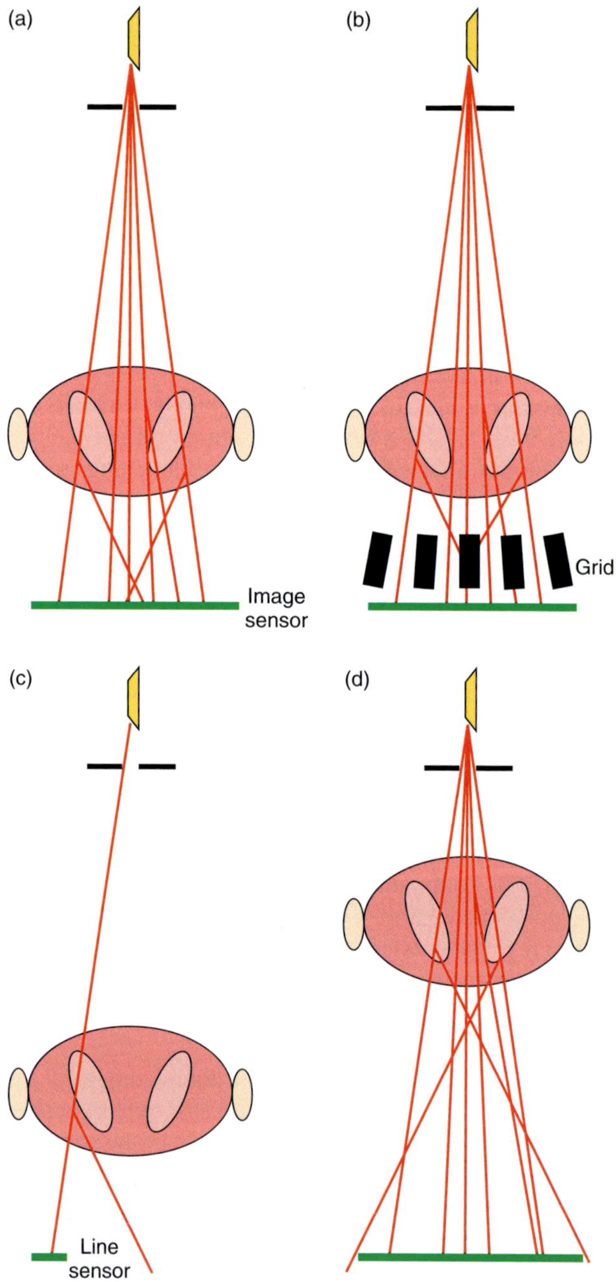

Figure 3.2. Reduction of scattered radiation in the image. (a) Radiation scattered in the object reaches the image detector. (b) An antiscatter grid eliminates most of the deflected photons, and part of the primary radiation, thus making it necessary to increase the patient dose. (c) Slit-scan technique. Most of the scattered radiation does not hit the detector row. (d) Increased distance between the object and the image detector leads to magnified images with a reduced portion of scattered radiation in the image and decreased geometrical sharpness.

also in two-dimensional orders) (Fig. 3.2b). Owing to the non-negligible cross section of these lamellas, not only unwanted scattered but also unscattered radiation will be absorbed, resulting in the need to increase the dose entering the patient in order to maintain the required detector dose. This dose increase can be on an order of magnitude from 3 to 8.

If the X-ray beam is narrowly collimated to a fan beam, and only one or a few lines of the image are registered simultaneously using a line shaped sensor (Fig. 3.2c), most of the scattered radiation passes by the sensor without the need to increase the entrance dose. The disadvantage of this method is a drastic increase in exposure time.

Increasing the distance between the object to be imaged and the image detector not only leads to magnified images but also—depending on the focus size—reduces sharpness. Magnifying the image in this manner does, however, have the inherent advantage of cutting out a significant amount of the scattered radiation, as this undesired radiation travels at an angle and will miss the image sensor (Fig. 3.2d).

Finally, since the amount of scattered radiation depends on the path length of the X-rays through the object, reducing the object thickness in several anatomic regions such as the abdomen or mammae is a way to reduce scatter, as well as entrance dose and overlay of anatomic structures.

3.2.1.3 Image Detection. The classic means of detection of X-ray images is the use of silver-bromide-based film. Owing to the low effectiveness of this medium, usually (except for the case of dental imaging) fluorescent screens are added. However, even if automated, the developing, fixation, and drying processes are quite laborious. Although in principle copies could be made, one film usually is available at exactly one place, which occasionally leads to logistic problems. This aspect, as well as technical issues, nowadays has allowed digital methods for the most part to replace the classical film-screen techniques.

Description of Image Quality. The quality of images—not only digital ones—can be described in a quantitative manner with just a few parameters and does not require too much familiarity with system theory.

The perceptibility of a structure in the image in front of a background is determined by the parameters image noise, contrast, and sharpness. Of great importance for the quality assessment of radiologic images is their Signal to Noise Ratio, SNR.

The noise is determined by the Poisson distribution of a number of independent events (e.g., the X-ray quanta registered by the image detector). For this reason, the standard deviation σ of the expected number of observed events (equal to the parameter λ of the Poisson distribution) equals the square root of the actuarial expectation, $\sigma = \sqrt{\lambda}$. This leads to the following equation for the SNR (Eq. 3.6)

$$SNR = \frac{\lambda}{\sigma} \approx \frac{\lambda}{\sqrt{\lambda}} = \sqrt{\lambda} \tag{3.6}$$

Of equal importance for the perception of structures in the image is the magnitude of the signal difference between the structure and the background compared to the image noise. This parameter is described by the Contrast to Noise Ratio, CNR. Here the contrast itself is used as a measure for the signal difference—a reasonable definition, as the noise contributions to S_A and S_B superimpose in an additive manner (Eq. 3.7):

$$CNR = \frac{S_A - S_B}{\sigma} \tag{3.7}$$

The impact of the sharpness on the perceptibility of structures, and in particular small structures, and hence on the quality of an image B, is usually described as convolution of an object function O (in the context of this chapter a nondistorted image) with a point spread function, P, which describes the imaging properties of the device (Eq. 3.8):

$$B = O \otimes P \tag{3.8}$$

In the case of an ideal distortion-free imaging system the point spread function is a δ function.

In the case of imaging systems with finite resolution, smaller structures shall always be pictured at inferior contrast. The dependence of the contrast on the size of the structures (more exactly on the spatial frequencies ν_x, ν_y along the coordinates x, y) is termed the Modulation Transfer Function (MTF). The MTF can be calculated from the point spread function as the absolute value of the corresponding Fourier transform $\boldsymbol{F}$.

The critical frequency ν_{max} is a measure for the minimal size of recognizable structures, and is determined by a minimum threshold value for the contrast, usually $MTF(\nu_{\text{max}}) = 5\%$.

The perceptibility of details is determined by the spatial resolution (given by MTF) and by the image noise. In X-ray diagnostics, the latter is controlled by the dose and how effectively the dose is utilized by the imaging system. While the dose applied to the patient is controlled by the user (and minimized with regard to the actual diagnostic question), the utilization of the dose is an attribute of the system. This attribute in general also depends on the size of the structure (described by the direction-dependent spatial frequencies ν_x, ν_y). In the case of smaller structures, blurring will lead to a cross-talking event (at the entry side X-ray quanta; at the outlet impulses e.g.) to neighboring pixels on the detector. Utilization of the dose can be defined as the percentage of X-ray quanta reaching the image detector that contributes to the SNR of the image. The utilization can be described by the parameters SNR_{in} and SNR_{out}, because of the relationship between the number of quanta and their random variation as given by the Poisson distribution (Eq. 3.6). Considering an incremental gain G for the description of nonlinear characteristics (i.e., dose-dependent sensitivities), the Detective Quantum Efficiency, DQE, can be described by the MTF, and the noise power spectra from the incoming beam, $S_{\text{f,in}}$, and the outgoing signal, $S_{\text{f,out}}$, at the input and output sides, respectively:

$$DQE = G^2 MTF^2 \frac{S_{\mathrm{f,in}}}{S_{\mathrm{f,out}}} \tag{3.9}$$

DQE is compromised by resolution power (MTF) and the utilization of the X-ray radiation $\left(\frac{S_{\mathrm{f,in}}}{S_{\mathrm{f,out}}}\right)$, two crucial parameters of any imaging system.

In the case of analog imaging systems, for example, film-screen systems, MTF approaches zero at high spatial frequencies. Digital systems, for example, computed radiographic systems or flat panel detectors, sample the object O at a spatial frequency determined by its design. According to the sampling theorem by Nyquist and Shannon, the sampling frequency has to be at least twice the spatial frequency of the smallest structure to be imaged. Violation of the sampling theorem causes artifacts by aliasing, that is, the fundamental frequency cannot be distinguished from its harmonics. In the case of a linear grating, aliasing causes brightness variations that show up as a beat in the signal and is related to the spatial frequencies of the grating and the pixel raster.

Film and Fluorescent Screen. The classical process of detection of X-rays is the formation of metallic silver grains of about 1 μm (compared to 0.02–0.7 μm for photographic films) in silver bromide crystals embedded in gelatin layers. Since the sensitivity (the so-called speed) increases with the areal density of AgBr, the thickness of these layers is about 0.03–0.04 mm, resulting in a silver content of about 5 g m^{-2}. The AgBr emulsion is mounted on a base that usually consists of polyester. The sensitivity of such films is quite limited, that is, rather high doses are required in order to reach a reasonable optical density. Therefore, fluorescent screens are mounted in film cassettes. Incident X-rays cause the emission of visible light, which causes additional blackening of the film. In practice, about 95% of the blackening is caused by fluorescent light and only 5% directly by the X-rays. To further improve the sensitivity of such film-screen systems, films with AgBr emulsions on both surfaces are used, as well as screens on both sides of the film.

The optical density D of an X-ray film is defined as the logarithmic ratio of incident light I_0 and transmitted light I (Eq. 3.10).

$$D_{\mathrm{opt}} = \log\left(\frac{I_0}{I}\right) \tag{3.10}$$

The optical density of a film depends on the energy of the incident photons and other effects, for example, the Schwarzschild effect. This holds true both with and without the application of intensifying screens. The characteristic of a film, that is, the relationship between dose and optical density, is described by an S-shaped curve. Only beyond a minimum dose is the density due to exposition able to be discriminated from the background (base and fog). On increasing the dose, the optical density depends almost linearly on the logarithm of the dose, until a saturation region (shoulder) is approached. In order to achieve an optimal exposure, the X-ray radiation dose together with the light emitted by the fluorescent foils have to be adjusted such that the object-related variability of the incident dose will be located on the linear part of the curve and hence best be transformed into a variability of the optical density. Film-screen systems of different sensitivities are available, depending on the thicknesses of both the emulsions of the film and the fluorescent screens. Owing to the varying sizes of the AgBr and phosphor crystals, as well as to different emulsion thicknesses, film-screen systems of higher sensitivity are less spatially resolving; for example, thicker layers ease the spreading of scattered light within the fluorescent screen (Fig. 3.3).

The sensitivity of film-screen systems (and the image detector dose used in the case of digital systems) is described by the speed, which in the case of X-ray films is defined as (Eq. 3.11)

$$S = \frac{1000\ \mu\text{Gy}}{\text{Dose(in }\mu\text{Gy) for opt. density 1 above base} + \text{fog}} \tag{3.11}$$

For an estimate it can be assumed that a film-screen system of twice the speed requires only half the radiation dose for the same optical density (usually at the expense of reduced lateral resolution).

Image Intensifier. The image intensifier is the traditional receiver used to depict time-dependent processes in the human body (Fig. 3.4). It consists of a vacuum vessel. A fluorescent layer at the entry side converts X-rays into visible light. The visible light subsequently hits a photocathode, which in turn generates an

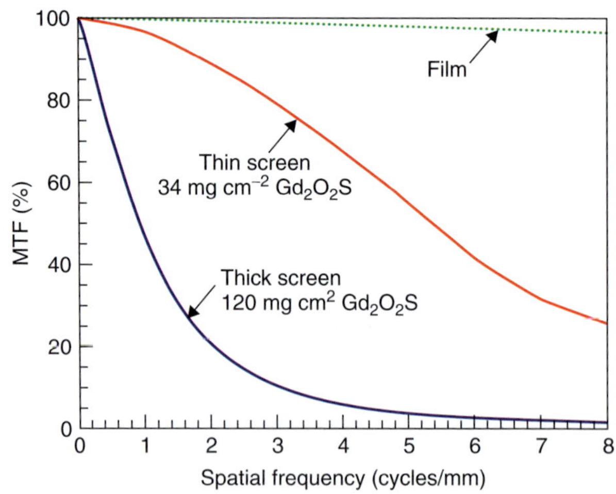

Figure 3.3. Modulation transfer function for film only as well as for films with fluorescent screen having two different thicknesses. *Source:* From Bushberg et al., 2002.

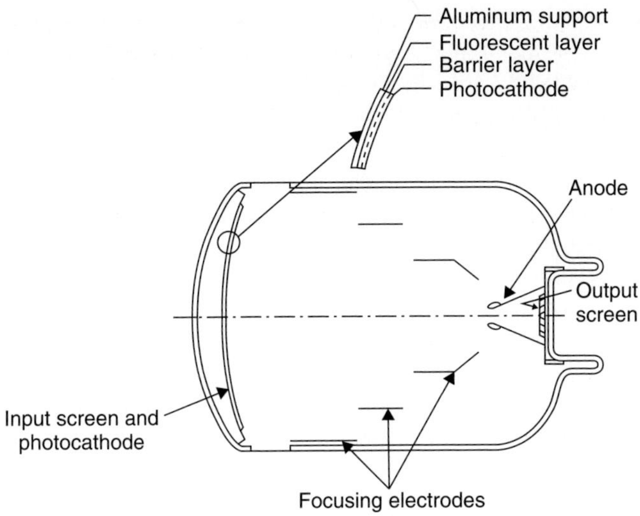

Figure 3.4. Structure of an image intensifier. *Source:* From Hendee and Ritenour, 2002.

amount of electrons proportional to the incident X-ray dose. The electrons are accelerated by a high voltage ranging from 25 to 35 kV and are usually focused by three focusing electrodes. The electrons gain energy in the high voltage field and generate an electron-optical copy of the initial image on the output screen, which converts it to visible light again. This visible image may now be transformed (historically by a TV camera, nowadays mainly by Charge-Coupled Device (CCD) chips) into an electronic signal. The input screen has to be bent in order to ensure a uniform voltage field gradient. However, the bent shape always causes pillow-shaped image distortions. The gain factor of an image intensifier, calculated as a ratio of the visible images on the input and output screens, is approximately 130. If the different sizes of the input and output screens are taken into consideration, the brightness gain ranges between 2500 and 7000.

An important characteristic quantity of an image intensifier is the conversion factor, defined as the ratio of luminance and dose rate (Eq. 3.12).

$$\frac{[\text{Luminance}]}{[\text{Dose rate}]} = \frac{Cd}{m^2} / \frac{mR}{s} = \frac{Cds}{mRm^2} \tag{3.12}$$

Dose rates of new image intensifiers are between 100 and 200 Cd s mR^{-1} m^{-2}. They fall continuously during the lifetime of the image intensifier. Another important characteristic quantity is the contrast ratio, which describes the ratio of the output signals when the center of the input screen is covered by a lead mask and when the input is unblocked, respectively. The contrast ratio should be in a range of 15–30. The main reason for the occurrence of a signal in the center of the input screen in spite of the lead cover is the propagation of scattered light within the output screen. Different zoom factors may be selected by simple electrostatic means, that is, by mapping a section of the input screen onto the output screen. The quantum efficiency of image intensifiers is usually inferior to flat screen detectors (see below). This inferiority is mainly caused by the aluminum cover on the input screen, which is needed for mechanical reasons.

Temporal Resolution and Signal to Noise Ratio. The SNR of an image is determined by both the number of image-forming X-ray quanta per pixel and the DQE of the imaging system. This results in a tight relationship between SNR and temporal resolution, if time-dependent phenomena are to be depicted. During fluoroscopic examinations using image intensifiers, the output image is usually calculated as a weighted average of the image intensifier signals at the current and previous times. More recent frames will be given higher weighting factors than previous ones. This procedure causes a certain lag in mobile structures in the image. An alternative approach can be chosen for pulsed irradiation (see below). Here the time resolution can be controlled by the pulse frequency and the sampling rate, which suppresses the image lag or replaces it by a controlled motion blur in the single images and/or by discontinuous movement displays.

Computed Radiography. Digital luminescence radiography, or Computed Radiography (CR), permits the registration of digital images on conventional X-ray instruments. The setup consists of a cassette-based work procedure similar to that of film-screen systems. The cassette contains a foil covered by a semiconductor material, for example, 85% BaFBr + 15% BaFI, doped with Eu. Interaction between the X-ray radiation and the semiconductor causes luminescence (luminescence releases visible light only after stimulation, in contrast to fluorescence). The X-ray quantum excites electrons from the valence band via the conducting band to trapping centers (doping-generated localized energy levels between the valence and conducting bands). Stimulation is achieved by sampling the storage foil using red laser light. These photons lift the electrons from the trapping centers into the conducting band. From there, the electrons relax via intermediate levels into the valence band. The excess energy is emitted as green light. The amount of emitted luminescence light is almost proportional to the amount of incident X-ray radiation. After reading, the storage foil is illuminated intensively again in order to transfer all possible remaining electrons from the trapping centers back into the conducting band, thus erasing all remaining image information. Afterward, the foil is ready for further X-ray recordings.

According to foil design, there are powder Imaging Plates (IPs) and needle IPs. Powder IPs are made of 3- to 10-μm phosphor grains embedded in binder. In needle IPs, the phosphor consists of needle-shaped crystals similar to those on the input screens of image intensifiers. They permit improved lateral resolution, that is, a higher cut-off frequency in the spatial domain (cf. MTF), and a superior digital quantum efficiency. In the conventional design, IPs are read sequentially pixel after pixel. The plate is moved row by row over a reading line, which in turn is scanned by laser light directed by a movable mirror. Quicker reading is achieved by reading whole rows at once. Readers of this type can be located next to the X-ray instrument, and the IP may already be read during the time it takes for the patient to be repositioned between two exposures.

Flat Panel Detectors. From the viewpoint of workflow, a more straightforward digital procedure can be achieved by application of flat panel detectors, that is, direct radiography. Three basically different designs are available for flat panel detectors, based on the direct or indirect conversion of X-rays into electrical signals. The latter is achieved by converting the X-rays into visible light by means of a scintillation layer with either a matrix of photodiodes located directly below or by light sensors coupled to the scintillator via fiber optics.

The most common implementation of flat panels employs an indirect method of detection based on a matrix of photodiodes or phototransistors on an amorphous silicon wafer, which in turn is covered by a scintillation layer (usually made of cesium iodide). Flat panel detectors of this type have wide applications in radiography devices and, for the past several years, in fluoroscopic and angiographic systems as well.

In another approach, the light emitted by the scintillator is forwarded via light-guiding fibers to CCD chips. The advantage of this design is its good value for money. The specifications concerning the DQE of such systems compared to the previously mentioned designs are nonuniform.

It should also be mentioned that pn-CCD sensors can be used without scintillators as well. With regard to the comparably low absorption of X-rays in silicon, systems of this kind can be used only at low X-ray energies (e.g., in stereotactic devices for breast diagnostics).

Typical implementations of direct conversion are selenium detectors. Initially a surface charge is deposited on the selenium layer. The charge is sustained because of the high electrical resistance of selenium. When the X-rays interact with this layer, electron–hole pairs emerge because of the inner photoelectrical effect. The electron–hole pairs moving in the applied electric field reduce the surface charge. After exposure to radiation, either the remaining surface charge is sampled or the resulting charge transfers are read off from the backside by suitable microelectronic units. Owing to the dependence of the cross section of the photoelectric effect on the forth power of the atomic number (Eq. 3.1), distinctly more X-ray radiation is absorbed in CsI than in selenium (50% absorption of 50-keV X-ray quanta requires a selenium layer of 270 μm thickness). The charge carriers generated by the radiation move parallel to the lines of electric flux. For the same lateral resolution, distinctly thicker layers can be used with selenium than with CsI powder. For this reason, selenium detectors exhibit a high DQE, but this disadvantage can be compensated for by using CsI needle crystals.

Finally, an inexpensive direct radiographic alternative for flat panel detectors is the connection of a scintillator layer (expediently also made of needle crystals) via a lens system to a CCD chip. This design provides reasonable lateral resolution but only a relatively low DQE.

Hybrid Systems. There are also systems on the market with an IP in a closed mechanical surrounding. The IP is read immediately after X-ray exposure. With these devices, a workflow similar to that with flat panel devices can be achieved, at equal image quality and only slightly higher dose requirements. Large and hence expensive silicon wafers are not needed, but moving mechanical parts have to be employed. The previous distinction between storage foil and flat panel devices became fuzzy after the appearance of the hybrid systems (Seibert, 2007).

Slit-Scan Technique. For a few application areas, the slit-scan technique is a direct radiographic alternative for flat panel detectors. Row-by-row scanning of the patient by a fan-shaped X-ray beam may be performed with parallel shifts of the X-ray tube, and a detector row during radiation exposition (cf. the registration of survey views for the interactive planning of Computed Tomographic (CT) cross sections) provides images of low geometric distortion of the whole skeleton, for example, for orthopedic purposes. If the required row sensor is made of ionization chambers, the recording of the whole skeleton requires 1–2 minutes scan time at a very low effective dose, on the order of 0.03 mSv. Another application of the slit-scan technique is found in mammography. In addition to the low distortion, this imaging technique has another advantage in that no antiscatter grid is required (Fig. 3.2). On the other hand, the relatively extended exposure time is a disadvantage, because it results in a much higher load on the X-ray tube than in the case of a cone beam exposition. For this reason, X-ray tubes used in slit-scan devices for mammography employ the thermally more stable tungsten anodes, instead of molybdenum or rhodium anodes, which emit a superior spectral composition of radiation.

3.3 CLINICAL APPLICATIONS

3.3.1 Diagnostic Devices

3.3.1.1 Projection Radiography. The basic layout of a workplace for X-ray imaging of a lying, standing, or sitting patient is shown in Figure 3.5. The machines have an automatic exposure system and allow a more or less free selection of generator parameters (one-parameter technology: preselection of only high voltage, definition of the integral of tube current over exposure time (the so-called mAs-product) by the automatic exposure system; two-parameter technology: preselection of high voltage and tube current, this mode is of interest as it allows for a certain amount of desired blurring in the image due to motion of body parts (e.g., blurring of the moving lower jaw in the case of cervical spine images) when extended exposure times are required; three-parameter technology: the automatic exposure system is fully abandoned). In the case of immobile X-ray workplaces, the distance between the detector and focus can be adjusted beyond a minimum of 1 m. When working with cassettes, the format of the cassette must be detected automatically in order to prevent regions of the patient outside the image area from being exposed to direct irradiation. Smaller cutouts using a light aperture are of course possible. Antiscatter grids of various

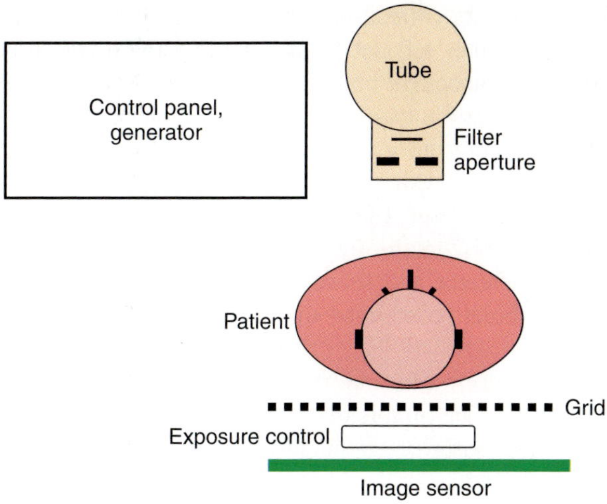

Figure 3.5. Layout of an X-ray workstation.

designs (see Section 2.1.2) must be removable in order to permit the registration of thin regions or the recording on infants with minimal radiation exposure and simultaneous sufficient image quality. Image detectors can be (i) cassettes, which contain either a film-screen system or a CR IP, or (ii) fully assembled detectors (flat panel detectors, CCD-based detectors, slit-scan units, drum detectors, CR automats).

The Automatic Exposure Control (AEC) system will shut off the beam generation after the optimal detector dose is reached. For this, sensors that monitor a measure that is correlated to the detector dose are needed. Two approaches are available. In the first, the measuring chambers are located directly in front of the image detector. The advantage of this approach is a radiation measurement independent of the design of the cassettes used; the disadvantage is a slight radiation loss due to absorption within the sensor. This approach requires an appropriate (although very small) enhancement of the patient dose. There might also be the risk of reproduction of the sensor in the image. Measurements behind the cassette provide the potential advantage of using the complete dose for image generation. Only radiation transmitted through the image detector will reach the exposure meter. This approach is preferentially used for mammography. As the sensitivities of both the image detector (i.e., the film-screen system, the CR IP or the flat panel detector) and the sensor of the automatic exposure system are dependent on the X-ray spectrum (that is, on high voltage, filtering, and beam hardening within the patient (specified, e.g., by the thickness of the patient, compression in mammography)), the corresponding detector dose measurements have to be interpreted with respect to these parameters. Alternatively, the beam quality can be recorded semiquantitatively using a tandem measuring chamber and utilized for the correction of the dosimeter data. In the case of flat panel detectors, an additional concept for data collection needs to be mentioned: a subset of all pixels of the detector is either left out from recording the image or their charge is initially only read via capacitive coupling for exposure control.

The two basic construction types are the Bucky table and the thorax wall stand, but an X-ray tube mounted to a floor stand or a ceiling stand may well supply both a Bucky table and a wall stand. The Bucky table is named after Gustav Peter Bucky (* 3. September 1880 in Leipzig; † 19. February 1963 in New York). The unit has a horizontally freely movable tabletop and ensures a distance between the image detector and sensor-facing side of the patient of maximum 7 cm. The Bucky cabinet (containing the antiscatter grid) can be relocated over a wide range.

In the case of a thorax wall stand, the recording unit may be relocated to very low levels and moreover be tiltable over a wide range of angles, which facilitates recordings in a sitting posture, examination of patients located on a transparent bed, imaging of feet, and so on.

The layout of X-ray machines with flat panel detectors is basically the same as that of cassette-based devices.

In dentistry and orthodontistry, more dedicated devices are used: dental radiographic or teleradiographic devices and orthopantomographs, which may even allow for the generation of CT-like images. Dental X-ray is the only medical application of analog imaging using films without fluorescent screens because of the limited space available. This approach is justified since the area of the patient that is irradiated is usually small. In the case of digital dental X-rays the detectors are usually CCD sensors or complementary metal-oxide semiconductor (CMOS) transistors. The dose savings compared to tooth film without screen amounts to between 10% and 90%.

The main applications of teleradiography are orthodontal and oral-surgical therapies, when crucial sizes and angles have to be obtained from the recordings. The required images of low distortion may be obtained employing distances of preferably more than 1.5 m between the detector and focus. Teleradiographic devices usually use film-screen systems or have CCD sensors installed and may combine orthopantomographs with tomographic features (conventional tomography, see below). In the case of Orthopantomography (OPG), the full dental region of the upper and lower jaws is imaged by stacking quasi-line registrations, which have been obtained using varying beam directions. This is achieved by moving the X-ray tube and the detector around the patient and registering, as in the case of slit-scan technique (Fig. 3.6), and results in images as seen in Figure 3.7. Some machines also permit the registration of conventional tomograms perpendicular to the orientation of the jaw (Fig. 3.8, see Section 3.3.3).

3.3.1.2 Mammography. Mammography instruments have to fulfill particular demands because of the required high contrast for soft tissue, which can be achieved with relatively low photon energy. For this reason, the working range for high voltage is between 28 and 40 kV. In this range, the anode material tungsten is inferior to molybdenum and rhodium because of radiation hygiene

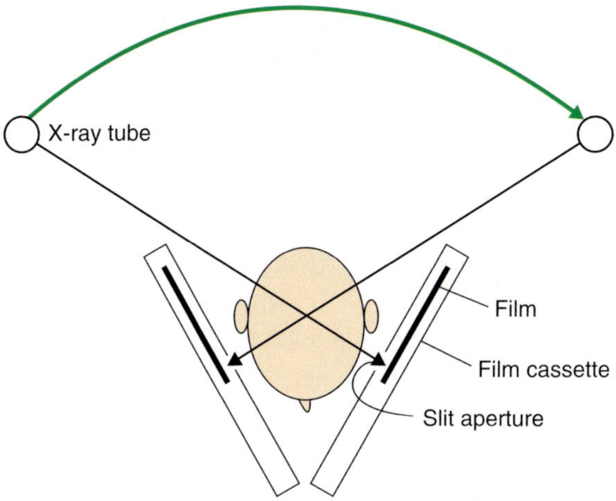

Figure 3.6. Principle of orthopantomography.

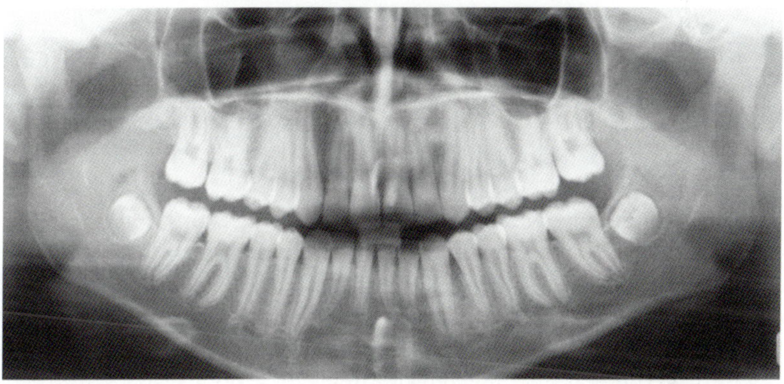

Figure 3.7. Orthopantomogram.

considerations. Mammography instruments employ tungsten anodes mainly when using the slit-scan technique (see Section "Slit-Scan Technique") in order to allow for the long exposure times and the resulting thermal tube load, which are necessary with this technique. The usual focal spot size is in the order of magnitude of 0.1–0.3 (which is a dimension-free nominal quantity describing the dimensions in millimeters under certain conditions). The benefits of compression also include the reduction of movement blur and superposition, as well as of scattered radiation due to the reduced path of the radiation through the tissue.

Another peculiarity of mammography instruments is the feature that allows recording of magnified images. In general, the distance between the object to be displayed and the image detector is minimized in order to reduce the geometrical blur. The extreme high contrast between soft parts and microcalcifications (in

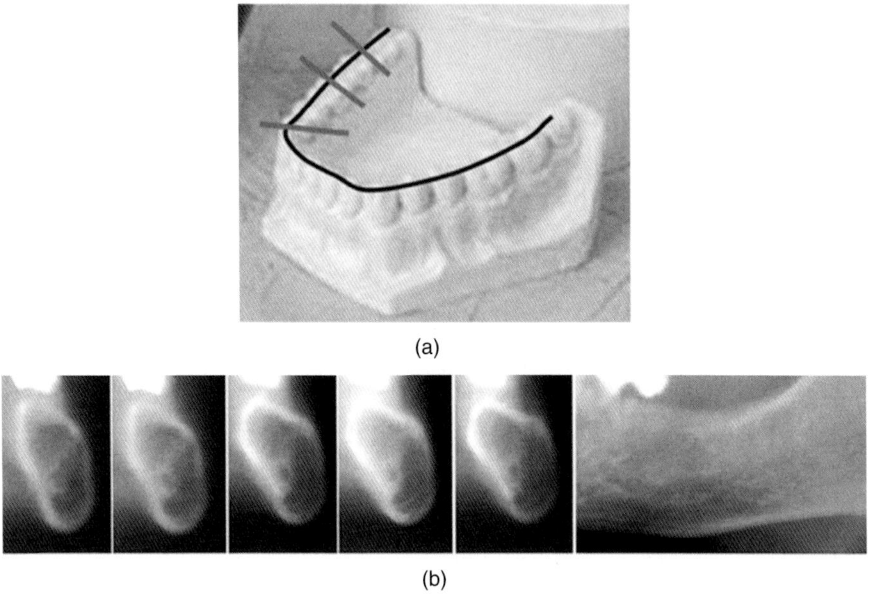

Figure 3.8. (a) Planning of the positions for classical tomographic images on a gypsum phantom. (b) Classical tomograms along and perpendicular to the row of teeth (Panorex-plus, 2006).

particular due to the low energy of the photons) induce an improved perception of the calcifications after magnification, as the blur due to magnification does not overly diminish the contrast between calcifications and their surroundings. Magnified images may be made using a small focus of 0.1 in order to limit the geometrical blur. This implies an upper limit of the tube current in the range of 25–30 mA, which results in exposure times of several seconds for optimally exposed images and the corresponding risk of motion blur. A geometrical blur due to magnification is of relevance only after the lateral resolution power of the subsequent detector is exceeded.

In the case of mamma diagnostic, imaging may be supplemented by selective biopsy or presurgical positioning of labels. Stereotactic punctures or labeling take advantage of the 3D information, which is always present in complementary images from different directions. If the structure to be labeled or punctured is located on two complementary images, the position of the instrument to be introduced on a flat or bent surface outside the mamma as well as the maximum penetration depth can be calculated and controlled by the computer. In addition to accessories that may be installed on instruments for mamma diagnosis, there are special instruments available to treat a lying patient. In this case, the image detectors, apart from flat panel detectors, are predominantly CCD detectors, since, in contrast to imaging diagnosis, the whole mammae do not need to be imaged.

3.3.1.3 Fluoroscopy. Instruments for fluoroscopic examinations are used to monitor time-dependent events, for example, the passage of contrast agents or functional imaging of moving joints. Common features and dissimilarities between imaging and fluoroscopic instruments are summarized in Table 3.1. Obviously, flat panel detectors or an assembly of image intensifiers and Bucky cabinet can be used for combined imaging and fluoroscopic instruments. In these cases, the scatter grid is a stationary grid. Fluoroscopic instruments allow the patient to adopt an inclined position if necessary for the required distribution of contrast agents in the body. Some of these instruments can be (partly) controlled from the patient's bed, which in turn requires suitable radiation protection for the employees. So far, image intensifiers are for the most part used as the image sensor, but they are increasingly being replaced by flat panel detectors.

The mechanical layout of the instruments can allow X-ray tubes above or below the table. There are also particularly flexible instruments, the so-called C-arm instruments, such as those used for angiography (see Section 3.3.1.4). The arrangement of the X-ray tube above the bed permits a relatively long distance between the focus and the detector and thus combines a relatively small geometrical distortion with good access to the patient. The arrangement of the X-ray tube below the bed can provide easier radiation protection. From a radiation-hygienic point of view, the below-bed arrangement offers safer manipulations of or at the patient within the ray path, as the hand of the examiner is not hit by the intense primary radiation but only by the distinctly less intense part of the radiation transmitted by the patient. For radiation-hygienic reasons, it is also required to leave the last image of a radioscopic sequence on the monitor after turning off the radiation. This allows a radiation-free thorough investigation of this image as well as readjustment of the opaque and/or semiopaque shutters without additional exposition.

Owing to occasional extended examination times, a radioscopic investigation may lead to relatively high radiation doses for the patient. To reduce this dose, keeping a small average tube current is recommended. This can be achieved by two approaches: reducing the continuous tube current and therefore smoothing the measured data over time (to preserve a certain SNR) or applying pulsed irradiation. Depending on the diagnostic question and the chosen compromise

TABLE 3.1. Detectors in Imaging and in Fluoroscopic Instruments

Detectors	Imaging	Fluoroscopy
Cassettes (film-screen systems, computed radiography)	x	
Flat panel detectors	x	x
CCD detectors	x	(x)
Image intensifiers		x

between patient dose and SNR, a certain loss of information on the time scale has to be accepted (see Section "Temporal Resolution and Signal to Noise Ratio"). If the same dose, the same time resolution, and the same SNR are compared, pulsed irradiation provides depiction with less blur at the expense of a continuous display of movement.

In fluoroscopic investigations, the AEC regulates parameters that directly influence the mean tube current (affecting either the tube current or the pulse width, in case of pulsed irradiation) and—in contrast to the exposure meters of cameras—the high voltage and therefore the image contrast. Devices based on image intensifiers are controlled by deflecting a part of the light emerging from the output screen. Flat panel detectors may permit signal collection by reading particular pixels, as discussed earlier, or are equipped with ionization chambers. The characteristic curves of AEC are optimized for different criteria: A control optimized for minimal radiation exposure shows a fast transition to high values of high voltage, and hence it provides a comparably low contrast image. In contrast, a characteristic curve optimized for high image contrast shows an extended region at lower values of high voltage but achieves high values of high voltage only in the region of maximum power deliverable by the generator. In the case of some fluoroscopic instruments, the information acquired by the exposure control during the last fluoro sequence can be used to calculate the default setting for a subsequent static imaging. It applies in particular for the specification of the high voltage according to a transfer characteristic, which may be specific for different organs. The tube current again is shot off after a particular detector dose is reached. This type of exposure control does not require any user intervention; hence, it is termed zero-parameter technology in analogy to the three-, two- and one-parameter technologies discussed earlier for static X-ray workplaces.

3.3.1.4 Angiography. The attenuation of X-ray radiation by blood or blood vessels is not very different from the attenuation by the surrounding tissue. For this reason, blood vessels are almost invisible in projection radiographic images. They can be distinguished after injecting a contrast agent, which basically raises the mean atomic number, for example, because of its content of iodine. Equations 3.1–3.3 indicate how the attenuation (composed of absorption and scattering) is enhanced. A concentration of the contrast agent that is sufficiently high for good contrast in the image of the vessels, but below toxic limits, is achieved by introducing a catheter in the vicinity of the vessels under investigation to administer the contrast agent during the recording using a motorized injector. The vessels containing the contrast agent together with other strongly attenuating structures are overlaid in the image. For investigations of some regions of the body, such as the skull, it might be desirable to avoid this kind of overlay. This can be achieved by collecting one or several native images (depending on the SNR) before administration of the contrast agent. The native image will be subtracted in real time from the series of images with the contrast agent. The result is basically an image

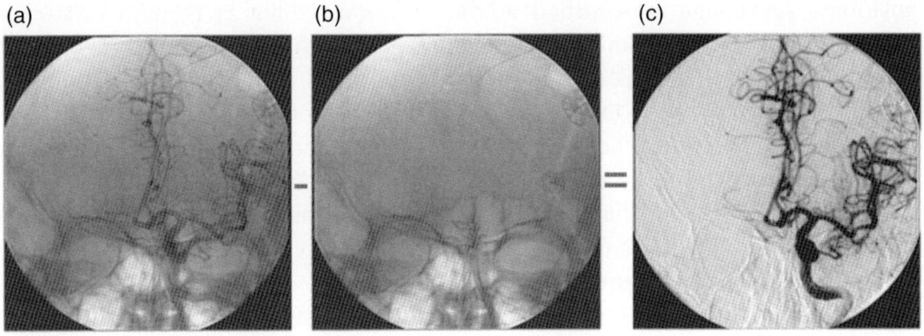

Figure 3.9. Digital subtraction angiography: the image series starts before injection of the contrast agent, and an image used as mask is obtained (b), which will be subtracted in real time from the images obtained during the injection of the contrast agent (a). The result is displayed in (c).

representing only the contrast agent containing vessels. This procedure is termed Digital Subtraction Angiography (DSA). By selection of appropriate weighting factors it is possible that anatomical landmarks may remain more or less visible in the image (Fig. 3.20). Moreover, 3D information may be obtained by varying the beam direction during a sufficiently prolonged administration of the contrast agent, for example, continuously by approximately 180°, thus providing a 3D display of the complete tree of the vessel. This procedure is termed rotational angiography. In structures of high contrast, this method may produce CT-like displays (see Section 3.3.1.5). Either image intensifiers or flat panel detectors can serve as image detectors in DSA, as was the case with the fluoroscopic instruments. The typical size of these image detectors is approximately 23 cm diameter for cardiologic applications (left heart catheterization), approximately 33 cm for neuroradiologic applications, and up to 40 cm for angiography in other regions of the body. Instruments with sufficiently large image detectors may be laid out as multifunctional instruments and used for radiographic investigations as well.

Pictures of blood vessels cannot always be unambiguously assessed. A contrast agent containing a structure beyond the lumen of the vessel may indicate an aneurysm, that is, expansion of the vessel wall that may potentially burst. A very similar picture may be obtained if a totally harmless loop of a vessel is imaged from an unfavourable direction. For this reason, angiography requires a very flexible beam geometry, which may be achieved by mounting the X-ray tube and the image receptor to a common C-arm. The rotational angiography mentioned earlier can also be easily accomplished by the C-arm geometry.

During the navigation of the catheter to the destination, the required dose of the contrast agent can be minimized by a procedure called road mapping. Small amounts of the contrast agent are released when the catheter rests at particular positions. An image is recorded at this position, which is then inverted and superimposed on subsequent radioscopic images. No further doses of the contrast agent are required in order to look up the position of the catheter within the vessel. As pulsations of the vessel or movements of the patient may hamper the correlation between the road map and the current radiographic image, the procedure may need to be repeated after some time.

Vessels may also be diagnosed using CT and Magnetic Resonance Imaging (MRI) (Chapters 4 and 5). These tomographic technologies provide slightly less information but employ much milder conditions for the patient. DSA is therefore of continuously decreasing importance as a diagnostic tool. At the same time, it gains interest as a therapeutic tool for vessel intervention, as it permits, for example, dilatation, thrombus removal, or stent placement through dedicated catheters.

3.3.1.5 Portable Devices. Portable X-ray devices are equipped with low output generators (20–35 kW) in order to limit the weight of the device and to ensure convenient power supply (AC mains power). Such devices can even be battery operated, and some of them can also be conveyed from place to place with motor drives. Some of these instruments are basically radiation generators consisting of a generator, an X-ray tube, and the necessary mechanics; others are complete digital portable devices with a flat panel detector as well as an image processing and display unit.

Portable radiographic devices usually have image intensifiers ranging from 14 to 24 cm in diameter. Similar devices using flat panel detectors are feasible as well. The layout of portable devices is based on the C-arm concept (see Section 3.3.1.4, Fig. 3.10). For mechanical reasons, computing equipment is often located

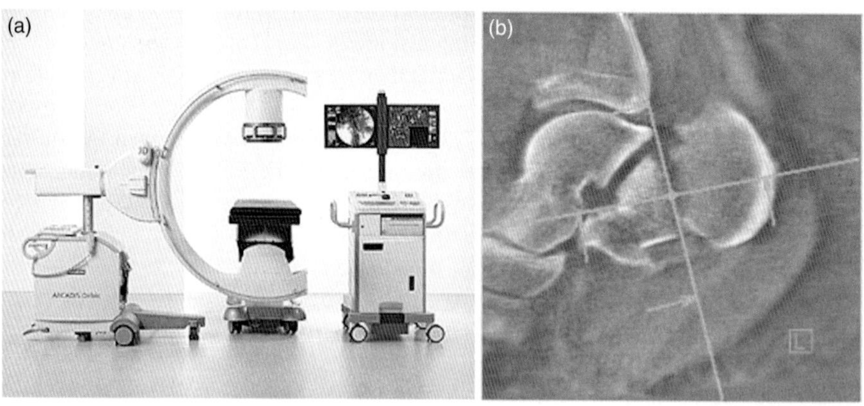

Figure 3.10. Portable fluoroscope (Siemens) for the operating room (a) permitting CT-like 3D image reconstructions (b).

on a separate trolley. Frequently used image processing tools are Multiplanar Reconstruction (MPR) and Maximum Intensity Projection (MIP). Depending on the configuration, these devices may be suitable for DSA, that is, they provide subtracted images in real time. High end devices even permit the rotation of the C-arm by at least 180° during irradiation and the calculation of CT-like images, which display structures of higher contrast (usually bones) in a quality acceptable for intraoperative application of these devices.

3.3.2 High Voltage and Image Quality

X-rays may be used to image practically all regions of the body. Depending on the requested or required contrast and thickness of the body parts to be investigated, a suitable X-ray spectrum has to be chosen for the available diagnostic devices. This can be done by selecting high voltage, choosing radiation filters where appropriate, and/or by selecting the optimal anode material. As the attenuation coefficient μ decreases on increasing photon energy (Eqs. (3.1)–(3.3)), higher energy radiation may be required for thicker body regions (increased high voltage) in order to ensure the required detector dose at sufficiently low irradiation dose for the patient (according to the current German guidelines, 75–85 kV for examinations of the lumbar spine in anteroposterior arrangement and 85–95 kV in lateral arrangement (BAeK, 2007; Fig. 3.11)). An immediate consequence of the reduced attenuation is images of lower contrast for structures either of varying area density or of varying mean atomic number. The high contrast for soft tissue necessary in case of mamma diagnostics requires a reduced high voltage. Appropriate diagnostic strategies (compression of the mamma) ensure a short path through the tissue and consequently sufficiently low irradiation.

Investigations of the chest may require images showing bony structures (ribs, spine) as well as soft tissue (e.g., lung parenchyma, mediastinal organs). Contrast between bones and soft tissue is determined by the photo effect; Eq. 3.1 indicates the forth power dependence of the photo effect on atomic number. But, the influence of the photo effect decreases faster than that of Compton scattering when photon energy is increased. This permits registration of images of both bones and soft tissue structures if hard radiation (high voltage above 100 kV) is used. On the other hand, application of high voltage below 100 kV, for example, typical for portable devices, permits superior diagnosis of the cortical and trabecular bones of the ribs (Fig. 3.12).

High contrast images of iodine-based contrast agents are obtained using high voltages at around 80 kV, which positions the focus of the intensity distribution of the spectrum close to the K-absorption edge of iodine (33 keV) depending on beam filtering. In the case of fluoroscopic devices (Fig. 3.13), these criteria may not be fulfilled because of the characteristic curve of the exposure control in the particular device (see Section 3.3.1.3).

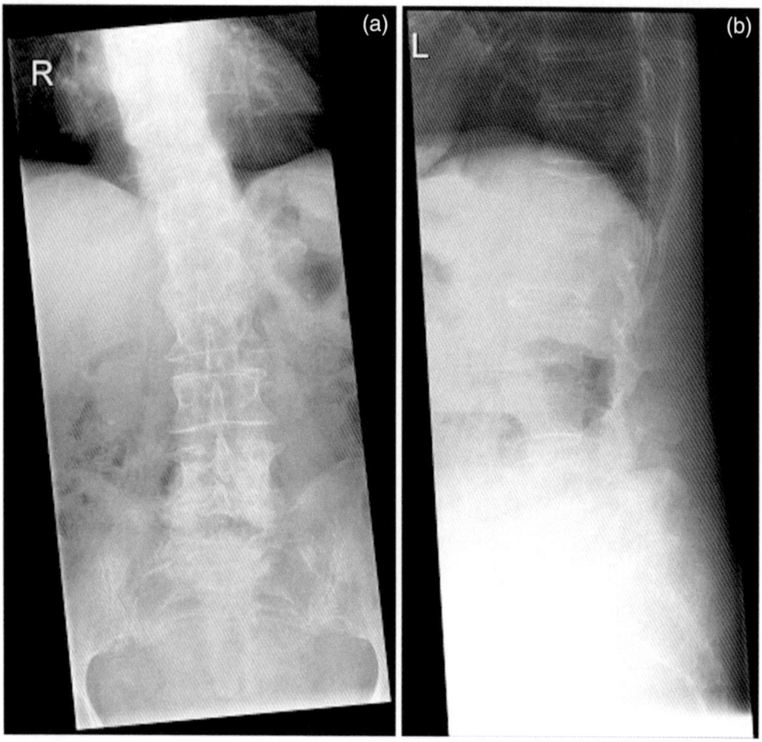

Figure 3.11. Images of the lumbar spine (a) in the anteroposterior projection at 81 kV and (b) in lateral projection at 90 kV.

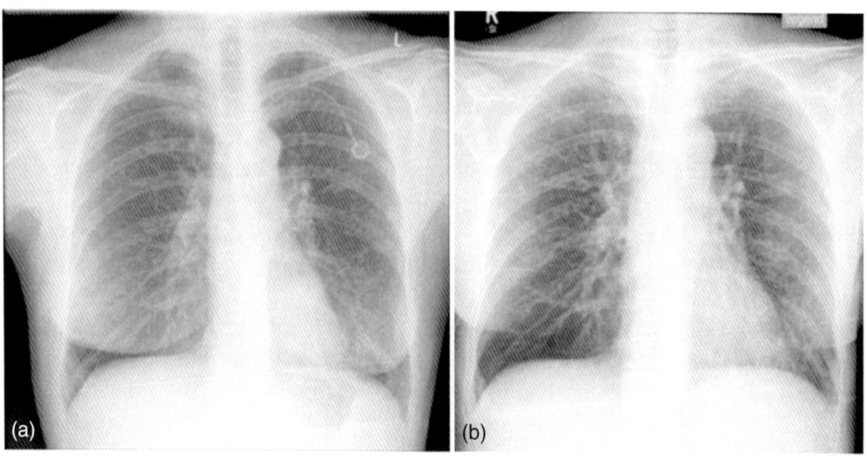

Figure 3.12. Thorax image (a) at 117 kV (hard X-ray technique) and (b) at 77 kV (soft X-ray technique). Higher contrasts at lower high voltage are observed among soft tissue parts, among bone tissue parts, as well as between soft and bone tissue parts.

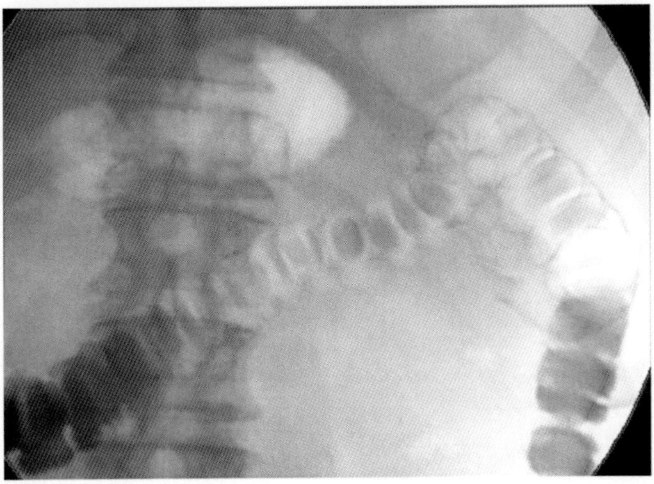

Figure 3.13. Fluoroscopic colon investigation at 96 kV after rectal administration of an iodine-containing contrast agent and subsequent administration of air ("double contrast").

3.3.3 Tomography/Tomosynthesis

The production of sharp images usually requires that, during exposure, the relative movement between the object and the optical system is smaller than the resolution of the imaging system. In classic tomography and its digital equivalent, termed as *shift-and-add tomosynthesis*, this condition is violated in a well defined way: radiation source and image detector move on (at least theoretically) parallel planes, while the center line between them always passes through a stationary point. This results in sharp and accentuated object structures in the plane of this point, while all other structures passed by the beam before and afterwards are blurred. In the case of digital imaging devices, the position of the intersection point, hence the location of the sharply displayed plane, can be shifted by appropriate displacement of the corresponding images (Figs. 3.14 and 3.15). In some devices, the radiation source and possibly the image detector move in a circular path. Procedures for tomographic reconstruction may be applied for processing larger quantities of measured angular positions and a wider range of covered angular segment (e.g., algebraic procedures, see Section 3.3.1.5).

3.3.4 Dual Energy Imaging

The dependence of the attenuation coefficient μ on both photon energy and material properties (density, mean atomic number) permits distinction between different materials. The classic dual energy absorptiometry used in Nuclear Medicine is based on two images acquired with monochromatic radiation of different energies, and the (surface) densities of both (supposed) components are calculated using a linear system of equations. The images discussed here may be taken

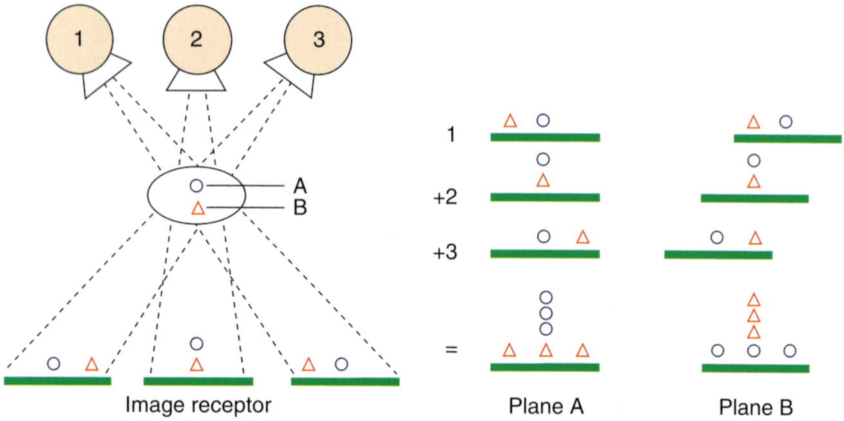

Figure 3.14. Shift-and-add tomosynthesis: depending on the shift of the individual images before overlay, either plane A or plane B is depicted sharply. *Source:* From (Dobbins and Godfrey, 2003).

by polychromatic radiation as well, but this requires approximations and calibrations. (Fig. 3.16). The two measurements may be performed using the same X-ray tube, but with different high voltages or using various radiation filtration at the detector side during one exposure.

The prevailing application of this approach in projectional radiography is osteodensitometry, where the mineral content of the bones is determined as area density. The same set of images can be used to estimate the ratio between muscle and fat tissue in the body, particularly, when (by slit-scan measurement, see Section "Slit-Scan" Technique) a whole-body scan is carried out.

Dual energy imaging is gaining increasing importance in CT as well (see Chapter 4).

3.3.5 Computer Applications

Technically more simple, but of high relevance clinically, is the utilization of the three-dimensional information in the case of stereotactic punctures and lesion marking in female breasts (see Section 3.3.1.2). The target region is marked in two subsequent images, which are obtained at different angles, and then the region's 3D position may be calculated. The guiding tool of the marking or puncture device is positioned above the calculated location of the lesion. In the case of movable lesions, the positioning of the guiding tool can be checked by additional images (Fig. 3.17).

Physicians can be assisted during diagnosis by digital image processing, for example, by emphasizing suspect structures or areas in mammograms, by using a multiscale local contrast measure defined in the wavelet domain, or even with knowledge-based classifiers. These procedures are not restricted to mammography.

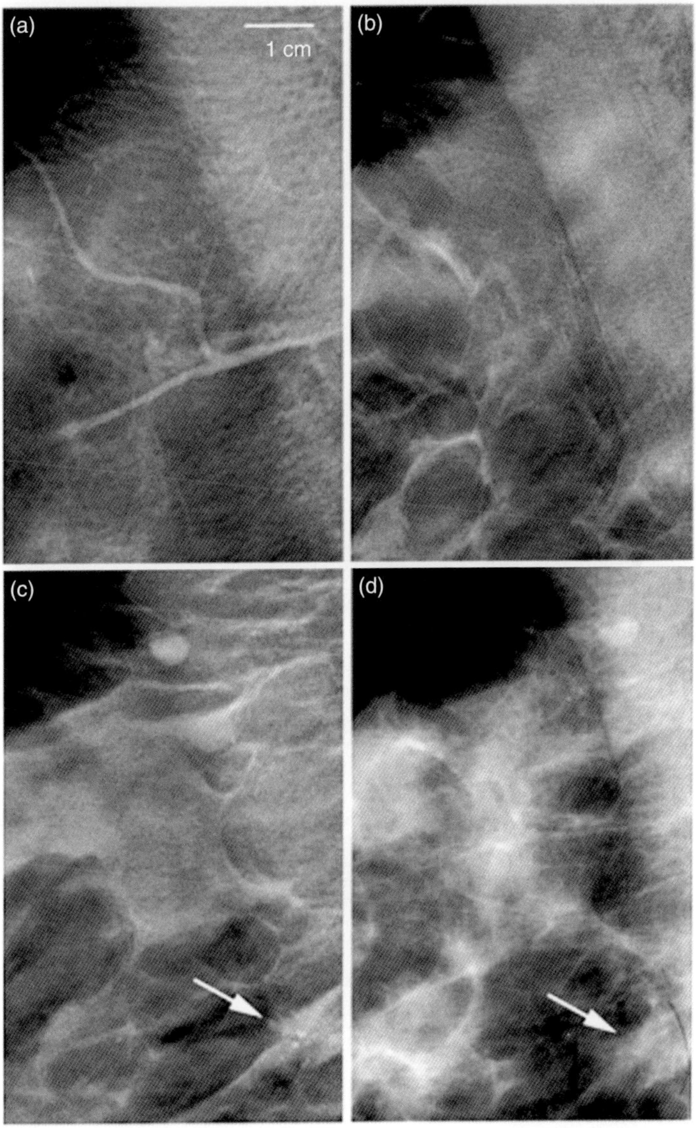

Figure 3.15. Mammographic tomosynthesis images of three different planes (a–c) and a conventional mammogram of the same region. The calcification of an invasive ductal carcinoma is detected more easily from the tomosynthesis (c) than from the projectional radiogram (d). *Source:* From (Dobbins and Godfrey, 2003).

(a)
(b)

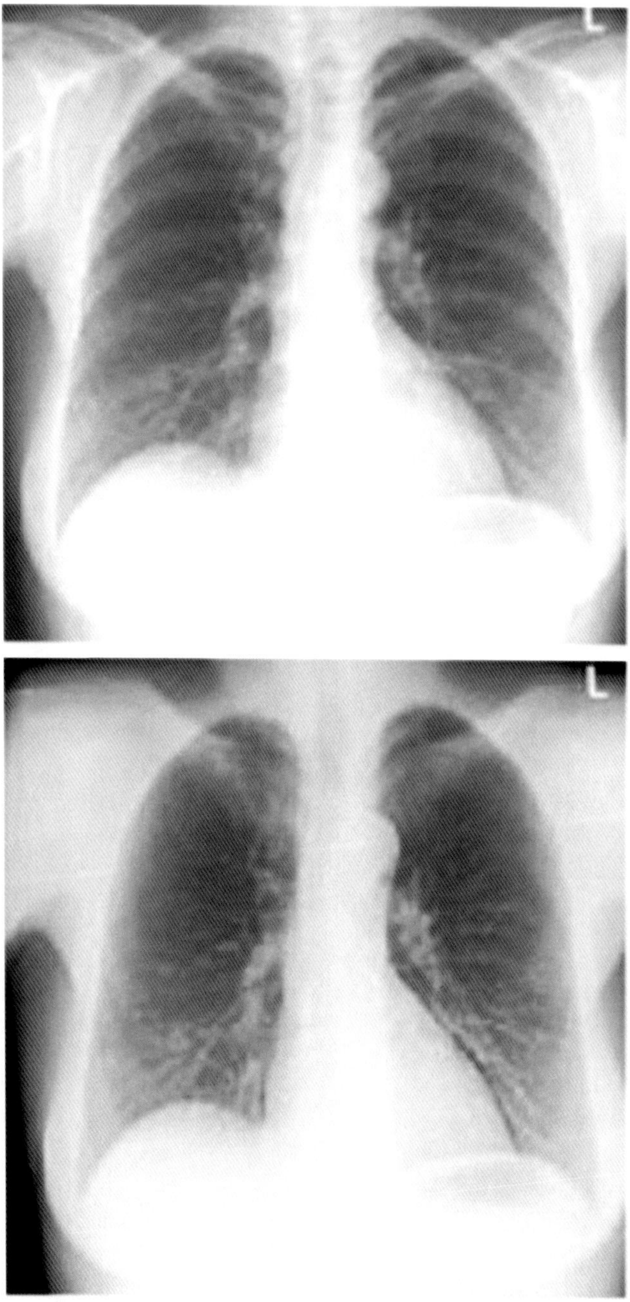

Figure 3.16. Dual energy images of the thorax: (a) classical image, (b) soft tissue image, (c) bone image. *Source:* From (GE, 2009).

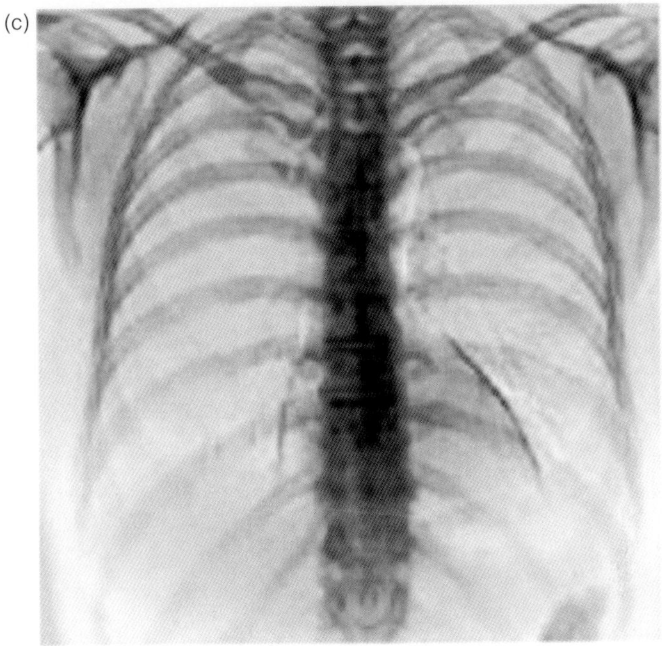

Figure 3.16. (*Continued*)

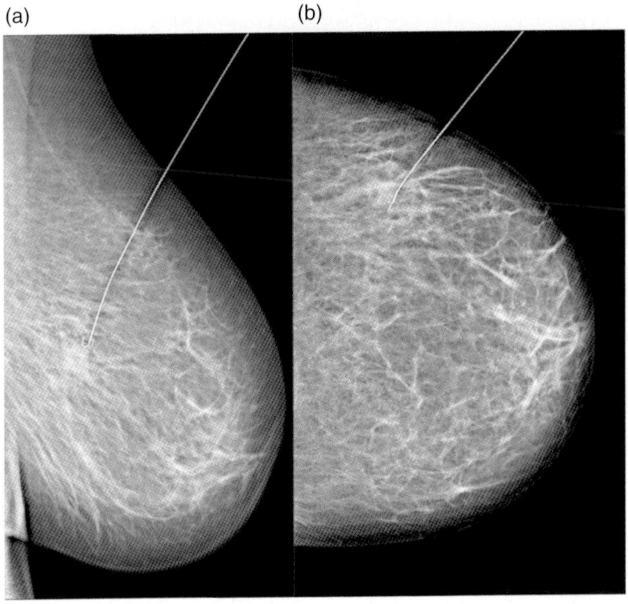

Figure 3.17. Stereotactic wire marking of ductal carcinoma *in situ* with hematoma after core needle biopsy. Imaging with 28 kV in mediolateral (a) and craniocaudal (b) projections.

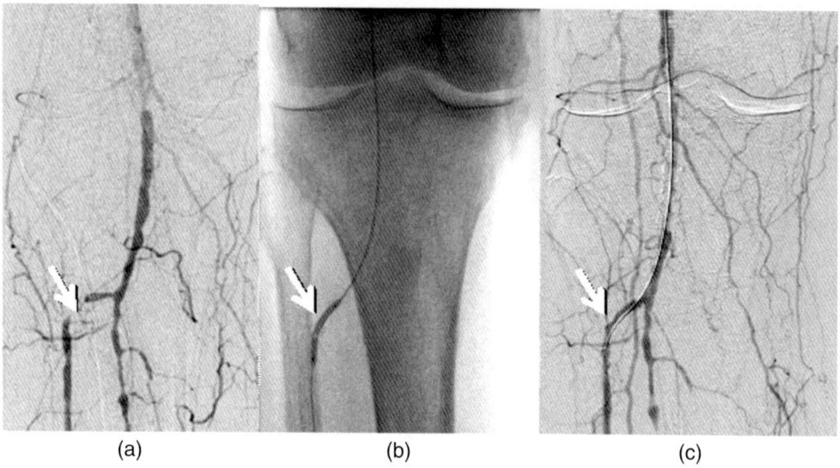

Figure 3.18. Stenosis of the anterior tibial artery (arrow). (a) Stenosed vessel (subtraction image), (b) balloon catheter positioned (unsubtracted), (c) status post balloon catheter dilatation.

3.3.6 Interventional Radiology

DSA may be used to display blood vessels for diagnostic purposes, but sectional views (see Section 3.3.1.4 and Chapters 4 and 5) are much gentler as compared to the former. For therapeutic purposes, however, the access to vessel lesions by X-ray-guided positioning of catheters is of considerable importance.

When indicated, thrombosed vessels may be recanalized by lysing drugs. In contrast to intravenous treatment, a high concentration of the drug may be achieved by local fibrinolysis via catheter, keeping side effects minimal. Stenosed or occluded regions may be dilated mechanically by a balloon catheter (Fig. 3.18) or be stabilized by insertion of a stent (Fig. 3.19).

Styptic materials such as tissue glue, metal coils, or particles sized between 50 and 1000 μm can be introduced by catheters into the vessels that feed the bleeding (Fig. 3.20).

Portal hypertension due to liver cirrhosis can be treated by creating an artificial connection between the hepatic portal vein and a liver vein and stabilizing it by a stent (*T*ransjugular *I*ntrahepatic *P*ortosystemic *S*hunt—TIPS).

Interventional radiology based on projectional radiography is also successfully applied for taking biopsies of tissue or for preoperative marking of lesions (see Section 3.3.5).

3.4 RADIATION EXPOSURE TO PATIENTS AND EMPLOYEES

A variety of methods for medical imaging based on X-rays is available. A similar wide range of radiation doses to patients corresponds to the different

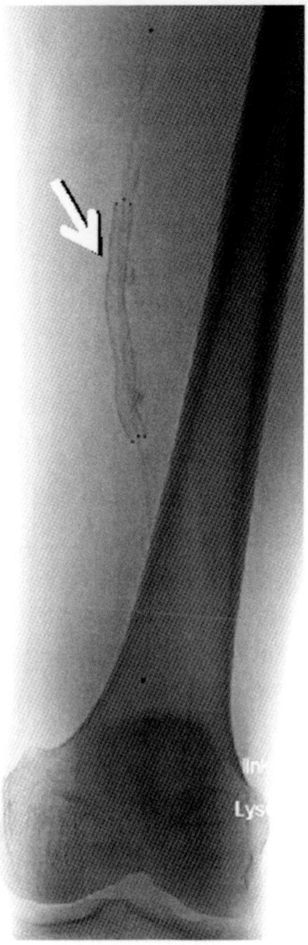

Figure 3.19. Stent in the arteria femoralis sinistra.

imaging methods. The required effective dose ranges from 0.01 mSv for extremity images to approximately 1 mSv for images of the spine and to several millisieverts for fluoroscopic examinations (and CT). The above-mentioned dose values correspond to 1.5 days to several years of mean natural radiation exposure in Germany (SSK, 2006). The patient dose required for a particular diagnostic procedure is primarily determined by the image detector. Actual values of DQE are above 50% for modern fluoroscopic devices; hence, a dose reduction to less than 50% is anticipated for the future. The radiation exposure documentation required by the German X-ray control law (Röntgenverordnung) usually refers to the dose–area product for several reasons: on one hand the product of the dose and irradiated area makes sense biologically, as the risk for damages caused by irradiation is approximately proportional both to the dose and to the number of involved cells. The latter corresponds roughly to the exposed area of the patient. On the other hand, the dose–area product can easily be measured. As the irradiated area increases with the squared distance to the radiation source and the dose decreases at the same rate, the product of area and dose remains independent of the distance. Thus a reliable value for the patient can easily be measured by

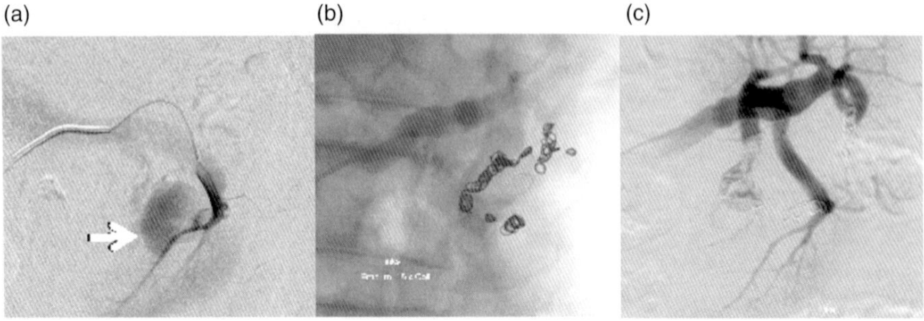

Figure 3.20. Embolization of bleeding in the renal pelvis-calyx system. (a) Extravasation of contrast indicates bleeding, (b) imaging of 18 coils placed, (c) bleeding supplying vessels are closed.

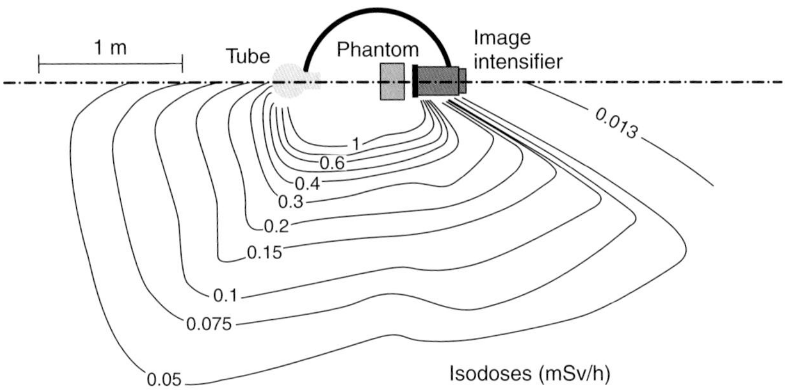

Figure 3.21. Dose distribution around surgical C-arm X-ray system in horizontal beam geometry. *Source:* Modified from Schulz, 2005.

a detector mounted on the protective case of the tube. The conversion of the dose–area products into effective doses requires additional information because of the varying radiation sensitivity between different tissue types.

The maximum allowed exposition per year in Germany for professionals in medicine is 20 mSv (effective dose with consideration of additional organ-specific limitations) (RöV, 2002). During 2005, this value was exceeded by 6 of the 239,178 monitored professionals in medicine. In the case of 99.99% of these professionals, the measured annual dose was $\leq$10 mSv (BfS, 2005). Such low exposure data can be achieved only by strict use of radiation protection gear and adherence to safety guidelines. According to (Naidu et al. 2005), abandonment of thyroid gland protection may lead to doses of 10 mSv or more in that organ for the endoscopist.

Attention must be paid during operations in the vicinity of the patient to whether body parts of the investigator are exposed to primary radiation, such as in applications of the over-table X-ray system (see Section 3.3.1.3). The spatial distribution of scattered radiation has to be taken into account, both for application of radiation protection gear and for positioning of the staff, for example, in the vicinity of an image intensifier in the operating room. Above a certain thickness of the radiation scattering body—as in case of an abdomen investigation—the expected exposure is higher on the side of the X-ray tube than on the side of the image detector (Fig. 3.21).

REFERENCES

BAeK. Leitlinie der Bundesärztekammer zur Qualitätssicherung in der Röntgendiagnostik. 2007. Available at http://www.drg.de/docs/anweisungen/leitlinie_baek_roev-2007.pdf.

BfS. Bundesamt für Strahlenschutz Jahresbericht 2005 Teil III: Berufliche Strahlenexposition; 2005.

Bushberg JT, Seibert JA, Leidholdt EM Jr, Boone JM. *The Essential Physics of Medical Imaging*. 2nd ed. Lippincott Philadelphia; 2002. ISBN 0-683-30118-7.

Dobbins JT, Godfrey DJ. Digital x-ray tomosynthesis: current state of the art and clinical potential. Phys Med Biol 2003;48: R65–R106.

GE. 2009. Available at http://www.gehealthcare.com/eude/radiography/products/applications/dual-energy-substraction.html.

Hendee WR, Ritenour ER. *Medical Imaging Physics*. Wiley-Liss New York; 2002. ISBN 0-471-38226-4.

Leicht H. Wilhelm Conrad Röntgen. Biographie. Ehrenwirth. München; 1994. ISBN 3-431-03354-7.

Morneburg H, editor. *Bildgebende Systeme für die medizinische Diagnostik*. Publicis MCD Verlag Erlangen; 1995. ISBN 89578-002-2.

Naidu LS, Singhal S, Preece DE, Vohrah A, Loft DE. Radiation exposure to personnel performing endoscopic retrograde cholangiopancreatography. Postgrad Med J 2005;81:660–662.

Panorexplus. 2006. Available at http://www.imagingsciences.com/html/products/panorexplus/panplusF.htm.

RöV. Verordnung über den Schutz vor Schäden durch Röntgenstrahlen. BGBII 1987, 114, zuletzt geändert; 2002.

Schedel A. Der Blick in den Menschen. Wilhelm Conrad Röntgen und seine Zeit. Urban & Schwarzenberg. München, Wien, Baltimore; 1995. ISBN 3-541-19501-0.

Schulz E. *Arten und Wirkung von Strahlenschutzzubehör*. Universität Lübeck, Institut für Radiologie; Lübeck:: 2005. Available at http://ikrweb.unimuenster.de/aptdir/veranstaltungen/vortraege/Goettingen/Schulz-Arten_Wirkung_Strahlenschutzzubehoer.pdf.

Seibert JA. Digital radiography: CR versus DR? Time to reconsider the options, the definitions, and current capabilities. Appl Radiol Suppl 2007;36:4–7.

Siemens ARCADIS Orbic 3D. Available at http://www.medical.siemens.com/webapp/wcs/stores/servlet/ProductDisplay~q_catalogId~e_-3~a_catTree~e_100010,1007660,12760,14264~a_langId~e_-3~a_productId~e_143790~a_storeId~e_10001.htm.

Sirona. 2008. Available at http://www.sirona.de/ecomaXL/index.php?site$=$SIRONA_roentgen_intraoral_sensoren.

SSK. *Orientierungshilfe für radiologische und nuklearmedizinische Untersuchungen. Berichte der Strahlenschutzkommission (SSK) des Bundesministeriums für Umwelt, Naturschutz und Reaktorsicherheit*. Heft 51. Berlin: H. HOFFMANN Fachverlag; 2006.

4

COMPUTED TOMOGRAPHY

STEFAN ULZHEIMER AND THOMAS FLOHR
Computed Tomography Department, Siemens Healthcare, Forchheim, Germany

4.1 BASICS

4.1.1 History

The first commercial medical X-ray Computed Tomography (CT) scanner was built in 1972 by the English engineer G.N. Hounsfield for the company EMI Ltd. as a pure head scanner with a conventional X-ray tube and a dual-row detector system moving incrementally around the patient.

It was able to acquire 12 slices, each 13 mm thick, and reconstruct the images with a matrix of 80 × 80 pixels in approximately 35 min. Figure 4.1 shows the image of the head on one of these early scanners and how it compares to the image quality of a state-of-the-art CT scanner today. Today, the whole brain can be visualized with high quality from a 10-s scan.

Until 1989 there were no principally new developments in conventional CT, although of course the performance of the CT scanners increased dramatically with the engineering progress. By then, the acquisition time for one image decreased from 300 s in 1972 to 1–2 s, slices as thin as 1 mm became possible, and the in-plane resolution increased from 3 line pairs per centimeter (lp/cm) to 10–15 lp/cm with typically 512 × 512.

As it was foreseen in the late seventies that acquisition times of mechanical CT scanners would be far too long for high quality cardiac imaging for the next years or even decades to come, a completely new technical concept for a CT scanner

Biomedical Imaging: Principles and Applications, First Edition. Edited by Reiner Salzer.

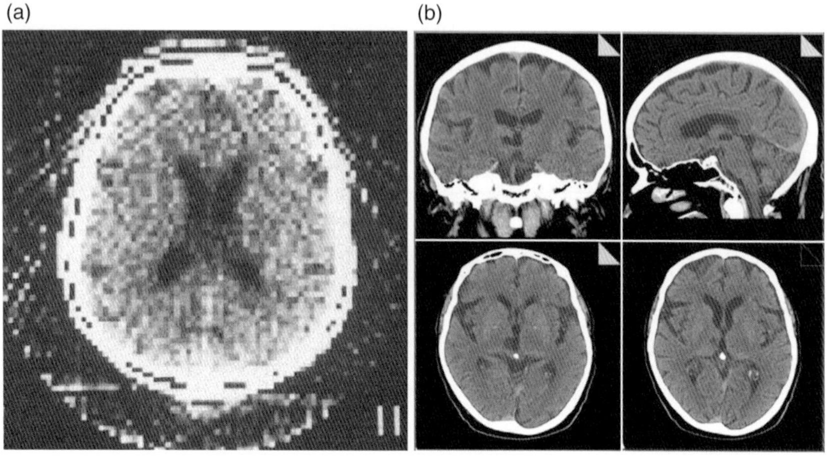

Figure 4.1. Development of computed tomography over time. (a) Cross-sectional image of a brain in the year 1971 and (b) the whole brain with sagital, coronal, and cross-sectional slices in the year 2007. Courtesy of Mayo Clinic, Rochester.

without moving parts for extremely fast data acquisition of 50 ms was suggested and promoted as Cardiovascular Computed Tomographic (CVCT) scanner. Later, these scanners were also called *ultrafast CT scanners* or, giving a hint about the scanning principle, "Electron Beam Computed Tomographic" (EBT or EBCTs) scanners. After the company "Imatron," which originally developed and produced these systems, was acquired by one of the major CT manufacturers several years ago, the development and production of these systems was stopped. High cost and limited image quality combined with low volume coverage prevented the wide propagation of the modality.

With the introduction of slip ring technology to get power to and data off the rotating gantry, continuous rotation of the X-ray tube and the detector became possible. The possibility of continuous rotation led to the development of spiral CT scanners in the early nineties (Crawford and King, 1990; Kalender et al., 1990), a method already theoretically proposed several years before (Mori, 1986; Nishimura and Miyazaki, 1988). Thus, volume data could be acquired without the danger of mis- or double-registration of anatomical details. Images could be reconstructed at any position along the patient axis (longitudinal axis, z-axis), and overlapping image reconstruction could be used to improve longitudinal resolution. Volume data became the very basis for applications such as CT angiography (Rubin et al., 1995), which has revolutionized noninvasive assessment of vascular disease. The ability to acquire volume data was the prerequisite for the development of three-dimensional image processing techniques such as Multiplanar Reformations (MPRs), Maximum Intensity Projections (MIPs), Surface Shaded Displays (SSDs), or Volume Rendering Techniques (VRTs), which have become a vital component of medical imaging today.

Main drawbacks of single-slice spiral CT are insufficient volume coverage within one breathhold time of the patient and missing spatial resolution in z-axis due to wide collimation. With single-slice spiral CT, the ideal of isotropic resolution, that is, of equal resolution in all three spatial axes, can be achieved only for very limited scan ranges (Kalender, 1995).

Larger volume coverage in shorter scan times and improved longitudinal resolution became feasible after the broad introduction of four-slice CT systems by all major CT manufacturers in 1998 (Klingenbeck-Regn et al., 1999; McCollough and Zink, 1999; Hu et al., 2000). The increased performance allowed for the optimization of a variety of clinical protocols. Examination times for standard protocols could be significantly reduced; alternatively, scan ranges could be significantly extended. Furthermore, a given anatomic volume could be scanned within a given scan time with substantially reduced slice width. This way, for many clinical applications the goal of isotropic resolution was within reach with four-slice CT systems. Multidetector Row Computed Tomography (MDCT) also dramatically expanded into areas previously considered beyond the scope of third-generation CT scanners based on the mechanical rotation of the X-ray tube and detector, such as cardiac imaging with the addition of Electrocardiographic (ECG) gating capability enabled by gantry rotation times as low as 0.5 s (Kachelriess et al., 2000; Ohnesorge et al., 2000). Despite all these promising advances, clinical challenges and limitations remained for four-slice CT systems. True isotropic resolution for routine applications had not yet been achieved for many applications requiring extended scan ranges, since wider collimated slices (4×2.5 mm or 4×3.75 mm) had to be chosen to complete the scan within a reasonable timeframe. For ECG-gated coronary Computed Tomographic Angiographies (CTAs), stents or severely calcified arteries constituted a diagnostic dilemma, mainly because of partial volume artifacts as a consequence of insufficient longitudinal resolution (Nieman et al., 2001), and reliable imaging of patients with higher heart rates was not possible because of limited temporal resolution.

As a next step, the introduction of an eight-slice CT system in 2000 enabled shorter scan times, but did not yet provide improved longitudinal resolution (thinnest collimation 8×1.25 mm). The latter was achieved with the introduction of 16-slice CT (Flohr et al., 2002a; Flohr et al., 2002b), which made it possible to routinely acquire large anatomic volumes with isotropic submillimeter spatial resolution. ECG-gated cardiac scanning was enhanced by both, temporal resolution was improved by gantry rotation times as low as 0.375 s, and spatial resolution was improved (Nieman et al., 2002; Ropers et al., 2003).

The generation of 64-slice CT-systems introduced in 2004 has become the established standard in the high end segment of the market. Two different scanner concepts were introduced by different vendors: the "volume concept" pursued by GE, Philips, and Toshiba aims at a further increase in volume coverage speed by using 64 detector rows instead of 16 without changing the physical parameters of the scanner compared to the respective 16-slice version. The "resolution concept" pursued by Siemens uses 32 physical detector rows in combination with double z-sampling, a refined z-sampling technique enabled by a periodic motion of the focal spot in the z-direction, to simultaneously acquire 64 overlapping slices with the goal of pitch-independent increase of longitudinal resolution and reduction of spiral artifacts. (Flohr et al., 2004; Flohr et al., 2005a). With this scanner generation, CT angiographic examinations with submillimeter resolution in the pure arterial phase become feasible even for extended anatomical ranges. The improved temporal resolution due to gantry rotation times as low as 0.33 s has the potential to increase clinical robustness of ECG-gated scanning at higher heart rates, thereby significantly reducing the number of patients requiring heart rate control and facilitating the successful integration of CT coronary angiography into routine clinical algorithms (Leschka et al., 2005; Raff et al., 2005). Today high end single source scanners offer rotation times of as low as 0.30 s and can acquire up to 128 slices with an isotropic resolution of down to 0.3 mm (Siemens SOMATOM Definion AS+, SOMATOM Definition Edge).

In 2005, the first Dual Source Computed Tomographic (DSCT) system, that is, a CT system with two X-ray tubes and two corresponding detectors offset by 90° was introduced by Siemens (Flohr et al., 2006). The key benefit of DSCT for cardiac scanning is improved temporal resolution. A scanner of this type provides temporal resolution of a quarter of the gantry rotation time, independent of the patient's heart rate and without the need for multisegment reconstruction techniques. DSCT scanners also show promising properties for general radiology applications. First, both X-ray tubes can be operated simultaneously in a standard spiral or sequential acquisition mode, providing high power reserves when necessary. In addition, both X-ray tubes can be operated at different kilovolt settings and/or different prefiltrations, allowing dual energy acquisitions. Applications of dual energy CT include tissue characterization, calcium quantification, and quantification of the local blood volume in contrast-enhanced scans. A second generation of dual source CT scanners (SOMATOM Definition Flash) enabled further improvements in Cardiac CT and Dual Energy CT through wider detectors with 128 slices and further increased rotation speed.

4.1.2 Basic Physics and Image Reconstruction

As described in Chapter 3, the photon intensity I behind an object depends on the primary photon intensity I_0, the distance d it traveled through the object, and a constant that depends on the material and the energy of the photons, the linear attenuation coefficient μ. For a homogeneous object and monoenergetic photons the physical law is a simple exponential relationship:

$$I = I_0 \cdot \mathrm{e}^{-\mu \cdot d} \tag{4.1}$$

The fact that μ depends on the attenuating material makes it possible to distinguish materials with different attenuation coefficients. Measuring the two-dimensional distribution of the attenuation coefficients $\mu(x, y)$ or $\mu(r, \varphi)$ in polar coordinates is the actual goal of CT. Each projection—in CT the measurement of intensities from one direction is called *projection*—is a superposition of the attenuation coefficients of all materials along one ray. From Eq. (4.1) we get for a single ray, that is, a fixed angle Θ and distance ξ from the center of rotation.

$$I = I_0 \cdot \mathrm{e}^{-\int_0^d \mu(r)\cdot \mathrm{d}r} \tag{4.2}$$

or

$$-\ln \frac{I}{I_0} = -\int_0^d \mu(r) \cdot \mathrm{d}r \tag{4.3}$$

To obtain a two-dimensional distribution of attenuation coefficients with n^2 values or an image with n^2 pixels we need at least n^2 independently measured intensities I in equation (4.3). I_0 is usually known from a calibration measurement using rays outside the actual field of measurement. For a 512^2 image matrix, a minimum of $512^2 = 262{,}144$ independent projection values are needed. If one tries to solve this problem iteratively as it was done in the early days of CT, this would result in a linear equation system of 512^2 equations with 512^2 unknown parameters.

For all practical purposes, this is even today not possible and therefore a numerical approach called *filtered backprojection* (Chapter 2) is used in all scanners to solve the problem. The applied filter or convolution kernel can be used to influence the image characteristics. For example, "sharp" kernels increase resolution and noise, whereas "soft" kernels decrease them.

The determined attenuation coefficient μ itself is an inconvenient measure, as it is not very descriptive and depends on the X-ray spectrum used. Therefore, the so-called CT value or CT number (CT#) given in Hounsfield units (HU; Chapter 2) was introduced. It is defined as

$$\mathrm{CT\#} = \frac{\mu - \mu_{\mathrm{water}}}{\mu_{\mathrm{water}}} \cdot 1000\ \mathrm{HU} \tag{4.4}$$

where μ_{water} is the attenuation coefficient of water for the respective tube voltage. It is determined by calibration measurements for each spectrum used. According to this definition, the CT value of water is zero and that of air is -1000 HU.

Unfortunately, the attenuation coefficient does not only depend on the material but also on the energy of the photons that interact with the material. Therefore, the spectrum changes on the X-ray's path through the material. For X-ray systems, this introduces a further integration over all photon energies E in Eq. (4.2):

$$I = \int_0^{E_{\mathrm{MAX}}} I_0(E) \cdot \mathrm{e}^{-\int_0^d \mu(E,r)\cdot \mathrm{d}r} \mathrm{d}E \tag{4.5}$$

This dependency is usually ignored in initial image reconstruction for all materials except water. This may result in so-called beam hardening artifacts, which can be corrected for in iterative processes. A more detailed overview of MDCT systems and image reconstruction techniques may be found in (Flohr et al., 2005b).

4.2 INSTRUMENTATION

The overall performance of an MDCT system depends on several key components. These components include the gantry, X-ray source, a high powered generator, detector and detector electronics, data transmission systems (slip rings), and the computer system for image reconstruction and manipulation.

4.2.1 Gantry

Third-generation CT scanners employ the so-called "rotate/rotate" geometry, in which both the X-ray tube and the detector are mounted onto a rotating gantry and rotated around the patient (Fig. 4.2). In an MDCT system, the detector comprises several rows of 700 and more detector elements, which cover a Scan Field of View (SFOV) of usually 50 cm. The X-ray attenuation of the object is measured by the individual detector elements. All measurement values acquired at the same angular position of the measurement system form a "projection" or "view".

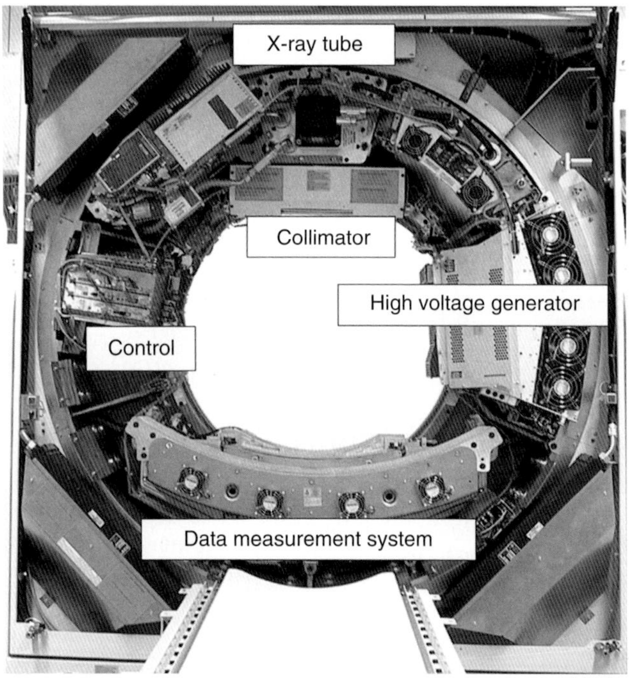

Figure 4.2. Basic system components of a modern "third-generation" CT system. First-generation systems used a collimated pencil beam and therefore required a translation of the pencil beam and the single detector element before each rotational step to scan the whole object. Second-generation scanners used a small fan beam but still required translational and rotational patterns of the X-ray source and the small detector array, whereas the fan beam of third-generation scanners covered the whole object the first time and allowed for a pure rotational motion of the tube and the detector around the patient.

Typically, 1000 projections are measured during each 360° rotation. The key requirement for the mechanical design of the gantry is the stability of both focal spot and detector position during rotation, in particular with regard to the rapidly increasing rotational speeds of modern CT systems (from 0.75 s in 1994 to 0.33 s in 2003). Hence, the mechanical support for the X-ray tube, tube collimator, and Data Measurement System (DMS) has to be designed such as to withstand the high gravitational forces associated with fast gantry rotation (~17G for 0.42 s rotation time, ~28G for 0.33 s rotation time). Rotation times of less than 0.25 s (mechanical forces >45G) appear to be beyond today's mechanical limits.

4.2.2 X-ray Tube and Generator

State-of-the-art X-ray tube/generator combinations provide a peak power of 55–100 kW, usually at various, user-selectable tube voltages, for example, 80, 100, 120, and 140 kV. Different clinical applications require different X-ray spectra and hence different kilovolt settings for optimal image quality and/or best possible signal to noise ratio at the lowest dose. Furthermore, the tube current (mA) can be freely selected to adjust the dose to the patient. Lower tube voltages require over-proportionately higher tube currents to achieve the same dose to the scanned object. In a conventional tube design, an anode plate of typically 160–220 mm diameter rotates in a vacuum housing (Fig. 4.3). The heat storage capacity of the anode plate and tube housing—measured in Mega Heat Units (MHU)—determines the performance level: the bigger the anode plate the larger the heat storage capacity and the more scan seconds can be delivered until the anode plate reaches its temperature limit. A state-of-the-art X-ray tube has a heat storage capacity of typically 5–9 MHU, realized by thick graphite layers attached to the backside of the anode plate. An alternative design is the rotating envelope tube (STRATON, Siemens, Forchheim, Germany, (Schardt et al., 2004)). The anode plate constitutes an outer wall of the rotating tube housing; it is therefore in direct contact with the cooling oil and can be efficiently cooled via thermal conduction (Fig. 4.3). This way, a very high heat dissipation rate of 5 MHU/min is achieved, eliminating the need for heat storage in the anode, which consequently has a heat storage capacity close to zero. Thanks to fast anode cooling, rotating envelope tubes can perform high power scans in rapid succession. Owing to the central rotating cathode, permanent electromagnetic deflection of the electron beam is needed to position and shape the focal spot on the anode. The electromagnetic deflection is also used for the double z-sampling technology of a 64-slice CT system (Flohr et al., 2004; Flohr et al., 2005a).

4.2.3 MDCT Detector Design and Slice Collimation

Modern CT systems use solid-state detectors in general. Each detector element consists of a radiation-sensitive solid state material (such as cadmium tungstate, gadolinium oxide, or gadolinium oxisulfide with suitable dopings), which

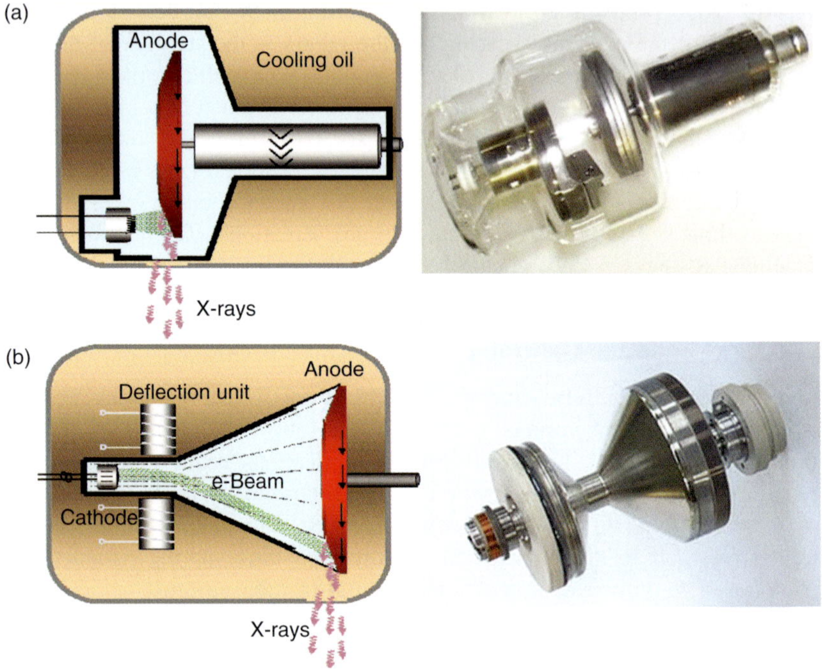

Figure 4.3. Schematic drawings and pictures of a conventional X-ray tube (a) and a rotating envelope tube (b). The electrons emitted by the cathode are represented by green lines; the X-rays generated in the anode are depicted as purple arrows. In a conventional X-ray tube, the anode plate rotates in a vacuum housing. Heat is mainly dissipated via thermal radiation. In a rotating envelope tube, the anode plate constitutes an outer wall of the tube housing and is in direct contact with the cooling oil. Heat is more efficiently dissipated via thermal conduction, and the cooling rate is significantly increased. Rotating envelope tubes have no moving parts and no bearings in the vacuum. (Images are not drawn to scale).

converts the absorbed X-rays into visible light. The light is then detected by a Si photodiode. The resulting electrical current is amplified and converted into a digital signal. Key requirements for a suitable detector material are good detection efficiency, that is, high atomic number, and very short afterglow time to enable the fast gantry rotation speeds that are essential for ECG-gated cardiac imaging.

A CT detector must provide different slice widths to adjust the optimal scan speed, longitudinal resolution, and image noise for each application. With a single-slice CT detector, different collimated slice widths are obtained by prepatient collimation of the X-ray beam. For a very elementary model of a two-slice CT detector consisting of $M = 2$ detector rows, different slice widths can be obtained by prepatient collimation if the detector is separated midway along the z-extent of the X-ray beam.

For $M > 2$ this simple design principle must be replaced by more flexible concepts requiring more than M detector rows to simultaneously acquire M slices.

Different manufacturers of MDCT scanners have introduced different detector designs. In order to be able to select different slice widths, all scanners combine several detector rows electronically to a smaller number of slices according to the selected beam collimation and the desired slice width.

For the four-slice CT systems introduced in 1998, two detector types have been commonly used. The fixed array detector consists of detector elements with equal sizes in the longitudinal direction. A representative example for this scanner type, the GE Lightspeed scanner, has 16 detector rows, each of them defining a 1.25-mm collimated slice width in the center of rotation (Hu et al., 2000; McCollough and Zink, 1999). The total coverage in the longitudinal direction is 20 mm at the isocenter; owing to geometrical magnification the actual detector is about twice as wide. In order to select different slice widths, several detector rows can be electronically combined to a smaller number of slices. The following slice widths (measured at the isocenter) are realized: 4 × 1.25 mm, 4 × 2.5 mm, 4 × 3.75 mm, 4 × 5 mm (Fig. 4.4a). The same detector design is used for the eight-slice version of this system, providing 8 × 1.25 mm and 8 × 2.5 mm collimated slice width.

A different approach uses an adaptive array detector design, which comprises detector rows with different sizes in the longitudinal direction. Scanners of this type, the Philips MX8000 four-slice scanner and the Siemens SOMATOM Sensation 4 scanner, have eight detector rows (Klingenbeck-Regn et al., 1999). Their widths in the longitudinal direction range from 1 to 5 mm (at the isocenter) and allow for the following collimated slice widths: 2 × 0.5 mm, 4 × 1 mm, 4 × 2.5 mm, 4 × 5 mm, 2 × 8 mm, and 2 × 10 mm (Fig. 4.4b).

Sixteen-slice CT systems have adaptive array detectors in general. A representative example of this scanner type, the Siemens SOMATOM Sensation 16 scanner, uses 24 detector rows (Flohr et al., 2002a) (Fig. 4.4c). By appropriate combination of the signals of the individual detector rows, either 16 slices with 0.75 mm or 1.5 mm collimated slice width can be acquired simultaneously. The GE Lightspeed 16 scanner uses a similar design, which provides 16 slices with either 0.625 or 1.25 mm collimated slice width. Yet another design, which is implemented in the Toshiba Aquilion scanner, allows the use of 16 slices with 0.5, 1, or 2 mm collimated slice width, with a total coverage of 32 mm at the isocenter.

The Siemens SOMATOM Sensation 64 scanner has an adaptive array detector with 40 detector rows (Flohr et al., 2004). The 32 central rows define a 0.6-mm collimated slice width at the isocenter; the four outer rows on both sides define a 1.2-mm collimated slice width (Fig. 4.4d). The total coverage in the longitudinal direction is 28.8 mm. Using a periodic motion of the focal spot in the z-direction (z-flying focal spot), 64 overlapping 0.6-mm slices per rotation are acquired. Alternatively, 24 slices with 1.2 mm slice width can be obtained. Toshiba, Philips, and GE use fixed array detectors for their 64-slice systems. The Toshiba Aquilion scanner has 64 detector rows with a collimated slice width of 0.5 mm. The total z-coverage at the isocenter is 32 mm. Both the GE VCT scanner and the Philips Brilliance 64 have 64 detector rows with a collimated

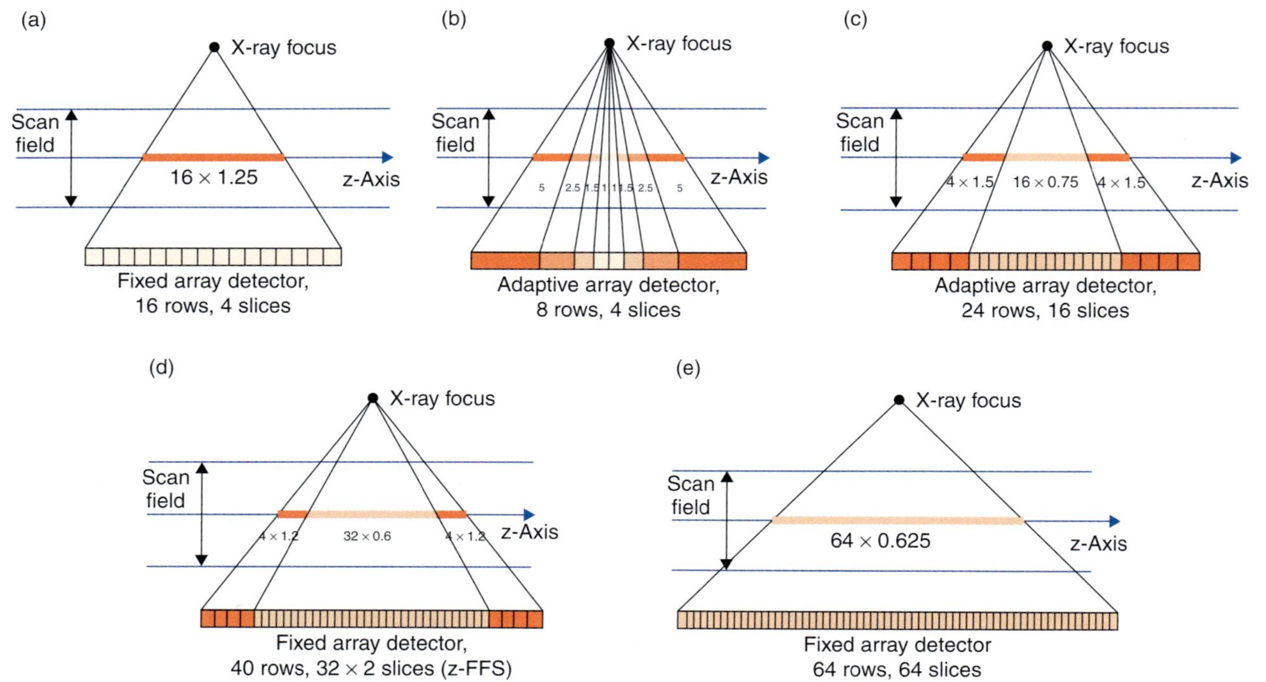

Figure 4.4. Examples of fixed array detectors and adaptive array detectors used in commercially available MDCT systems.

slice width of 0.625 mm, enabling the simultaneous readout of 64 slices with a total coverage of 40 mm in the longitudinal direction (Fig. 4.4e).

4.2.4 Data Rates and Data Transmission

With increasing number of detector rows and decreasing gantry rotation times, the data transmission systems of MDCT scanners must be capable of handling significant data rates: a four-slice CT system with 0.5 s rotation time roughly generates 1000 (projections) $\times$ 700 (detector channels) $\times$ 4 (detector rows) $\times$ 2 bytes (per detector) = 5.6 MB of data per rotation, corresponding to 11.2 MB/s; a 16-slice CT scanner with the same rotation time generates 45 MB/s; and a 64-slice CT system can produce up to 180–200 MB/s. This stream of data is a challenge for data transmission off the gantry and for real-time data processing in the subsequent image reconstruction systems. In modern CT systems, contactless transmission technology is generally used for data transfer, either laser transmission or electromagnetic transmission with a coupling between a rotating transmission ring antenna and a stationary receiving antenna. In image reconstruction, computer images are reconstructed at a rate of up to 40 images per second for a 512 $\times$ 512 matrix using special array processors.

4.2.5 Dual Source CT

A recently introduced DSCT system is equipped with two X-ray tubes and two corresponding detectors (Flohr et al., 2006). The two acquisition systems are mounted onto the rotating gantry with an angular offset of 90°. Figure 4.5 illustrates the principle. Using the z-flying focal spot technique (Flohr et al.,

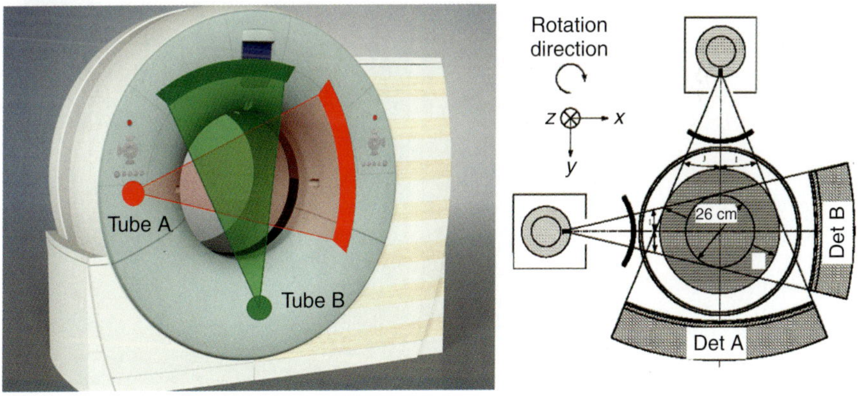

Figure 4.5. Schematic illustration of a dual source CT (DSCT) system using two tubes and two corresponding detectors offset by 90°. A scanner of this type provides temporal resolution equivalent to a quarter of the gantry rotation time, independent of the patient's heart rate. In a technical realization, one detector (A) covers the entire scan field of view with a diameter of 50 cm, while the other detector (B) is restricted to a smaller, central field of view.

2004; Flohr et al., 2005a), each detector acquires 64 overlapping 0.6-mm slices per rotation. The shortest gantry rotation time is 0.33 s. The key benefit of DSCT for cardiac scanning is improved temporal resolution. In a DSCT scanner, the halfscan sinogram in parallel geometry needed for ECG-controlled image reconstruction can be split up into two quarter scan sinograms, which are simultaneously acquired by the two acquisition systems in the same relative phase of the patient's cardiac cycle and at the same anatomical level because of the 90° angle between both detectors. Details of cardiac reconstruction techniques can be found in Section 3.3.

With this approach, constant temporal resolution equivalent to a quarter of the gantry rotation time, $T_{rot}/4$, is achieved in a centered region of the scan field of view. For $T_{rot} = 0.33$ s, the temporal resolution is $T_{rot}/4 = 83$ ms, independent of the patient's heart rate.

DSCT systems show interesting properties for general radiology applications, too. If both acquisition systems are simultaneously used in a standard spiral or sequential acquisition mode, up to 160 kW X-ray peak power is available. These power reserves are beneficial not only to examine morbidly obese patients, whose number is dramatically growing in Western societies, but also to maintain adequate X-ray photon flux for standard protocols when high volume coverage speed

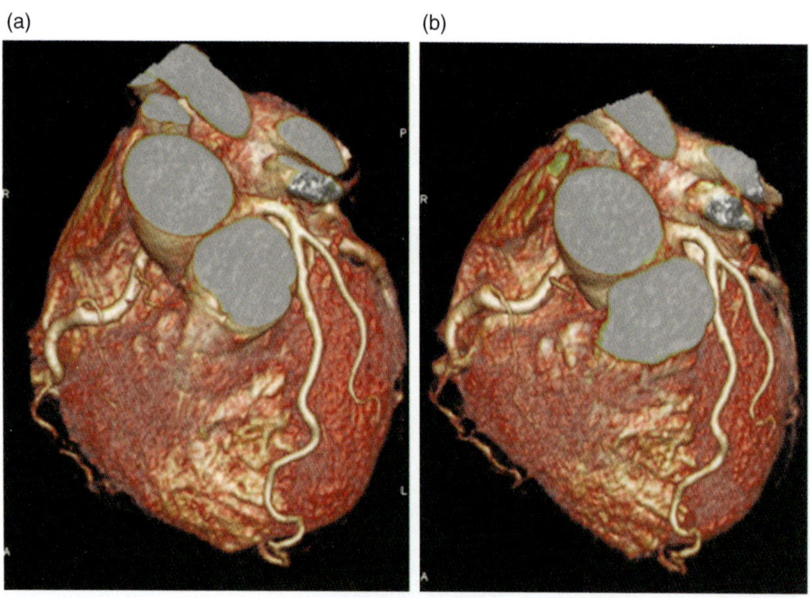

Figure 4.6. Case study illustrating the clinical performance of dual source CT (DSCT) for ECG-gated cardiac imaging. VRT renderings of a 59-year-old male patient with suspicion of Right Coronary Artery (RCA) stenosis. The mean heart rate of the patient during the scan was 85 bpm. (a) Diastolic reconstruction at 65% of the cardiac cycle. (b) End systolic reconstruction at 28% of the cardiac cycle. In both cases the coronary arteries are clearly depicted with little or no motion artifacts.

is necessary. In addition, both X-ray tubes can be operated at different kilovolt and milliampere settings, allowing the acquisition of dual energy data. While dual energy CT was already evaluated 20 years ago (Kalender et al., 1986; Vetter et al., 1986), technical limitations of the CT scanners at those times prevented the development of routine clinical applications. On the DSCT system, dual energy data can be acquired nearly simultaneously, with subsecond scan times. The ability to overcome data registration problems should provide clinically relevant benefits. The use of dual energy CT data can in principle add functional information to the morphological information based on X-ray attenuation coefficients that is usually obtained in a CT examination.

With the DSCT system, the depiction of the moving coronary artery phantom is nearly free of artifacts, thereby allowing for a reliable evaluation of the in-stent lumen. Figure 4.6 shows a clinical example to illustrate the clinical performance of DSCT for ECG-gated cardiac scanning.

4.3 MEASUREMENT TECHNIQUES

The two basic modes of MDCT data acquisition are axial and spiral (helical) scanning.

4.3.1 MDCT Sequential (Axial) Scanning

Using sequential (axial) scanning, the scan volume is covered by subsequent axial scans in a "step-and-shoot" technique. Between the individual axial scans, the table is moved to the next z-position. The number of images acquired during an axial scan corresponds to the number of active detector slices. By adding the detector signals of the active slices during image reconstruction, the number of images per scan can be further reduced and the image slice width can be increased. A scan with 4×1 mm collimation as an example provides either four images with 1 mm section width, two images with 2 mm section width, or one image with 4 mm section width. The option to realize a wider section by summation of several thin sections is beneficial for examinations that require narrow collimation to avoid partial volume artifacts and low image noise to detect low contrast details, such as examinations of the posterior fossa of the skull or the cervical spine.

With the advent of MDCT, axial "step-and-shoot" scanning has remained in use for only few clinical applications, such as head scanning, high resolution lung scanning, perfusion CT, and interventional applications. A detailed theoretical description to predict the performance of MDCT in the step-and-shoot mode has been given in (Hsieh, 2001).

4.3.2 MDCT Spiral (Helical) Scanning

Spiral/helical scanning is characterized by continuous gantry rotation and continuous data acquisition while the patient table moves at a constant speed (Fig. 4.7).

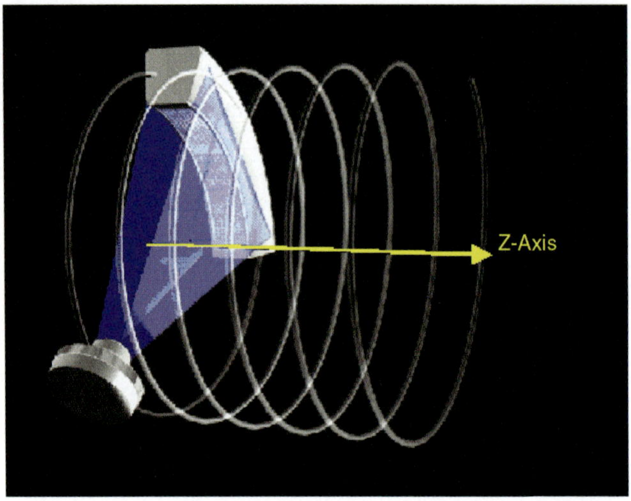

Figure 4.7. Principle of spiral/helical CT scanning: the patient table is continuously translated while multiple rotations of scan data are acquired. The path of the X-ray tube and detector relative to the patient is a helix. An interpolation of the acquired measurement data has to be performed in the z-direction to estimate a complete CT data set at the desired image position.

4.3.2.1 ***Pitch.*** An important parameter to characterize a spiral/helical scan is the pitch p. According to IEC (International Electrotechnical Comission) specifications p is given by

$$p = \text{tablefeed per rotation}/\text{total width of the collimated beam}$$

This definition holds for single-slice CT as well as for MDCT. It shows whether data acquisition occurs with gaps ($p > 1$) or with overlap ($p < 1$) in the longitudinal direction. With 4×1 mm collimation and a tablefeed of 6 mm per rotation, the pitch is $p = 6/(4 \times 1) = 6/4 = 1.5$. With 16×0.75 mm collimation and a tablefeed of 18 mm per rotation, the pitch is $p = 18/(16 \times 0.75) = 18/12 = 1.5$, too. For general radiology applications, clinically useful pitch values range from 0.5 to 2. For the special case of ECG-gated cardiac scanning, very low pitch values of 0.2–0.4 are applied to ensure gapless volume coverage of the heart during each phase of the cardiac cycle.

4.3.2.2 ***Collimated and Effective Slice Width.*** Both single-slice and multislice spiral CT require an interpolation of the acquired measurement data in the longitudinal direction to estimate a complete CT data set at the desired plane of reconstruction. As a consequence of this interpolation, the slice profile changes from the trapezoidal, in some cases almost rectangular, shape known from axial scanning to a more bell-shaped curve (Fig. 4.8). Z-axis resolution is no longer determined by the collimated beam width s_{coll} alone (as in axial scanning), but

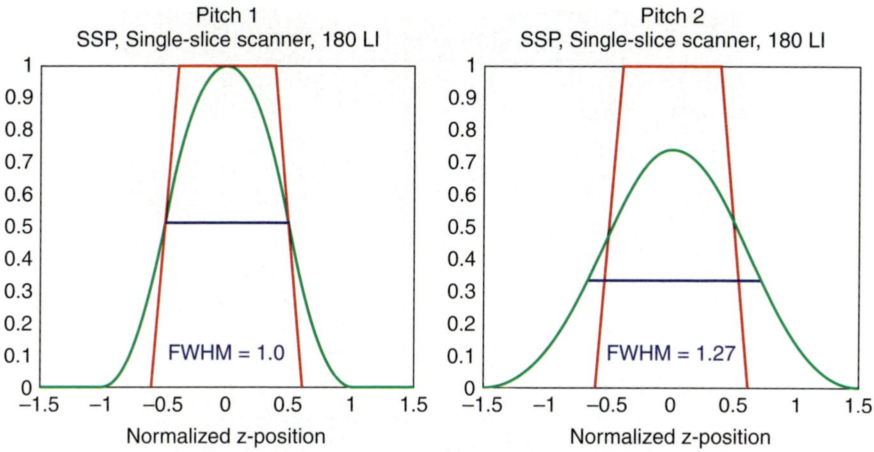

Figure 4.8. Effective slice width in spiral/helical CT: the collimated slice profile, which is a trapezoid in general, is indicated in red. The SSPs after spiral/helical interpolation are bell shaped; see the blue curves for the most commonly used single-slice approach (180-LI) at different pitch values. This approach (180-LI) relies on a projection-wise linear interpolation of direct and complementary data. In spiral/helical CT, z-axis resolution is no longer determined by the collimated slice width alone, but by the effective slice width, which is defined as the full width at half maximum (FWHM) of the SSP.

by the effective slice width s, which is established in the spiral interpolation process. Usually, s is defined as the Full Width at Half Maximum (FWHM) of the Slice Sensitivity Profile (SSP). The wider s gets for a given collimated beam width s_{coll}, the more the longitudinal resolution degrades. In single-slice CT, s increases with increasing pitch (Fig. 4.9). This is a consequence of the increasing longitudinal distance of the projections used for spiral interpolation. The SSP is not only characterized by its FWHM, but by its entire shape: an SSP that has far-reaching tails degrades longitudinal resolution more than a well-defined, close to rectangular SSP, even if both have the same FWHM and hence the same effective slice width s. For a further characterization of spiral SSPs, the Full Width at Tenth Area (FWTA) is often considered in addition.

*4.3.2.3 **Multislice Linear Interpolation and z-Filtering.*** Multislice linear interpolation is characterized by a projection-wise linear interpolation between two rays on either side of the image plane to establish a CT data set at the desired image z-position. The interpolation can be performed between the same detector slice at different projection angles (in different rotations) or different detector slices at the same projection angle. In general, scanners relying on this technique provide selected discrete pitch values to the user, such as 0.75 and 1.5 for 4-slice scanning (Hu, 1999) or 0.5625, 0.9375, 1.375 and 1.75 for 16-slice scanning (Hsieh, 2003). The user has to be aware of pitch-dependent effective slice widths s. For low pitch scanning (at $p = 0.75$ using 4 slices and at $p = 0.5625$ or 0.9375

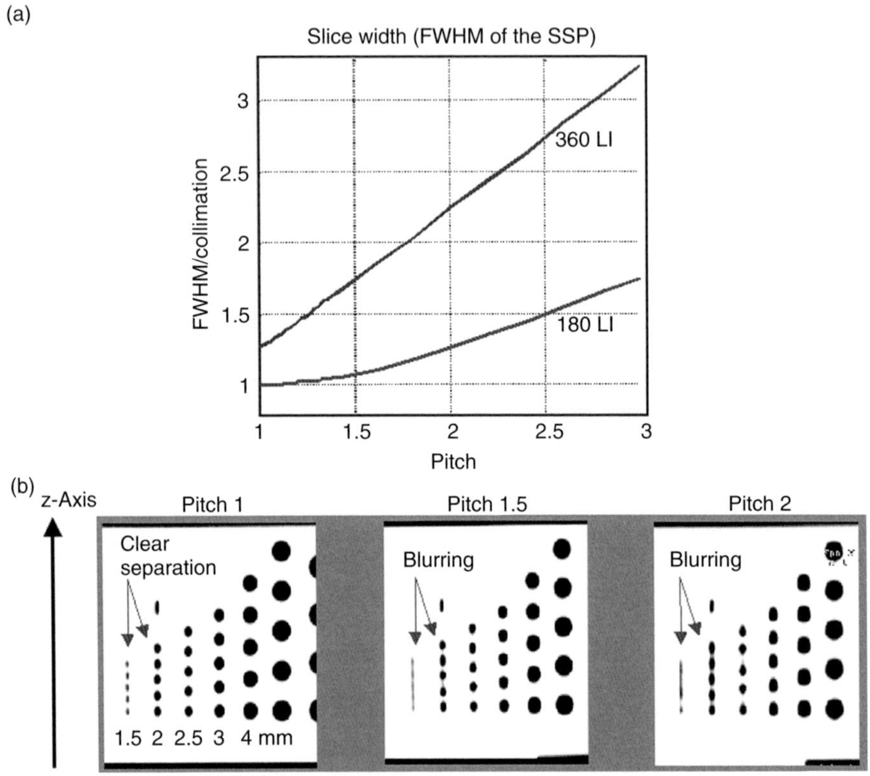

Figure 4.9. (a) FWHM of the SSP as a function of the pitch for the two most commonly used single-slice spiral interpolation approaches, 180° linear interpolation (180-LI) and 360° linear interpolation (360-LI). For both, the slice significantly widens with increasing pitch as a result of the increasing distance of the interpolation partners. (b) MPRs of a spiral z-resolution phantom scanned with 2 mm collimation (180-LI) show increased blurring of the 1.5-mm and 2-mm cylinders with increasing pitch as a consequence of the increasing effective slice width.

using 16 slices), $s \sim s_{coll}$ and for a collimated 1.25-mm slice the resulting effective slice width stays at 1.25 mm. The narrow SSP, however, is achieved by conjugate interpolation at the price of increased image noise (Hu, 1999; Hsieh, 2003). For high pitch scanning (at $p = 1.5$ using 4 slices and at $p = 1.375$ or 1.75 using 16 slices), $s \sim 1.27 s_{coll}$ and a collimated 1.25-mm slice results in an effective 1.5- to 1.6-mm slice. To obtain the same image noise as in an axial scan with the same collimated slice width, 0.73–1.68 times the dose depending on the spiral pitch is required, with the lowest dose at the highest pitch (Hsieh, 2003). Thus, as a "take home point," when selecting the scan protocol for a particular application, scanning at low pitch optimizes image quality and longitudinal resolution at a given collimation, yet at the expense of increased patient dose. To reduce patient dose, either milliampere settings should be reduced at low pitch or high pitch values should be chosen.

In a more advanced z-filter multislice spiral reconstruction (Taguchi and Aradate, 1998; Schaller et al., 2000), the spiral interpolation for each projection angle is no longer restricted to the two rays in closest proximity to the image plane. Instead, all direct and complementary rays within a selectable distance from the image plane contribute to the image. A representative example for a z-filter approach is the adaptive axial interpolation (Schaller et al., 2000) implemented in Siemens CT-scanners. Another example is the MUSCOT algorithm (Taguchi and Aradate, 1998) used by Toshiba. Z-filtering allows the system to trade-off z-axis resolution with image noise (which directly correlates with required dose). From the same CT, raw data images with different slice widths can be retrospectively reconstructed. Only slice widths equal to or larger than the sub-beam collimation can be obtained. With adaptive axial interpolation, the effective slice width is kept constant for all pitch values between 0.5 and 1.5 (Klingenbeck-Regn et al., 1999; Schaller et al., 2000; Fuchs et al., 2000). Therefore, longitudinal resolution is independent of the pitch (Fig. 4.10). As a consequence of the pitch-independent

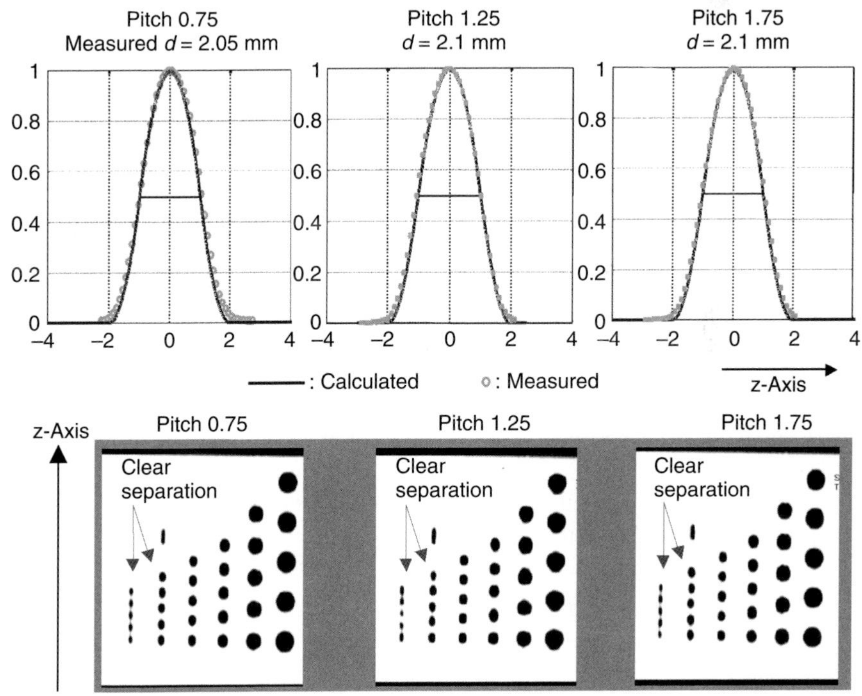

Figure 4.10. Adaptive axial interpolation for a four-slice CT system: SSP of the 2-mm slice (for 4 × 1 mm collimation) at selected pitch values. The functional form of the SSP, and hence the effective slice width, are independent of the pitch. Consequently, MPRs of a spiral z-resolution phantom scanned with 2-mm slice width show clear separation of the 1.5- and 2-mm cylinders for all pitch values.

spiral slice width, the image noise for fixed "effective" milliampere-second (mAs) (that is mAs divided by the pitch p) is nearly independent of the pitch. For 1.25-mm effective slice width reconstructed from 4×1 mm collimation, 0.61–0.69 times the dose is required to maintain the image noise of an axial scan at the same collimation (Fuchs et al., 2000). Radiation dose for fixed effective mAs is independent of the pitch and equals the dose of an axial scan at the same mAs. Thus, as a "take-home point," using higher pitch does not result in dose saving at a fixed effective mAs, which is an important practical consideration with CT systems relying on adaptive axial interpolation and the "effective" mAs concept.

With regard to image quality, narrow collimation is preferable to wide collimation, because of better suppression of partial volume artifacts and a more rectangular SSP, even if the pitch has to be increased for equivalent volume coverage. Similar to single-slice spiral CT, narrow collimation scanning is the key to reduce artifacts and improve image quality. Best suppression of spiral artifacts is achieved by using both narrow collimation relative to the desired slice width and reducing the spiral pitch.

4.3.2.4 Three-Dimensional Backprojection and Adaptive Multiple Plane Reconstruction (AMPR). For CT scanners with 16 or more slices, modified reconstruction approaches accounting for the cone-beam geometry of the measurement rays have to be considered: the measurement rays in MDCT are tilted by the so-called cone angle with respect to a plane perpendicular to the z-axis. The cone angle is largest for the slices at the outer edges of the detector, and it increases with increasing number of detector rows if their width is kept constant. Some manufacturers (Toshiba, Philips) use a 3D filtered backprojection reconstruction (Feldkamp et al., 1984; Grass et al., 2000; Hein et al., 2003; Wang et al., 1993). With this approach, the measurement rays are backprojected into a 3D volume along the lines of measurement, this way accounting for their cone-beam geometry. Other manufacturers use algorithms that split the 3D reconstruction task into a series of conventional 2D reconstructions on tilted intermediate image planes. A representative example is the Adaptive Multiple Plane Reconstruction (AMPR) used by Siemens (Flohr et al., 2003a; Schaller et al., 2001b). Multislice spiral scanning using AMPR in combination with the "effective" mAs concept is characterized by the same key properties as adaptive axial isnterpolation. Thus, all recommendations regarding selection of collimation and pitch that have been discussed there also apply to AMPR.

4.3.2.5 Double z-Sampling. The double z-sampling concept for multislice spiral scanning makes use of a periodic motion of the focal spot in the longitudinal direction to improve data sampling along the z-axis (Flohr et al., 2004; Flohr et al., 2005a). By continuous electromagnetic deflection of the electron beam in a rotating envelope X-ray tube, the focal spot is wobbled between two different positions on the anode plate. The amplitude of the periodic z-motion is adjusted in a way that two subsequent readings are shifted by half a collimated slice width in the patient's longitudinal direction (Fig. 4.11). Therefore, the measurement

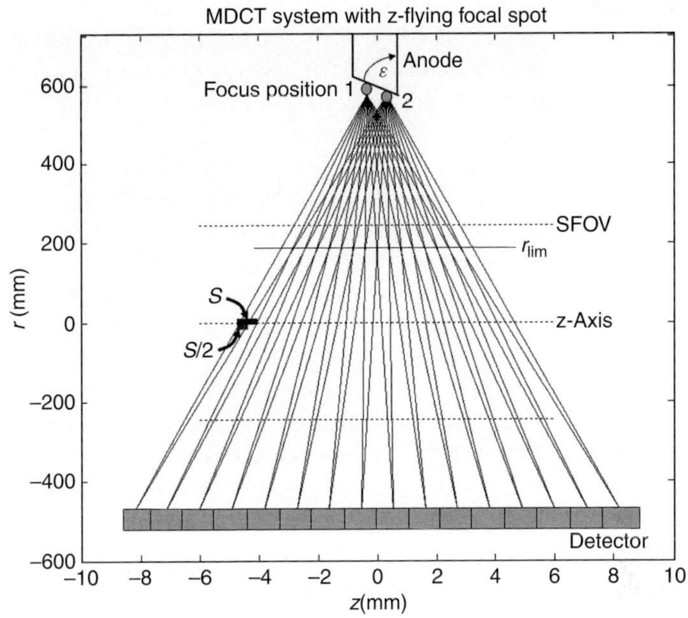

Figure 4.11. Principle of improved z-sampling with the z-flying focal spot technique. Owing to a periodic motion of the focal spot in the z-direction two subsequent M-slice readings are shifted by half a collimated slice width $s_{coll}/2$ at the isocenter and can be interleaved to one $2M$-slice projection.

rays of two subsequent readings with collimated slice width s_{coll} interleave in the z-direction and every two M-slice readings are combined to one $2M$-slice projection with a sampling distance of $s_{coll}/2$.

In the SOMATOM Sensation 64 (Siemens, Forchheim, Germany) as an example of an MDCT system relying on double z-sampling, two subsequent 32-slice readings are combined to one 64-slice projection with a sampling distance of 0.3 mm at the isocenter. As a consequence, spatial resolution in the logitudinal direction is increased, and objects <0.4 mm in diameter can be routinely resolved at any pitch (Fig. 4.12). Another benefit of double z-sampling is the suppression of spiral "windmill" artifacts at any pitch (Fig. 4.13).

4.3.3 ECG-Triggered and ECG-Gated Cardiovascular CT

4.3.3.1 Principles of ECG-Triggering and ECG-Gating. For ECG-synchronized examinations of the cardiothoracic anatomy, either ECG-triggered axial scanning or ECG-gated spiral scanning can be used. A technical overview on ECG-controlled CT scanning may be found in (Flohr et al., 2003b).

In ECG-triggered axial scanning, the heart volume is covered by subsequent axial scans in a "step-and-shoot" technique. The number of images per scan corresponds to the number of active detector slices. In between the individual

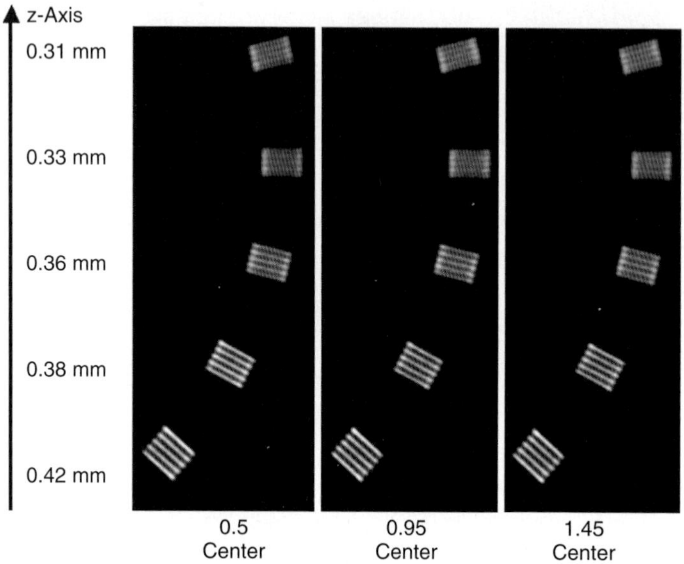

Figure 4.12. Demonstration of z-axis resolution for a MDCT system using the z-flying focal spot technique. MPRs of a z-resolution phantom (high resolution insert of the CATPHAN, the Phantom Laboratories, Salem, NY, turned by 90°) in the isocenter of the scanner as a function of the pitch. Scan data has been acquired with 32 × 0.6 mm collimation in a 64-slice acquisition mode using the z-flying focal spot and reconstructed with the narrowest slice width (nominal 0.6 mm) and a sharp body kernel. Independent of the pitch, all bar patterns up to 16 lp/cm can be visualized. The bar patterns with 15 lp/cm are exactly perpendicular to the z-axis, corresponding to 0.33 mm longitudinal resolution.

axial scans the table moves to the next z-position. Owing to the time necessary for table motion, only every second heart beat can be used for data acquisition, which limits the minimum slice width to 2.5 mm with four-slice or to 1.25 mm with eight-slice CT systems if the whole heart volume has to be covered within one breath-hold period. Scan data are acquired with a predefined temporal offset relative to the R-waves of the patient's ECG-signal, which can be either relative (given as a certain percentage of the RR-interval time) or absolute (given in milliseconds) and either forward or reverse (Flohr and Ohnesorge, 2001; Ohnesorge et al., 2000) (Fig. 4.14).

To improve temporal resolution, modified reconstruction approaches for partial scan data have been proposed (Flohr and Ohnesorge, 2001; Ohnesorge et al., 2000), which provide a temporal resolution up to half the gantry rotation time per image in a sufficiently centered region of interest. Gantry rotation times as short as 0.4 s, 0.37 s, or even 0.33 s are offered by 16-slice and 64-slice CT systems. In this case, temporal resolution can be as good as 200 ms, 185 ms, or 165 ms.

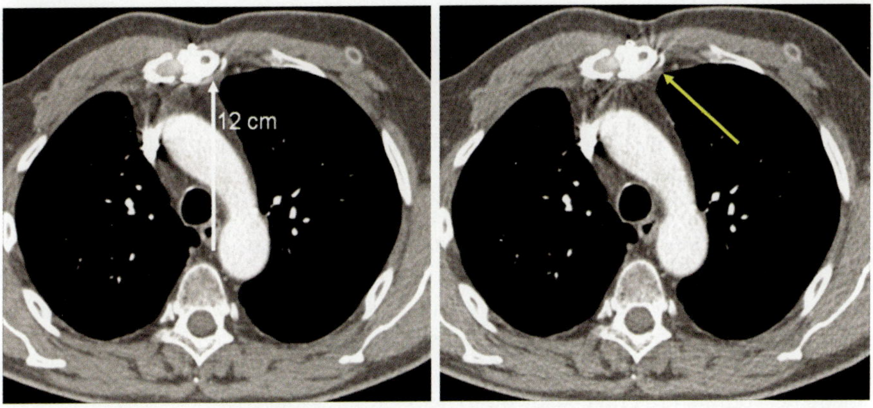

Figure 4.13. Reduction of spiral artifacts with the z-flying focal spot technique. Left: Thorax scan with 32 × 0.6 mm collimation in a 64-slice acquisition mode with z-flying focal spot at pitch 1.5. Right: Same scan, using only one focus position of the z-flying focal spot for image reconstruction. This corresponds reasonably well to evaluating 32-slice spiral data acquired without z-flying focal spot. Owing to the improved longitudinal sampling with z-flying focal spot (left) spiral interpolation artifacts (windmill structures at high contrast objects) are suppressed without degradation of z-axis resolution.

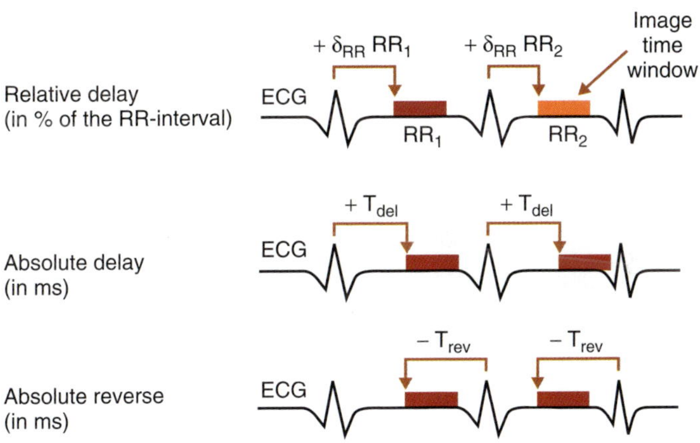

Figure 4.14. Schematic illustration of absolute and relative phase setting for ECG-controlled CT examinations of the cardiothoracic anatomy.

With retrospective ECG gating, the heart volume is covered continuously by a spiral scan. The patient's ECG signal is recorded simultaneously to data acquisition to allow for a retrospective selection of the data segments used for image reconstruction. Only scan data acquired in a predefined cardiac phase, usually the diastolic phase, is used for image reconstruction (Flohr and Ohnesorge, 2001; Kachelriess et al., 2000; Ohnesorge et al., 2000; Taguchi and Anno, 2000). The data segments contributing to an image start with a user-defined offset relative to the onset of the R-waves, similar to ECG-triggered axial scanning (Fig. 4.15).

Image reconstruction generally consists of two parts: multidetector row spiral interpolation to compensate for the continuous table movement and to obtain scan data at the desired image z-position, followed by a partial scan reconstruction of the axial data segments (Fig. 4.15).

4.3.3.2 ECG-Gated Single-Segment and Multisegment Reconstruction. In a single-segment reconstruction, consecutive multislice spiral data from the same heart period are used to generate the single-slice partial scan data segment for an image (Fig. 4.15). At low heart rates, a single-segment reconstruction yields the best compromise between sufficient temporal resolution on one hand and adequate volume coverage with thin slices on the other.

The temporal resolution of an image can be improved up to $T_{\mathrm{rot}}/(2N)$ by using scan data of N subsequent heart cycles for image formation in a so-called multisegment reconstruction (Cesmeli et al., 2001; Flohr and Ohnesorge, 2001; Kachelriess et al., 2000; Taguchi and Anno, 2000); T_{rot} is the gantry rotation time of the CT scanner. With increased N, better temporal resolution is achieved but at the expense of slower volume coverage: every z-position of the heart has to be seen by a detector slice at every time during the N heart cycles. As a consequence, the larger the N and the lower the patient's heart rate, the more the spiral pitch has to be reduced. With this technique, the patient's heart rate and the gantry rotation time of the scanner have to be properly desynchronized to allow for improved temporal resolution. Depending on the relationship between the rotation time and the patient heart rate, the temporal resolution is generally

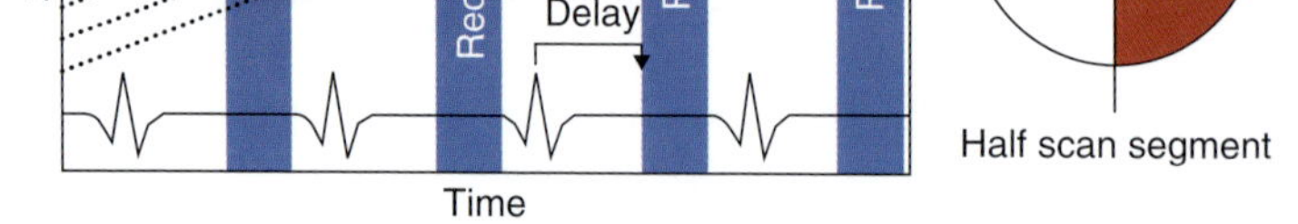

Figure 4.15. Principle of retrospectively ECG-gated spiral scanning with single-segment reconstruction. The patient's ECG signal is indicated as a function of time on the horizontal axis, and the position of the detector slices relative to the patient is shown on the vertical axis (in this example for a four-slice CT system). The table moves continuously, and continuous spiral scan data of the heart volume are acquired. Only scan data acquired in a predefined cardiac phase, usually the diastolic phase, are used for image reconstruction (indicated as red boxes). The spiral interpolation is illustrated for some representative projection angles.

not constant, but varies between one half and $1/(2N)$ times the gantry rotation time in an N-segment reconstruction. There are "sweet spots," heart rates with optimal temporal resolution, and heart rates where temporal resolution cannot be improved beyond half the gantry rotation time. Multisegment approaches rely on complete periodicity of heart motion, and they encounter their limitations in patients with arrhythmia or patients with changing heart rates during examination. They may improve image quality in selected cases, but the reliability of obtaining good-quality images with N-segment reconstruction goes down with increasing N. In general, clinical practice suggests the use of one segment at lower heart rates and $N \geq 2$ segments at higher heart rates (Flohr and Ohnesorge, 2001; Flohr et al., 2003b). Image reconstruction during different heart phases is feasible by shifting the start points of the data segments used for image reconstruction relative to the R-waves. For a given start position, a stack of images at different z-positions covering a small subvolume of the heart can be reconstructed because of multislice data acquisition (Flohr and Ohnesorge, 2001; Ohnesorge et al., 2000).

Prospective ECG triggering combined with "step-and-shoot" acquisition of axial slices has the benefit of smaller patient dose than ECG-gated spiral scanning, since scan data is acquired in the previously selected heart phases only. However, it does not provide continuous volume coverage with overlapping slices, and misregistration of anatomical details cannot be avoided. Furthermore, reconstruction of images in different phases of the cardiac cycle for functional evaluation is not possible. Since ECG-triggered axial scanning depends on a reliable prediction of the patient's next RR-interval by using the mean of the preceding RR-intervals, the method encounters its limitations for patients with severe arrhythmia. To maintain the benefits of ECG-gated spiral CT but reduce patient dose, ECG-controlled dose modulation has been developed (Jakobs et al., 2002). During the spiral scan, the output of the X-ray tube is modulated according to the patient's ECG. It is kept at its nominal value during a user-defined phase of the cardiac cycle, in general the mid to end -diastolic phase. During the rest of the cardiac cycle, the tube output is typically reduced to 20% of its nominal values although not switched off entirely to allow for image reconstruction throughout the entire cardiac cycle. Depending on the heart rate, dose reduction of 30–50% has been demonstrated in clinical studies (Jakobs et al., 2002).

The major improvements from 4-slice to 64-slice scanners include improved temporal resolution due to shorter gantry rotation times, better spatial resolution owing to submillimeter collimation and considerably reduced examination times (Flohr and Ohnesorge, 2001; Flohr et al., 2003b) (Fig. 4.16).

4.4 APPLICATIONS

4.4.1 Clinical Applications of Computed Tomography

Even though the driving force for the development of CT in the past years was cardiac CT with a strong focus on reducing temporal resolution and effective scan times, cardiac CT examinations still only account for a very small amount

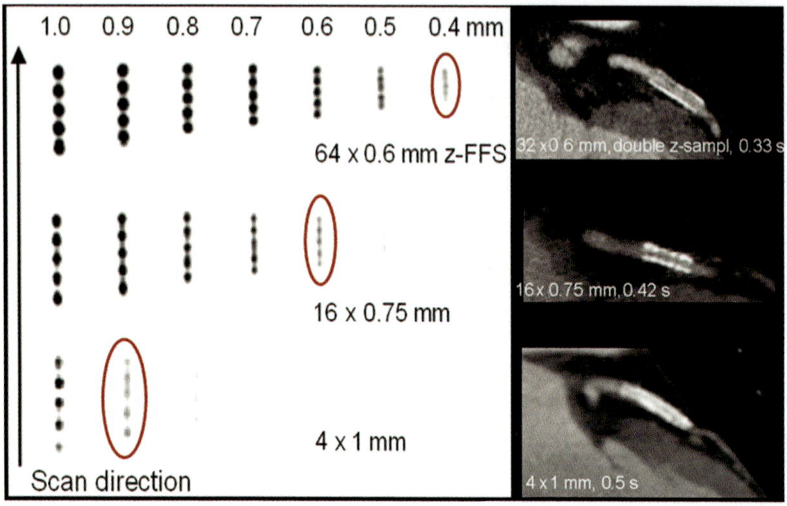

Figure 4.16. Progress in longitudinal resolution for ECG-gated cardiac scanning from 4-slice CT to 64-slice CT. The four-slice CT scanner with 4 × 1 mm collimation (bottom) can resolve 0.9- to 1.0-mm objects. With 16 × 0.75 mm collimation, 0.6-mm objects can be delineated (center). The 64-slice CT scanner with 64 × 0.6 mm collimation and double z-sampling can routinely resolve 0.4-mm objects (top). The corresponding patient examples depict similar clinical situations (a stent in the proximal Left Anterior Descending Artery (LAD)). With the 64-slice system, an in-stent re-stenosis (arrow) can be evaluated. Four-slice case courtesy of Hopital de Coracao, Sao Paulo, Brasil; 16-slice case courtesy of Dr A. Küttner, Tübingen University, Germany; and 64-slice case courtesy of Dr C. M. Wong, Hong Kong, China.

of all CT examinations. Figure 4.16 shows an impressive example of small and fast moving coronary arteries with a diameter of 5 mm in proximal segments down to 2 mm in distal segments depicted within state-of-the-art systems.

Of course, all traditional applications benefited from the tremendous improvements of scanner and data postprocessing technology in the past years.

Today, CT is the technique of choice for evaluating head injury; assessing spinal, pelvic, or abdominal trauma; characterizing parenchymal lung diseases; in combination with other techniques staging of almost all solid tumors, including lymphoma; and treatment planning for most solid tumors. Figure 4.17 shows an example where CT is used for tumor staging, in this case a lymphoma.

During the past years, CT angiography became increasingly important to depict the inner opening of blood filled structures, especially arteries. As blood itself is not clearly visible in CT images, because of its low contrast with respect to other soft tissue structures in the body, iodinated contrast material is injected intravenously for CTA examinations.

CTA is used to examine blood vessels in key areas of the body, including the abdominal aorta and arteries to the kidneys and intestines, the brain, kidneys, pelvis, legs, lungs, heart and neck. Figure 4.18 shows an example of a CTA of the abdominal aorta and the peripheral vessels displayed in VRT and an MIP.

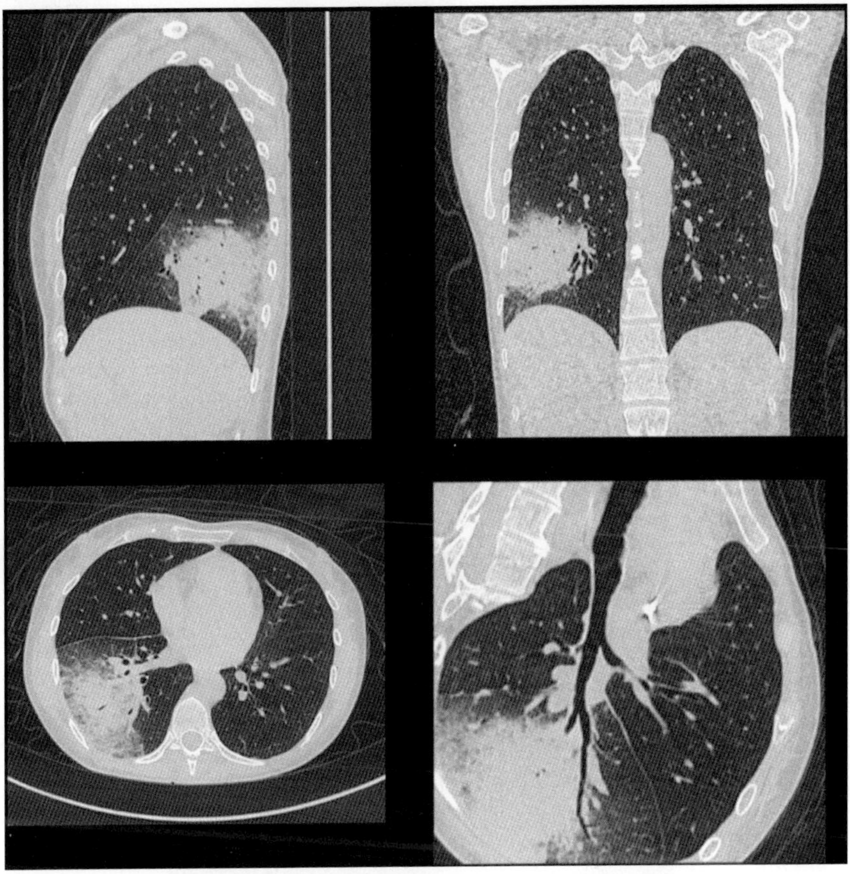

Figure 4.17. Example of a lung scan used for tumor staging.

The procedure is used to identify disease and aneurysms in the aorta or in other major blood vessels; detect atherosclerosis disease in the carotid artery of the neck, which may limit blood flow to the brain and cause a stroke; identify aneurysms or arteriovenous malformation inside the brain; or detect atherosclerotic disease that has narrowed the arteries to the legs.

It can be used to diagnose disease in the renal artery or visualize blood flow to help prepare for a kidney transplant, guide surgeons making repairs to diseased blood vessels, such as implanting or evaluating a stent, detect injury to one or more arteries in trauma patients, or evaluate the details of arteries feeding a tumor before surgery.

CTA can identify dissection in the aorta or its major branches; show the extent and severity of atherosclerosis in the coronary arteries; help plan for a surgical operation, such as coronary bypass; screen individuals for arterial disease, especially patients with a family history of arterial disease or disorders; and evaluate prospective kidney donors.

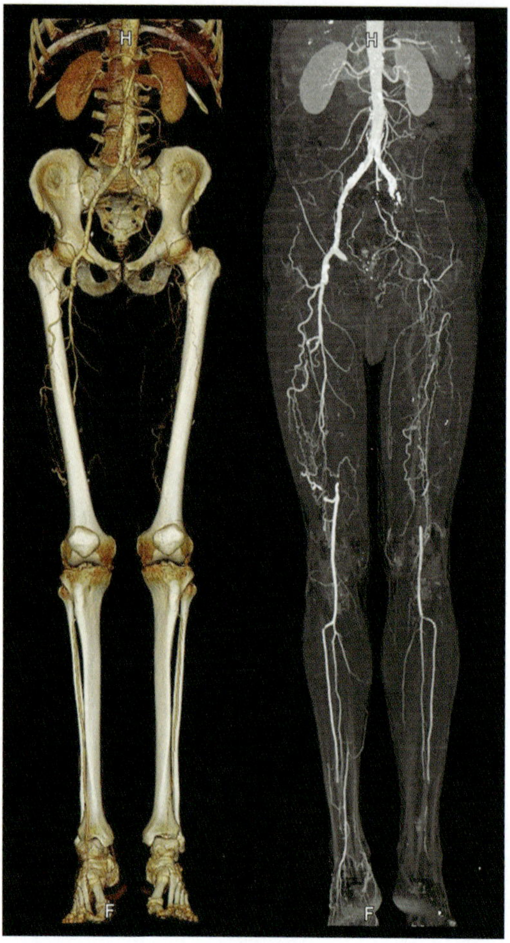

Figure 4.18. Example of CTA of the abdominal aorta and peripheral arteries in the legs that shows strong calcifications in the MIP representation (right) and occlusions of both the femoral arteries and the thick collateral vessels that were formed to bypass that occlusion.

In the past years, CTA became the primary choice to examine pulmonary arteries in the lungs to rule out Pulmonary Embolism (PE). This short selection of areas where CTA is used shows the wide applicability of the examination.

4.4.2 Radiation Dose in Typical Clinical Applications and Methods for Dose Reduction

Exposure of the patient to radiation during CT and the resulting potential radiation hazard has recently gained considerable attention both in the public and scientific literature (Brenner et al., 2001; Nickoloff and Alderson, 2001). Typical values for the effective patient dose of selected CT protocols are 1–2 mSv (millisievert) for a head examination, 5–7 mSv for a chest CT, and 8–11 mSv for CT of the abdomen and pelvis (McCollough, 2003; Morin et al., 2003). This radiation exposure must be appreciated in the context of the average annual background radiation, which is 2–5 mSv (3.6 mSv in the United States).

CT is considered to be a "high dose" examination because compared to a typical chest X-ray with an effective dose of approximately 0.1 mSv it exposes the patient to 20–100 times of the radiation. Moreover, because of its undoubted diagnostic benefits the percentage of CT examinations compared to other diagnostic examinations is continuously rising. In 1989, the National Radiological Protection Board in the United Kingdom showed that despite comprising only 2% of all examinations, CT contributed around 20% of the collective dose to the UK population from diagnostic X-ray imaging (Shrimpton et al., 1991). The use of CT has been steadily increasing, and more recent data indicate that CT now accounts for 40% of the collective dose to the US population from medical X-rays (Mettler et al., 2000). This is a global trend, especially pronounced in the United States where CT became the almost universal initial diagnostic tool. It must be emphasized that the dose of single CT examinations is still low compared to radiation dose ranges with proven health hazards. There is no study that can associate CT with additional cancer incidence in the examined patients. Nevertheless, even though the risk is small but not exactly known, the ALARA principle (As Low As Reasonably Achievable) must be applied in all examinations involving the exposure of patients to X-rays and there must be a clear clinical indication for the examination.

In CT, the average dose in the scan plane is best described by the weighted computerized tomographic dose index $\mathrm{CTDI_w}$ (McCollough, 2003; Morin et al., 2003), which is determined from $\mathrm{CTDI_{100}}$ measurements both in the center and at the periphery of a 16-cm lucite phantom for head and a 32-cm lucite phantom for body. For the $\mathrm{CTDI_{100}}$ measurements, a 100-mm-long ionization chamber is used. $\mathrm{CTDI_w}$ is a good estimate for the average patient dose as long as the patient size is similar to the size of the respective phantoms. $\mathrm{CTDI_w}$ is defined according to the following equation (Morin et al., 2003)

$$\mathrm{CTDI_w} = 1/3\mathrm{CTDI_{100}}(\mathrm{center}) + 2/3\mathrm{CTDI_{100}}(\mathrm{periphery})$$

$\mathrm{CTDI_w}$, given in milligray (mGy), is always measured in an axial scan mode. It depends on scanner geometry, slice collimation and beam prefiltration as well as on X-ray tube voltage, tube current mA, and gantry rotation time T_{rot}.

The product of tube current in mA and T_{rot} is the mAs value of the scan. To obtain a parameter characteristic for the scanner used, it is helpful to eliminate the mAs dependence and to introduce a normalized $(\mathrm{CTDI_w})_n$ given in mGy per mAs:

$$\mathrm{CTDI_w} = \mathrm{mA} \times T_{\mathrm{rot}} \times (\mathrm{CTDI_w})_n = \mathrm{mAs} \times (\mathrm{CTDI_w})_n$$

$(\mathrm{CTDI_w})_n$ still depends on X-ray tube voltage and on slice collimation. Both parameters are needed to specify $(\mathrm{CTDI_w})_n$. Scan protocols for different CT scanners should always be compared on the basis of $\mathrm{CTDI_w}$ and never on the basis of mAs, since different system geometries can result in significant differences of the radiation dose applied at identical mAs.

To represent the dose in a spiral scan, it is essential to account for gaps or overlaps between the radiation dose profiles from consecutive rotations of the X-ray source (Morin et al., 2003). For this purpose, $\mathrm{CTDI_{vol}}$, volume $\mathrm{CTDI_w}$, has been introduced

$$\begin{aligned}\mathrm{CTDI_{vol}} &= 1/p \times \mathrm{CTDI_w}\\ &= \mathrm{mAs} \times 1/p \times (\mathrm{CTDI_w})_\mathrm{n} = \mathrm{mA} \times T_\mathrm{rot} \times 1/p \times (\mathrm{CTDI_w})_n\end{aligned}$$

where p is the spiral pitch. The factor $1/p$ accounts for the increasing dose accumulation with decreasing spiral pitch due to the increasing spiral overlap. In principle, this equation holds for single-slice CT as well as for MDCT. Some manufacturers such as Siemens and Philips have introduced an "effective" mAs concept for spiral/helical scanning, which includes the factor $1/p$ into the mAs definition:

$$(\mathrm{mAs})_\mathrm{eff} = \mathrm{mA} \times T_\mathrm{rot} \times 1/p = \mathrm{mAs} \times 1/p$$

For spiral/helical scans, $(\mathrm{mAs})_\mathrm{eff}$ is indicated on the user interface. The dose of a multidetector row spiral/helical scan is simply given by

$$\mathrm{CTDI_{vol}} = (\mathrm{mAs})_\mathrm{eff} \times (\mathrm{CTDI_w})_n$$

Some other manufacturers, such as Toshiba and GE, have not introduced the effective mAs concept and decided to keep the original the conventional mAs definition. When comparing the scan parameters for CT systems of different manufacturers, the underlying mAs definition has to be taken into account and the correction for pitch has to applied manually when this is not done automatically through effective mAs. This is of particular importance for scan protocols relying on very low pitch settings such as in ECG-gated cardiac CT.

$\mathrm{CTDI_w}$ is a physical dose measure and therefore does not provide full information on the radiation risk associated with a CT examination. For this purpose, the concept of "effective dose" has been introduced by ICRP (International Commission on Radiation Protection). The effective dose is given in millisievert. It is a weighted sum of the dose applied to selective radiation-sensitive organs in a CT examination and includes both direct and scattered radiation. The weighting factors depend on the biological radiation sensitivities of the respective organs. The effective patient dose depends on the scanned range and scanned body region. For a comparison of effective dose values for different protocols or different scanner types, scan ranges should be similar.

The most important factor for reducing radiation exposure is an adaptation of the dose to patient size and weight (Donelly et al., 2001; Frush et al., 2002; Wildberger et al., 2001). This is of particular importance in pediatric imaging. Dose reduction can also be achieved by mAs reduction and lower kV settings.

Another means to reduce radiation dose is to adapt the X-ray tube voltage to the intended application. In contrast-enhanced studies, such as in CTA, the contrast to noise ratio for fixed patient dose increases with decreasing X-ray tube voltage. As a consequence, to obtain the desired contrast to noise ratio, patient dose can be reduced by choosing lower kV settings. Ideally, 80 kV should be used for CTA in order to reduce patient dose. Clinical studies (Schaller et al., 2001a) have demonstrated a potential for dose reduction of about 50% when using 80 kV instead of 120 kV for performing CTA. In reality, however, the maximum X-ray tube current available at 80 kV is generally not sufficient to scan bigger patients, which limits the routine application of this approach. Use of 100 kV appears as a suitable compromise and the method of choice for performing CTA. A recent study recommends 100 kV as the standard mode for aortoiliac CTA and reports a dose saving of 30% without loss of diagnostic information (Wintersperger et al., 2005).

An approach that finds increased implementation in clinical practice is anatomical tube current modulation. In this technique, the tube output is adapted to the patient geometry during each rotation of the scanner to compensate for strongly varying X-ray attenuations in asymmetrical body regions such as the shoulders and pelvis. The variation of the tube output is either predefined by an analysis of the localizer scan (topogram, scout view) or determined online by evaluating the signal of a detector row. With the use of this technique, dose can be reduced by 15–35% without degrading image quality, depending on the body region (Greess et al., 2000). In more sophisticated approaches, the tube output is modified according to the patient geometry not only during each rotation but also in the longitudinal direction to maintain adequate dose when moving to different body regions, for instance, from thorax to abdomen (automatic exposure control). Automatic adaptation of the tube current to patient size prevents both over- and underirradiation, considerably simplifies the clinical workflow for the technician, and eliminates the need for lookup tables of patient weight and size for adjusting the mAs settings.

4.5 OUTLOOK

In future, the trend toward a larger number of slices will not be driven by the need to increase scan speed in spiral acquisition modes, but rather by the desire to increase volume coverage in nonspiral dynamic acquisitions, for example, by the introduction of area detectors large enough to cover entire organs, such as the heart, the kidneys or the brain, in one axial scan (~120 mm scan range). With these systems, dynamic volume scanning will become feasible, opening up a whole spectrum of new applications, such as functional or volume perfusion studies. Area detector technology is currently under development, but no commercially available system so far fulfills the requirements of medical CT with regard to contrast resolution and fast data read-out. A scanner with 256 × 0.5 mm detector elements has been proposed by one manufacturer and appears conceptually promising, but has not left the prototype stage so far (Mori et al., 2004; Mori et al., 2006). Prototype systems by other vendors use CsI-aSi flat panel detector technology, originally used for conventional catheter angiography, which is limited in low contrast resolution and scan speed. Short gantry rotation times <0.5 s, which are a prerequisite for successful examination of moving organs such as the heart, are beyond the scope of such systems. Spatial resolution is excellent, however, because of the small detector pixel size (Gupta et al., 2006). In preclinical installations, potential clinical applications of flat-panel volume CT systems are currently being evaluated (Knollmann and Pfoh, 2003; Gupta et al., 2003). The application spectrum ranges from ultrahigh resolution bone imaging to dynamic CT angiographic studies and functional examinations. Figure 4.19 shows an example of a dynamic CTA of a living rabbit.

The combination of area detectors that provide sufficient image quality with fast gantry rotation speeds will be a promising technical concept for medical CT systems. Yet, a potential increase in spatial resolution to the level of flat-panel CT will be associated with increased dose demands, and the clinical benefit has to be carefully considered in the light of the applied patient dose. Reduction of patient dose, in general, will remain a big topic in CT. Especially iterative reconstruction (IR) techniques will become more important in the future. IR uses iterative loops to improve image quality and lower image noise and can potentially help to

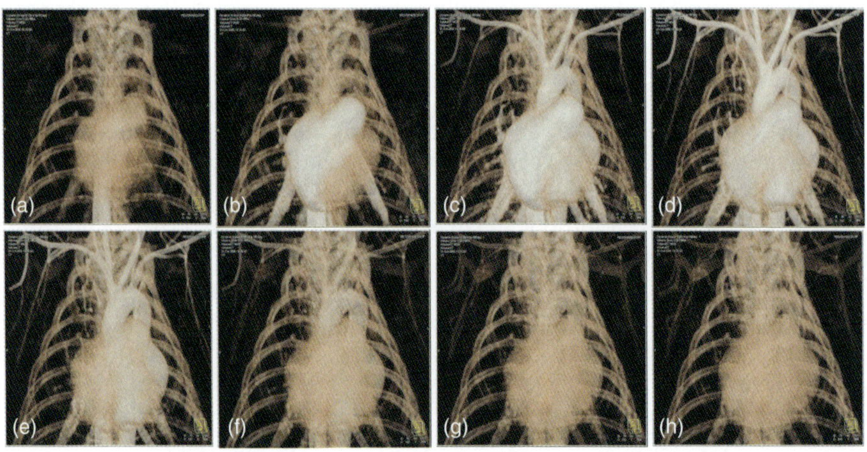

Figure 4.19. Study illustrating the performance of a prototype CT system with CsI-aSi flat-panel detector. Perfusion of the heart and the thoracic vasculature in a rabbit is shown; notice the evolution of first-pass contrast transit from the Inferior Vena Cava (IVC) (a) to the right side of the heart (b), to the left side (c–f), and then finally to the venous system (g, h); frame rate, 30 frames per second; tube voltage 100 kV; tube current 30 mA; time shift between subsequent images 2.5 s; rotation time 5 s. Courtesy of Dr Rajiv Gupta, MGH, Boston, USA.

reduce dose in CT and remove remaining artifacts. A detailed description of IR is beyond the scope of this book chapter.

For further reading, very useful up-to-date information regarding CT is readily available on the Internet, for example at the UK MDA CT website www.medical-devices.gov.uk or at www.ctisus.org.

REFERENCES

Brenner D, Elliston C, Hall E, Berdon W. Estimated risks of radiation-induced fatal cancer from pediatric CT. Am J Roentgenol 2001;176:289–296.

Cesmeli E, Edic M, Iatrou M, Pfoh A. A novel reconstruction algorithm for multiphasic cardiac imaging using multislice CT. Proc SPIE Int Symp Med Imaging 2001;4320:645–654.

Crawford CR, King KF. Computed tomography scanning with simultaneous patient translation. Med Phys 1990;17:967–982.

Donelly LF, Emery KH, Brody AS. Minimizing radiation dose for pediatric body applications of single-detector helical CT: strategies at a large children's hospital. Am J Roentgenol 2001;176:303–306.

Feldkamp LA, Davis LC, Kress JW. Practical cone-beam algorithm. J Opt Soc Am A 1984;A1:612–619.

Flohr T, Ohnesorge B. Heart rate adaptive optimization of spatial and temporal resolution for ECG-gated multi-slice spiral CT of the heart. J Comput Assist Tomogr 2001;25(6):907–923.

Flohr T, Stierstorfer K, Bruder H, Simon J, Schaller S. New technical developments in multislice CT, part 1: approaching isotropic resolution with sub-mm 16-slice scanning. Röfo Fortschr Geb Rontgenstr Neuen Bildgeb Verfahr 2002a;174:839–845.

Flohr T, Bruder H, Stierstorfer K, Simon J, Schaller S, Ohnesorge B. New technical developments in multislice CT, part 2: sub-millimeter 16-slice scanning and increased gantry rotation speed for cardiac imaging. Röfo Fortschr Geb Rontgenstr Neuen Bildgeb Verfahr 2002b;174:1022–1027.

Flohr T, Stierstorfer K, Bruder H, Simon J, Polacin A, Schaller S. Image reconstruction and image quality evaluation for a 16-slice CT scanner. Med Phys 2003a;30(5):832–845.

Flohr T, Schoepf UJ, Kuettner A, Halliburton S, Bruder H, Suess C, Schmidt B, Hofmann L, Yucel EK, Schaller S, Ohnesorge B. Advances in cardiac imaging with 16-section CT-systems. Acad Radiol 2003b;10:386–401.

Flohr T, Stierstorfer K, Raupach R, Ulzheimer S, Bruder H. Performance evaluation of a 64-slice CT-system with z-flying focal spot, Röfo Fortschr Geb Rontgenstr Neuen Bildgeb Verfahr 2004;176:1803–1810.

Flohr TG, Stierstorfer K, Ulzheimer S, Bruder H, Primak AN, McCollough CH. Image reconstruction and image quality evaluation for a 64-slice CT scanner with z-flying focal spot. Med Phys 2005a;32(8):2536–2547.

Flohr TG, Schaller S, Stierstorfer K, Bruder H, Ohnesorge B M, Schoepf UJ. Multi-detector row CT systems and image-reconstruction techniques. Radiology 2005b;235:756–773.

Flohr T, McCollough C, Bruder H, Petersilka M, Gruber K, Süß C, et al. First performance evaluation of a dual-source CT (DSCT) system. Eur Radiol 2006;16:256–268.

Frush DP, Soden B, Frush KS, Lowry C. Improved pediatric multidetector body CT using a size-based color-coded format. Am J Roentgenol 2002;178:721–726.

Fuchs T, Krause J, Schaller S, Flohr T, Kalender WA. Spiral interpolation algorithms for multislice spiral CT–part 2: measurement and evaluation of slice sensitivity profiles and noise at a clinical multislice system, IEEE Trans Med Imaging 2000;19(9):835–847.

Grass M, Köhler T, Proksa R. 3D cone-beam CT reconstruction for circular trajectories. Phys Med Biol 2000;45(2):329–347.

Greess H, Wolf H, Baum U, et al. Dose reduction in computed tomography by attenuation-based on-line modulation of the tube current: evaluation of six anatomical regions. Eur Radiol 2000;10:391–394.

Gupta R, Grasruck M, Süß C, Bartling SH, Schmidt B, Stierstorfer K, Popescu S, Brady T, Flohr T. Ultra-high resolution flat-panel volume CT: fundamental (2006) principles, design architecture, and system characterization. Eur Radiol 2006;16(6):1191–205.

Gupta R, Stierstorfer K, Popescu S, Flohr T, Schaller S, Curtin HD. Temporal bone imaging using a large field-of-view rotating flat-panel CT scanner. Abstract Book of the 89th Scientific Assembly and Annual Meeting of the RSNA, Chicago 2003. p. 375.

Hein I, Taguchi K, Silver M D, Kazarna M, Mori I. Feldkamp-based cone-beam reconstruction for gantry-tilted helical multislice CT. Med Phys 2003;30(12):3233–3242.

Hsieh J. Investigation of the slice sensitivity profile for step-and-shoot mode multi-slice computed tomography. Med Phys 2001;28:491–500.

Hsieh J. Analytical models for multi-slice helical CT performance parameters. Med Phys 2003;30(2):169–178.

Hu H. Multi-slice helical CT: scan and reconstruction. Med Phys 1999;26(1):5–18.

Hu H, He HD, Foley WD, Fox SH. Four multidetector-row helical CT: image quality and volume coverage speed. Radiology 2000;215:55–62.

Jakobs TF, Becker CR, Ohnesorge B, Flohr T, Suess C, Schoepf UJ, Reiser MF. Multislice helical CT of the heart with retrospective ECG gating: reduction of radiation exposure by ECG-controlled tube current modulation. Eur Radiol 2002;12:1081–1086.

Kachelriess M, Ulzheimer S, Kalender W. ECG-correlated image reconstruction from subsecond multi-slice spiral CT scans of the heart. Med Phys 2000;27:1881–1902.

Kalender W. Thin-section three-dimensional spiral CT: is isotropic imaging possible? Radiology 1995;197:578–580.

Kalender WA, Perman WH, Vetter JR, Klotz E. Evaluation of a prototype dual-energy computed tomographic apparatus. I. Phantom studies. Med Phys 1986;13(3):334–339.

Kalender W, Seissler W, Klotz E, Vock P. Spiral volumetric CT with single-breath-hold technique, continuous transport and continuous scanner rotation. Radiology 1990;176:181–183.

Klingenbeck-Regn K, Schaller S, Flohr T, Ohnesorge B, Kopp AF, Baum U. Subsecond multi-slice computed tomography: basics and applications. Eur J Radiol 1999;31:110–124.

Knollmann F, Pfoh A. Image in cardiovascular medicine. Coronary artery imaging with flat-panel computed tomography. Circulation. 2003;107(8):1209.

Leschka S, Alkadhi H, Plass A, Desbiolles L, Grunenfelder J, Marincek B, Wildermuth S. Accuracy of MSCT coronary angiography with 64-slice technology: first experience. Eur Heart J 2005;26(15):1482–1487.

McCollough C. Patient dose in cardiac computed tomography. Herz 2003;28:1–6.

McCollough CH, Zink FE. Performance evaluation of a multi-slice CT system. Med Phys 1999;26:2223–2230.

Mettler FA Jr, Wiest PW, Locken JA, Kelsey CA. CT scanning: patterns of use and dose. J Radiol Prot 2000;20:353–359.

Mori I. Computerized tomographic apparatus utilizing a radiation source. US patent 4,630,202. 1986.

Mori S, Endo M, Obata T, Tsunoo T, Susumu K, Tanada S. Properties of the prototype 256-row (cone beam) CT scanner. Eur Radiol 2006;16(9):2100–2108.

Mori S, Endo M, Tsunoo T, Kandatsu S, Tanada S, Aradate H, et al. Physical performance evaluation of a 256-slice CT-scanner for dour-dimensional imaging. Med Phys 2004;31(6):1348–1356.

Morin R, Gerber T, McCollough C. Radiation dose in computed tomography of the heart. Circulation 2003;107:917–922.

Nickoloff E, Alderson P. Radiation exposure to patients from CT: reality, public perception, and policy. Am J Roentgenol 2001;177:285–287.

Nieman K, Cademartiri F, Lemos PA, Raaijmakers R, Pattynama PMT, de Feyter PJ. Reliable noninvasive coronary angiography with fast submillimeter multislice spiral computed tomography. Circulation 2002: 106; 2051–2054.

Nieman K, Oudkerk M, Rensing B, van Oijen P, Munne A, van Geuns R, de Feyter P. Coronary angiography with multi-slice computed tomography. The Lancet 2001;357:599–603.

Nishimura H, Miyazaki O. Temporal bone imaging using a large field-of-view rotating flat-panel CT scanner. Abstract Book of the 89th Scientific Assembly and Annual Meeting of the RSNA, Chicago 2003. p. 375.

Ohnesorge B, Flohr T, Becker C, Kopp A, Schoepf U, Baum U, Knez A, Klingenbeck Regn K, Reiser M. Cardiac imaging by means of electrocardiographically gated multisection spiral CT–initial experience. Radiology 2000;217:564–571.

Raff GL, Gallagher MJ, O'Neill WW, Goldstein JA. Diagnostic accuracy of non-invasive coronary angiography using 64-slice spiral computed tomography. J Am Coll Cardiol 2005;46(3):552–557.

Ropers D, Baum U, Pohle K, et al. Detection of coronary artery stenoses with thin-slice multi-detector row spiral computed tomography and multiplanar reconstruction. Circulation 2003;107:664–666.

Rubin GD, Dake MD, Semba CP. Current status of three-dimensional spiral CT scanning for imaging the vasculature. Radiol Clin N Am 1995;33(1):51–70 (Review).

Schaller S, Flohr T, Klingenbeck K, Krause J, Fuchs T, Kalender WA. Spiral interpolation algorithm for multi-slice spiral CT—part I: theory. IEEE Trans Med Imaging 2000;19(9):822–834.

Schaller S, Niethammer MU, Chen X, Klotz E, Wildberger JE, Flohr T. Comparison of signal-to-noise and dose values at different tube voltages for protocol optimization in pediatric CT. Abstract Book of the 87th Scientific Assembly and Annual Meeting of the RSNA, 2001a. p. 366.

Schaller S, Stierstorfer K, Bruder H, Kachelrieß M, Flohr T. Novel approximate approach for high-quality image reconstruction in helical cone beam CT at arbitrary pitch. Proc SPIE Int Symp Med Imaging 2001b;4322:113–127.

Schardt P, Deuringer J, Freudenberger J, Hell E, Knuepfer W, Mattern D, Schild M. New X-ray tube performance in computed tomography by introducing the rotating envelope tube technology. Med Phys 2004;31(9):2699–2706.

Shrimpton PC, Jones DG, Hillier MC, Wall BF, Le Heron JC, Faulkner K. Survey of CT practice in the UK. Part 2: dosimetric aspects. Report nr NRPB R249. Chilton: NRPB; 1991.

Taguchi T, Aradate H. Algorithm for image reconstruction in multi-slice helical CT, Med Phys 1998;25(4):550–561.

Taguchi K, Anno H. High temporal resolution for multi-slice helical computed tomography. Med Phys 2000;27(5):861–872.

Vetter JR, Perman WH, Kalender WA, Mazess RB, Holden JE. Evaluation of a prototype dual-energy computed tomographic apparatus. II. Determination of vertebral bone mineral content. Med Phys 1986;13(3):340–343.

Wang G, Lin T, Cheng P. A general cone-beam reconstruction algorithm, IEEE Trans Med Imaging 1993;12:486–496.

Wildberger JE, Mahnken AH, Schmitz-Rode T, Flohr T, Stargardt A, Haage P, Schaller S, Guenther RW. Individually adapted examination protocols for reduction of radiation exposure in chest CT. Invest Radiol 2001;36(10):604–611.

Wintersperger B, Jakobs T, Herzog P, Schaller S, Nikolaou K, Suess C, Weber C, Reiser M, Becker C. Aorto-iliac multidetector-row CT angiography with low kV settings: improved vessel enhancement and simultaneous reduction of radiation dose. Eur Radiol 2005;15:334–341.

5

MAGNETIC RESONANCE TECHNOLOGY

Boguslaw Tomanek and Jonathan C. Sharp
Institute for Biodiagnostics (West), National Research Council of Canada, Calgary, AB, Canada

5.1 INTRODUCTION

Magnetic resonance technology comprises the hardware, software, and imaging techniques used in Magnetic Resonance Imaging (MRI) and Magnetic Resonance Spectroscopy (MRS). MRI has become one of the most useful imaging techniques used in medical diagnosis. Thousands of MRI systems have been produced and installed in clinics since the first introduction to hospitals in the early 1980s. In recognition of the importance of MRI to the practice of medicine, Dr Paul Lauterbur and Sir Peter Mansfield were awarded the 2003 Nobel Prize in Medicine for their discoveries concerning MRI. The Nuclear Magnetic Resonance (NMR) phenomenon, on which MRI is based, was discovered in 1945 by Purcell, Torrey, and Pound at Harvard (1) and independently by Bloch, Hansen, and Packard at Stanford (2). This followed the discovery of electron paramagnetic resonance by J. Zawoysky in 1944. Their work was continued by Hahn (3), who discovered the Spin Echo (SE), and Gabillard (4, 5), who showed that a magnetic field gradient can be used to obtain the spatial distribution of a sample of spins. These discoveries were used exclusively in chemistry until the 1950s, when NMR began to find an application in medicine with the discovery of the relationship between relaxation times and water content in tissue. This was confirmed by Damadian in 1971 (6), who showed that the relaxation times of cancerous and normal tissues

Biomedical Imaging: Principles and Applications, First Edition. Edited by Reiner Salzer.

may differ. The early 1970s saw the development of diverse MRI approaches by Mansfield (7–9), Hinshaw (10), Andrew (11), Lauterbur (12), Garroway (13), Hoult (14), Kumar (15), and many others.

MRI allows the visualization of internal structures of a body containing water and fat molecules. Since the human body consists of more than 50% water (about 90% in brain), MRI could be used to image practically any organ. Clinically, MRI is used for early disease diagnosis, while research areas cover new fast imaging techniques, high resolution human and animal anatomy, and details of physiology and pathology. Although the detected signal comes from water or fat molecules, MRI is sensitive to much more than simple Proton Density (PD). The contrast in MR images can come from blood flow, blood oxygenation, water diffusion, or specific properties of tissues, and is called *relaxation times*. The contrast in an MR image depends on the specific imaging technique used, allowing many types of image appearances, thus giving many options for the clear visualization of specific tissues or physiology. This makes the technique superior in flexibility to other imaging modalities such as Computed Tomography (CT, Chapter 4) or Ultrasound (US, Chapter 11), which use only radiation absorption, reflection, or scattering to obtain an image. Because MR uses only magnetic and radiofrequency (rf) fields, unlike CT, it does not expose the patient to harmful ionizing radiation. MRI can easily provide isotropic 2D or 3D images in any plane, whereas both CT and US techniques are more limited geometrically. Furthermore, MRI suffers from neither heavy absorption in bone (as do X-rays) nor strong reflections from bone (as does US) and thus is ideal for brain and spine imaging—the Central Nervous System (CNS) being encased within bony structures. MRI offers excellent contrast between soft tissues also superior to other modalities.

Owing to this impressive set of advantageous features, the application of MRI has become very broad and includes the diagnosis of many diseases, such as cancer, stroke, brain disorders, and heart conditions. MRI continuously expands into other areas and finds new applications such as the assessment of surgery using intraoperative MRI (16) or image-guided procedures such as biopsy or laparoscopy. The combination of MRI with the specific biochemical information provided by MRS provides potentially a powerful tool for clinical management of problems such as stroke, tumor classification, and monitoring and assessment of other diseases.

To produce an MR image, a strong magnetic field (order of 1 T), time-variable magnetic field gradients, and a rf field are used. As the Signal to Noise Ratio (SNR), and thus image resolution available, increases with the magnetic field strength, as explained in the following sections, there is an industry trend toward the use of stronger magnets. The standard clinical system is equipped with a 1.5-T magnet, but 3-T systems have recently been granted approval by the US Food and Drug Administration (FDA) for clinical use. While stronger magnets (above 3 T) are technically feasible, their possible, yet not proven, harmful side effects and high costs (usually $1M per 1 T for each unit) are the limiting factors. However, new pulse sequences and new types of rf coils are being continuously introduced, improving image quality and extending applications of MRI and MRS.

Many books have been published explaining the principles of MRI (17) and the details of MRI techniques (18, 19).

5.2 MAGNETIC NUCLEI SPIN IN A MAGNETIC FIELD

Atoms with an odd number of nucleons (neutrons + protons) have net non-zero spin, caused by the rotation of charged nuclei. Such spinning nuclei can be imaged with MRI (Table 5.1). Among such atoms are hydrogen (^{1}H), carbon (^{13}C), fluorine (^{19}F), phosphorus (^{31}P), nitrogen (^{15}N), oxygen (^{17}O), and sodium (^{23}Na). These occur in varying abundance within the human body. Owing to the overwhelmingly high content of protons in the tissues (due to water), MRI of hydrogen atoms is predominant in clinical MRI. Some gases, for example, xenon (^{129}Xe) or helium (^{3}H), also possess spin and thus can be imaged after inhalation. However, because of their low density, they must be hyperpolarized (pumped with "extra" energy using laser light) to provide sufficient signal for imaging.

The physics of NMR is described in detail by quantum mechanics, but the classical approach is much easier to understand; therefore, it is herein presented. Following this approach, the spin can be envisioned as a very small rotating magnet, denoted frequently as an arrow (vector). Spins placed in an external magnetic field precess around that field (Fig. 5.1). The frequency of that precession

TABLE 5.1. Properties of Some NMR Sensitive Nuclei

Nucleus	Natural Abundance (%)	Spin (I)	Resonance Frequency (MHz at 1 T)	Relative NMR Sensitivity[a]
^{1}H	99.98	1/2	42.57	1.0000
^{2}H	1.5×10^{-2}	1	6.54	0.0628
^{13}C	1.108	1/2	10.71	0.0632
^{14}N	99.63	1	3.08	0.0139
^{15}N	0.37	1/2	4.31	0.0103
^{17}O	3.7×10^{-2}	5/2	5.77	0.2144
^{19}F	100	1/2	40.05	0.8851
^{23}Na	100	3/2	11.26	0.3498
^{29}Si	4.6832	1/2	8.46	0.0395
^{31}P	100	1/2	17.23	0.1639
^{35}Cl	75.53	3/2	4.17	0.0480
^{37}Cl	24.47	3/2	3.47	0.0333
^{39}K	93.10	3/2	1.99	0.0109
^{41}K	6.88	3/2	1.09	0.0033
^{43}Ca	0.145	7/2	2.86	0.0951
^{57}Fe	2.19	1/2	1.38	0.0010

[a]Calculated for the same amount of nuclei.

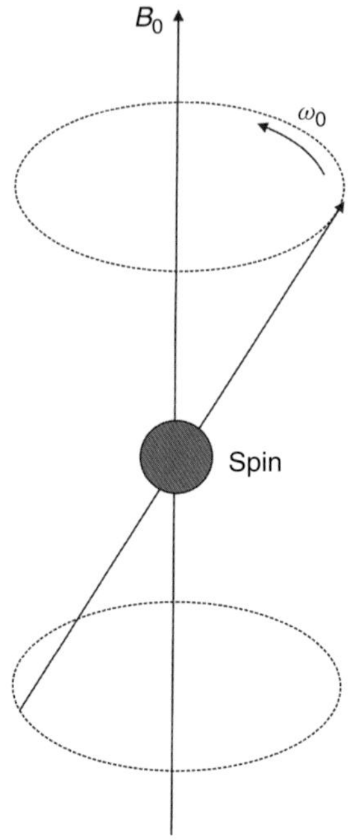

Figure 5.1. Rotation of the spin in the external magnetic field B_0.

is proportional to the magnetic field and is described by the Larmor equation:

$$\omega_0 = \frac{\gamma}{2\pi} B_0 \tag{5.1}$$

where ω_0 is Larmor frequency (in Hz), γ is a gyromagnetic ratio that depends on the nuclei, B_0 is the externally applied magnetic field (in tesla). As can be seen from Eq. (5.1), different nuclei precess with different frequencies in the same magnetic field. The frequency of the precession of the most commonly used NMR nuclei and their NMR sensitivities are shown in Table 5.1. Because of the linear relationship between the frequency of rotation and the external field, both ω_0 and B_0 values are used interchangeably in the literature. For example, one can hear about 1.5 T or 64 MHz MRI system, because 1.5 T corresponds roughly to the proton frequency of 64 MHz ($\gamma_H = 2.675$ rad/sT) and vice versa; 3 T corresponds to 128 MHz. The magnetization created by a nucleus depends also on the type of nuclei because the difference in the energy of the system spins up and down depends on its magnetic moment, which is different for different nuclei. The sensitivity shown in Table 5.1 (last column) shows the signal that could be received from a particular element, assuming the same number of nuclei. The sensitivity of ^1H is assumed to be one.

Equation (5.1) describes the behavior of a single spin, whereas in imaged objects there are many spins (order of 10^{24}). When such an object is placed in a

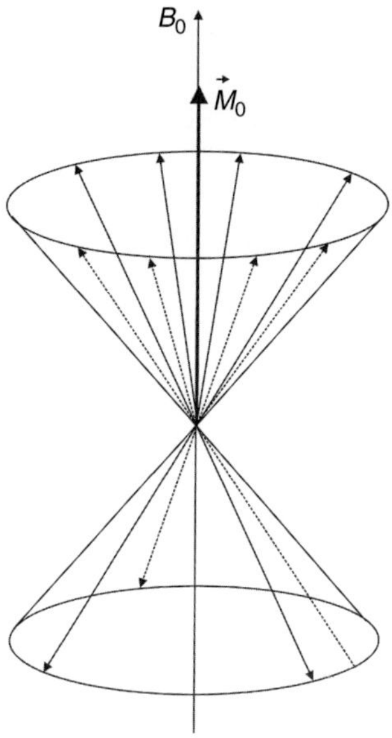

Figure 5.2. Spins placed in the external magnetic field B_0 create net magnetization $\vec{M}_0$ along the direction of the field.

magnetic field, its spins align either parallel or anti-parallel to the field (Fig. 5.2). There is only a very small difference, about one per million, between the number of spins aligned parallel to the field and those aligned antiparallel. This small difference makes MR less sensitive than other imaging methods, such as infrared spectroscopy (Chapter 9). This excess of spins creates a net magnetization, which is detected by MR systems as the NMR signal. The amplitude of the magnetization depends on the strength of the external magnetic field. For instance, in the Earth's magnetic field the magnetization is practically undetectable. Therefore, very strong magnetic fields must be generated by specially designed magnets (most frequently superconductive) to be able to produce enough signal. The magnetic fields used in present clinical MRI systems vary from 0.2 to 3 T (the Earth's magnetic field is about 50 μT, i.e., about 500,000 times lower). Experimental MRI systems currently reach 14 T, while systems for NMR spectroscopy approach 20 T (almost 1 GHz for protons).

5.2.1 A Pulsed rf Field Resonates with Magnetized Nuclei

As explained above, there is a net magnetization created when magnetic nuclei are placed in a magnetic field. In other words, the patient becomes magnetized. The application of an external rf field (or precisely its magnetic component B_1) in the plane perpendicular to the external magnetic field, crucially at the rf corresponding to the frequency of the rotating spins, "flips" some or all of them from up to down position (Fig. 5.3). This phenomenon is known as *nuclear magnetic resonance* (NMR).

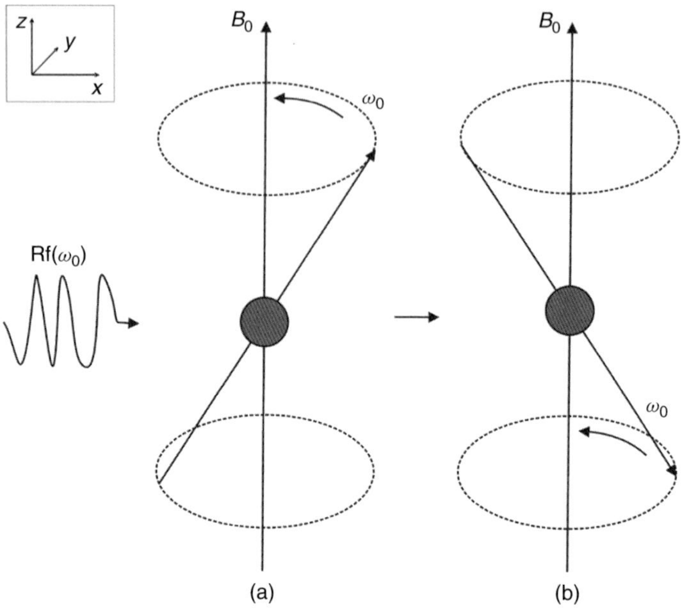

Figure 5.3. (a) Spin rotates around the magnetic field B_0. (b) Application of the rf pulse, corresponding to the frequency of the spin rotation, flips the spin.

To understand what happens after the rf pulse is applied, let us assume that the external magnetic field is applied in the z direction and the rf pulse is applied in x-y plane. Before the pulse is applied, $\vec{M}_0$ (the sum vector of all spins) is in equilibrium and is aligned along the external $\vec{B}_0$ magnetic field (Fig. 3a). Following the application of the rf pulse, the net magnetization $\vec{M}_0$ flips away from its equilibrium position (Fig. 5.4). This tilt is called the *flip angle* (φ)

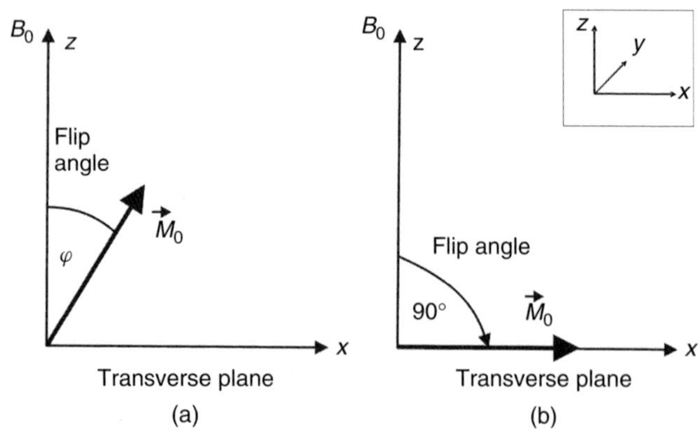

Figure 5.4. (a) Application of the φ degree rf pulse tilts the magnetization $\vec{M}_0$ from its equilibrium position along the z direction by the angle φ. (b) Magnetization lies along the x direction after the 90° rf pulse is applied.

and depends on the product of the amplitude and duration of the rf pulse. For a rectangular pulse of duration t_p, and rf amplitude B_1, the flip angle can be expressed as $\varphi = \gamma B_1 t_p$ or more generally for a pulse of any shape:

$$\varphi = \int_0^{t_p} \gamma B_1(t)\mathrm{d}t \tag{5.2}$$

where $B_1(t)$ is the envelope of the rf pulse of duration t_p.

As can be seen from Eq. (5.2), the stronger the rf field applied or the longer it lasts the larger the flip angle. An rf pulse that flips the magnetization 90° from the equilibrium position is termed 90° (or $\pi/2$) pulse, and similarly for other flip angles (45°, 180°, etc.). The maximum NMR signal available from a sample is obtained after a 90° pulse.

5.2.2 The MR Signal

To produce the rf field and detect the signal, rf coils (often referred to as *rf probes* or resonators or incorrectly as antennas) are used. The simplest rf coil is a solenoid. The coils are designed to produce their rf field in x-y plane (Fig. 5.5). After the application of a 90° rf pulse, the magnetization $\vec{M}_0$ rotates along the z direction in the x-y plane. The M_{xy} component of the magnetization induces a voltage in the coil that can be amplified and detected. The rf pulse not only flips the spins but also imposes the phase coherence of the spins. Immediately after, the rf pulse (Fig. 5.6b) spins have the same phase, but soon after they dephase because each spin rotates in a slightly different magnetic field due to

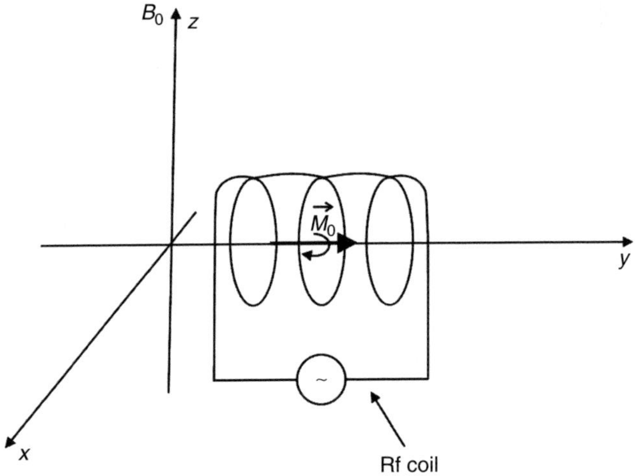

Figure 5.5. Rotating magnetization $\vec{M}_0$ induces current in the receiving rf coil.

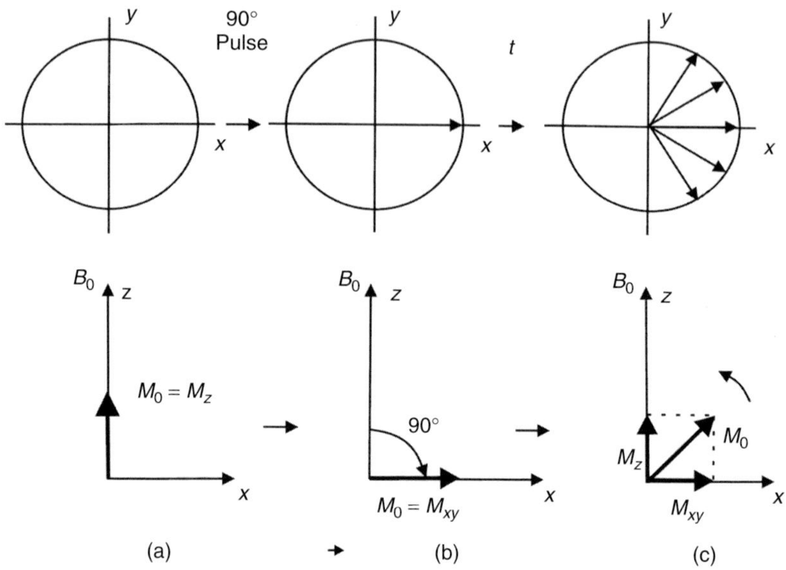

Figure 5.6. Behavior of the magnetization $\vec{M}_0$ in the external magnetic field B_0 along the z direction: x-y plane (top row), z-x plane (bottom row): (a) Magnetization in equilibrium; (b) magnetization just after 90° rf pulse; (c) magnetization returns to equilibrium after time t from the application of the 90° rf pulse; spins dephase in x-y plane.

inhomogeneities of the magnetic field (order of 10^{-6} of the main field in standard MRI magnets). Inhomogeneous magnetic field means that there is a different field at each point. Thus, spins within the same field rotate with slightly different frequencies that depend on their position ($\omega(\vec{r}) \sim B_0(\vec{r})$), causing an overall spin vector dephasing. As spins lose their phase coherence, the amplitude of the induced MR signal decreases. This natural process is known as *Free Induction Decay* (FID), and its exponential decrease is described by time called T_2^* ("t 2 star").

5.2.3 Spin Interactions have Characteristic Relaxation Times

As mentioned above, the signal induced in the rf coil (caused by M_{xy}) decreases with time because of the inhomogeneity of the external magnetic field. This is, however, not the only reason that causes the signal to decay. Before the 90° pulse is applied, there is a net magnetization along the z direction ($\vec{M}_z = \vec{M}_0$) (Fig. 5.6a). The 90° rf pulse flips magnetization $\vec{M}_0$ to the x-y plane, creating a net magnetization in the x-y plane (M_{xy}) (Fig. 5.6b). At that point, the M_z component is zero. After the rf pulse is removed, the net magnetization M_z returns, like all natural processes, to equilibrium (Fig. 5.6c); this process of rebuilding M_z is called *longitudinal or spin-lattice relaxation*. The time constant describing the recovery of the magnetization is known as the T_1 *relaxation time*. The decay of the magnetization M_{xy} in the x-y plane is called *transverse or spin-spin relaxation* or

T_2 *decay*. One can show that (for a Lorentzian spectral function) $\frac{1}{T_2^*} = \frac{\gamma \Delta B_0}{2} + \frac{1}{T_2}$ thus $T_2^* \leq T_2 \cdot T_1$ and T_2 are defined exactly as the time needed for 63% of the M_z to recover and M_{xy} to decay, respectively. The details of the processes causing the relaxation can be found, for example, in Reference (20). Generally, the longitudinal relaxation is caused by the rotational and translational molecular motion, which creates a small time-varying magnetic field as seen by the spin, and which causes spins to flip and transfer their energy to the surrounding molecules (lattice). Therefore, this type of relaxation is particularly efficient in the presence of paramagnetic substances (such as O_2). Thus, pure, degasified water has a T_1 of about 4 s (the exact value depending on the external magnetic field and temperature), whereas water in brain or blood has a T_1 of about 100 ms because of dissolved ions creating fluctuating magnetic fields. As a result, the energy of the spins dissipates as heat (although a very small amount). Conversely, the transverse relaxation (T_2) is caused by interactions among spins themselves. Each flip of a spin changes the local magnetic field, which in turn affects surrounding spins and accelerates the transition of spin from one position to the other. Contrary to longitudinal relaxation, there is no net heat created in this process. As in all natural processes, the relaxations have exponential behavior and can be mathematically described, following the 90° pulse, as $M_z(t) = 1 - M_0 \exp(-t/T_1)$, $M_{xy}(t) = \exp(-t/T_1^*)$. Both processes, the return of M_z to its equilibrium and the decay of M_{xy} to zero, can be probed by an MR system and exploited to obtain image contrast.

5.3 IMAGE CREATION

To create an MR image, the main magnetic field, three gradients of the magnetic field, and an rf field are all required. This section describes mathematically how an image can be created if all these requirements are provided.

5.3.1 Slice Selection

One of the advantages of MRI over other imaging techniques is the possibility of selection of the slice of interest. To understand how the slice is selected, we will first consider the rf pulses used in MRI. As mentioned before, rf pulses are needed to generate an MR signal. There are two types of rf pulses: non-selective and selective (Fig. 5.7). Each pulse used in MRI is "filled" with an rf field corresponding to the Larmor frequency. Therefore, its shape is called an *envelope function*. A detailed analysis of the rf pulses, for example (21), reveals that each pulse has its own frequency spectra. It means that an rf pulse "contains" not only one particular frequency but rather a band of frequencies, the distribution of which depends on the shape (envelope function) of the rf pulse. For example, a very long (infinite) sinusoidal pulse in the time domain ($s(t) = \sin \omega_0 t$) produces only one frequency (ω_0) in the frequency domain, but a rectangular pulse has a spectrum of frequency distributed around the central frequency ω_0 and decreasing with the

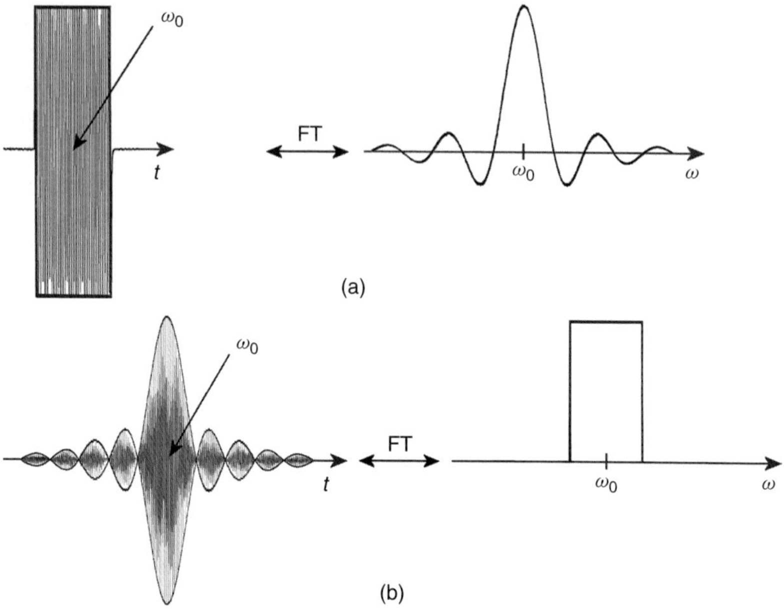

Figure 5.7. (a) Selective (soft) rf pulse and its Fourier transform. (b) Nonselective (hard) rf pulse and its Fourier transform.

frequency offset from ω_0 (Fig. 5.7a). The most commonly used selective pulses in MRI are pulses with so-called sinc ($\mathrm{sinc}(x) = \sin x/x$) envelope (Fig. 7b), because their frequency spectra is nearly rectangular, leading to a rectangular slice profile. Other complex pulses, for example, based on Hermite function, are also used, as their slice profile is even closer to rectangular than the sinc function.

The mathematical formula describing the relationship between the time and frequency domains is called a *Fourier Transform* (FT): $F(\omega) = \int_{-\infty}^{+\infty} S(t)\exp(2i\pi\omega t)\mathrm{d}t$, where $F(\omega)$ is the frequency domain of the signal $S(t)$ in the time domain (22). Interestingly, the inverse FT links $F(\omega)$ with $S(t) : S(t) = \int_{-\infty}^{+\infty} F(\omega)\exp(-2i\pi\omega t)\mathrm{d}t$. The FT is of fundamental importance in MRI, where it is used to process the MR signal to obtain an MR image. FT was first applied in NMR by Richard Ernst in 1966 (23). The application of FT to NMR later allowed the extension to MRI and the subsequent development of other imaging techniques. The simultaneous application of the constant gradient ($G_z = \frac{\mathrm{d}B}{\mathrm{d}z} = \mathrm{const}$) of the magnetic field and the selective rf pulse allows slice selection (Fig. 5.8). When the gradient is applied, for example, along the z direction ($B(z) = z\frac{\mathrm{d}B}{\mathrm{d}z}$), the frequency of the spins (Eq. 5.1) depends on their position along that direction ($\omega(z) = z\frac{\Delta\omega}{\Delta z}$). The stronger the gradient and/or the narrower the rf pulse bandwidth (BW) the thinner the selected slice, according to the formula: $\Delta z = \Delta\omega/\gamma G_z$, where G_z is a constant gradient in the z direction,

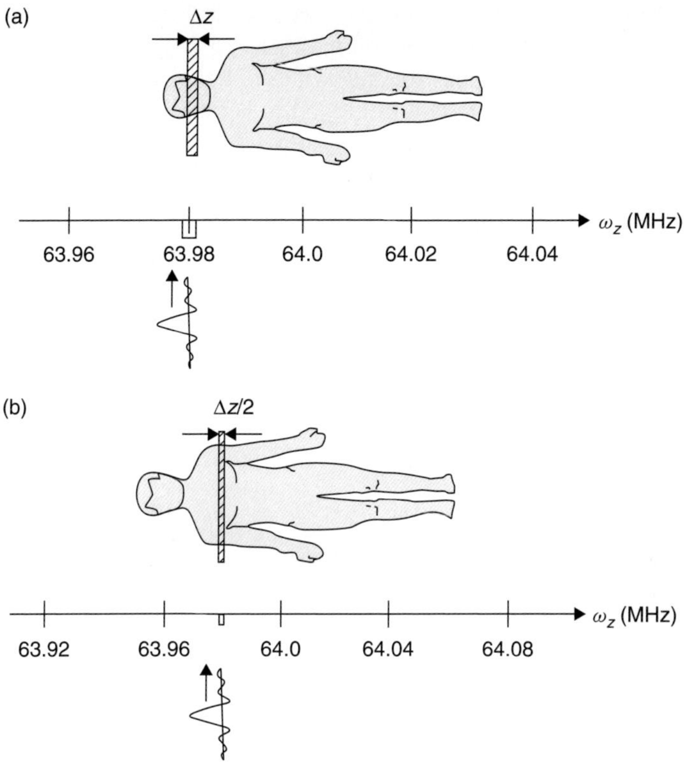

Figure 5.8. Process of slice selection using gradient of the magnetic field and selective rf pulse. (a) Selective rf pulse corresponding to the frequency 63.98 ± 0.01 MHz selects a slice of Δz thickness. (b) The same rf pulse as in (a), but the gradient is two times stronger: slice thickness is now half as wide as above.

$\Delta\omega$ is the BW of the rf pulse, and Δz is the slice thickness. In modern MRI systems, gradient coils can generate field gradients up to 40 mT/m, which along with the application of a standard selective rf pulse of several kHz BW allows submillimeter slice thicknesses.

To analyze in detail the slice selection process shown in Figure 5.8, let us assume that a patient is lying in the 1.5-T magnet and both the main field and the gradients are applied along the z direction. And let us also assume that the frequency in the center of the magnet is exactly 64.00 MHz. If we add a magnetic field gradient to the main field, the precession frequency of the spins in a patient's body will depend on their position: spins will precess faster in the legs and slower in the head. If we now apply a selective rf pulse, with the spectrum width $\Delta\omega = \omega_0 \frac{\Delta z}{z} = 0.02$ MHz and with frequency ω_0 corresponding to the frequency of the spins rotating in the head (63.98 MHz) (Fig. 8a) we excite, thus select, only spins in the slice Δz that spins rotate at the frequency 63.98 ± 0.01 MHz. What happens is that the band of frequencies presents in the rf pulse matches the resonant frequencies of the spins within a thin slice of the patient.

In a second experiment, we use the same selective rf pulse but double the strength of the gradient (Fig. 5.8b) and thus select a different slice (e.g., through a chest), because now the spins rotating with the frequency matching that of the rf pulse are "shifted" (to the right in Fig. 5.8b) because of the stronger gradient. Furthermore, the selected slice Δz_{new} in now only half as wide, because now the same $\Delta\omega$ corresponds to half the thickness of the previous slice: $\Delta z_{\text{new}} = \Delta\omega/\gamma 2G_z$. In other words, we have narrowed the frequency window. In this way, slice thickness could be controlled.

The other way of changing the slice thickness is to use a selective pulse with a narrower spectrum. This could be accomplished, for example, by using longer, thus more selective rf pulses or by changing their shape. To select a different slice but of the same thickness, an rf pulse with different center rf frequency is used. Unfortunately, selective pulses do not have perfect rectangular spectra; therefore, spins may experience slightly different rf fields across the slice and their flip angles may be different. Such "slice profile" effects can be the source of artifacts.

5.3.2 The Signal Comes Back—The Spin Echo

To understand how an MR image is created, first we will explain the spin (or Hahn) echo. The SE was discovered by Erwin Hahn in 1950 (3). As we already know, the application of a 90° rf pulse with frequency corresponding to the frequency of the rotating spins creates a net magnetization in x-y plane (Fig. 5.9). Owing to the inhomogeneities of the magnetic field and the relaxation T_2, the spins dephase after the rf pulse is removed, leading to decay of the MR signal. This process is detected by the rf receiver coil as the FID with the T_2* time. Because FID occurs just after the rf pulse and is usually very short, its detection is rather difficult. Therefore, often additional rf pulses are used to collect the MR data. The most common is the application of the 180° pulse after the 90° pulse. The 180° pulse, also called a *refocusing pulse*, flips all spins vectors by 180° about some axis. Specifically, a 180°_y pulse (180° with y phase) flips the spins about the y axis. (The 180°_x pulse would flip the spins along x axis.) As can be seen from Figure 5.9, the spins dephasing will now rephase again, and exactly after the same time (t) as 180° pulse was applied after 90° pulse, they will all align along the y axis. In other words, after the 180° pulse is applied, the spins that rotated fast (dephased faster) will continue to rotate faster, but now they will chase the slower rotating spins to catch them up on the y axis, exactly after the same time as the time interval between 90° and 180° pulses. To explain the SE phenomenon, many authors bring an analogy of the sprinters beginning the race at the same start point and then, at any point during the race, they suddenly (180° pulse) move back with the same speed (as in a move played backwards). As one can easily imagine, all sprinters will reach the starting point at the same time (they will be in phase again). Fortunately, in real life, the time cannot be set backwards, so there is a sense of running fast if you want to win!

The application of a series of 180° pulses following the 90° pulse creates a series of SEs (Fig. 5.10), as each 180° keeps refocusing spins. If there were

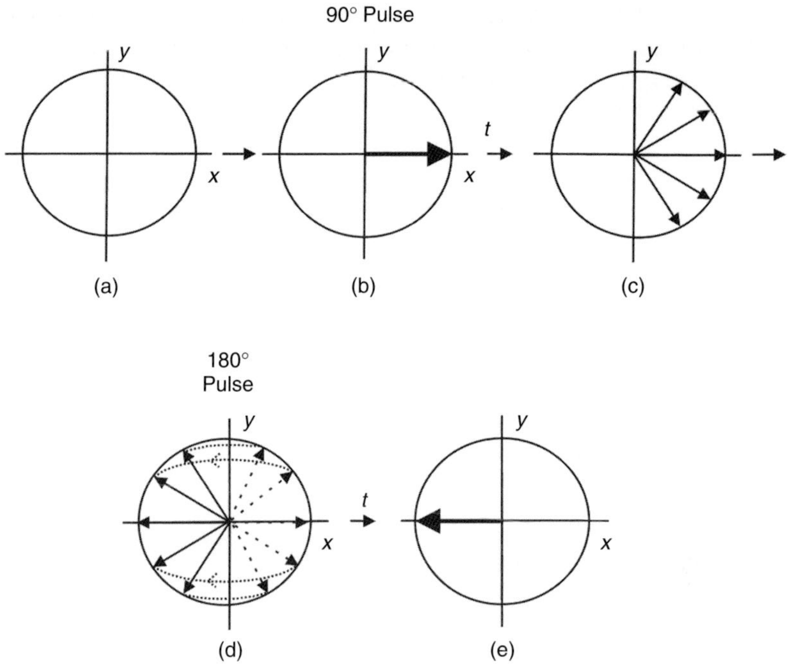

Figure 5.9. Spin echo: (a) magnetization in equilibrium; (b) 90° rf pulse applied; (c) spins dephasing for time t; (d) 180° rf pulse applied, spins rephasing; and (e) spins align along the y axis as in (b) after time t.

no relaxation processes, as assumed above, the amplitude of each echo would remain constant. However, in reality, between the application of a 90° pulse and the detection of each SE, spins interact with each other (T_2 relaxation), causing some of them "to be lost" in this time, thus reducing the amplitude of the echoes. Therefore, echo train amplitude will be decreasing with T_2 constant. The application of a 90°_x pulse followed by a series of 180°_y pulses is called the *CPMG pulse sequence*, from the name of its discoverers in 1954: Carr, Purcell, Meiboom, and Gill (24). This is the most frequently used method of measurement of the T_2 relaxation time in MR.

5.3.3 Gradient Echo

The other method of obtaining an MR signal in the form of an echo is the so-called Gradient Echo (GE). This method allows a much faster acquisition of the signal because it does not require the application of 180° rf pulses. Instead of the refocusing rf pulses, typically lasting about 2–5 ms, a gradient reversal is used (Fig. 5.11). Following the low angle rf pulse (usually 5–15°) for the fast data acquisition, a negative gradient is applied, followed by the reverse gradient of the same duration and amplitude. The negative gradient causes the spins to

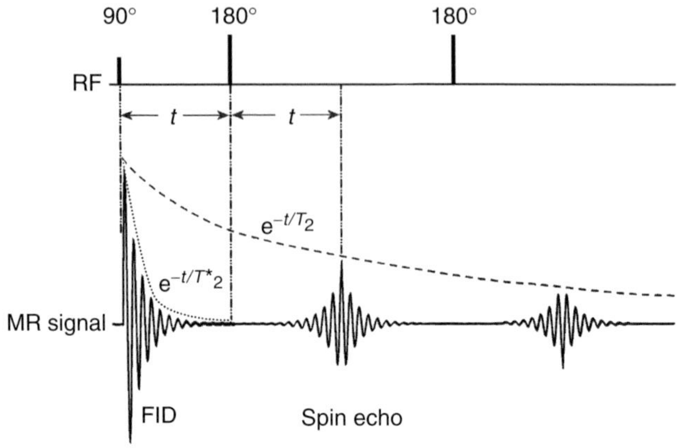

Figure 5.10. MR signal created by a 90° pulse and a series of 180° pulses (CPMG pulse sequence). The FID of the signal following the 90° pulse depends on T_2*; the curve connecting peaks of echoes created by series of 180° pulses is T_2 dependent.

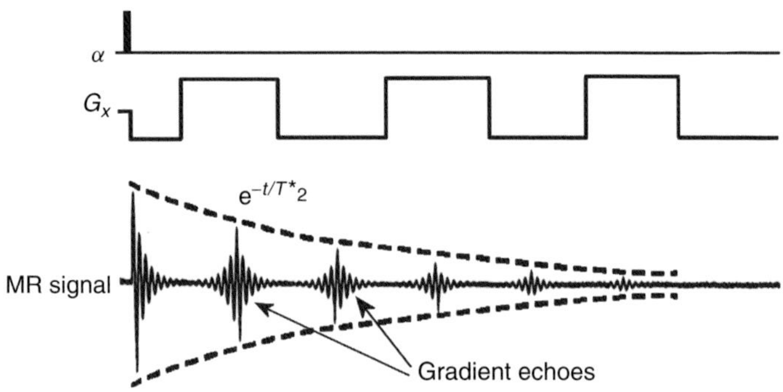

Figure 5.11. Gradient echoes created by a switching gradient. The decay curve is T_2* dependent.

rotate with different frequencies that depends on the spins' spatial position ($\omega = \gamma G_x x$), causing their dephasing with time. Following the negative gradient, the positive one is applied, causing spins to refocus, as now the faster defocusing ones are faster to refocus. However, unlike SE, GE is affected by the main field inhomogeneities, because this effect is not cancelled by the rf refocusing pulses. The rf refocusing 180° pulse, in contrary to the switching gradients, reverses the effects of the inhomogeneous field. As a consequence, the GEs are T_2* dependent. The switching gradients, as refocusing pulses, can be repeated to obtain a GE train (Fig. 5.11) and used in GE imaging (Section 5.8).

Advanced readers may be interested in the so-called stimulated echo, which is created by three rf pulses. Because of the need for three rf pulses and an amplitude of only half that of an SE, the stimulated echo is not commonly used in MRI (3). In addition, stimulated echoes may present as image artifacts in sequences using more than two rf pulses for the single excitation. However, the stimulated echo has found an application in localized MR spectroscopy.

5.4 IMAGE RECONSTRUCTION

Now that basic MR terminology and phenomena have been covered, we can proceed with the details of the nature of the MR image creation.

To understand how an MR image is created, we shall consider a pulse sequence based on SE, as shown in Figure 5.12. The general principles of other pulse sequences are similar. Section 5.3.1 discussed how a slice is selected using simultaneously the selective rf pulse and the gradient of the magnetic field. As shown in Figure 5.12a gradient in the z direction and a selective rf pulse are used to excite spins in the desired slice. The application of two additional orthogonal gradients in x and y directions allows information about the spatial position of the spins.

The y gradient (G_y) applied after the first rf pulse for a short time t causes the spins to rotate with a different frequency along y, thus accumulating a final phase ($\varphi(y) = \gamma G_y yt$) that depends on the position of the spins along the y direction (Fig. 5.13). This gradient is called *phase encoding*. (The gradient with the same amplitude and duration is also applied after SE sequence to begin the next acquisition from the same spin settings; this is omitted in Fig. 5.12 for simplicity.)

The application of the second gradient along the x direction (the so-called read gradient) during the acquisition of the SE causes spins to rotate with a frequency dependent on the x position of the spins. This way, each spin has a different frequency or phase depending on its spatial position. The electronics used in MR can detect the phase and frequency of the MR signal. The pulse sequence has to be

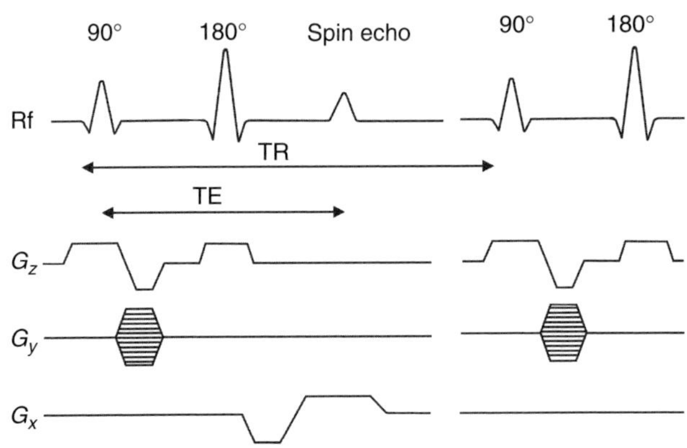

Figure 5.12. Slice-selective spin echo (SE) pulse sequence: G_z, slice selection gradient; G_y, phase encoding gradient; G_x, frequency encoding gradient, TR, repetition time, and TE, echo time.

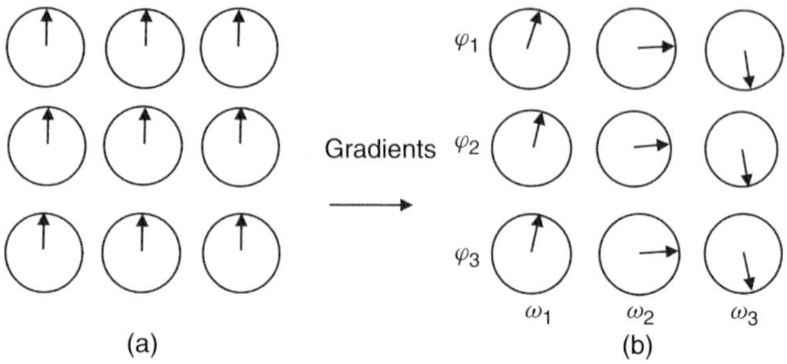

Figure 5.13. (a) Spins of the object placed in the perfectly homogenous magnetic field. (b) Spins change phase and frequency after the application of two perpendicular gradients.

repeated with different amplitudes of the phase encoding gradient to reconstruct an image in two dimensions, as the multiple phases in a single data acquisition cannot be resolved. The acquired data (SE) is digitized using an Analog to Digital Converter (ADC) and stored in the computer memory, and then the 2-dimensional (2D) FT converts frequency into position, first along read direction and then along the phase direction to reconstruct a 2D image. The details of the FT procedure can be found, for example, in Reference 19. The time interval between data points collected along the read direction is called sampling rate, which is the inverse of the receiver sampling BW. The raw data collected by an MRI system and an image created after FT is applied are shown in Figure 5.14. The top picture shows the data (sampled echo) collected with different phase encoding gradients starting from its positive maximum value (first row) down to maximum negative value (last row). The maximum MR signal, and the most valuable information about an imaged object, is collected in the center of the data matrix (center line), where phase encoding gradient is close to zero. The raw data is often referred to as *k-space*. An introduction of the k-space concept simplified the mathematical description of MRI methods; however, its analysis is beyond the scope of this chapter, but can be found, for example, in References 19, 21.

The described method applies to all MRI techniques, as one direction is always frequency encoding and the other phase encoding, and 2D FT is used for image reconstruction.

As mentioned earlier, phase encoding must be repeated to be able to obtain 2-dimensional information about the object. Therefore, the spins must be excited more times, thus the rf pulses, 90° and 180°, as well as all the gradients are applied repetitively, but each time the amplitude of the phase encoding gradient varies.

5.4.1 Sequence Parameters

The time between each consecutive 90° rf pulse is called *Repetition Time* (TR), while the time between a 90° pulse and the maximum amplitude of the echo is called *Echo Time* (TE) (Fig. 5.12). The time required to obtain data to create an

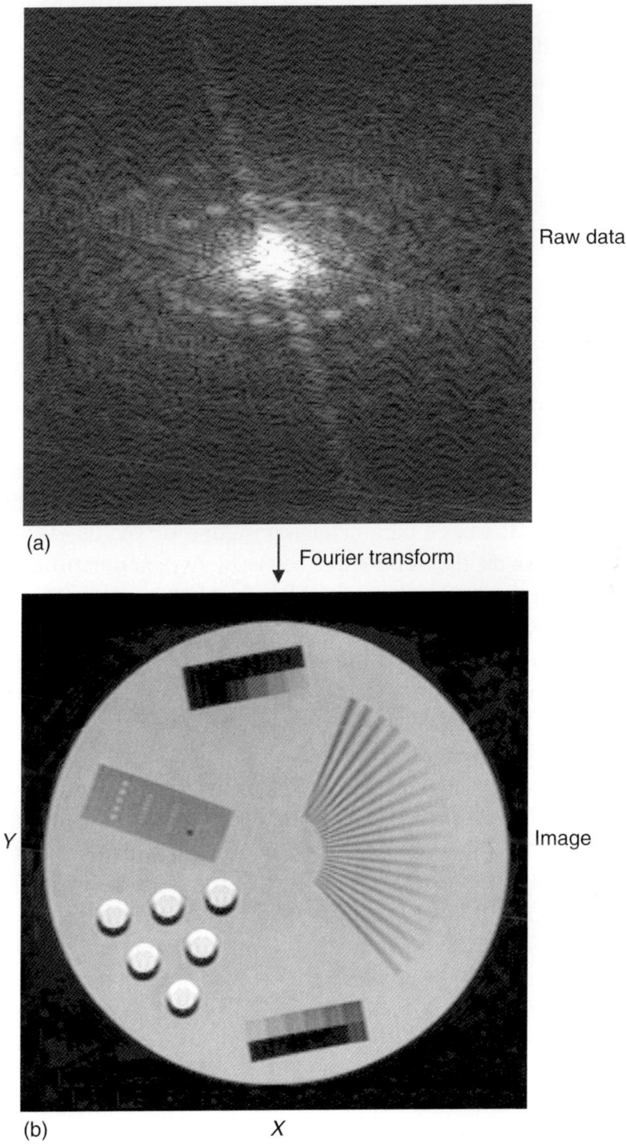

Figure 5.14. (a) The raw data acquired by the MRI system. Each horizontal line corresponds to echo obtained at different phase gradients. The read gradient is constant for each line. (b) Image obtained after 2D FT is applied to the raw data.

image is called the *total acquisition time* (or *scan time*). For pulse sequences that require multiple excitations, the total acquisition time is equal to TR multiplied by number of phase encoding steps. To increase SNR and image quality, the pulse sequence may be repeated and data co-added, but at the expense of an extended total acquisition time.

Proper selection of such sequence parameters allows different MR image contrast to be obtained. This selectable image contrast is a major difference between MRI and other imaging techniques. This unique feature dramatically enhances diagnostic capabilities of MRI, as tissue contrast can be tailored to the disease under investigation. This also makes MRI interpretation more complex because a tissue, for example, fat or blood, may be bright on one image but dark on another, depending on a pulse sequence and parameters used.

5.5 IMAGE RESOLUTION

As explained in Section 5.3.1, the imaged slice in MRI is selected by the gradients and the selective rf pulse. In medical practice, the most commonly used slice thickness, an important MR image parameter, is around 1 mm. While a thinner slice would ideally provide more precise diagnostic information, thinner slices also require longer scan times to produce image with high enough quality. An equally important MR image parameter is in-plane or spatial resolution. Spatial resolution is defined as the separation between two neighboring points of the imaged object, which can be distinguished. In MRI, spatial resolution depends on the Field of View (FOV) and the number of points (pixels) along each direction (Chapter 2). The number of pixels in the read direction depends on the number of collected (sampled) data points. The number of phase encoding gradient steps used to collect each row of data determines the image resolution in the phase encoding direction. However the raw data matrix may be different from the image matrix because of postprocessing methods such as zero filling (increasing the size of the data matrix by filling the data with zeros before FT), which are used to improve displayed image quality (while remaining the same scan time).

The image resolution depends on the size of the imaged object and the matrix size. For example, for human head imaging, FOV is usually 24 cm and data matrix 256 × 256. These parameters give in-plane resolution of 0.94 mm × 0.94 mm (FOV/matrix size = 0.94 mm). For a smaller object, say a finger, FOV may be 2 cm and matrix, 256 × 256, which gives an in-plane resolution of 78 μm × 78 μm.

The question arises: what are the limits of resolution? Couldn't we just increase the number of sampling points and phase encoding steps to increase the resolution indefinitely? Unfortunately, there is no simple answer, as there are important trade-offs that limit the resolution: signal-to-noise ratio (SNR), gradients strength, rf power, and diffusion. The limits of gradient strength and rf power are due to hardware limitations and subject safety (see Section 14), diffusion is a property of a living tissue, while SNR limit as associated with both physics and hardware.

The FOV and hence the image resolution limit due to the gradients strength is described by Nyquist theorem:

$$FOV \sim \frac{1}{G\Delta t} \tag{5.3}$$

where Δt is the sampling rate in the read direction or the duration of the phase gradient and G is the amplitude of the gradient. As can be seen from the equation, the FOV is inversely proportional to the gradient strength. The amplitude of the gradients is limited by the construction of the gradient coils, by the gradient amplifiers, and ultimately by safety concerns. Currently, gradient amplifiers producing 2 kV and a few hundred amperes are used to generate a 40-mT/m gradient in clinical systems, while smaller experimental MRI systems can provide a gradient stronger than 1000 mT/m, allowing resolution of about 10 μm. An additional safety issue in human systems is the regulatory limits on gradient rise time (dB/dt) imposed to avoid nerve stimulation.

Water molecules in biological objects move with the speed of about 2 μm/ms due to diffusion. This process is yet another limitation of the resolution in MRI, and in particular in MR microimaging, where resolution reaches 10 μm or even less. Diffusive motion in the presence of the strong and long gradient required for high resolution leads to signal loss from irreversible dephasing.

5.6 NOISE IN THE IMAGE—SNR

There are a few different definitions of SNR. In MRI, SNR is usually defined as the ratio of the averaged signal intensity over the imaged object (or part of it) to the average noise intensity, calculated over a small area outside the imaged object (i.e., noise background). It can also be defined as the ratio of the mean signal intensity within the imaged object to the standard deviation of the background noise selected outside the object. Both definitions describe how strong the signal is in relation to the noise. In MRS, SNR is usually defined as the ratio of the signal amplitude to the average baseline noise. Of course, the higher the SNR the better image quality, which in turn can allow higher resolution. Without high SNR, high resolution images, although technically feasible, cannot provide meaningful images. Frequently the term *Contrast-to-Noise Ratio* (CNR) is also used to describe image quality and its value in detecting pathology. CNR is a measure of the difference in contrast between two tissues, relative to overall SNR. CNR can be improved by the selection of proper parameters of the pulse sequence, to best emphasis the difference in relaxation times, as described in Section 5.7.

Quantum mechanics shows that the MR signal is proportional to the square of the strength of the main magnetic field ($S \sim B_0^2$) and to the number of spins, namely, the volume of the sample (20). The undesired noise comes from the random thermal motion of water (and other) molecules of the sample and electronic noise of the MR system, including the noise of the receiver coil and the preamplifier. Therefore, SNR depends on many factors such as the strength of the magnetic field, resistance and quality factor (Q) of the coil, its geometry, sample volume, filling factor of the coil, and so on.

Experience has lead to a rule of thumb that says that, if all other aspects of the experiment are held constant, SNR is proportional to the main magnetic field strength. This formula holds for human systems up to 3 T. The detail analysis of SNR was first presented by Hoult (25). A relatively easy way of improving SNR is multiple acquisitions of the same data. This is accomplished by repeating the pulse sequence with identical parameters and adding the collected data. This is called *repetition*, or averaging (N), or number of excitations (N_{ex}). It may be proved that SNR increases with the root square of the repetitions ($SNR \sim \sqrt{N}$). Because each repetition increases the total scan time twofold to double SNR requires a fourfold longer acquisition time, so this approach clearly has its practical limits. The linear relationship between the field strength and the SNR explains the tendency to introduce stronger magnets as an effective, yet expensive, way of increasing SNR.

5.7 IMAGE WEIGHTING AND PULSE SEQUENCE PARAMETERS TE AND TR

The signal induced by the magnetization in an rf coil is proportional to the number of excited protons in the imaged object, thus regions with higher PD exhibit a stronger signal. These signal differences can be observed using PD-weighted (PD or ρ) MRI; however in general, the variation in PD between healthy and diseased tissue is rather small. Fortunately for MRI's clinical diagnostic applications, there are better alternatives.

Abnormal tissues vary in a number of parameters including T_1, T_2 and T_2* relaxation times, also diffusion, blood flow, susceptibility, and various other effects that influence the MR signal in detectable ways.

While MRI does allow the precise quantification of these parameters, it is more common to use the "weighted" MR techniques. As an example, T_1-weighted imaging means that the image contrast is created mostly (although not entirely) based on the differences in T_1 values of the tissues. A similar terminology applies to T_2, PD, or Diffusion-Weighted (DW) MRI. In this way, tissues with generally rather similar proton densities but differing in some other tissue property can be better visualized (Fig. 5.15). For instance, cancerous tissues can be better identified using T_1 or T_2 than PD. So how is this achieved in practice?

5.7.1 T_2-Weighted Imaging

As explained in Section 5.2.3, the decay of the echo amplitudes in an SE pulse sequence depends on the T_2 relaxation time. Therefore, the longer the TE the lower the amplitude of the echo due to T_2 relaxation. For example, consider two tissues (Fig. 5.16): A with short T_2 (for example, fat or muscle tissue) and B with long T_2 (e.g., cyst or blood). If we chose a very short TE, little T_2 weighting will develop, and the difference in the amplitudes of echoes from both tissues will be small. However, if we use a longer TE (typically of the order of T_2 or longer), the difference in the echo amplitudes increase and become detectable. To totally avoid any T_1 contribution, TR must be rather long ($5T_1$ or longer).

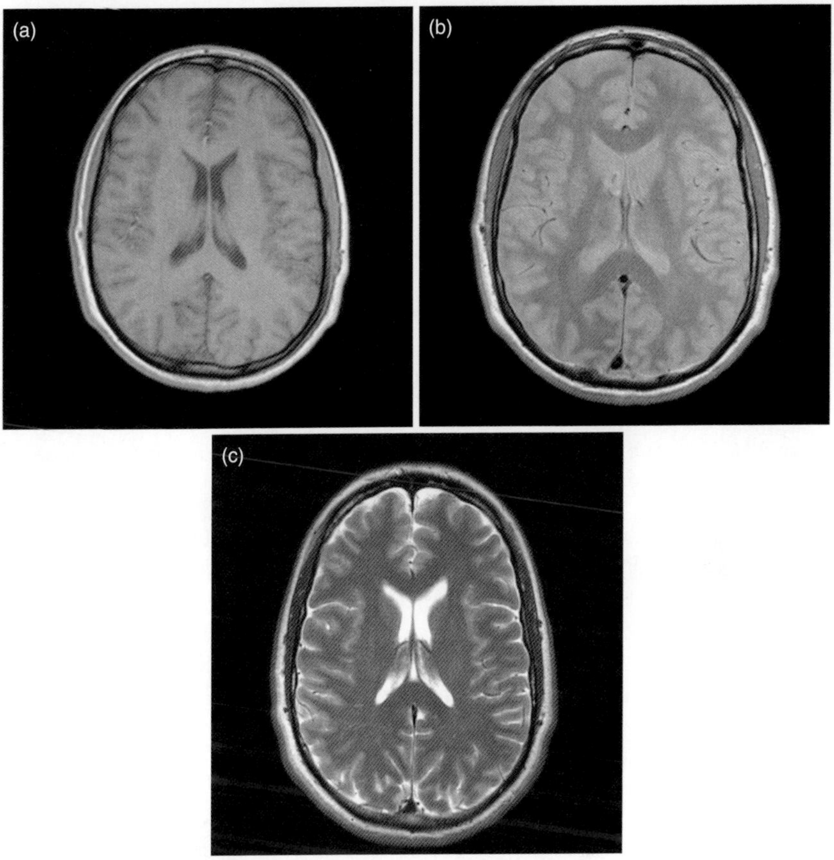

Figure 5.15. MR images of the brain. (a) T_1 weighted (GE pulse sequence: TR = 475 ms, TE = 2.46 ms; slice thickness 4 mm, FOV = 25 cm). (b) PD weighted (SE pulse sequence: TR = 3000 ms, TE = 20 ms, slice thickness 4 mm, FOV = 22 cm). (c) T_2 weighted (SE pulse sequence: TR = 6000 ms, TE = 90 ms, FOV = 22 cm; slice thickness 4 mm).

Because relaxation times depend on both the imaged tissue and the main magnetic field strength, the optimal TE and TR values parameters vary. However, the standard parameters for clinical T_2-weighted MRI are TE > 80 ms and TR > 2000 ms. A longer TR increases total scan time; therefore, often T_2-weighted images have some contribution of T_1. To avoid T_1 weighting, TR should be longer than 5 s, as T_1 of tissues is in the order of 0.5–2.0 s.

5.7.2 T_2*-Weighted Imaging

T_2*-weighted images can be obtained similarly; however, instead of an SE, a GE pulse sequence is used. To allow fast imaging, usually a small flip angle is applied. A low flip angle avoids T_1 weighting (even at short TR values) because

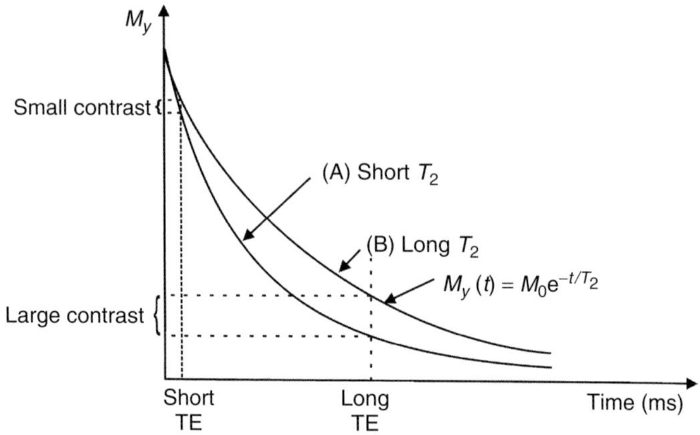

Figure 5.16. Return of magnetization after a 90° pulse in the y direction for tissues with (a) short T_2 and (b) long T_2.

the magnetization remains closely aligned along the z-axis. Of course, a lower flip angle decreases the SNR, as only part ($M_0 \sin\varphi$) of the available magnetization becomes transverse and thus detectable. The typical T_2*-weighted parameters for GE are TR = 100–500 ms, flip angle = 5–20°, and TE = 20–50 ms. Note that the TR and flip angle are coupled; smaller flip angle allows shorter TR, and larger flip angle requires longer TR to avoid T_1 contribution.

5.7.3 Proton-Density-Weighted Imaging

PD-weighted images can be obtained, in both SE and GE, using an as short as possible TE and long TR, to minimize both T_2 and T_1 weightings. Spins of each tissue have no time to relax in the x-y plane (short TE) but return to maximum value along the z direction (long TR). To obtain PD image using GE, typical parameters are TR > 300 ms, TE < 10 ms, and flip angle <10°.

5.7.4 T_1-Weighted Imaging

In T_1-weighted imaging, the contrast mostly depends on the T_1 values of tissues. To obtain a T_1-weighted image and avoid T_2 contribution, both TR and TE should be short. A short TR (order of 200–400 ms) allows only partial recovery of the net magnetization along the z direction. Therefore, fast relaxing (short T_1) tissues appear brighter. T_1-weighted images are usually used for anatomy. However, many tumors have T_1 values different from those of normal tissue; therefore, T_1 is also used for the detection of pathology.

5.8 A MENAGERIE OF PULSE SEQUENCES

MRI was established about 30 years ago, but hundreds of imaging techniques have since been invented. However, practically all of them are modifications of

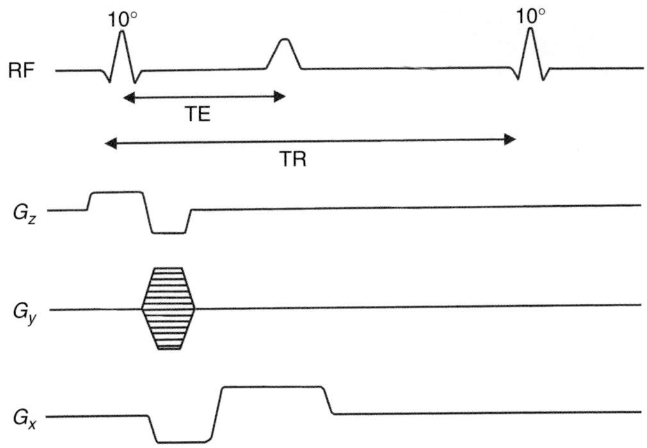

Figure 5.17. Gradient echo (GE) pulse sequence: TE, echo time; TR, repetition time; G_z, slice selection gradient; G_y, phase encoding gradient; G_x, frequency encoding gradient. The phase encoding gradient is repeated after the echo to destroy transverse magnetization before the next excitation.

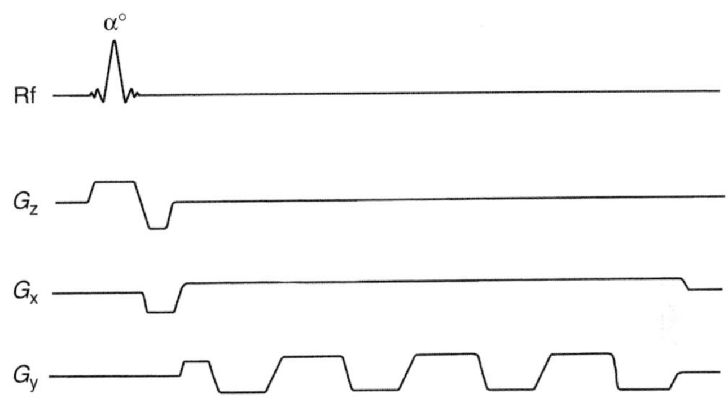

Figure 5.18. Gradient echo echo planar imaging (GE–EPI) pulse sequence: G_z, slice selection gradient; G_x, frequency encoding gradient, and G_y, phase encoding gradient.

SE, GE or Echo Planar Imaging (EPI). Since MR images are created using a series of gradient and rf pulses, this has led to imaging techniques known as *pulse sequences*.

Both SE (Fig. 5.17) and GE (Fig. 5.18) pulse sequences require spins to be excited multiple times.

The application of a single low flip angle pulse per repetition in GE allows the collection of an image in the order of a few seconds, which is much faster than SE. The first description of GE, including an application of the gradients and low flip angles to obtain a fast image was presented by Hasse in 1989 (26) and called *FLASH* (Fast Low Angle Shot). This sequence uses so-called spoiling gradients and/or rf spoiling (27) after the acquisition of the echo to destroy the transverse magnetization before the next excitation. When balanced (refocusing) gradients instead of spoiling gradients are used to keep magnetization tilted by the same angle throughout the pulse sequence using the series of rf pulses, the sequences are the so-called Steady-State Free Precession (SSFP) (28). Pulse sequences based on SSFP are, for example, Gradient Refocused Acquisition in the Steady-State (GRASS) or Fast Imaging with Steady-State Precession (FISP or True-FISP) (29, 30). FISP is more sensitive to T_2 than the standard GE pulse sequence, which is mostly T_2* sensitive.

5.8.1 EPI

The fastest MRI technique, *echo planar imaging* (EPI), was first introduced by Mansfield in 1977 (31). In the standard version of this technique (single-shot GE-EPI), spins are excited only once (Fig. 5.18), which allows an MR image to be obtained within 50–100 ms. Because GE is used, this pulse sequence is T_2* or PD (very short TE) weighted. Very short TE (order of 2–5 ms) can be used. This technique uses low rf power (low flip angle) and very rapidly switching gradients, which create significant acoustic noise due to the gradient coil vibrations. Because the spins are excited only once, there must be enough echo signal available throughout the entire sequence. Therefore, very good shimming of the magnetic field to prolong T_2* has to be achieved before the execution of the sequence, as the amplitude of echoes decreases with T_2*. The T_2* decay also reduces the resolution of EPI in comparison to SE or GE. The image resolution can be increased using multiple-shot EPI, but at the expense of an increased scan time. Since in EPI, spins are excited only once (single-shot EPI), EPI is T_2 (SE-EPI) or T_2* (GE-EPI) weighted. There is also some PD weighting that depends on the TE value; the shorter the TE the more PD weighting and less T_2 and vice versa: longer TE, more T_2 and less PD weighting.

To reduce T_2* decay effect and the noise generated by the gradient coils, so-called spiral EPI (32) was introduced. The sequence uses sinusoidal gradient waveforms with increasing amplitude in phase and read directions, that creates a spiral trajectory in the k-space (hence the name).

The modification of EPI, SE-EPI, uses 90° and 180° pulses followed by switching gradients as shown in Figure 5.19. In this way, T_2 weighting is introduced to EPI.

5.8.2 FSE

Another commonly used pulse sequence is the *Fast Spin Echo* (FSE), which uses a series of 90°–180°–180°–180°–... selective rf pulses, similar to the CPMG pulse sequence (Fig. 5.10), along with the appropriate gradients. Each 180° pulse allows collection of an SE, which thus speeds up the acquisition. For instance, for an Echo Train Length (ETL) of 8, only $256/8 = 32$ repetitions are needed, instead of 256. FSE is very significant clinically because it allows strong T_2

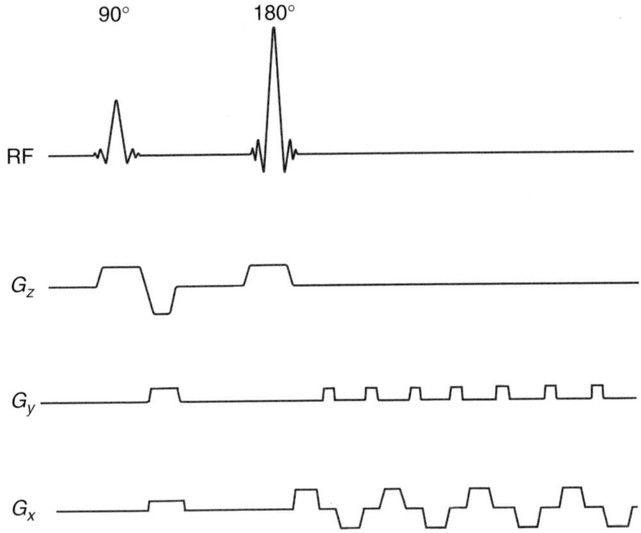

Figure 5.19. Spin echo echo planar imaging (SE-EPI) pulse sequence: G_z, slice selection gradient; G_y, phase encoding gradient; and G_x, frequency encoding gradient.

weighting in a short acquisition time. Recall that for SE both long TR and TE are required for T_2 weighting—this is slow. FSE can achieve a very long TE for the later echoes in the train, and also a very long TR, as the number of repetitions is reduced by the factor ETL, decreasing the overall acquisition time drastically.

5.8.3 Inversion-Recovery

Inversion Recovery (IR) is an alternative method for the introduction of T_1 image weighting. It involves the application of a 180° inversion pulse before the imaging sequence (Fig. 5.20), followed by a variable interval called the *Inversion Time* (TI). The effect of the inversion pulse is to flip all spins to the $-z$ axis. The spins then relax back toward the $+z$ axis with time constant T_1. At some point, they must pass though the origin, that is, zero M_z. This is known as the *null point*. If the 90° excitation pulse (for any sequence) is applied at this point in time, then spins at the null will not be excited and will appear black in the image. In this way, unwanted signal (e.g., from tissue A) can be suppressed. In practice, tissue A is usually blood or fat.

There are many combinations of IR with other imaging techniques. Fast inversion recovery is a combination of IR and FSE and allows T_1 and/or T_2 weighting depending on the selected parameters. STIR (Short Ti Inversion Recovery) is used mostly for fat suppression and applies short TI (100–200 ms) to null the signal from fat, as TI is comparable to fat's T_1. To suppress signal from fluids that have long relaxation times ($\sim$2 s), such as Cerebrospinal Fluid (CSF), TI corresponding to T_1 of CSF is selected. Therefore, a pulse sequence with a long

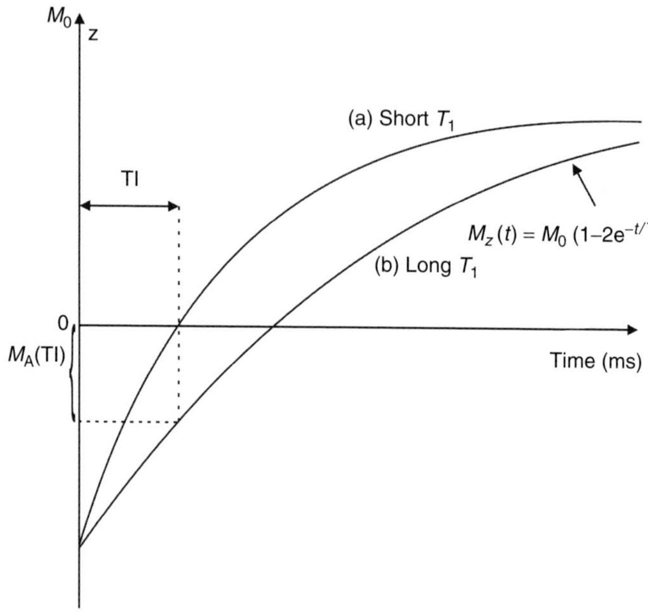

Figure 5.20. Return of magnetization after 180° pulse for the tissue with short (A) and long (B) T_1. Magnetization after inversion time (TI) for tissue with short T_1 is zero ($M_A(T_I) = 0$), but there is a net magnetization for tissue with long $T_1 : M_B(T_I) \neq 0$. An imaging sequence may start after time TI to avoid signal from tissue A.

TI (over 1500–2500 ms) called *Fluid Attenuated Inversion Recovery* (FLAIR) (33–36) is frequently used for brain and spinal cord imaging to null bright CSF.

5.8.4 DWI

In some diseases, for example, stroke, water diffusion is reduced because of cell swelling and their disruption; therefore, *diffusion-weighted* (DW) MRI is often used (37, 38). DW-MRI can be added to most standard pulse sequences by adding diffusion-sensitizing gradients along one or more directions (depending on the application). The principle is that if a pair of gradients is used, first a dephase gradient, followed after a delay by a rephase gradient, then all static spins will see no net effect. However, moving spins will be at different locations for the two pulses, so will not fully rephase. For random motion (i.e., diffusion), this results in signal loss due to the partially randomized spin phases. The signal reduction depends on the diffusion speed of the spins, amplitude, and duration of the gradients. To obtain stronger diffusion weighting, stronger and/or longer duration gradients must be used.

For SE sequences, DW is implemented by adding two identical gradient pulses, one before and one after the 180° pulse. For GE sequences, a positive polarity pulse is followed by a negative polarity one. Areas of reduced diffusion, such as stroke, appear bright in DW-MRI.

While standard DW-MRI techniques suffer from motion artifacts, the recent application of fast imaging (EPI) along with high magnetic field (3 T and above) can generate fast, high quality DW-MRI. Moreover, multiple diffusion weightings in different directions can be measured to study the directionality of diffusion. The three gradients x, y, z may be combined to create a gradient along combined directions, for example, x-z or x-y. This is the basis of Diffusion Tensor Imaging (DTI) technique, which shows diffusion coefficients in nine directions. Because neurons exhibit faster diffusion along the nerve fibers that surround tissues, points along the maximum diffusion can be connected in three dimensions, using a software program, to create fiber tracking MRI showing spatial distribution of neuronal tissues in brain and recently in spinal cord (Fig. 5.21).

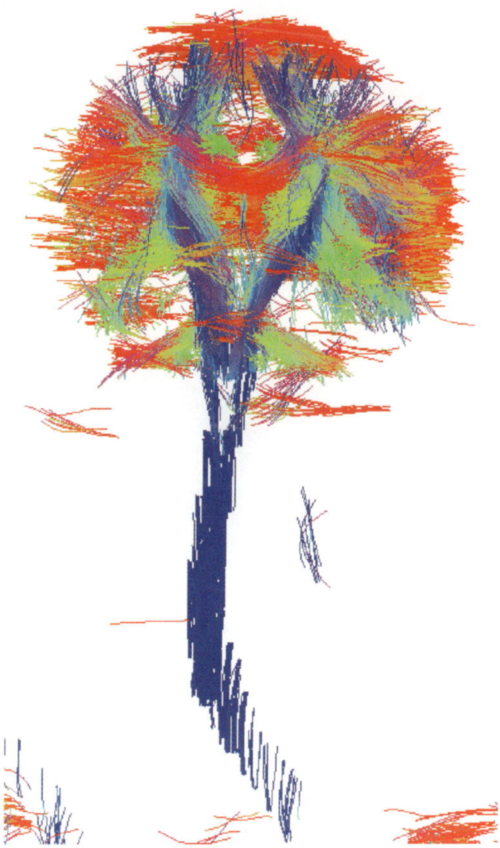

Figure 5.21. Fiber tracts of the human brain and cervical spinal cord. Red color represents fibers running left-right, green represents fibers running anterior-posterior, and blue represents fiber tracts running inferior-superior (3 Tesla Siemens Trio, IBD/NRC, Winnipeg, MB, Canada).

5.8.5 MRA

The ability of MRI to measure flow (39) is used in *Magnetic Resonance Angiography* (MRA) to visualize vasculature, arteries and veins (Fig. 5.22) (40, 41). There are two basic MR methods that make MRI flow sensitive: Time of Flight (TOF) (42, 43) and Phase-Contrast (PC) MRA (44, 45).

TOF MRA usually uses a GE pulse sequence with short TR and TE. It uses to its advantage the fresh, full magnetization flowing into the imaged slice, which is larger than the magnetization of the stationary spins. The short TR (shorter than T_1 of the stationary tissue) does not allow the stationary spin to fully recover; therefore, fresh, in-flowing spins have a stronger signal and appear bright.

PC MRA is accomplished by including bipolar gradients in the pulse sequence: a pair of gradients of the same amplitude but opposite direction is applied one after another. Such gradients affect only the phase of moving spins. This technique, unlike TOF MRA, is sensitive to both incoming spins and spins flowing within the imaged area.

There are 2D and 3D versions of MRA. To obtain a 3D image of blood vessels, a postprocessing method called *Maximum Intensity Projection* (MIP) is used. The MIP method combines multislice 2D data into one 3D data set by assuming that the strongest signal comes from the vessels. Multiple projections of only the areas of maximum signal (41) onto the image are performed, creating a 3D image of blood vessels. This 3D dataset can then be visualized from different angles by rotation.

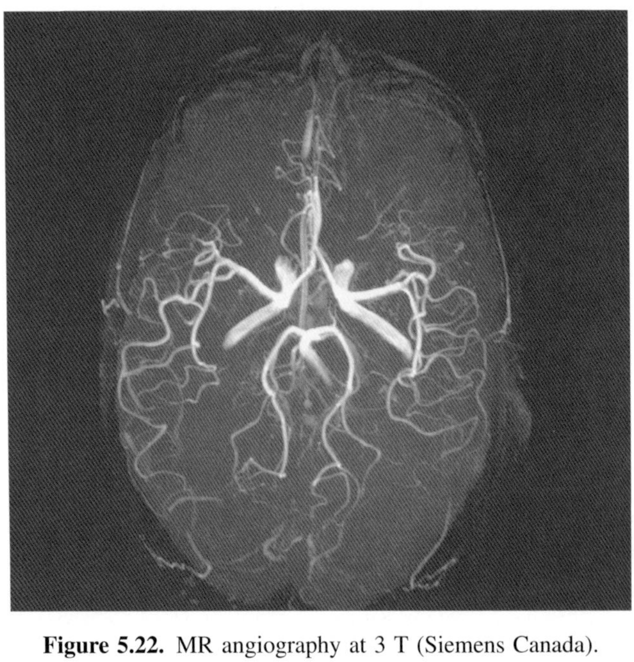

Figure 5.22. MR angiography at 3 T (Siemens Canada).

To improve the quality of MRA, contrast agents to reduce T_1 of the blood are often used, allowing short TR and increasing the blood signal. This technique is called *contrast-enhanced MRA* (46).

5.8.6 Perfusion

An MRI technique called *perfusion MRI* allows the measurement of cerebral (or other) blood volume (CBV). The technique uses a short T_2 intravenous bolus injection (e.g., Gd based) along with a fast T_2 or T_2* pulse sequence. The flowing contrast agent causes a transient decrease in the signal from the blood vessels. Data postprocessing analyzes the decay in the signal with time to calculate the volume and speed of the blood. This information is particularly useful in ischemia or in diseases causing metabolic disorders.

Other MRI techniques, still under development, allow for temperature and elastic properties of the tissue to be imaged.

5.9 ENHANCED DIAGNOSTIC CAPABILITIES OF MRI—CONTRAST AGENTS

Abnormal tissues are observed with MRI mostly because of their different relaxation times in comparison to healthy tissues. However, the differences are often too small to be readily detectable. To increase the difference, and thus improve CNR, agents that decrease T_1 and/or T_2 are used. They decrease the tissue proton relaxation times because of their paramagnetic properties, which cause enhanced magnetic field fluctuations in their vicinity, which act to increase proton relaxation. Contrast agents are injected intravenously (~0.1 mmol/kg). Because tumors have better vasculature than the surrounding tissue, the density of contrast agents is higher within the tumor. This causes a stronger decrease in the relaxation times within the tumor and results in better tumor contrast. Contrast agents are also particularly useful in the diagnosis of CNS tumors, as they pass through the ruptures in the Blood–Brain Barrier (BBB).

The most common contrast agents are gadolinium(Gd) based. Because Gd ions are toxic if used without a shell, chelates, such as Diethylene Triaminepentaacetic Acid (DTPA), are used to ensure Gd biocompatibility. Gd-DTPA shortens mostly T_1. Other contrast agents, such as iron oxide, shorten T_2.

5.10 MOLECULAR MRI

Experimental MRI systems using very high fields (9.4 T and above) allow imaging with in-plane resolution below 20 μm (47, 48). Nonetheless, even this resolution does not allow for true *in vivo* observation of single cells or molecules. Standard human MRI allows detection of tumors of the order of millimeters in diameter (~10^8 cells) but no smaller.

However, the recent developments in nanotechnology and molecular biology (49, 50) have allowed this limit to be overcome, and cellular or even molecular MRI was recently established. Molecular MRI uses strong paramagnetic or superparamagnetic Nanoparticles (NPs) (such as FeCo nanocrystals) that decrease relaxation times more than standard contrast agents (such as Gd-DTPA). Biologically active entities such as stem cells or antibodies can then be labeled with these NPs and be tracked with MRI. Owing to their strong paramagnetic properties, even small amounts of NPs can allow imaging of small numbers of specific cells, targeted by the appropriate biological vehicles. The development of this method allows the detection of cancer and other diseases at a very early stage, which is extremely important to achieve successful treatment. In addition, NPs used in MRI can also be synthesized with a shell that can be detected with other imaging modalities, such as infrared spectroscopy (Chapter 9), expanding MRI into multimodal diagnostic imaging (49). A very recent study showed that it may also be possible to not only diagnose the disease but also treat by thermoablation of the abnormal tissues using rf-generated heat absorbed by certain types of NPs (51–53) attached to the target.

5.11 READING THE MIND—FUNCTIONAL MRI

Functional Magnetic Resonance Imaging (fMRI) is a technique that has introduced imaging into new areas of neuroscience, psychology, and clinical applications. fMRI allows for noninvasive, indirect observation of the neuronal activity in the brain (54) and, very recently, in the spinal cord (55, 56). With fMRI, it is possible to dynamically image blood oxygenation levels during the synaptic activity. This mechanism is called *Blood Oxygen Level Dependent* (BOLD) MRI and was first observed with MRI in 1990 by Ogawa et al. (57). Deoxyhemoglobin (a paramagnetic substance) shortens T_2* (and to a lesser extent T_2). During brain activation, the amount of oxyhemoglobin increases and deoxyhemoglobin decreases, increasing T_2*, detectable as an increase in GE signal intensity. Since the changes in the signal intensity are rather small (2–5%), in order to increase the statistics, an fMRI study usually comprises 2–3 rest and 2 active periods. This pattern of stimulation is called the *paradigm*. Therefore, subjects under fMRI examination are requested to repeat the task (e.g., finger tapping or a mental task) two or more times. During the fMRI experiments, serial MR images are obtained continuously and at as high a rate as possible. Statistical analysis (58) of the collected images is used to determine voxels of *activation*, by correlating their signal intensity changes over time with the paradigm. The paradigm for the correlation analysis is usually designed as a ramped step increase/decrease in signal intensity when the stimulation comes on and off during the experiment. Voxels undergoing signal intensity changes that correlate with the defined paradigm (with a correlation coefficient threshold of $p \leq 0.01$ or better) are assumed to represent regions of neuronal activation corresponding to the applied stimulation. The activated voxels are then overlaid with a color

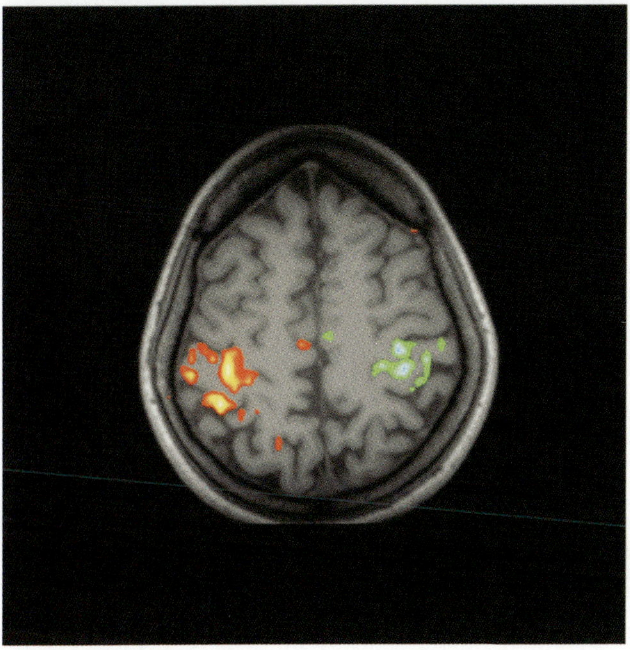

Figure 5.23. fMRI image showing areas of neuronal activity caused by a movement of the left (red) and right (yellow) hands.

scale corresponding to level or correlation to the paradigm, onto high resolution anatomical images (Fig. 5.23). To optimize fMRI sensitivity to T_2* relaxation, GE or EPI pulse sequences are used with TE $\approx T_2$* (about 30 ms at 1.5 T).

There are other possible mechanisms that may also be involved in fMRI based on changes in diffusion (59) and extravascular proton content (60) during neuronal activation.

5.12 MAGNETIC RESONANCE SPECTROSCOPY

MR spectroscopy (MRS) represents a whole new dimension to biological MR. Historically, MRS (or NMR spectroscopy) preceded MRI as a simpler technique *ex vivo* and found an application in biochemistry in the 1960s. Spectroscopy provides information about the chemical composition of the object studied.

As mentioned in Section 5.2, the Larmor frequency (frequency of the spins rotating in the magnetic field) depends on the strength of the external field. Electrons orbiting the nucleus shift the main field by a few parts per million (ppm). Thus, the frequency of the nuclei depends on the local electron environment, that is, on the position of the nuclei within the molecule, in other words, on the chemistry. For this reason, this effect is called *chemical shift* (δ), and it is the principle that gives MRS the ability to locate MR-sensitive atoms within

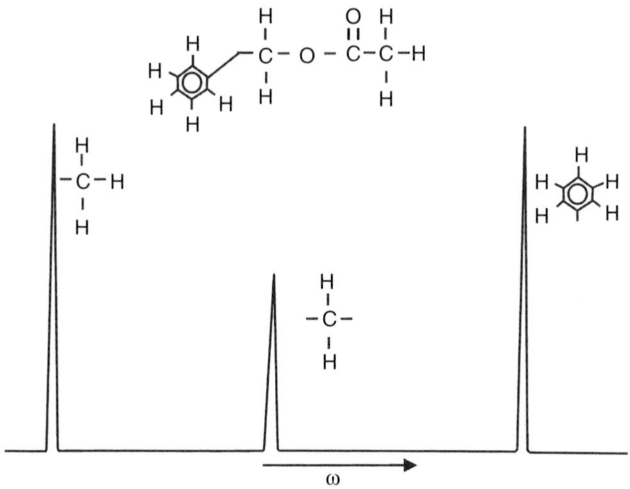

Figure 5.24. MR spectrum of benzyl acetate. The peaks correspond to different positions of ^{1}H in the compound.

a molecule. Because each compound has a unique chemical structure, its MR spectra can be used for identification. For example, the spectra of benzyl acetate $C_6H_5CH_2COOCH_3$ (Fig. 5.24) reveals three peaks corresponding to the three different proton locations within the compound. The amplitude of the peaks corresponds to the number of protons within the compound. Note the smaller peak in Figure 5.24 from CH_2 (two protons), relative to CH_3 (three protons).

In vitro MR spectra are obtained by applying an rf pulse (usually nonselective 90°), followed by FT of the collected data. No gradients are required. The stronger the external field, the easier it is to separate peaks in the spectra, therefore the use of strong magnets (up to about 20 T) for high resolution spectroscopy. Critical, however, is making the main field as homogenous as possible (so-called shimming), as the FID decreases faster with the field inhomogeneities and the spectral signals (lines) become broader and overlap. To be able to identify spectra independently of the strength of the external field, chemical shift (δ) is expressed in ppm as $\delta = \frac{\omega_{\text{nuclei}} - \omega_{\text{calib}}}{\omega_0}$, where ω_{calib} is the Larmor frequency of the external marker (usually water) and ω_0 is the frequency of the spectrometer.

MR spectra used as a "fingerprint" of a compound allows identification of metabolites and monitoring of metabolic processes in tissues. As the content and the ratio of specific metabolites, such as choline, creatine, N-acetyl-aspartate (NAA), glucose, or lactate, change with pathology (e.g., in cancer or stroke), MRS can be used to identify the disease (61) or its stage. The same principles apply to other NMR nuclei; however, their MR sensitivity is usually lower than ^{1}H, thus a longer acquisition time is needed to collect valuable data. Of particular interest is phosphorus (^{31}P), which is important in energy storage and energy exchange processes within cells. For example, ^{31}P MRS shows changes in the ratio between Phosphocreatine (PCr) and Inorganic Phosphate (Pi) during muscle exercise, as well as the shift in the peaks frequency due to changes in pH (62). The ratio PCr/Pi can be diagnostic, as it varies in certain diseases (64).

5.12.1 Single Voxel Spectroscopy

Single voxel localized MRS allows the collection of MR spectra from a selected region of interest (voxel) within a patient. To define the voxel, three selective pulses, along with slice selection gradients, are applied in three directions. The signal is collected from the spins in the intersection of the three planes. The two most common of these methods are Stimulated Echo Acquisition Mode (STEAM) and Point Resolved Spectroscopy (PRESS). STEAM uses stimulated echoes to collect the data (63, 64). PRESS uses SEs and results in double the signal strength in comparison to STEAM (65).

MRS requires very good field shimming before the collection of data. An example of an *in vivo* spectrum from a selected voxel at 9.4 T is shown in Figure 5.25. In practice, because spectral resolution and SNR increases with the field, MRS benefits greatly from higher field strengths (3 T or higher); however; it is not uncommon to see good spectra at 1.5 T.

5.12.2 Spectroscopic Imaging

An interesting combination of MRS and MRI is MR Spectroscopic Imaging (SI or MRS imaging) or Chemical Shift Imaging (CSIs). SI shows the spectra from each voxel (usually 16 × 16 or 32 × 32) overlaid on anatomical MR images. In this way, observations of differences in metabolite content between, for example, left and right hemispheres, or abnormal spectra in dubious areas, can be made and used for enhanced diagnosis. A disadvantage of SI is the long time required

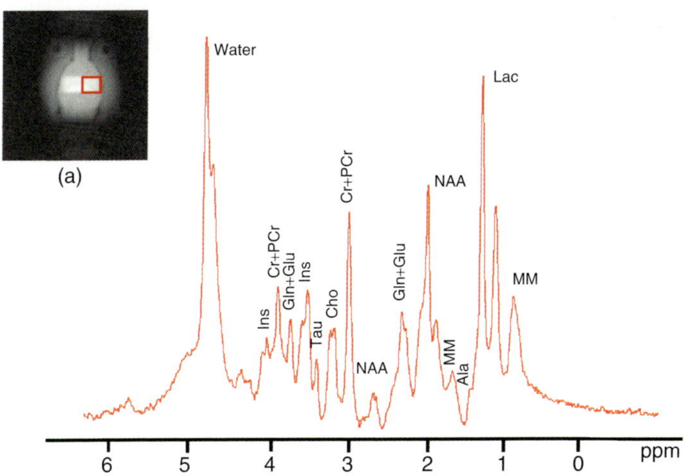

Figure 5.25. MR spectrum of metabolites from VOI shown in (a) at 9.4 T using STEAM.

to collect data from all, usually small (~5 mm × 5 mm × 5 mm), voxels. The distribution of a selected metabolite within the subject may be displayed as an image. This is achieved by selecting a particular peak of the spectrum from each voxel, calculating the total area under that peak and assigning a pixel intensity or color at each point.

5.13 MR HARDWARE

To the patient, CT and MRI systems look much alike—resembling a tube or ring. However, this is the only similarity between the techniques, as both the principles and equipment are very different.

As described in the previous sections, to obtain an MR image, an external static, variable magnetic gradients, rf field, data acquisition, and postprocessing are all needed. To achieve all this, each MRI system consists of a set of subsystems with distinct functions: magnet and shim system, gradient system, rf system, and the user interface and control system. Alternatively, the system can be broken down by physical assemblies: magnet, gradient coils, rf coils, power amplifiers, and console. The schematic diagram of an MRI system is shown in Figure 5.26. The components are described in detail by Chen and Hoult (66).

5.13.1 Magnets

The basic parameters of a magnet are the *strength* of the magnetic field (expressed in tesla (SI) or Gauss; 1 T = 10,000 Gs), the *homogeneity* of the field within the Volume of Interest (VOI) (ppm over Diameter of Spherical Volume (DSV)),

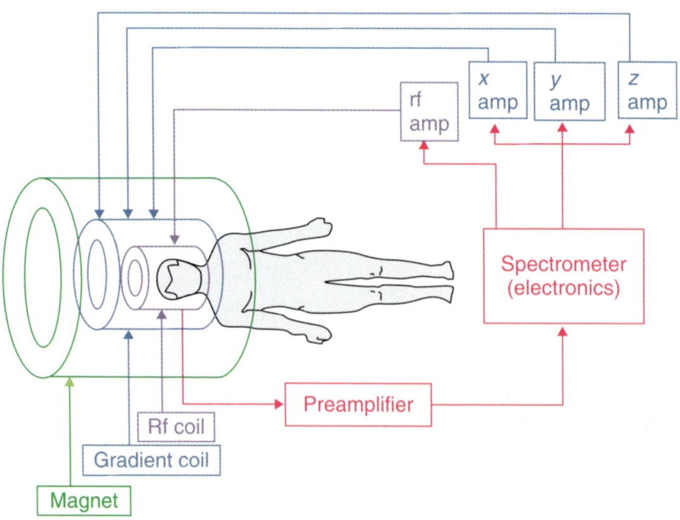

Figure 5.26. Schematic of major components of an MRI system.

and the *fringe field* that describes the distribution of the field around the magnet. The edge of the fringe field is usually defined at the 5 Gs line. This denotes the distance from the center of the magnet to the location where the field has fallen to 5 Gs.

MR magnets must generate a field stronger than 0.1 T. Currently, most clinical systems generate 1.5 T. However, human 3 T magnet systems, which recently obtained FDA approval, are more and more common. Seven-tesla whole-body magnets are used in human research systems, and even higher field whole-body systems are under construction. Experimental animal systems, with a magnet bore of 30 cm or less, are usually equipped with magnets of 4.7 T (200 MHz), 7 T (300 MHz), 9.4 T (400 MHz), and 11.7 T (500 MHz) (Fig. 5.27), whereas stronger (14 T) magnets are under construction. Magnets generating a magnetic field of 20 T or above are used for *ex vivo* MRS. Stronger magnets are not common yet not only due to the technical challenges associated with the construction of magnet but also due to safety issues. There are three types of magnets used in MRI depending on the manufacturing process: permanent, electromagnets, and superconductive.

The majority of human and all high field experimental MRI systems are equipped with *superconductive magnets*. These can produce very stable and strong magnetic fields up to about 20 T. Their shape usually resembles a vertical (Fig. 5.27a) or horizontal (Fig. 5.27b) cylinder. All human and most animal MRI systems are horizontal. The most important geometric parameter of the superconductive magnet is the diameter of its inner tube ("the bore") of the magnet. Shimming coils, gradients coils, and body rf coils (in humans systems) are placed within the bore of the magnet.

Construction of superconductive magnets became possible following the discovery of the phenomenon of superconductors, which carry electrical current without any resistance. Superconductive materials (e.g., alloy niobium–titanium)

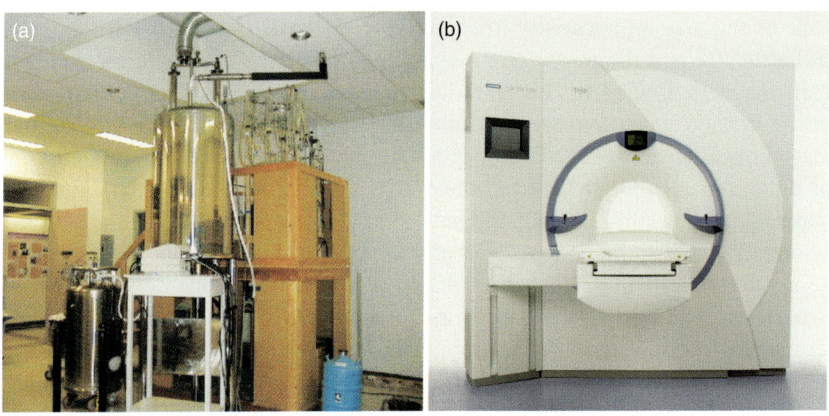

Figure 5.27. Vertical experimental 11.7-T MRI system (IBD/NRC), magnet (Magnex Scientific, England), and console (Bruker, Germany). (b) 3-T Siemens Trio MRI system.

have no resistance at a very low temperature (~4 K). Superconductive magnets are made of many turns of superconductive solenoidal wire, submersed in liquid helium at its boiling point of a temperature of 4.2 K (−269°C). The magnet is charged with an electrical current of hundreds of amperes into the superconductive wire. As long as the wire is submersed in liquid helium, the current remains constant—forever. To prevent excessive boiling, the liquid helium is separated from the warm air in the magnet room with layers of liquid nitrogen (77K = −196°C) and vacuum. Most magnets produced before the year 2000 require filling with liquid hydrogen every 5–6 weeks and with liquid helium every few months. However, most twenty-first century magnets are equipped with helium cryocoolers, thus liquid nitrogen is not required. Should the liquid helium level become too low, the magnet may disastrously and expensively "quench," as the wire temperature becomes too high to sustain superconductivity. The wire becomes resistive, generating a large amount of heat, causing rapid helium boiling and evaporation. So each system must be also equipped with a fat quench line to vent the helium gas outside to prevent oxygen depletion in the magnet room.

Human superconductive 1.5- and 3-T magnets, with bore diameter of about 1 m, despite so-called active shielding (superconductive wires around the main wire restraining the outside field), have a rather large fringe field: the 5-Gs line extends about 2–4 m from the center of the magnet. This can be a distinct siting issue for 3-T magnets in particular. At the time of writing, large bore magnets over 4 T are not actively shielded; thus, their fringe field is much larger (order of 10 m). In that case, an iron cage around the magnet is often used to reduce the fringe field. The price for the MRI system based on a superconductive magnet is roughly \$1M per 1 T, that is, a 1.5-T system costs about \$1.5M.

Permanent magnets are constructed with hundreds of brick-shaped (about 5 cm × 5 cm × 10 cm each), very strong permanent magnets, supported by a steel structure with high magnetic permeability, which becomes part of the magnetic circuit. The small magnets are made of iron-rare-earth elements (Nd-Fe-B). The shape of the magnet is usually four post (Fig. 5.28) or C-shaped. The supporting steel structure and the posts (or the arm) shape the magnetic field created by the small magnets. Owing to the open design, children and claustrophobic patients can be imaged with less stress. Motion of joints (e.g., knee) can also be easily imaged because of the legroom afforded by the open design. The maximum field for human imaging is 0.35 T, so the acquisition time required to obtain an MR image of 1.5-T quality is much longer. However, for many practical applications, the exquisite 1.5-T image quality is unnecessary, and permanent magnet systems are a viable alternative. Recent advantages in pulse sequence development such as parallel imaging, allowing decrease of the acquisition time, however, make permanent magnets more appealing. The fringe field is very small, and a 5-Gs line is usually about 0.5 m from the magnet's edge. Permanent magnets are maintenance free, as they require no power supply or cryogens to operate; however, their weight is about 10 tonnes (10,000 kg). As the field strength of permanent magnets drifts down with increasing temperature, thermal stabilization

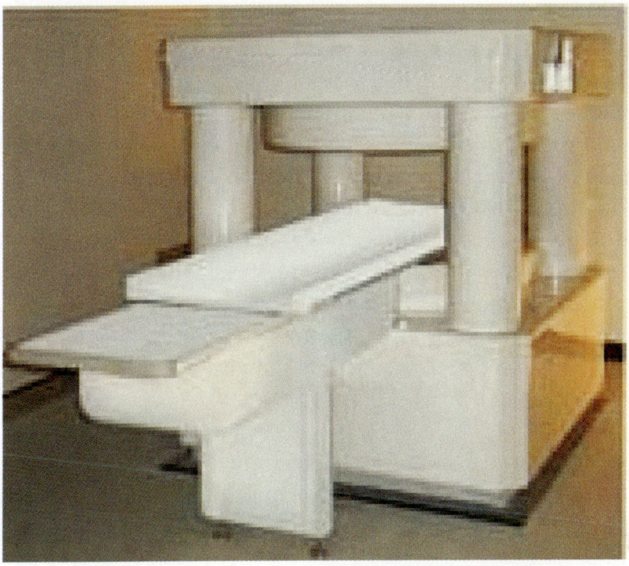

Figure 5.28. A 0.2T four-post MRI system (MRI-Tech, Canada).

(about $\pm 1^{\circ}$C) or field drift compensation systems are required in the magnet room. Modern air conditioning systems can easily meet this requirement. Field compensation system, called B_0 *compensation*, is also simple to implement by using an additional pair of circular wires on magnet poles.

Electromagnets (resistive magnets) are rather uncommon in MRI. They use conductive wires to produce the magnetic field and generate fields up to 0.5 T. They require huge amounts of electrical power provided by a water-cooled power supply. As small variations in the wire current cause changes in both the field strength and homogeneity, dedicated field stabilization systems are needed. Short-term instabilities can be dealt with by flux stabilizers, while long-term drift is minimized using additional field coils.

5.13.2 Shimming

Shimming is the process of fine-tuning the magnet field uniformity. There are three methods: passive, active with resistive coils, and active with superconductive coils.

The use of iron pieces for shimming is called *passive shimming* and is used for shimming to about 10 ppm. Washer-like iron pieces of about 1-cm diameter are placed on both poles of the magnet in very specific locations, as determined by computerized field analysis.

For high field human MRI, the homogeneity should be about 10 ppm over 30–50 cm DSV, while for MRS, local homogeneity should be in the order of 1 ppm over a voxel volume. (It can be proved that for MRS the variation in field frequency should not be larger than $1/\pi T_2$ over the sample volume (67).)

Although superconductive magnets produce highly uniform fields, homogeneity improvement of the field is often needed. Passive shimming, using iron pieces placed on the inner surface of the bore of the magnet, is used. Superconductive wires (cryoshims) submersed in liquid helium are also used in some magnets for active shimming. The shims are charged after the main wire is charged.

As a sample or a subject changes the magnetic field because of their magnetic properties, additional shimming is often needed before each imaging session. This fine shimming is accomplished by resistive, Room Temperature (RT) shims. These shims are usually incorporated into the gradient coils on their external surface. As each field can be mathematically expressed in spherical harmonics, the process of shimming aims at the minimization of specific harmonics, denoted as x, y, z, $2xy$, $z^2 - y^2$, and so on. RT shims are particularly useful in MRS and multiecho pulses (such as GE-EPI), as they are very sensitive to any field inhomogeneity.

A permanent magnet has a "raw" homogeneity of about 300–500 ppm over 30–50 cm DSV. Passive shimming allows improvement of homogeneity to about 10 ppm. Of course, there are no cryoshims available for permanent or electromagnets.

5.13.3 Rf Shielding

The NMR signal is very weak, so the magnet is placed in an rf-shielded room to prevent any external rf interferences that could cause spurious signals to be detected by the system. The shielding efficiency should be about 100 dB. There must be special conductive doors installed to make sure that the room is "rf sealed" during imaging. All cables coming into and out of the magnet room must go through an rf filter panel to block unwanted signals, while nonconductive tubes may go through waveguides that prevent rf leakage.

5.13.4 Gradient System

Gradients provide spatial information in MRI. The gradient system consists of: waveform generation, gradient power amplifiers, high power cables and filters, and finally the gradient coils within the magnet. To generate a time-variable gradient, needed for spatial spin encoding, the magnetic field gradient coils are made of resistive wires overlaid on the surface of a fibreglass tube. As three perpendicular gradients are needed, usually six layers of wire are used: three inner layers generating gradients within the VOI and three layers used as a magnetic shield to prevent eddy currents being induced in the cryostat. Of course, each layer must be electrically separated and water or air cooling must be provided, as large currents are generated when gradients are working. The gradients are wired on the surface of a fibreglass tube and immobilized and electrically separated with an epoxy resin or a similar substance. The tube is then placed inside the bore of the magnet. Important parameters of the gradients coils are linearity over VOI, efficiency, maximum strength, and rise time or slew rate. The linearity defines how constant the gradient is over the VOI (usually better than 5%). This is a very important parameter, as any deviation from linearity distorts an image. The maximum gradient produced by the gradient coils can be calculated by multiplying the coil efficiency (in mT/m/A) by the maximum current provided by gradient amplifiers. Modern MRI clinical systems provide a maximum gradient of about 40 mT/m, while experimental MR systems provide gradients over 1000 mT/m. Gradient amplifiers generate hundreds of amperes and hundred of volts. Minimum rise time is the minimum time required to achieve maximum gradient amplitude. This time varies from system to system and depends on inductance and resistance of the coil and the gradient amplifiers used. In clinical systems, minimum rise times vary from 100–500 μs, while it is less than 100 μs in experimental MR systems. Another frequently used parameter is the *slew rate*, which combines maximum gradients strength and their rise times, expressed in mT/m/s.

5.13.5 MR Electronics—The Console

The rack of low power electronics and the computers used to run the system is termed the *console*. A typical breakdown of a console would be into a Graphical User Interface (GUI), a synchronous high speed control assembly, and a low speed asynchronous control assembly.

The main tasks of the high speed synchronous control are to generate the gradient, rf, and timing waveforms and to acquire and digitize the NMR signals. Modern systems may have a large number of receiver channels, such as 32. Low speed control is used for tasks such as configuration of gains, switches, shim currents, temperature monitoring, and so on.

There is no console standardization in the industry—each major and minor manufacturer, both clinical and otherwise, have their own designs. Thus, it can be a major task to transfer experience from one to another. On the bright side, however, all clinical manufacturers do comply to a standard clinical image data format (DICOM).

The three largest commercial suppliers of human MRI systems are GE, Siemens, and Philips. Two major suppliers of experimental MRIs are Bruker and Varian. There are many smaller suppliers around the world.

Most commercial MR consoles are based on dedicated and sophisticated computers. However, recent progress in personal computers allowed their application to MRI. A few smaller commercial suppliers (e.g., ONI Corp, Maran (Oxford Instruments)) and even research institutions have created systems based on PCs. For example, the National Research Council of Canada has designed a console system that integrates simulation of the MR experiment with the acquisition of experimental data. The device consists of a magnetic resonance (MR) research console with a full-function hardware-independent pulse programming environment and a parallel computer cluster running Bloch equation MR physics simulations on a 3D digitally defined spin phantom. The system is designed to allow precise side-by-side comparisons of experimental against theoretical predictions for real world, complex pulse sequences and is in operation on both 0.2T and 9.4 T systems (67).

5.13.6 Rf Coils

The rf coils (rf probes) generate the rf (B_1) pulse fields and receive the MR signals. The basic construction principles are simple, based on the L-C resonance circuit. There are transmit (T_X)-only, receive (R_X)-only, and combined transmit and receive (T_X/R_X) rf coils. Most clinical systems are equipped with a T_X-only large rf coil (body rf coil) and a selection of local R_X-only coils. The parameters of the rf coil are B_1 (rf) field homogeneity, quality factor (Q), and the coil's FOV. MRI and MRS require both maximal SNR and homogeneous B_1 field. Unfortunately, these requirements usually conflict: the better the SNR the worse the B_1 and vice versa.

An inhomogeneous B_1 transmit field causes variations in the MR image intensity because of the spatial dependence of the flip angles (compare Eq. 5.2). This is particularly inconvenient when more than one pulse is used for MRI or MRS. In quantitative MRS, metabolite concentration cannot be properly evaluated when the rf coil produces an inhomogeneous B_1 field. Therefore, the application of rf coils producing a spatially uniform B_1 field is preferred.

The best SNR is produced over a small FOV by a local (surface), single loop coil (Figs 5.29c and 5.30), which, however, produces a very inhomogeneous B_1 field, dropping rapidly with distance from the coil. Various designs of small R_X-only coils are used for particular body parts such as the knee, arm, or head.

Volume coils produce a homogenous B_1 field over a large area, such as the body or the head. The most common volume coils are saddle coil, the solenoidal coil, the Alderman-Grant, the Helmholtz pair, and birdcage (Fig. 5.29). Unfortunately, they suffer from low sensitivity (as receiver coils) and high power requirements (up to 30 kW) compared to the surface coil (68). Examples of various rf coils are shown in Figure 5.30.

Coil sensitivity depends on the geometry, quality factor (Q), material used for the coil construction, electric circuit used to couple the coil (inductive or capacitive), filling factor of the coil (ratio between the volume of B_1 and the volume of the imaged object), and type of polarization (linear or circular).

Almost all volume coils and some surface coils use quadrature detection (so-called Circular Polarized (CP) coil) (69, 70). The quadrature detection allows SNR increase by up to $\sqrt{2}$ when compared to the Linear Polarized (LP coil) coil. The quadrature rf coil requires the creation of two equal and orthogonal B_1 fields. This can be easily achieved in the birdcage coils using proper driving system and two of its modes. The quadrature coil requires less power when compared to the LP coil.

Surface coils produce high SNR but within limited FOV. To extend the FOV over the sample a phased array technology was introduced (71). Each element of the array, coupled to an independent receiver channel, works as an independent surface coil maximizing SNR and increasing FOV.

Advanced MRI systems allow multinuclear studies to be performed. Quantification of tissue metabolites by heteronuclear MRS can be achieved using dual-frequency rf coils. The dual-frequency coils allow simultaneous measurement of two nuclei frequencies, such as ^{1}H and phosphorus (^{31}P). The proton signal is

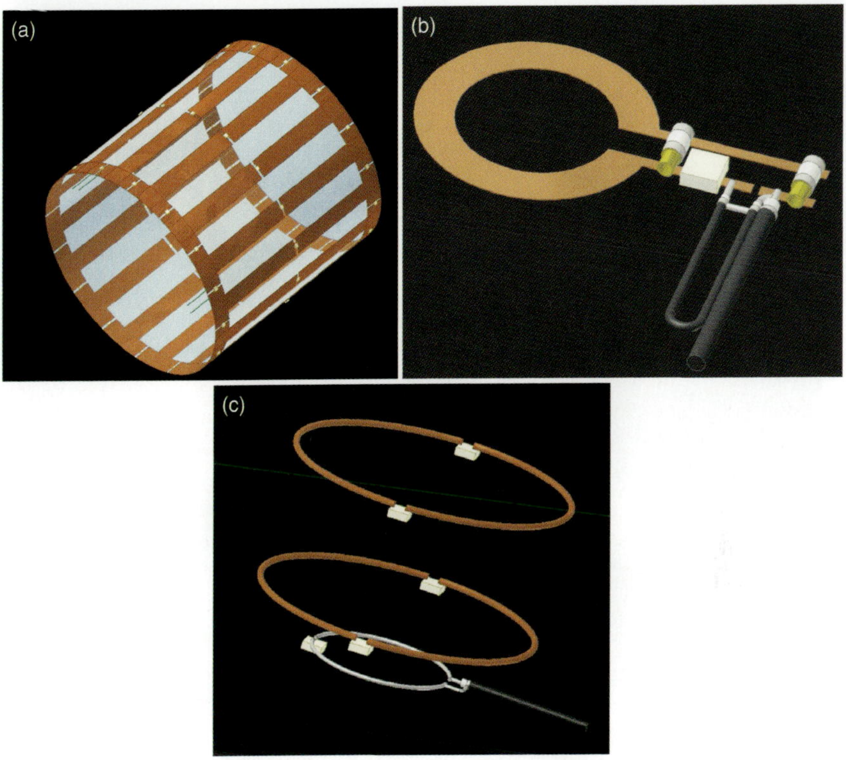

Figure 5.29. Inner structure of rf coils. (a) Birdcage, (b) surface, (c) inductively coupled Helmholtz pair (NRC, Canada).

usually used for high resolution imaging, whereas the other frequency is used for spectroscopy. The proton frequency also provides the sensitivity needed for shimming. Dual-frequency coils have to deliver the SNR of the single-frequency rf coil as well as produce homogenous rf field over the sample volume. To achieve these needs, double-tuned quadrature birdcage coils were developed (72).

5.14 MRI SAFETY

MRI is a noninvasive imaging technique with no long-term side effects observed. However, there are a few potential safety issues that should be considered when working with MRI systems or as a subject of MR examination: static magnetic field, rf power absorbed by the subject, and variable gradients of the magnetic field.

5.14.1 Magnet Safety

While long-term effects of the static magnetic field on living organisms have not been observed, the FDA, as a precaution, set up a limit of 3 T for human clinical

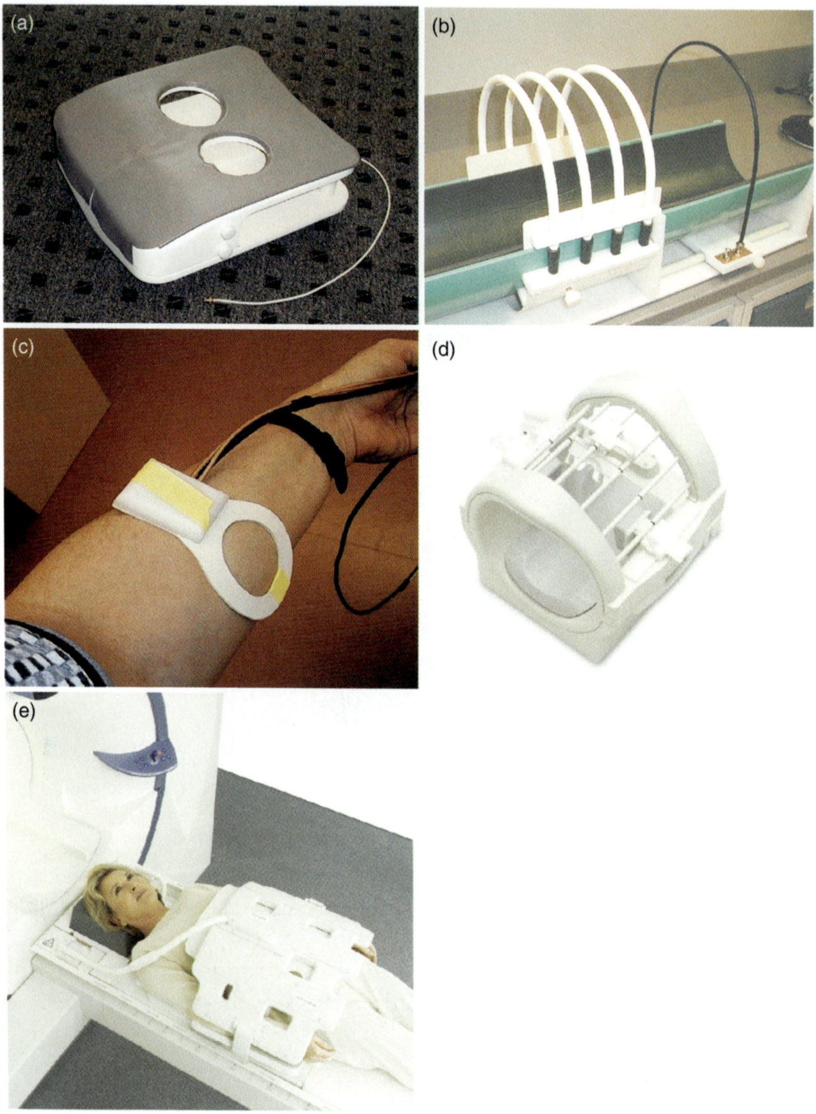

Figure 5.30. Examples of rf coils. (a) Breast coil (IBD/NRC), (b) solenoidal volume coil (IBD/NRC), (c) surface coil (IBD/NRC), (d) head coil (Siemens, Germany), and (e) phase array torso coil (Siemens, Germany).

MRIs. Other countries followed that limit. Potential subtle, long-term biological effects aside, there is always an immediate danger—projectiles.

Magnetic fields attract ferromagnetic objects, such as oxygen tanks, scissors, carts, computers, and so on. Such objects can become projectiles and injure or kill anyone between the magnet and the object. Therefore, there *must* be no ferromagnetic objects *within* the 5-Gs line. Some surgical clips, prosthesis, and implants may also be attracted by the magnet. However, some of them, made of nonferrous material, are MRI compatible and can be safely imaged. Nonetheless, in most cases they create artefacts in MR images. Of course, under no circumstance can patients with pacemakers be imaged. It is considered that the region *outside* the 5-Gs line is safe for practically all objects, including cardiac pacemakers, but it may be worth to remember that magnetic cards (such a credit card or hotel magnetic key) may be erased by the field around 5 Gs.

In very rare cases, moving in the magnet may cause a temporal discomfort, depending on the individual's sensitivity, because of the eddy currents induced in the brain due to the motion in the magnetic field.

Clinical MRI systems are equipped with rf power amplifiers capable of generating up to 30 kW rf power in short pulses, which heat up tissues and can be potentially harmful. Therefore, the regulations do not allow the use of rf power that would heat the tissue by more than 1°C. However, this definition is not convenient in MRI; therefore, *Specific Absorption Rate* (SAR) is used. This is defined as rf power absorbed in tissue per unit mass, and is expressed in watts per kg (W/kg). The SAR limits vary from 3 W/kg to 12 W/kg depending on the total exposure time and on the part of the body. Clinical MRI systems calculate the SAR value before the pulse sequences are run and lock-out the imaging in case SAR exceeds the allowed value. It also should be noted that SAR increases with ${B_0}^2$ for fields below 4 T.

5.14.2 Gradient Safety

Gradient coils produce a time-varying magnetic field (dB/dt) that can cause peripheral nerve stimulation and involuntary muscle contraction. Therefore dB/dt is also limited.

In addition, fast switching current in the gradient coils causes acoustic noise due to coil vibrations, which depends on the pulse sequence used. The more demanding the pulse sequence from the point of view of the gradient strength and rise time, the noisier the sequence is. Therefore, fast pulse sequences such as EPI are usually very noisy. However, spiral EPI, which reduces the gradients' rise time, makes the sequence quieter. DW-MRI is also often noisy because of strong diffusion gradients. Because the gradient strength required increases with the field strength, the stronger the magnet, the noisier the pulse sequences are. But this is also the reason why there is practically no noise in low field MRI, such as 0.2 T.

5.15 IMAGING ARTEFACTS IN MRI

MRI allows imaging of many different tissue properties depending on the technique used. The variety of techniques is possible because of the sensitivity of MRI to different phenomena. This sensitivity, however, may cause a lot of artefacts due to the hardware imperfections, improper pulse sequence tuning, or some external factors. Hardware imperfections may include inhomogeneous main field, nonlinear gradients, inhomogeneous rf field, or eddy currents induced in the cryostat, to mention a few. Improper optimization of pulse sequences may cause a lot of artefacts depending on the pulse sequence used, for example, multiecho pulse sequences may produce unwanted stimulated echoes, improper rf spoiling or refocusing may create unwanted MR signals, etc. The most common artefacts are susceptibility artefacts, flow, phase wrapping (aliasing), or motion ghosting. Phase wrapping occurs when the FOV is smaller than the object size along the phase encoding direction, because of the impossibility of distinguishing between ϕ and $\phi + 360^\circ$ phase of the signal. This artefact manifests itself when a part of an image shows on the opposite side of the imaged object. The FOV is increased to rectify this problem.

However, there is no good remedy for the susceptibility artefact caused by the variation in the magnetic field between two different tissues or image objects, such as lungs and blood or bone and implants. The images can be badly distorted in such areas, especially for sensitive sequences such as EPI.

Motion artefact (ghosting) is the most common artefact caused by the motion of the subject during data acquisition. It is observed as a blurring or multiplication of the object, depending on the degree of movement, along the phase encoding direction, due to phase misregistration. The remedy is obvious but not always possible, as not all patients can stay motionless for the imaging session. This is particularly important in fMRI, when series of images are compared and any misregistration can lead to incorrect data analysis; therefore, software programs are used to realign the images.

Flow artefact may cause areas of flowing spins to enhance or reduce image intensity. Artefacts from pulsatile flow in arteries may also cause periodic ghosting.

5.15.1 High Field Effects

Serious problems with image homogeneity and SAR occur when the size of the imaged object becomes comparable with the half wavelength (in this object) of the rf field used for imaging. This occurs, for instance, for whole-body imaging at field strengths above 3 T. As described and explained by Hoult (73), even a perfectly made rf coil, producing a homogenous rf field, will not provide a homogeneous image because of this interaction between the rf field and the tissue. As a result, images may be, for example, dark in the center and bright at the edges, or vice versa, depending on the power of the rf pulse used. Maybe of even more importance than image inhomogeneities, is the local SAR that may exceed SAR limits in certain areas of the body, because of the uneven distribution of the electrical field. This problem is a major challenge in very high (>3 T) human MRI. One approach to deal with this problem, the use of multiple transmit systems, was recently introduced (74) and is a subject of research.

5.16 ADVANCED MR TECHNOLOGY AND ITS POSSIBLE FUTURE

A major direction in MR technique development is the reduction of imaging time without any decrease in image resolution. Probably the biggest advancement in this area recently was triggered by the introduction of the parallel imaging technique (75–78). This is a technique requiring MRI systems equipped with multiple receivers. Parallel imaging works by using knowledge of the spatial sensitivity response of multiple receiver coils to decode under-sampled data to produce images.

There are two basic approaches to parallel imaging with different mathematics, but which fundamentally achieve the same result. They are the Simultaneous Acquisition of Spatial Harmonics (SMASH) (75) and its modifications, Sensitivity Encoding (SENSE) (77) and Generalized Autocalibrating Partially Parallel Acquisitions (GRAPPA) (78). Parallel imaging allows reduction of the acquisition time without any loss in data-acquisition efficiency.

The challenges associated with image homogeneity at high field spurred the development of multi-transmit systems (transmit array), which allow control of both phase and amplitude in each independent transmit channel. While such a design has been primary used for B_1 shimming it may possibly also be used for new MRI techniques, which can reduce some gradient requirements to obtain an MR image (79). The possible combination of receive and transmit phase array systems, should it be successful, may overcome the image resolution limits caused by the standard way of data collection (with gradients). Such a system of the future may push the resolution limits and at the same time avoid acoustic noise generation and safety issues associated with dB/dt and SAR.

In summary, new MRI techniques, new discoveries, and new applications keep broadening the MRI horizons. The information provided by MRI allows better and better diagnosis, more timely treatments, and better outcomes.

ACKNOWLEDGMENTS

We thank Nancy Anderson and Rudy Sebastian for the great assistance and dedication with drawing the pictures. We also thank Dr Dorota Bartusik for help with literature search.

REFERENCES

1. Carr HY, Purcell EM. Effects of diffusion on free precession in nuclear magnetic resonance experiments. Phys Rev 1954;94(3):630–638.
2. Bloch F. Nuclear induction. Phys Rev 1946;70:460–474.
3. Hahn EL. Spin echoes. Phys Rev 1950;80:580–594.

4. Gabillard R. Résonance nucléaire mesure du temps de relaxation T2 en presence d'une inhomogenéité de champ magnétique supérieure à la largeur de raie. C R Acad Sci (Paris) 1951;232:1551–1553.
5. Gabillard R. A steady state transient technique in nuclear resonance. Phys Rev 1952;85:694–695.
6. Damadian R. Tumor detection by nuclear magnetic resonance. Science 1971;171:1151–1153.
7. Mansfield P, Grannell PK, Garroway AN, Stacker DC. Proceedings of the 1st Specialised Colloque Ampere; Krakow, Poland; 1973.
8. Mansfield P, Grannell PK. NMR 'diffraction' in solids? J Phys 1973;C6:L422.
9. Mansfield P, Maudsley AA. Proceedings of the 19th Colloque Ampere; Heidelberg; 1976. p.247.
10. Hinshaw WS. Spin mapping: the application of moving gradients to NMR. Phys Lett 1974;48A:87–88.
11. Andrew ER, Bottomley PA, Hinshaw WS, Holland GN, Moore WS, Simaroj C. NMR images by the multiple sensitive point method: application to larger biological systems. Phys Med Biol 1977;22:971–974.
12. Lauterbur PC. Image formation by induced local interactions: Examples employing nuclear magnetic resonance. Nature 1973;242:190–191.
13. Garroway AN, Grannell PK, Mansfield P. Image formation in NMR by a selective irradiation process. J Phys 1974;C7:L457.
14. Hoult DI. Zeugmatography: a criticism of the concept of a selective pulse in the presence of a field gradient. J Magn Reson 1977;26:165.
15. Kumar A, Welti D, Ernst RR. NMR fourier zeugmatography. J Magn Reson 1975;18:69–83.
16. Hoult DI, Saunders JK, Sutherland GR, Sharp J, Gervin M, Kolansky HG, Kripiakevich DL, Procca A, Sebastian RA, Dombay A, Rayner DL, Roberts FA, Tomanek B. The engineering of an interventional MRI with a movable 1.5 Tesla magnet. J Magn Reson Imaging 2001;13:78–86.
17. Westbrook C. *MRI at a Glance*. Osney Mead, Oxford: Blackwell Publishing Ltd; 2002.
18. Bernstein MA, King KF, Zhou JX. *Handbook of MRI Pulse Sequences*. London: Elsevier Academic Press; 2004.
19. Liang Z, Lauterbur PC. *Principles of Magnetic Resonance Imaging: A Signal Processing Perspective*, IEEE Press Series in Biomedical Engineering. New York: IEEE Press.
20. Abragam A. *Principles of Nuclear Magnetism*. New York: Oxford University Press; 1989.
21. Haacke EM, Brown RW, Thompson MR, Venkatesan R. *Magnetic Resonance Imaging: Physical Principles and Sequence Design*. New York: John Wiley & Sons; 1996.
22. Bracewell RN. *The Fourier Transform (FT) and its Applications*. New York: McGraw-Hill; 1986.
23. Ernst RR, Anderson WA. Application of Fourier transform to magnetic resonance spectroscopy. Rev Sci Instrum 1966;37:93–102.
24. Carr HY, Purcell EM. Effects of diffusion on free precession in nuclear magnetic resonance experiments. Phys Rev 1954;94:630–638.

25. Hoult DI, Richards RE. The signal-to-noise ratio of the nuclear magnetic resonance experiment. J Magn Res 1976;24:71.

26. Haase A, Frahm J, Matthaei D, Hänicke W, Merboldt KD. FLASH imaging: rapid NMR imaging using low flip angle pulses. J Magn Reson 1989;67:388–397.

27. Wehrli FW. *Fast-Scan Magnetic Resonance: Principles and Applications*. New York: Raven Press; 1991.

28. Haacke EM, Wielopolski PA, Tkach JA, Modic MT. Steady-state free precession imaging in the presence of motion: application for improved visualization of the cerebrospinal fluid. Radiology 1990;175:545–552.

29. Oppelt A, Graumann R, Barfuss FisherH, Hartl W, Schajor W. FISP: eine neue schnelle Pulssequenz für die Kernspintomographie. Electromedica 1986;54:15–18.

30. Scheffler K, Henning J. T_1 quantification with inversion recovery True-FISP. Magn Reson Med 2001;45:72–723.

31. Mansfield P. Multi-planar image formation using NMR spin echoes. J Phys C: Solid State Phys 1977;10:L55–L58.

32. Ahn AB, Kim JH, Cho ZH. High-speed spiral-scan echo planar NMR imaging. IEEE Trans Med Imaging 1986;MI-5:1–6.

33. Hajnal JV, De Coene B, Lewis PD, Baudouin CJ, Cowan FM, Pennock JM, Young IR, Bydder GM. High signal regions in normal white matter shown by heavily T_2-weighted CSF nulled IR sequences. J Comput Tomogr 1992;16:506–513.

34. De Coene B, Hajnal JV, Gatehouse P, Longmore DB, White SJ, Oatridge A, Pennock JM, Young IR, Bydder GM. MR of the brain using fluid-attenuated inversion recovery (FLAIR) pulse sequences. Am J Neuroradiol 1992;13:1555–1564.

35. Rydberg JN, Hammond CA, Grimm RC, Erickson BJ, Jack CR Jr, Huston J III, Rieder SJ. Initial clinical experience in MR imaging of the brain with a fast fluid-attenuated inversion recovery pulse sequence. Radiology 1994;193:173–180.

36. Noguchi K, Ogawa T, Inugami A, Toyoshima H, Okudera T, Uemura K. MR of acute subarachnoid hemorrhage: a preliminary report of fluid-attenuated inversion-recovery pulse sequences. Am J Neuroradiol 1994;15:1940–1943.

37. Stejskal EO, Turner JE. Spin-diffusion measurements: spin-echoes in the presence of a time-dependent field gradient. J Chem Phys 1965;42:288–292.

38. Hoehn-Berlage M. Diffusion-weighted NMR imaging: application to experimental focal ischemia. NMR Biomed 1995;8:345–358.

39. Moran PR. A flow velocity zeumatographic interlace for NMR imaging in humans. Magn Reson Imaging 1982;1:197–203.

40. Anderson C, Edelman R, Turski P. *Clinical Magnetic Resonance Angiography*. New York: Raven Press; 1993. pp. 309–314.

41. Laub G, Gaa J, Drobitzky J. Magnetic resonance angiography techniques. Electromedica 1998;66(2):68–75.

42. Masaryk TJ, Modic MT, Ruggieri PM, Ross JS, Laub G, Lenz GW, Tkach JA, Haacke EM, Selman WR, Harik SI. Three-dimensional (volume) gradient-echo imaging of the carotid bifurcation: preliminary clinical experience. Radiology 1989;171:801–806.

43. Keller PJ, Drayer BP, Fram EK, Williams KD, Dumoulin CL, Souza SP. MR angiography with two-dimensional acquisition and three-dimensional display. Radiology 1989;173:527–532.

44. Axel L, Morton DMR. flow imaging by velocity-compensated/uncompensated difference images. J Comput Tomogr 1987;11:31–34.

45. Pernicone JR, Siebert JE, Potchen EJ, Pera A, Dumoulin CL, Souza SP. Three-dimensional phase contrast MR angiography in the head and neck: preliminary report. Am J Neuroradiol 1990;11:457–466.

46. Lin W, Haacke EM, Smith AS, Clampitt ME. Gadolinium-enhanced high-resolution MR angiography with adaptive vessel tracking: preliminary results in the intracranial circulation. J Magn Reson Imaging 1992;2:277–284.

47. Bowtell RW, Peters A, Sharp JC, Mansfield P, Hsu EW, Aiken N, Horsman A, Blackband SJ. NMR microscopy of single neurons using spin-echo and line-narrowed 2DFT imaging. Magn Reson Med 1994;32:199–205.

48. Jacobs RE, Fraser SE. Magnetic resonance microscopy of embryonic-cell lineages and movements. Science 1994;263:681–684.

49. Seo WS, Lee JH, Sun X, Suzuki Y, Mann D, Liu Z, Terashima M, Yang PC, McConnell MV, Nishimura DG, Dai H. FeCo/graphitic-shell nanocrystals as advanced magnetic-resonance-imaging and near-infrared agents. Nature 2006;5:971–976.

50. Weissleder R. Molecular imaging in cancer. Science 2006;312:1168–1171.

51. Hirsch LR, Stafford RJ, Bankson JA, Sershen SR, Rivera B, Price RE, Hazle JD, Halas NJ, West JL. Nanoshell-mediated near-infrared thermal therapy of tumors under magnetic resonance guidance. Proc Natl Acad Sci U S A 2003;100:13549.

52. Ito A, Shinkai M, Honda H, Kobayashi T. Medical application of functionalized magnetic nanoparticles. J Biosci Bioeng 2005;100:1–11.

53. Vargas HI, Dooley WC, Gardner RA, Gonzalez KD, Venegas R, Heywang-Kobrunner SH, Fenn AJ. Focused microwave phased array thermotherapy for ablation of early-stage breast cancer: results of thermal dose escalation. Ann Surg Oncol 2004;11:139–146.

54. Heeger DJ, Ress D. What does fMRI tell us about neuronal activity? Nat Rev Neurosci 2002;3:142–151.

55. Stroman PW, Tomanek B, Krause V, Malisza KL. Functional magnetic resonance imaging of the human brain based on signal enhancement by extravascular protons (SEEP fMRI). Magn Reson Med 2003;49(3):433–439.

56. Majcher K, Tomanek B, Jasinski A, Foniok T, Stroman PW, Tuor UI, Kirk D, Hess G. Simultaneous functional magnetic resonance imaging in the rat spinal cord and brain. Exp Neurol 2006;197:458–464.

57. Ogawa S, Lee TM, Kay AR, Tank D. Brain magnetic resonance imaging with contrast dependent on blood oxygenation. Proc Natl Acad Sci U S A 1990;87:9868–9872.

58. Baumgartner R, Ryner L, Richter W, Summers R, Jarmasz M, Somorjai R. Comparison of two exploratory data analysis methods for fMRI: fuzzy clustering vs. principal component analysis. Magn Reson Imaging 2000;1:89–94.

59. Darquie A, Poine JB, Poupon C, Saint_Jalmes H, Le Bihan D. Trnasient transient decrease in water diffusion onbserved in human occipital cortex during visual stimulation. Proc Natl Acad Sci U S A 2001;98:9391–9395.

60. Stroman PW, Tomanek B, Malisza K. Functional magnetic resonance imaging of the human brain and spinal cord by means of signal enhancement by extravascular protons. Concepts Magn Reson Part A 2003;16A(1):28–34.

61. Stanwell P, Gluch L, Clark D, Tomanek B, Baker L, Giuffrè B, Lean C, Malycha P, Mountford C. Specificity of choline metabolites for *in vivo* diagnosis of breast cancer using ^{1}H MRS at 1.5T. Eur Radiol 2005;15:1037–1043.
62. Hoult DI, Busby SJ, Gadian DG, Radda GK, Richards RE, Seeley PJ. Observation of tissue metabolites using 31P nuclear magnetic resonance. Nature 1974;252:285–287.
63. Frahm J, Merboldt KD, Hänicke W. Localized proton spectroscopy using stimulated echoes. J Magn Reson 1987;72:502–508.
64. Merboldt KD, Chien D, Hänicke W, Gyngell ML, Bruhn H, Frahm J. Localized 31P NMR spectroscopy of the adult human brain *in vivo* using stimulated echo (STEAM) sequences. J Magn Reson 1990;89:343–361.
65. Dujin JH, Matson GB, Maudsley AA, Hugg JW, Weiner MW. Human brian infarction: proton MR spectroscopy. Radiology 1992;183:711–718.
66. Chen CN, Hoult DI. *Biomedical Magnetic Resonance Technology*. Bristol, New York: Adam Hilger; 1989. (new edition by Hoult in preparation).
67. Sharp JC, Yin D, Bernhardt RH, Deng Q, Procca AE Tyson RL Lo K Tomanek B. The integration of real and virtual magnetic resonance imaging experiments in a single instrument. Rev Sci Instrum. 2009 Sep;80(9):093709.
68. Tomanek B. Radio frequency coils for magnetic resonance spectroscopy, "Medical Uses". In: Mountford C, Himmelreich U, Webb G, editors. Volume 2, *Modern Magnetic Resonance*. London: Springer; 2006. pp. 1–8.
69. Chen CN, Hoult DI, Sank VJ. Quadrature detection coils–a further $\sqrt{2}$ improvement in sensitivity. J Magn Reson 1983;54:324–327.
70. Hyde JS, Jesmanowicz A, Grist TM, Froncisz W, Kneeland JB. Quadrature detection surface coil. Magn Reson Med 1987;4:179–184.
71. Roemer PB, Edelstein WA, Hayes CE, Souza SP, Mueller OM. The NMR phased array. Magn Reson Med 1990;16:192–225.
72. Fitzsimmons JR, Beck BL, Brooker HR. Double resonant quadrature birdcage. Magn Reson Med 1993;30:107–114.
73. Hoult DI. Sensitivity and power deposition in a high-field imaging experiment. J Magn Reson Imaging 2000;12:46–67.
74. Setsompop K, Wald LL, Alagappan V, Gagoski B, Hebrank F, Fontius U, Schmitt F, Adalsteinsson E. Parallel RF transmission with eight channels at 3 Tesla. Magn Reson Med 2006;56:1163–1171.
75. Sodickson DK, Mannig WJ. Simultaneous acquisition of spatial harmonics (SMASH): fast imaging with radiofrequency coil arrays. Magn Reson Med 1997;38:591–603.
76. Blaimer M, Brueer F, Mueller M, Heidemann RM, Griswold MA, Jackob PM. SMASH, SENSE, PILS, GRAPPA: how to choose the optimal method. Top Magn Reson Imaging 2004;15:223–236.
77. Pruessmann KP, Weiger M, Scheidegger MB, Boesiger P. SENSE: sensitivity encoding for fast MRI. Magn Reson Med 1999;42:952–962.
78. Griswald MA, Jackob PM, Heidemann RM, Nittka M, Jellus V, Wang J, Kiefer B, Haase A. Generalized autocalibrating partially paralell acquisition (GRAPPA). Magn Reson Med 2003;47:1202–1210.
79. King S, Yin D Thingvold S, Sharp J, Tomanek B. Transmit array spatial encoding (TRASE): a new data acquisition method in MRI. 2007 Submitted to ISMRM Annual Meeting; Berlin. 2007.

6

TOWARD A 3D VIEW OF CELLULAR ARCHITECTURE: CORRELATIVE LIGHT MICROSCOPY AND ELECTRON TOMOGRAPHY

JACK A. VALENTIJN, LINDA F. VAN DRIEL, KAREN A. JANSEN, KARINE M. VALENTIJN, AND ABRAHAM J. KOSTER

Department of Molecular Cell Biology, Leiden University Medical Center, Leiden, The Netherlands

6.1 INTRODUCTION

The terms "multimodality imaging" and "correlative microscopy" are employed in the biomedical literature to designate any combination of two or more microscopic techniques applied to the same region in a biological specimen. "Correlative microscopy" should not be confused with "fluorescence correlation microscopy," which is a method to measure diffusion of fluorescent molecules in cells (Brock and Jovin, 1998). The purpose of multimodality imaging is to obtain complementary data, each imaging modality providing different information on the specimen that is under investigation. Correlative Light and Electron Microscopy (CLEM) is by far the most widespread form of multimodality imaging.

CLEM makes use of the fact that imaging with photons on one hand, and electrons on the other, offers specific advantages over one another. For instance, the low magnification range inherent to Light Microscopy (LM) is particularly well suited for the rapid scanning of large and heterogeneous sample areas, while the high resolution that can be achieved by Electron Microscopy (EM)

Biomedical Imaging: Principles and Applications, First Edition. Edited by Reiner Salzer.

allows for the subsequent zooming in on selected areas of interest to obtain ultrastructural detail. A further advantage of LM is that it can be used to study dynamic processes, up to the molecular level, in living cells and tissues. The recent surge in live-cell imaging research has catalyzed a renewed interest in CLEM methodologies, as the interpretation of the dynamic processes observed by LM often requires high resolution information from EM data. CLEM is also gaining in momentum in the field of cryoelectron microscopy where the low contrast conditions and low electron dose requirements put a constraint on the detection efficacy.

Current CLEM procedures face a number of challenges. First, sample preparation methods for LM and EM can be quite divergent because of different requirements for preservation, embedding, sectioning, and counterstaining. Therefore, alternative sample preparation protocols that are suitable for both LM and EM need to be devised. Second, CLEM often requires the correlated localization of specific molecules in cells or tissues, for which specialized detection systems need to be developed. Standard detection methods are based on tagging of molecules either with fluorochromes for LM or with gold particles for EM and are thus less suitable for CLEM where the tag should ideally be visible in both modalities. Third, the transition from imaging by LM to EM may involve handling and additional processing of samples, which can lead to changes in orientation and morphology of the sample. This in turn can hamper the finding back of and correlation with previously established areas of interest.

This chapter discusses past, present, and prospective strategies for CLEM. Special emphasis is given to 3D imaging methods, in particular electron tomography.

6.2 HISTORICAL PERSPECTIVE

When Porter, Claude, and Fullam published in their 1945 landmark article the earliest transmission electron microscopic images of an intact cell, describing for the first time the endoplasmic reticulum, they made a side-by-side comparison with light microscopic images (Porter et al., 1945). Although they did not perform genuine CLEM—the light and electron micrographs were not taken from the same cells—the authors clearly felt the need to correlate their electron microscopic observations with the more familiar light microscopic data as a means to validate their novel findings. Thus, in a sense, CLEM is as old as the earliest applications of EM to biological samples. In the 1950s–1980s, numerous "correlated light and electron microscopic" studies were published based on the same concept of comparing structures observed by LM with similar structures visualized by EM. True CLEM emerged in the early 1970s and culminated in the 1980s with the publication of a dedicated book in the authoritative Hayat series on EM techniques (Hayat, 1987), and with the development of instrumentation such as a combined instrument for LM and scanning EM (Wouters and Koerten, 1982) and the commercial LEM 2000 (Akashi Seisakusho Ltd., Tokyo, Japan) for LM and transmission EM. Interestingly, and perhaps ironically, among the first genuine CLEM applications were studies that combined EM with live-cell imaging

(Buckley, 1971), the latter being again responsible for the recent revival of CLEM. Neuroanatomy was another field of research that pioneered CLEM techniques to facilitate sampling of central nervous tissue for EM (Hollander, 1970).

The 1990s saw a steady decrease in the use of EM for life science studies (Geuze, 1999). Several factors were responsible for this decline. First, the genomics era was in full bloom, and the inherent emphasis on functional/mechanistic studies overshadowed the static images and descriptive data that EM produced. Second, there had been major developments in LM, the most important of which was the introduction of "turnkey" systems for confocal laser scanning microscopy (Paddock, 1996). These systems offered improved resolution up to the subcellular level, while requiring less investment, infrastructure, and expertise than a typical EM setup. Hence, confocal microscopes replaced the electron microscopes in many cell biology laboratories. Last but not least, the discovery of Green Fluorescent Protein (GFP; see Section 6.4.1.1) and the demonstration that it could be used to tag proteins genetically stirred a revolution in biomedical research, as it allowed for the tracking of specific proteins in living cells by means of fluorescence microscopy.

In the present postgenomics climate, EM is coming back with a vengeance. Despite the dip in EM-based research during the previous decade, the development of novel EM technologies moved forward at a steady pace, resulting in several breakthrough applications. Among them are electron tomography (see Section 6.5.4) and cryoelectron tomography (see Section 6.5.5), which are techniques for high resolution 3D visualization and which are gradually becoming mainstream tools in structural molecular biology. As discussed in more detail later, (cryo)electron tomography is often hampered by the lack of landmarks in the 2D views used to select areas of interest. CLEM has the potential to play an important role here by facilitating the search for such areas of interest. In addition, CLEM is taking front stage in live-cell imaging, where there is growing demand for fine structural information on processes whose dynamics have been recorded light microscopically.

6.3 STAINS FOR CLEM

Biological specimens are notorious for their high intrinsic translucency and electron permeability. As a result, images produced by LM and Transmission Electron Microscopy (TEM) exhibit poor contrast. Specialized imaging techniques can be used to enhance contrast, such as differential interference contrast (DIC) for LM (Salmon and Tran, 2003), energy filtering for TEM (de Bruijn et al., 1993), and Z-contrast imaging for Scanning Transmission Electron Microscopy (STEM) (Carlemalm and Kellenberger, 1982). Alternatively, contrast enhancement can be achieved by means of chemical staining. Despite the obvious drawback of possible structural and chemical sample alteration that is inherent to such staining procedures, histochemical and cytochemical techniques are still widely employed and will remain popular because of their relative ease of use and the high level of morphologic detail they can reveal. Stains for LM are mostly dye based (chromophores and fluorophores), whereas EM stains employ electron-dense heavy atoms (osmium, uranium, and lead compounds). Thus, usually, the same stain cannot be visualized both by LM and EM. There are, however, a few exceptions, such as the Golgi-impregnation procedure, which is based on a silver-precipitation reaction and used to stain neurons (Fairen, 2005). In general, LM and EM stains can be combined, but the thinness of ultrathin sections required for EM reduces the uptake of LM dyes thereby diminishing the intensity of the stain. Jones et al., reported that toluidine blue is a suitable LM stain for epoxy sections of osmicated tissue if the section thickness is above 100 nm (Jones et al., 1982). The toluidine blue stain is useful in surgical histopathology, as it allows for the LM detection of areas of diagnostic importance in thin sections of human biopsies.

An alternative approach for staining biological samples for CLEM is the inclusion of low molecular weight fluorescent dyes, such as acridine orange and saffranin O, in the substitution medium used during freeze substitution (the principle of freeze substitution is discussed in Section 6.5.6) (Biel et al., 2003; Pfeiffer et al., 2003). The rationale for this method is that just as molecules with a molecular weight up to 700 Da are washed out of the sample during freeze substitution (Pfeiffer et al., 2000), small molecules can also infiltrate the sample. Originally, the technique was developed for staining of high pressure frozen samples (see Section 6.5.5 for the principle of high pressure freezing), and the fluorescence signal was recorded by confocal laser scanning microscopy through the block face of a specimen block. Ultrathin sections were subsequently cut from the same block face, and EM images were correlated with the corresponding slices in three-dimensional reconstructions of confocal image stacks (Biel et al., 2003). The protocol was therefore rather cumbersome and laborious. In our laboratory, we have successfully labeled nuclei of chemically fixed cells and tissues with acridine orange and visualized the fluorescence directly in ultrathin sections, thus allowing for the correlation of LM and EM in the exact same slice (Fig. 6.1) (van Driel et al., 2008).

6.4 PROBES FOR CLEM

While the histo- and cytochemical stains discussed earlier provide visual clues of gross features that can be used as landmarks in a multimodal coordinate system, molecular probes or indicators can be employed to label and detect specific molecules in and around cells. In addition, there are probes that can detect ions, pH, membrane potential, enzymatic activities, and molecular interactions.

6.4.1 Probes to Detect Exogenous Proteins

6.4.1.1 Green Fluorescent Protein. Genetically encoded indicators have become extremely popular among cell and molecular biologists as a tool to study the spatiotemporal expression of proteins in living cells. For this purpose, cells or whole organisms are genetically altered so that they express one or

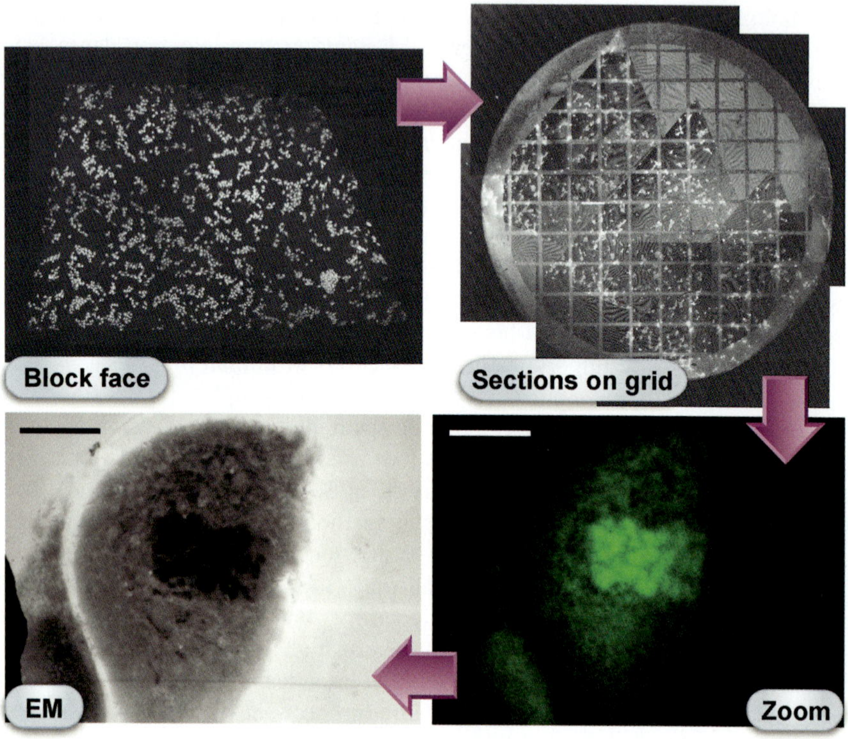

Figure 6.1. CLEM in action. African green monkey kidney epithelial cells (Vero) grown under standard cell culture conditions were plunge frozen in liquid-nitrogen-cooled ethane, freeze substituted, and flat embedded in Lowicryl HM20 resin. Acridine orange, a fluorescent label for DNA and RNA, was added to the acetone/uranyl acetate mixture used as solvent and fixative, respectively, during the freeze-substitution step. After trimming of the specimen block, fluorescently labeled cells could be observed in the block face, viewed with a confocal laser scanning microscope. The fluorescence was retained in ultrathin sections of 100 nm, cut from the block face and collected on an electron microscope grid. The fluorescence micrographs of the block face and sections on grid each represent a montage of 16 individual images acquired with a 10X objective and stitched with the help of image processing software. As demonstrated in the zoom image taken at higher magnification (63X objective), acridine orange enabled the selection of a rare mitotic event. By means of a coordinate system, the same cell was easily retrieved in the electron microscope. The electron micrograph was acquired at a relatively low magnification to allow for direct comparison with the fluorescence micrograph. In addition to facilitating the search for dividing cells, acridine orange can also help identify cells with characteristic nuclear patterns in complex tissues (e.g. neutrophils, Langerhans cells, and tumor cells). The block face in the upper left panel measures about 2×1 mm, the grid in the upper right panel has a diameter of 3 mm, and the scale bars in the bottom panels represent 10 μm.

more proteins of interest ectopically with a built-in amino acid sequence that serves as the indicator. The most widely used sequence is 238 amino acids long and encodes for GFP (Chalfie et al., 1994). The gene for GFP, which is a naturally occurring fluorescent protein, was isolated from the jellyfish *Aequorea victoria* (Prasher et al., 1992). GFP emits green light when illuminated with blue light. In the jellyfish, the blue light is generated upon the binding of Ca^{2+} ions to the luminescent protein aequorin (Shimomura, 2005). In the laboratory, the blue light is generated by lasers or mercury or xenon vapor lamps. Several mutants of GFP that emit stronger fluorescence and at different wavelengths have been engineered (Tsien, 2005), the latter allowing for the detection of molecular interactions by means of specialized microscopic techniques such as Fluorescence Energy Resonance Transfer (FRET) and Fluorescence Lifetime Imaging (FLIM).

Unfortunately, GFP cannot be observed directly by EM, thus restricting somewhat its usefulness for CLEM. Nevertheless, several procedures have been established for correlated LM and EM detection of GFP. A number of these procedures are based on the principle of 3,3′-Diaminobenzidine (DAB) oxidation by free oxygen radicals. The free radicals can be formed during the enzymatic conversion of peroxide by Horseradish Peroxidase (HRP) or during photobleaching of fluorochromes by means of intense illumination and with oxygen present. When DAB is oxidized, it polymerizes and precipitates at the site of oxidation. The osmiophilic DAB precipitate becomes electron dense when treated with osmium tetroxide and can thus be visualized by EM (Hanker, 1979; Maranto, 1982).

In principle, the fluorescence of GFP itself could be used to photo-oxidize DAB. However, this is currently a matter of debate in the literature. On one hand, Because the GFP chromophore is buried inside the protein, and because of the lack of an aqueous environment, it would not be able to generate sufficient free radicals for efficacious photoconversion of DAB (Gaietta et al., 2002; Mironov et al., 2000). On the other, Monosov et al. demonstrated that GFP targeted to peroxisomes in yeast cells was able to photo-oxidize DAB at sufficient levels to permit EM localization (Monosov et al., 1996); Grabenbauer et al. recently reported on an improved method for GFP-mediated photo-oxidation (Grabenbauer et al., 2005). The improvements of the method, which they termed *GRAB* for Gfp Recognition after Bleaching, consisted in the reduction of background by quenching of autofluorescence and blocking of endogenous enzyme activities and in the use of elevated oxygen content throughout the photoconversion reaction. To this date, and to the best of our knowledge, only the two studies mentioned here have employed photo-oxidation by GFP. Additional studies will be needed to further validate the practicability and universality of the approach, and the development of GFP derivatives with higher sensitivity for illumination-based EM detection may be needed to unleash its full potential.

An alternative method that also uses DAB oxidation to reveal GFP by EM, one that appears more widely accepted, is based on the detection of GFP by GFP antibodies that in turn are decorated by HRP-conjugated secondary antibodies (Mironov et al., 2000; Mironov et al., 2005). In a typical experiment, the GFP signal is first monitored in living cells by means of time-lapse fluorescence microscopy, that is, live-cell imaging. When at a given point in time the GFP signal develops an interesting pattern that merits EM clarification, the cells are rapidly fixed to immobilize the GFP pattern and underlying structures. Thereafter, the cells are permeabilized to allow access of the antibodies to the GFP epitopes, the DAB precipitation reaction is carried out, and cells are postfixed with osmium tetroxide and embedded in a resin to permit ultramicrotomy. The GFP-HRP approach has been used successfully to identify and characterize transport intermediates along the secretory pathway (Polishchuk et al., 2000). A drawback of the procedure is that the requirements for immunolabeling (mild fixation and cell permeabilization) are antithetical to optimal conditions for ultrastructural preservation. This limitation could be overcome by adapting the GFP immunodetection strategy for use with ultrathin cryosections (Tokuyasu method; see also Section 6.5.6), which is advertised for its superior ultrastructural preservation while retaining immunogenicity. In this scenario, detection of GFP should be carried out using immunogold rather than immunoperoxidase labeling (Koster and Klumperman, 2003; Polishchuk et al., 2006; Verdijk et al., 2005; Westbroek et al., 2003). Usually, the preparation of cells for cryosectioning involves enzymatic or mechanic dispersion and centrifugation to obtain a cell pellet that is suitable for freezing. However, these steps will obliterate the spatial coordinates needed for correlating cells at the LM and EM level. To circumvent such problems, Oorschot et al. have developed a flat-embedding method that allows for ultracryotomy of cultured cells while preserving their topology (Oorschot et al., 2002).

The aforementioned procedures for the detection of GFP at the EM level suffer from limitations with regard to the precision of correlation that can be achieved between the LM and EM images. This is because the LM image represents an optical section through a cell layer, which cannot be exactly matched with the EM image that is taken from an ultrathin section cut through the same cell layer. Using high resolution (i.e., high numerical aperture) objectives in combination with image deconvolution, the optical section thickness that can be attained is typically around 200 nm, whereas an ultrathin section usually varies in thickness from 50 to 70 nm. In addition to this mismatch between optical and ultrathin section thickness, there may be a discrepancy between the relative depths in the cells at which the sections are taken. Furthermore, there may be differences in the planar angle of the light optical and electron optical section because of the realignment of the cell or tissue block in the ultramicrotome.

6.4.1.2 Tetracysteine Tags. Although GFP and its derivatives have been successfully incorporated into many different proteins without detectably interfering with the functions of these proteins, the considerable size of the GFP analogs (approximately 30 kDa) can pose a problem when coupled to smaller proteins (Evans and Martin, 2002; Frischknecht et al., 2006). This was elegantly demonstrated in a study by Andresen et al., which showed that the genetic tagging of GFP to β-tubulin was nonviable in haploid yeast cells, while tagging with shorter sequences did not interfere with the formation and dynamics of microtubules (Andresen et al., 2004). For this reason, alternative genetically encoded markers that are smaller and thus less likely to interfere with the biological function of the tagged protein are sought. A method that is becoming increasingly popular is based on protein tagging with a tetracysteine (4C) motif, which is a small peptide sequence of 10–20 amino acids containing two pairs of cysteine residues that flank a pair of spacer amino acids (Cys-Cys-Xaa-Xaa-Cys-Cys, where Xaa represents a noncysteine amino acid) (Giepmans et al., 2006; Tsien, 2005). This motif can bind to fluorescent biarsenical derivatives, each arsenic interacting with one of the cysteine doublets. The most widely employed biarsenical dyes are the green light emitting FlAsH (Fluorescein-Based Arsenical Hairpin Binder) and the red light emitting ReAsH (Resorufin-Based Arsenical Hairpin Binder) (Machleidt et al., 2007; Tsien, 2005). These dyes are membrane permeable and can therefore be used to label 4C tags in living cells (Gaietta et al., 2002; Rudner et al., 2005). Because arsenics are potentially cytotoxic, FlAsH and ReAsH need to be administered to the cells in combination with an antidote, such as 1,2-ethanedithiol or β-mercaptoethanol. In addition to reducing the toxicity of the biarsenical dyes, the antidote diminishes the fluorescence of the dyes before their binding to a 4C motif. Nevertheless, background fluorescence is an issue in this technique that can hamper the detection of weak signals. Part of this background fluorescence can be due to nonspecific binding of biarsenicals to endogenous proteins that are cysteine-rich (Stroffekova et al., 2001). Considerable effort has been directed toward optimizing the 4C/biarsenical labeling technique, and the future is likely to hold further improvements. Already, new biarsenical probes that produce less background have been devised, and novel 4C motifs that display higher affinity and stronger fluorescence have been found (Adams et al., 2002; Martin et al., 2005; Spagnuolo et al., 2006).

The 4C/biarsenical detection system can also be employed for CLEM. Gaietta et al., showed that ReAsH bound to tetracysteine motifs and immobilized by chemical fixation was able to photoconvert DAB (Gaietta et al., 2002). This technique allowed the authors to demonstrate differences in the intracellular trafficking route between newly synthesized and older connexins, which are the building blocks of gap junctions (Sosinsky et al., 2003).

6.4.1.3 Theme Variations: Split GFP and GFP-4C. As discussed in Sections 6.4.1.1 and 6.4.1.2, the currently available toolbox of genetic probes for live-cell imaging and CLEM has a number of limitations. Thus GFP and GFP analogs can cause functional interference and may produce only weak photoconversion reactions, while nonspecific reactions, cytotoxic effects, and the need for a reducing environment can plague the 4C/biarsenical system. Indeed, establishing a procedure for live-cell imaging and CLEM always implies that one needs to find a compromise between functional integrity and experimental feasibility. And for as long as the ideal probe remains to be discovered, there is merit in developing adaptations of existing detection systems that may remedy some of the side effects.

Ghosh et al., showed that when GFP is split into two polypeptides they will not fluoresce independently, but when coexpressed in bacteria they will reconstitute and fluoresce (Ghosh et al., 2000). However, in order for the reconstitution to occur, the polypeptide sequences needed to be linked to antiparallel leucine zipper domains. Cabantous et al., extended this research and engineered self-assembling GFP fragments (Cabantous et al., 2005). They showed that small GFP fragments (16 amino acids long), coupled to the protein of interest via a linker peptide, could self-assemble with the complementary GFP fragment that was expressed separately. Because the split GFP approach involves the coming together of two GFP fragments, it has been proved to be useful to study protein–protein interactions, coexpression, and conformational changes in proteins (Magliery et al., 2005; Zhang et al., 2004). In the future, it may also become a powerful alternative to the 4C/biarsenical system by displaying the same advantage as the latter (small tag attached to protein of interest) but without the disadvantages. It would be conceivable then to expand the complementary GFP fragment with an HRP sequence (~44 kDa) to achieve optimal DAB oxidation for CLEM.

In a different adaptation published recently, part of the Golgi resident enzyme α-mannosidase II was fused to a hybrid tag containing both a GFP and a 4C sequence (Gaietta et al., 2006). This construct was used to study by means of CLEM the reassembly of the Golgi apparatus in daughter cells formed during mitosis. Live-cell imaging was carried out by monitoring the GFP fluorescence, while 4C/ReAsH was used to photoconvert DAB for visualization at the EM level. The advantage of this procedure lies in the fact that the photoconversion of DAB was not triggered by direct excitation of ReAsH but by FRET between GFP and ReAsH. Because FRET occurs only when the participating fluorochromes are less than ~8 nm apart, the DAB precipitation becomes more specific as background fluorescence of ReAsH is virtually eliminated.

6.4.2 Probes to Detect Endogenous Proteins

The genetic approaches outlined in Section 6.4.1 can be very powerful for studying a protein's dynamic function, localization, and interactions. However, since a genetically tagged protein is always overexpressed in cells or tissues, it may affect in unpredictable ways its own behavior and that of its endogenous counterpart (Andresen et al., 2004; Hanson and Ziegler, 2004). Therefore, there is a constant necessity to obtain feedback from nontransformed cells or tissues. The most widespread detection system is based on the recognition of unique epitopes in proteins by monospecific antibodies. The antibodies can be visualized by fluorochromes, gold particles, or the product of an enzymatic reaction (e.g., HRP/DAB) (Sternberger, 1986). Often, the label is not conjugated to the primary antibody but to a secondary detection molecule that recognizes the primary antibody; the secondary molecule can be an antibody as well or the bacterially derived protein A and protein G. The advantages of indirect immunobased detection are that (i) the cross-linking of the label does not compromise the specificity of the primary antibody, (ii) it opens up the possibility of signal amplification, and (iii) the same secondary probe can be used to detect different primary antibodies.

Immunocytochemical procedures usually require prior chemical fixation of the biological material, and to ensure accessibility of intracellular epitopes to the detection molecules, membranes have to be permeabilized. Paradoxically, only mild chemical fixatives can be used, as the stronger fixatives suppress the immunogenicity of the specimen. Weak fixation and permeabilization have a negative impact on the ultrastructural preservation. It follows that protocols for immuno-EM necessitate a careful balance of antigenicity and preservation.

In addition to antibody-based detection systems, there are a number of compounds that display high affinity for specific proteins and that can be conjugated to fluorescent or other types of indicators. Classic examples are the cytoskeletal markers, phalloidin and paclitaxel. Phalloidin is a toxin derived from the death cap mushroom, *Amanita phalloides*, and binds specifically to filamentous actin (Small et al., 1999; Vetter, 1998; Wulf et al., 1979). Paclitaxel, better known by its trade name Taxol, is a compound derived from the bark of the Pacific yew tree, *Taxus brevifolia*, and labels microtubules (Manfredi et al., 1982). Eosin-labeled phalloidin is not only fluorescent but also suitable for photo-oxidation, ergo for CLEM (Capani et al., 2001). Because phalloidin and eosin are both small molecules, they can easily penetrate fixed cells and tissues.

6.4.2.1 Antifluorochrome Antibodies. Antibodies raised against fluorochromes can be used to bring a gold label in the vicinity of a fluorescent label. The feasibility of this approach was first demonstrated in the early 1990s by van Dam et al., who used gold-conjugated antibodies against Fluorescein Isothiocyanate (FITC) to detect at the ultrastructural level a protein (gut-associated circulating cathodic antigen) in the worm *Schistosoma mansoni* (van Dam et al., 1991). Hence the technique is potentially useful for CLEM studies. Recently, Coleman et al., reported that the fluorochrome Alexa Fluor 488 remains immunoreactive even after fixing with glutaraldehyde and osmium tetroxide, embedding in epoxy resin, and etching with sodium ethoxide (Coleman et al., 2006). They demonstrated that it was thus possible to perform pre-embedding immunolocalizations of a transporter and an ion channel in rat kidney and to detect the Alexa Fluor 488 label subsequently in semithin and thin plastic sections with anti-Alexa Fluor 488 antibodies. These antibodies were in turn detected by secondary antibodies conjugated either to a fluorophore for LM or to colloidal gold for EM.

6.4.2.2 Combined Fluorescent and Gold Probes. The ideal CLEM probe is self-contained and visible by LM as well as by EM. One possible design that has received reasonable attention in the literature is to conjugate to the same antibody or antibody fragment both a fluorochrome and a gold particle. Early attempts to generate such a probe led to the notion that fluorescence is quenched by colloidal gold, presumably by FRET from the fluorochrome to the gold particle (Powell et al., 1998). Despite that, secondary antibodies with both a fluorochrome conjugate and 5- or 10-nm colloidal gold are still commercially available. Kandela and Albrecht recently demonstrated that these are actually a mixture of antibodies carrying either fluorochromes only or both fluochromes and colloidal gold. They went on to show that the fluorescence of the colloidal-gold-conjugated antibodies was almost completely quenched (Kandela and Albrecht, 2007).

These probes are therefore not suitable for a 1:1 colocalization as is ideally required for correlation between LM and EM, especially when taking into account the difference in penetration rate between antibodies with and without a gold label.

The problem of fluorescence quenching by gold can be overcome by using small gold cluster complexes, that is, nanogold, instead of colloidal gold (Robinson and Vandre, 1997). Owing to the smaller size of the gold particle, there is an additional advantage, namely, the probe can penetrate cells and tissues more readily. The accessibility of antigenic sites to FluoroNanogold probes is further increased by coupling the fluorochrome and nanogold to only that portion of an antibody (the Fab′ fragment) that binds to the antigen. However, nanogold particles are too small and display too little contrast to be observed by EM at the normal magnification range for heavy-metal-stained biological specimens. An enlargement step is therefore required to increase the size and contrast of the gold particles. This can be achieved either by gold toning or by silver enhancement (Baschong and Stierhof, 1998; Sawada and Esaki, 2000). Both techniques are prone to artifacts, ranging from ultrastructural modifications to nonspecific precipitations (Baschong and Stierhof, 1998). They also eliminate the fluorescent properties of the fluorochrome, so that fluorescence microscopy needs to be performed before the enlargement step. It is possible, however, to view the silver-enhanced immunogold signal by means of brightfield LM, thus allowing for precise correlation between the fluorescence and electron microscopic images. Notwithstanding the pitfalls associated with the use of FluoroNanogold, a number of studies have emphasized its potential for CLEM applications. Most notably, Takizawa and Robinson applied FluoroNanogold to ultrathin cryosections of human placental tissue and were thus able to investigate by CLEM the subcellular distribution of markers of caveolae and endosomes (Takizawa and Robinson, 2003). A spin-off of this research was the realization that because of their thinness, ultrathin cryosections yield very sharp fluorescence micrographs that lack z-axis blur (Mori et al., 2006).

6.4.2.3 Quantum Dots. Quantum Dots (Qds) are inorganic fluorescent semiconductor nanocrystals. They possess unique properties that are extremely advantageous for biomedical applications in general, and CLEM in particular: (i) QDs can be tuned to emit light at a wide spectrum of wavelengths by changing their composition and size; (ii) in comparison with organic fluorophores, QDs possess a long Stoke's shift and a narrow emission spectrum, thus allowing for superior spectral separation and improved detection sensitivity; (iii) QDs of different emission wavelengths can be excited by the same excitation wavelength, which facilitates imaging of multiple labels; (iv) unlike organic fluorophores, QDs can be illuminated over extended periods of time without showing any noticeable photobleaching; (v) because they are inorganic, QDs are resistant to biodegradation and can therefore be used for *in vivo* imaging over extended periods of time; (vi) QDs possess elevated two-photon absorptivity (up to 47,000

Goeppert-Mayer units), making them ideal for multiphoton fluorescence microscopy; and (vii) QDs are electron dense, and their sizes are within the range of immunogold particles, so that they can be detected by EM (Bruchez, 2005; Giepmans et al., 2005; Jaiswal and Simon, 2004; Larson et al., 2003; Nisman et al., 2004).

QDs are rapidly finding applications in many areas, ranging from nanotechnology to consumer electronics. The composition of QDs varies accordingly, and many laboratories are working on new and improved flavors. QDs that are employed in fluorescent probes typically possess a core–shell structure, the core consisting of cadmium selenide (CdSe) and the shell of zinc sulfide (ZnS). This core–shell configuration results in enhanced quantum yield and photostability. The size of the core determines the wavelength of the emitted light. Without modifications, QDs are toxic and hydrophobic, properties that are incompatible with studies in living cells, tissues, or whole organisms and that render difficult their conjugation to biomolecules. Therefore, QDs for biomedical research are encapsulated with a polymer to prevent leaking of the toxic metals and to permit binding of biomolecules. Nevertheless, the potential toxic effects of QDs remain an area of concern among many investigators (Chang et al., 2006; Hardman, 2006; Ryman-Rasmussen et al., 2007). It is a complicated matter because QDs can have such different compositions and consequently display very different degrees of toxicity.

QDs have been used and are commercially available as conjugates with secondary antibodies or streptavidin for indirect detection methods, but they can also be labeled directly to the primary detection molecule. Owing to their size and properties, QDs cannot traverse the membrane of cells, thus limiting their usefulness for live-cell imaging. It is therefore a challenge for current research to devise protocols that allow passage of QDs across the membrane of living cells. Hoshino et al., took a step in this direction by demonstrating that QDs conjugated with peptides that encode either a nuclear localization signal or a mitochondrial localization signal are rapidly targeted to nuclei or mitochondria, respectively, of cells in culture (Hoshino et al., 2004). Another strategy involves the uptake of QDs via endocytosis, allowing, for instance, monitoring of the dynamics of receptor internalization (Chang et al., 2006; Genovesio et al., 2006; Michalet et al., 2005; Seleverstov et al., 2006; Sundara Rajan and Vu, 2006). Recently, Duan and Nie reported that a surface coating of QDs with polyethylene glycol grafted polyethylimine allows the QDs to escape from endosomes via endosomolysis (Duan and Nie, 2007). Although it is a stretch to name these QDs "cell penetrating," they represent promising candidates for intracellular delivery of QDs. Further data will be needed to assess their cytotoxicity and their ability to be stably conjugated to biological detection molecules such as antibodies.

6.4.2.4 Dendrimers. Dendrimers constitute an exciting new class of nanocarriers. They are named after their dendritic architecture, which consists of branched subunits attached to a central core. The surface of dendrimers can be modified to confer special properties pertaining to their biocompatibility (Najlah and D'Emanuele, 2006). Dendrimers have already found numerous applications in pharmaceutics. Their ability to encapsulate drugs allows for site-specific and controlled drug delivery, protection of drugs against premature biodegradation, decreased toxicity, and improved solubility. In addition to the entrapping of molecules within the dendritic structure, it is possible to conjugate molecules, such as antibodies, to surface groups of dendrimers (Roberts et al., 1990). Of special interest is the ability of dendrimers to enter cells, which renders them very useful as carriers for intracellular delivery (Najlah and D'Emanuele, 2006). As a matter of fact, dendrimers are already used quite successfully as gene carriers, that is, transfection agents, and are commercially available for that purpose (SuperFect reagent from Qiagen).

At the time of writing, there are no known CLEM applications yet that employ dendrimer nanotechnology. However, it is in the line of expectation that this will change soon, as there is growing awareness of the potential benefits of using dendrimers as nanoprobes. A particularly promising area of research involves the coating of QDs with dendrimers (Liu et al., 2006). In doing so, Wisher et al. recently demonstrated that dendrimer-coated QDs, with a total diameter of 11 nm, were internalized by NT2 cells and that these fluorescent nanocarriers could cotransport the calcium-binding protein, S100A4 (Wisher et al., 2006). The mechanism via which dendrimers are internalized appears to involve endocytosis. Escape of the dendrimers and their cargo from endosomal compartments are likely to represent a major obstacle for efficient cytosolic delivery. If future research unequivocally demonstrates that dendrimer-based nanoprobes can effectively translocate from endosomal compartments to the cytosol, they will become extremely powerful tools for live-cell imaging and CLEM detection of endogenous proteins and other molecules.

6.4.3 Probes to Detect Nonproteinaceous Molecules

In principle, all of the indicators discussed in Section 6.4.2 can also be employed to visualize biomolecules that are nonproteinaceous (e.g., lipids, nucleic acids, sugars). To this effect, they need to be conjugated to specific bioprobes. To name a few, lectins derived from either plants or animals are used to detect various sugar residues, oligonucleotides can be designed and synthesized to detect specific RNA and DNA sequences, and cholera toxin binds to plasma membrane ganglioside GM1, which partitions into lipid rafts. Some probes for nonproteinaceous molecules display intrinsic fluorescent properties, thereby obviating the need for conjugation to a separate fluorochrome. A widely used example of such a probe is FM 1-43, an amphipatic molecule that intercalates into the outer leaflet of lipid bilayers, after which its fluorescence increases greatly. FM 1-43 is often employed to visualize activity-dependent membrane recycling, that is, the coupled process of endocytosis and exocytosis, in nerve terminals (Cochilla et al., 1999). Of particular interest for CLEM, it has been shown that FM 1-43 can be detected at the EM level via photo-oxidation of DAB (Darcy et al., 2006; Henkel et al., 1996; Nishikawa and Sasaki, 1996).

6.5 CLEM APPLICATIONS

6.5.1 Diagnostic Electron Microscopy

The advent of Enzyme-Linked Immunosorbent Assay (ELISA) and nucleic acid amplification tests has led to a considerable diminution in the diagnostic use of EM (Biel and Gelderblom, 1999). Nevertheless, there are still numerous clinically important diseases where EM excels as a diagnostic tool. These include skin and renal diseases involving structural defects of components of the extracellular matrix, in particular collagen; ciliary disorders such as Kartagener's syndrome where dynein arms and other components of the axoneme are absent or defective; lysosomal storage diseases; and pulmonary conditions caused by intrapulmonary deposits, especially asbestos (Alroy and Ucci, 2006; Carlen and Stenram, 2005; Foster et al., 2005; Howell et al., 1998; Suzuki et al., 2005). Diagnostic EM is also a vital and powerful tool for the identification of infectious agents such as viruses. When combined with a negative stain procedure, it is a more rapid method for viral diagnosis than other diagnostic tests that are currently available (Biel and Gelderblom, 1999). Moreover, and in contrast to other tests, diagnostic EM does not require any prior assumptions about the nature of the infectious agent, so that even unexpected pathogens can be detected. It is this same undirectedness that renders EM also important as a tool for assessing tumor cell lineage in the course of tumor diagnosis. Examples of ultrastructural determinants for cell lineage are Birbeck granules (Langerhans cells), lamellar bodies (alveolar epithelial type II cells), Weibel-Palade bodies (endothelial cells), and intercellular junctions (epithelial cells).

CLEM can complement diagnostic EM techniques as a means to facilitate the search in biopsies for areas of disease that require ultrastructural analysis. Thus, at the LM level, tissue samples can be surveyed to obtain rapidly relevant information on the orientation, architecture, and location of tissue components (Jones et al., 1982). It is then a matter of selecting areas of interest, which can be zoomed into at the EM level. To give an example, thin basement membrane nephropathy and X-linked Alport syndrome are glomerular disorders that are characterized by diffuse thinning of the glomerular basement membrane. Ultrastructural examination of renal biopsies is considered an essential step toward the final diagnosis of these diseases. However, the thickness of the glomerular basement membrane varies greatly, and to obtain accurate measurements, care must be taken that the methods for tissue preparation and morphometry are standardized. For instance, it is common practice to measure the thickness of the basement membrane in at least 2 glomeruli and at random sites in different capillary loops with the same orientation (Foster et al., 2005). It would be much less time consuming if the selection of areas to be measured could be done at the LM level.

The now defunct LEM 2000 combined light and electron microscope (Akashi Seisakusho Ltd., Tokyo, Japan) was equipped with a microprocessor that enabled the recording of coordinates for multiple areas of interest selected in LM mode. The coordinates could then be retrieved in EM mode to permit precise correlation with the LM fields of view. The LEM 2000 used a larger grid size (7 mm in diameter; for comparison, standard grid size is 3 mm), allowing for the observation of larger sample areas (Nelson, 1986). These features made the LEM 2000 an instrument of choice for diagnostic CLEM (Jones et al., 1982). It is therefore puzzling that the LEM 2000 has not become more of a mainstream microscope in pathology departments. Maybe it was introduced ahead of its time when its true potential could not yet be appreciated (the Commission of the European Communities decided on July 6, 1981, that the LEM 2000 may not be imported free of common customs tariffs duties because "apparatus of scientific value equivalent to the said apparatus, capable of being used for the same purposes, are currently being manufactured in the Community"). At present, it would be the right time to resurrect a combined light and electron microscope system, taking advantage of modern digital imaging techniques, microscope automation, and ever increasing computing resources. The LM mode of the LEM 2000 allowed only widefield images to be taken. Therefore, it was necessary to generate contrast by staining the ultrathin sections with toluidine blue. A modern version of an integrated CLEM system should also include the possibility of visualizing fluorescent signals in order to increase the palette of stains and probes that can be applied to specimens. As a matter of fact, such an integrated system has recently been developed. Named LEM, for light and electron microscope, it comprises a laser scanning fluorescence microscope built into a commercially available TEM (Agronskaia et al., (2008)). The principle of the LEM is illustrated schematically in Figure 6.2. The laser scanning fluorescence microscope of the LEM is a retractable unit mounted on one of the TEM's side ports. Imaging in LM and EM mode is done sequentially, using the original sample stage and specimen holder of the TEM. Intermodal coordinate retrieval is fully automated via software implementation. The lateral optical resolution of the Fluorescence Laser Scanning Microscope (FLSM) is estimated at 0.55 μm for an excitation wavelength of 470 nm. The power of the LEM system has been demonstrated already using several different biological samples. This integrated approach obliterates the disadvantages that accompany conventional CLEM procedures. It will be useful in many areas of biomedical research, such as diagnostic EM.

6.5.2 Ultrastructural Neuroanatomy

Neuroscientists have embraced and developed CLEM techniques to elucidate the intricate microcircuits formed by neuronal connections in the central nervous system and to correlate (electro)physiological data with morphological characteristics. Owing to their considerable size, neurons are readily classified at the LM level, while EM resolution is required to characterize their synaptic connectivity (Valentijn et al., 1989). For a long time, CLEM was performed by means of the combined Golgi-EM technique (Fairen, 2005; Peters, 2002). Central to this technique was the Golgi impregnation method, which randomly impregnated in tissue blocks a subset of neurons and glial cells with a metallic deposit. At the LM level, impregnated cells appeared dark, and cell bodies with their processes (dendrites and axons) could be viewed in three dimensions. The metallic impregnation was electron dense, so that the same neurons could be identified at the

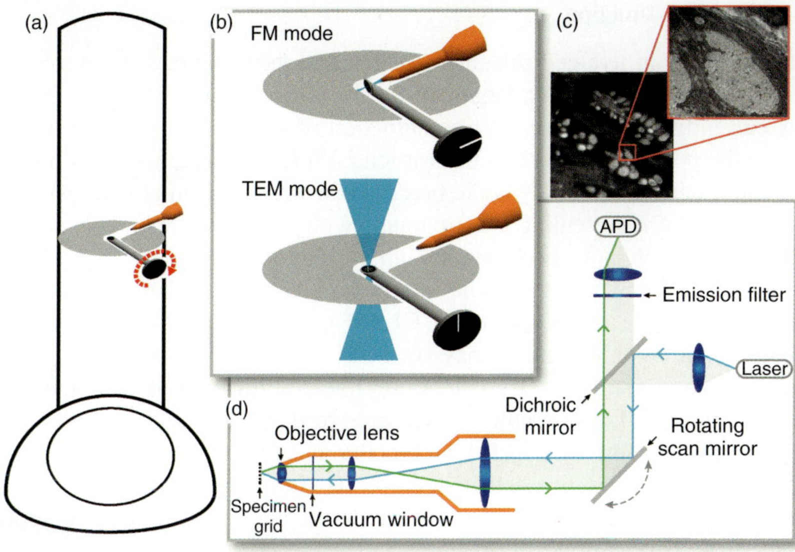

Figure 6.2. Schematic representation of the integrated light and electron microscope (LEM), which was recently developed as a novel approach to CLEM. The LEM comprises a Fluorescence Laser Scanning Microscope (FLSM) that is mounted as a retractable unit (depicted in orange) on one of the side ports of a commercial TEM (a). The FLSM is positioned perpendicular to the TEM specimen holder. In fluorescence microscopy mode (FM mode), the specimen and specimen holder are rotated 90° so that the specimen can be scanned by the laser beam of the FLSM unit (b). In TEM mode, the FLSM unit is retracted and the specimen tilted to the 0° position, allowing for imaging with the electron beam. (c) A typical fluorescence micrograph of a 300 μm × 300 μm area taken with the LEM in FM mode and a zoom of the boxed area acquired in TEM mode. The sample was a thin plastic section of rat duodenum in which the mucous granule fields of goblet cells were fluorescently labeled with Alexa Fluor 488 conjugated wheat germ agglutinin. The optical module of the FLSM (d) was designed to fit in the limited space available in the TEM column and to be vacuum compatible. For this reason, the objective consists of a single aspherical lens, shielded from the rest of the optical system by a thin, flat vacuum window. The fluorescence emission is detected by an Avalanche Photo Diode (APD). (With thanks to Dr Sasha Agronskaia for help with the recording of the fluorescence micrograph in (c)).

EM level. Several enhancements to the technique, such as deimpregnation and gold toning, resulted in finer ultrastructural detail (Fairen, 2005).

Today, the Golgi-EM technique has fallen from grace; as alternatives, more predictable methods are available. These include intracellular or juxtacellular injection of fluorescent tracers (e.g., lucifer yellow) and loading of synaptic vesicles with FM 1-43 or one of its spectral variants (Cochilla et al., 1999; Stewart, 1981). Photoconversion of DAB can then be used to obtain an electron-dense label for EM analysis (Maranto, 1982; Nikonenko et al., 2005). Another approach is to perform pre-embedding labeling of the tracer with silver-enhanced ultrasmall gold (Morozov et al., 2002).

6.5.3 Live-Cell Imaging

The recent surge in live-cell imaging research and the concomitant development of genetic probes account in a large part for the renaissance of CLEM techniques that is currently taking place. The combination of CLEM and live-cell imaging opens up the possibility to obtain ultrastructural information at a chosen moment during the progression of a dynamic process that was captured at LM resolution. Hence, instead of representing a static image with features of unknown pedigree, an EM micrograph now becomes a high resolution "snapshot" in which the features have a known history. The interpretational gain is therefore immense. An elegant example of the power of CLEM combined with live-cell imaging is the work of Svitkina and Borisy on actin dynamics (Svitkina and Borisy, 1998; Svitkina et al., 2003). By combining live-cell imaging of GFP-actin with platinum replica EM, these authors were able to develop models explaining the molecular mechanisms by which lamellipodia and filipodia are formed. This is also a demonstration of live-cell imaging at its simplest: making use of unique features to detect actin filaments at the EM level, there was no need to apply a label for EM visualization.

The studies by Svitkina and Borisy took advantage of the fact that the cellular protrusions they investigated were thin enough to be imaged in toto. It is a commonly encountered problem, however, that the cells in which a dynamic process is observed are too thick for subsequent EM analysis. The current remedy is embedding of the cells in either ice or a resin, followed by ultrathin sectioning. The drawback of this strategy, as discussed in Section 6.4.1.1, is that an optical section recorded by LM can never be matched exactly with an ultrathin section because of differences in section thickness and section angle. In the worst-case scenario, it could result in a fluorescent signal being attributed erroneously to an ultrastructural feature that is not at all present in the optical section from which the fluorescence was recorded. A prospective solution that depends on the implementation of image processing routines is to perform multimodal alignment of three-dimensional reconstructions of both LM image stacks and EM tilt series (see Section 6.5.4).

When the fluorescent signal under investigation stems from a genetically tagged protein that does not display any particular structural feature recognizable at the EM level, additional processing is required to convert the fluorescent label in an electron-dense label. Photoconversion of DAB and (silver-enhanced) immunogold labeling are the currently available options. Photoconversion appears to yield the best results when the DAB precipitation is confined to a fully or partially membrane-enclosed space, such as the lumen of a Golgi cisterna, a synaptic vesicle, or a dendritic spine (Capani et al., 2001; Darcy et al., 2006; Grabenbauer et al., 2005). Owing to the nature of the reaction, DAB staining is rather diffuse. As a consequence, there is limited high resolution information available in DAB-labeled structures. Immunogold labeling, on the other hand, can be capricious, as several parameters pertaining to sample preparation (e.g., fixation, permeabilization) influence the efficacy and uniformity of the label. In this regard, when one scrutinizes published examples, the correlation between fluorescent and immunogold signals can sometimes be quite obscure.

6.5.4 Electron Tomography

Analogous to the miscellaneous forms of tomography used in modern diagnostic medicine—several of which are discussed in the present volume—electron tomography is a technique that generates a 3D reconstruction, that is, a tomogram, from a series of 2D images taken of a 3D object at different viewing angles (Koster et al., 1997; McEwen and Marko, 2001). As its name indicates, electron tomography deals with 2D images that are acquired with an electron microscope. The high resolution of EM enables electron tomography to model structures that are as small as macromolecules. The different 2D viewing angles are obtained by tilting the specimen in the electron beam while acquiring images at discrete tilt angles (McIntosh et al., 2005). With increasing tilt angles, the path length of the electron beam through the specimen increases gradually, up to a point where the majority of the electrons are scattered and image detail is lost. In practice, this means that the maximum usable range of tilt angles goes from -70 to 70°. As a consequence, tomograms display a so-called missing wedge artifact due to the lack of 3D information at higher tilt angles. The missing wedge is characteristic for electron tomography, that is, it is not found in medical tomographies. It causes a distortion along the viewing axis perpendicular to the tilt axis, which results in the fading of linear structures such as membranes and fibers. Fortunately, the missing wedge artifact can be greatly reduced by tilting the specimen around two orthogonal axes, resulting in a dual-axis tomogram (Marsh, 2005; McIntosh et al., 2005).

The development and implementation of electron tomographic techniques goes hand in hand with the ongoing progress in computer-assisted microscope automation, digital image acquisition, and computing resources (Leapman, 2004). A powerful computing environment is important not only to display the large data sets tomograms consist of but also to calculate the 3D reconstructions from the 2D data. Several algorithms are available to generate tomograms, but the most commonly used are based on the principle of back projection (Fig. 6.3).

With an appropriate viewer program, tomograms can be browsed slice by slice, and along any of the three axes. Each tomographic slice represents an image that is just a few nanometers thick. The resolution is comparably high on all three axes. Conversely, in a conventional 2D electron micrograph the lateral resolution is also in the order of a few nanometers, but the z-axial resolution is limited by the section thickness (typically 50–70 nm; Fig. 6.4) (McIntosh et al., 2005). The fine structural detail in three dimensions revealed by a tomogram can be overwhelmingly complex. It is therefore common practice to generate graphic models in which features of interest are accentuated by different colors; shadows and color gradients are applied to simulate lighting and perspective (for some colorful examples, see References Marsh, 2005; McIntosh et al., 2005; Trucco et al., 2004). These graphic representations can be drawn by hand or generated with the assistance of image processing routines such as an edge detection filter.

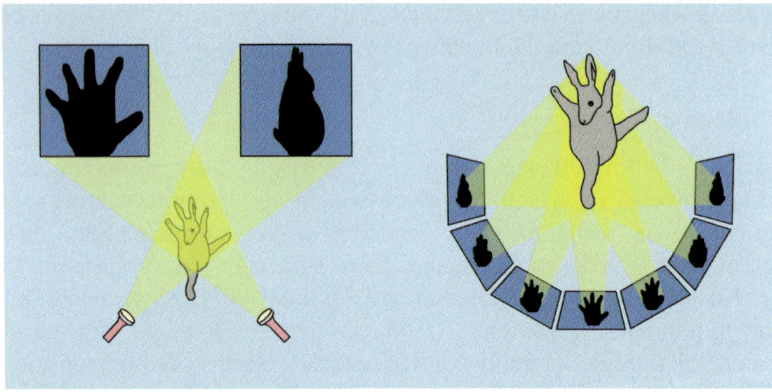

Figure 6.3. The principle of electron tomography. Depending on the projection angle of the light source, the 3D rabbit will cast a different 2D shadow. By analogy, a 3D biological sample will generate varying 2D projections when it is tilted in the electron microscope. By back projection of a series of 2D images into a virtual 3D space, the source 3D object can be reconstructed. (Based on a cartoon by John O'Brien, which appeared in *The New Yorker* magazine).

Electron tomography is still too time consuming to allow for live 3D browsing of a specimen. For this reason, areas of interest need to be selected in 2D views. If the electron-accelerating voltage of the electron microscope is sufficiently elevated or if an energy filter is used, high resolution electron tomograms can be made from specimens that are up to 400 nm thick, and yet thicker specimens have been imaged with special high voltage electron microscopes. Even at more standard specimen sizes (around 200 nm thick) for electron tomography, it can be difficult to find areas of interest in a 2D image because of the stacking of electron-dense features that obscure the image. In this respect, CLEM has the potential to facilitate the search for areas of interest, as the section thickness will not obscure photon-based imaging. Crucial for this application is the availability of fluorescent labeling protocols that are compatible with thin plastic sections and EM processing. An alternative approach that is interesting to highlight here is the GRAB technique by Grabenbauer et al., already mentioned in Section 6.4.1.1, which allowed the authors to study by means of CLEM and electron tomography the Golgi distribution of the glycosylation enzyme *N*-acetylgalactosaminyltransferase (Grabenbauer et al., 2005).

Apart from aiding in the retrieval of areas of interest, CLEM techniques are also invaluable for electron tomography in combination with live-cell imaging. Thus McEwen et al. used video LM to track chromosome movement in living cells and subsequently employed CLEM to perform electron tomography on the kinetochores of the same chromosomes (McEwen et al., 1997).

6.5.5 Cryoelectron Microscopy

Electron microscopists working in the life sciences have always been concerned with possible side effects of chemical fixation, dehydration, embedding, and

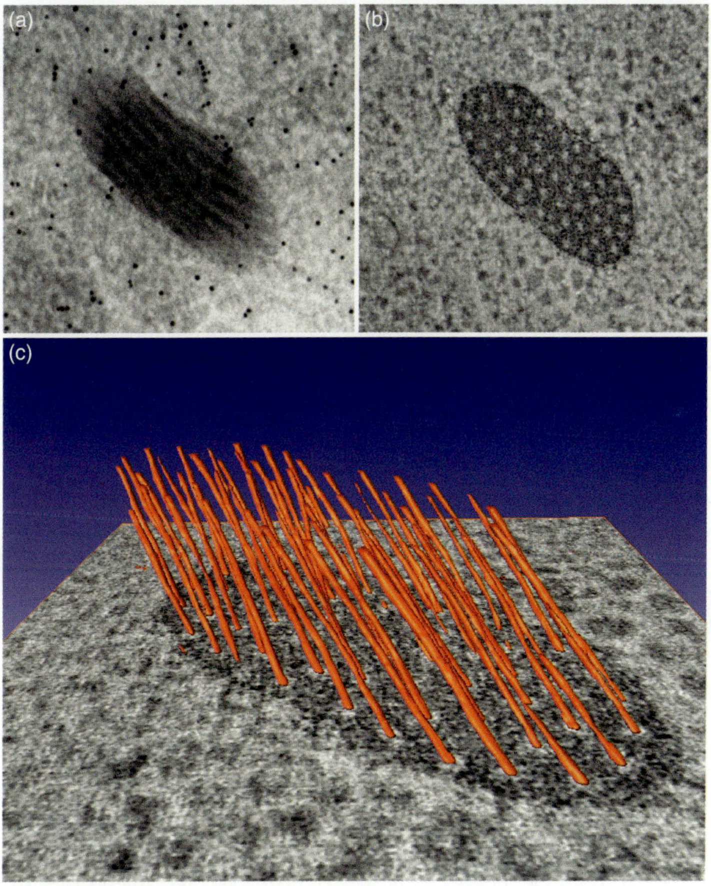

Figure 6.4. The power of electron tomograpy. Images illustrate alternative views of a Weibel-Palade body, a specialized secretory granule, in a human umbilical vein endothelial cell. The Weibel-Palade body measures approximately 450 × 200 nm. (a) A standard 2D electron micrograph. Note the ill-defined boundaries of the Weibel-Palade body, which appears to contain seven longitudinal striations running in parallel. The black dots correspond to 10-nm gold particles; they were applied on the section as fiducial markers to aid in the alignment of the tomographic images. (b) A tomographic slice 4 nm thick taken from the reconstruction of the Weibel-Palade body after imaging by dual-axis tomography. Note that the boundaries are much sharper and that the organelle now contains 58 cross-sectioned tubules. (c) A 3D model of the internal organization of the Weibel-Palade body, superimposed on a tomographic slice. Evidently, the tomography data reveal important features that are masked in the 2D micrograph.

contrasting on the ultrastructural preservation of tissues, cells, or isolated macromolecular complexes (see, e.g., Murk et al., 2003). Thus, the question arises as to what extent structural and molecular interactions observed in heavily processed specimens reflect the functioning in living cells. Cryoelectron microscopy emerged out of an urge to address this very question (Lucic et al., 2005; McIntosh, 2001). Central to cryoelectron microscopic techniques is the preservation of biological specimens in their native, that is, hydrated, state. This is done via vitrification, a process whereby the specimen is cooled very rapidly to liquid nitrogen temperatures, so that the water in and around the specimen becomes vitreous, that is, an amorphous or noncrystalline liquid (Costello, 2006). In the process, all molecules become immobilized without any alteration in their location or chemical composition. This is sometimes referred to as *cryofixation*, which is a confusing term because it wrongly suggests that the molecules are cross-linked.

The most commonly used vitrification methods are plunge freezing and high pressure freezing (Braet et al., 2007; McDonald and Auer, 2006; McIntosh et al., 2005). The former consists in the plunging of the specimen into a cryogen, ethane or propane, that is cooled by liquid nitrogen, and the latter uses high pressure (around 2100 bar) combined with rapid freezing to prevent ice crystal formation. Plunge freezing is limited by a vitrification depth of just a few micrometers and is therefore suitable only for thin cells and suspensions of macromolecules. High pressure freezing, on the other hand, permits cryoimmobilization of samples up to 0.2 mm thick and is therefore also suitable for tissue fragments such as biopsies.

There is a price to be paid when studying biological samples in their native state. First, samples need to remain cooled at all times after vitrification to avoid ice crystal formation, which will occur if the temperature rises to -135°C or higher (Al-Amoudi et al., 2004). This requires highly specialized equipment and techniques for handling and imaging. Second, cryoelectron micrographs display an elevated signal to noise ratio because of the lack of image contrast. The reason for this is that the samples cannot be stained and they can only be viewed under low electron dose conditions in order to avoid radiation damage. Third, when the specimen thickness reaches 1μm or above, it cannot be observed anymore by a regular TEM. This restriction can be overcome by cutting ultrathin vitreous sections of the objects that are too large for direct observation (Al-Amoudi et al., 2004). This approach, termed *CEMOVIS* for Cryoelectron Microscopy of Vitreous Sections, adds to the complexity and required skills of the whole sample preparation procedure. Despite all the limitations mentioned here, several laboratories around the world perform cryo-EM and CEMOVIS routinely and successfully.

Cryo-EM is most rewarding when combined with tomography. Cryoelectron tomography allows for the 3D imaging of cellular components in a close-to-native state, with a resolution of 4–5 nm, high enough to detect macromolecular complexes (Grunewald et al., 2003; Steven and Aebi, 2003). There is increasing awareness that many of a cell's molecules are organized in larger macromolecular complexes or machines (Chiu et al., 2006; Nogales and Grigorieff, 2001), of which the ribosome is the quintessential example (Medalia et al., 2002); other examples are the nuclear pore complex (Beck et al., 2004) and the proteasome (Nickell et al., 2007; Walz et al., 1998). One of the most exciting applications of cryoelectron tomography is to map the cellular distribution of such macromolecular complexes. The mapping is achieved with the help of computational methods, in particular, pattern-recognition algorithms such as template matching via cross-correlation. This field of research, which was baptized "visual proteomics" by one of its front-runners, the Baumeister group at the Max Planck Institute in Martinsried, Germany, aims at establishing 3D atlases of supramolecular structures in cells (Nickell et al., 2006). Once available, these atlases would have the potential to provide novel insights into the spatial regulation of protein interactions.

The aforementioned low contrast conditions and low electron dose requirements for cryo-EM make it particularly difficult to retrieve areas of interest. Quite frequently, one only knows if the selected areas are interesting after the final image or tilt series is collected and enhanced by image processing routines. Several laboratories are currently developing cryo-CLEM methods as a tool to identify areas for subsequent cryo-EM analysis (Leis et al., 2005; Sartori et al., 2005). The technical challenge these laboratories are facing is that fluorescence microscopy needs to be performed on specimens kept at liquid nitrogen temperatures, while using optics that yield sufficient resolution to obtain subcellular detail. Furthermore, labeling with a fluorescent marker needs to be carried out before the cryoimmobilization procedure. This is an additional complication, because many fluorescent probes cannot penetrate the plasma membrane of living cells without additional treatment, such as microinjection, lipofection, or electroporation.

6.5.6 Immuno Electron Microscopy

Ultrastructural studies emanating from a cell biological question often call for the localization of a specific protein. Immunogold detection is the most widely used method. There are several strategies for decorating the protein of interest with an immunogold tag. Pre-embedding immunogold labeling is carried out on chemically fixed material before resin embedding. To enhance penetration of the antibodies and gold particles, the specimen is usually permeabilized. This can be done by using a detergent to extract membranes or by using a number of freeze-thaw cycles to puncture membranes with ice crystals (Stirling, 1990); some investigators even go as far as smashing tissue fragments in a homogenizer (Michalet et al., 2005). It will come as no surprise that these techniques yield poor ultrastructural preservation.

Much better preservation can be obtained with postembedding immunogold labeling on ultrathin sections. The Tokuyasu method, named after its inventor, utilizes ultrathin sections of chemically fixed material, cut by means of cryoultramicrotomy (Liou et al., 1996; Tokuyasu, 1973); the labeling and microscopy, however, is performed at room temperature. This technique can be combined with electron tomography, and as such, it has enabled Zeuschner et al., to analyze COPII-coated transport carriers between the endoplasmic reticulum and the Golgi apparatus (Zeuschner et al., 2006). Immunogold labeling can also be performed on ultrathin sections of resin-embedded specimens. Acrylate- and methacrylate-based resins can be directly labeled, while epoxy resins require additional treatment, such as surface etching with sodium ethoxide, for antigen retrieval (Groos et al., 2001; Newman and Hobot, 1999). Freeze substitution is the preferred method for specimen infiltration with resin, as it results in improved morphology and immunoreactivity (Shiurba, 2001. The principle behind freeze substitution is to replace the ice in a cryoimmobilized specimen by an organic solvent (e.g., acetone or methanol) while a low temperature is maintained (-80 to -90°C) (Giddings, 2003; Shiurba, 2001). As the temperature is slowly raised, fixatives added to the solvent will start to cross-link biomolecules in the sample. Subsequently, the sample is infiltrated with resin, and the resin is polymerized either by UV illumination at low temperatures (-30°C) or by warming (60°C).

The postembedding immunostaining techniques can be adapted for CLEM by using bifunctional probes, such as antibodies conjugated to FluoroNanogold, HRP/DAB, or QDs (Groos et al., 2001; Robinson et al., 2001). Alternatively, probes that only provide visual clues at the LM level to reveal histoarchitectural features can be used, which can aid in general orientation and identification of specific areas (McNary et al., 1964). In a number of studies, CLEM has been carried out on adjacent ultrathin and semithin sections cut by cryoultramicrotomy (Mironov et al., 2003; van der Wel et al., 2005). The rationale for this approach is that the semithin cryosectioning technique allows for the sampling of larger tissue areas, typically 2×2 mm; this facilitates the pinpointing of areas of interest, which can then be isolated by further trimming of the specimen block to an area, typically 300×200 μm, suitable for ultrathin sectioning and immunogold labeling for immuno-EM (van der Wel et al., 2005).

6.6 FUTURE PERSPECTIVE

The ultimate CLEM experiment would yield a 3D reconstruction that combines perfectly aligned fluorescence microscopic and electron tomographic data taken throughout a whole cell or tissue fragment, with a resolution in all three planes of 100–200 nm and 3–4 nm, respectively. The apotheosis would be complete if such a CLEM image volume could in turn be correlated with a 3D volume obtained by a type of medical tomography, for instance, computer tomography (CT). The main ingredients for achieving these goals are already available. Thus confocal laser scanning microscopy followed by deconvolution-based image restoration allows for optical sectioning of a cell with a z-resolution that is nearly as good as the lateral resolution of 100–200 nm (Agard et al., 1989; Hell et al., 1997). Methods for serial section electron tomography have been developed together with algorithms to join multiple tomograms (Marsh, 2005; Soto et al., 1994). The bottleneck at present is that such an endeavor would take many months if not years to complete. This is mainly due to a lack of computational tools for high throughput analysis of complex 3D data sets.

Another consideration for future directions in CLEM is the development of universally applicable protocols. Presently, many different recipes for CLEM are described in the literature, and especially for the novice venturing in this field of research, the information and available options may be daunting. This is well illustrated in Figures 6.5–6.7, which recapitulate the various CLEM strategies

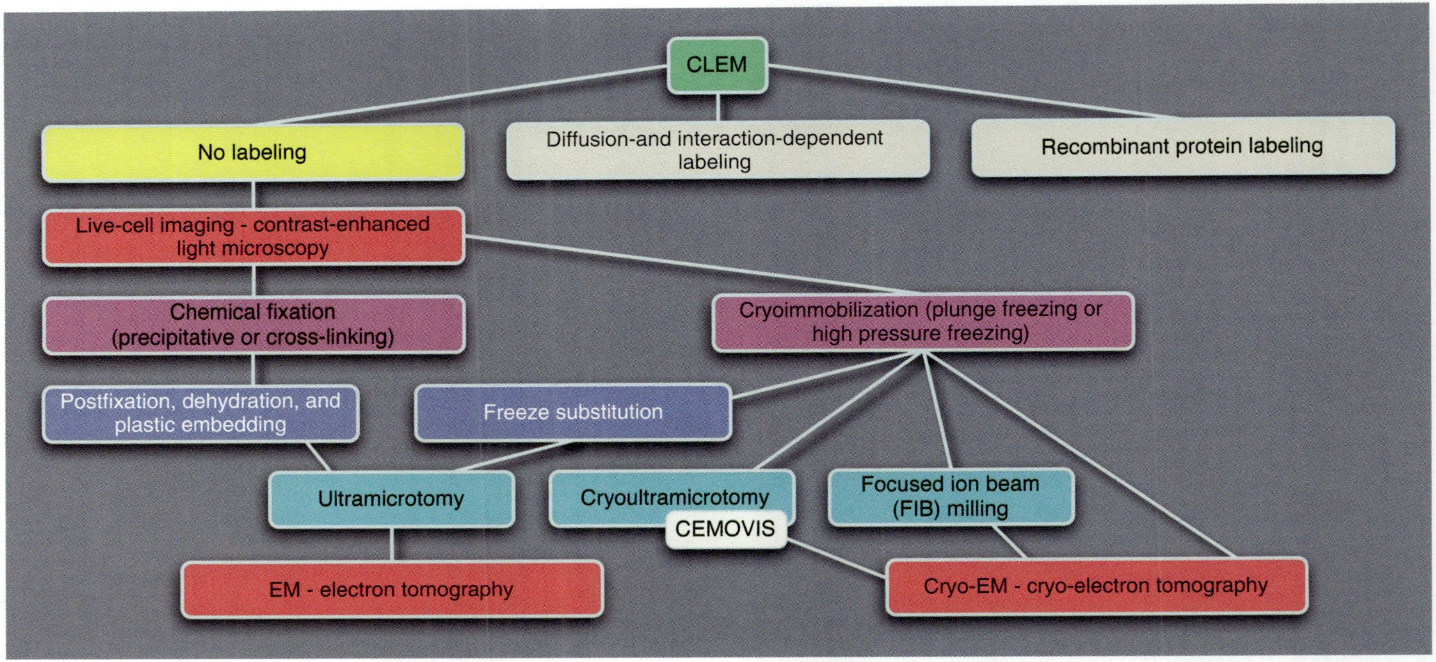

Figure 6.5. Schematic representation of possible CLEM strategies. For the sake of clarity, the flowchart has been broken down into three parts on the basis of labeling methods. This figure deals with CLEM without any labeling.

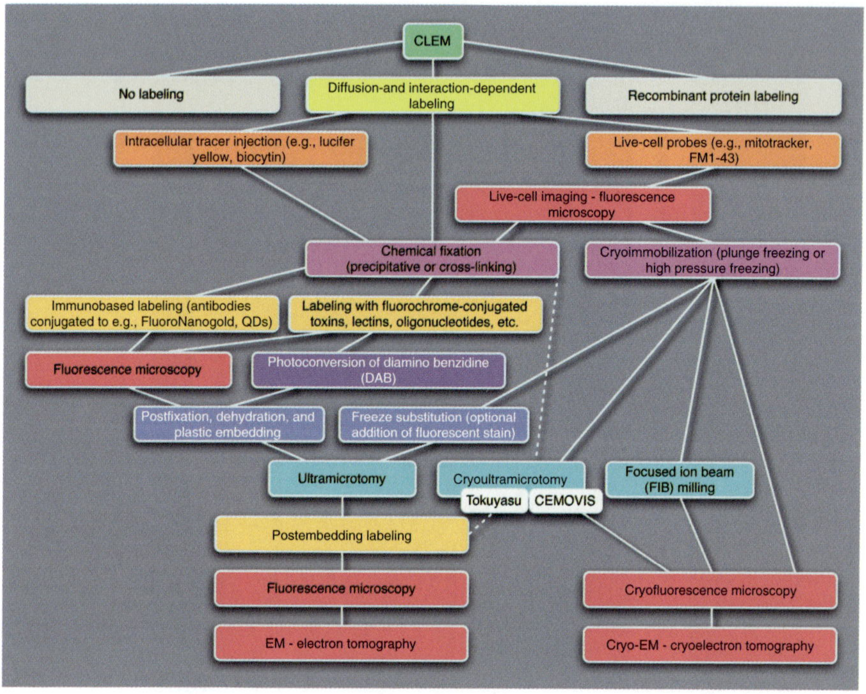

Figure 6.6. Schematic representation of possible CLEM strategies using diffusion- and interaction-dependent labeling techniques.

discussed here. Clearly, an important reason for this amalgam of methods is the lack of a multifunctional probe that can be used ubiquitously. QDs are promising, but currently their applicability is restricted by their difficulty to traverse cell membranes. The same problem haunts fluoronanogold probes, albeit to a lesser extent, but their need for silver enhancement is not without complications as well. Future developments in the field of multimodal indicators are therefore eagerly awaited. A new generation of reporters that have the potential to form multifunctional probes is represented by infrared up-converting phosphors (Corstjens et al., 2005).

New developments in instrumentation for EM and LM will also have a great impact on CLEM applications. Notably, Focused Ion Beam (FIB) technology is showing promise as a tool to thin whole frozen-hydrated cells so that they can be imaged by cryo-EM (Marko et al., 2006; Marko et al., 2007). It would be extremely helpful if a fluorescence microscopic signal could be used as a guide for the FIB procedure. In parallel, light microscopic techniques that exceed the diffraction limit of resolution by at least fivefold (e.g., Total Internal Reflectance Fluorescence Microscopy (TIRFM) and 4Pi microscopy) (Egner and Hell, 2005; Schneckenburger, 2005) have been developed. Recent advances in wet EM, also referred to as *Environmental Scanning Electron Microscopy* (ESEM), are likely to boost CLEM applications as well (Timp et al., 2006). Unlike conventional

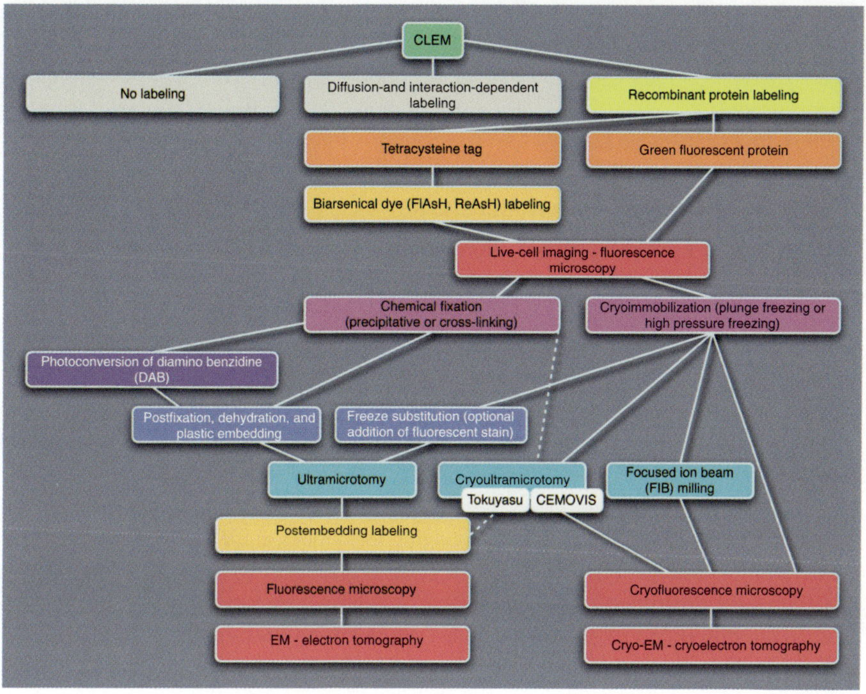

Figure 6.7. Schematic representation of possible CLEM strategies using recombinant protein labeling. Note that the tetracysteine method actually uses a combination of genetic tagging and diffusion-/interaction-dependent labeling.

EM, wet EM permits the observation of hydrated samples without the need for specimen preparation (Muscariello et al., 2005).

Unquestionably, there are interesting times ahead for EM and LM techniques in general, and for CLEM in particular.

REFERENCES

Adams SR, Campbell RE, Gross LA, Martin BR, Walkup GK, Yao Y, Llopis J, Tsien RY. New biarsenical ligands and tetracysteine motifs for protein labeling in vitro and in vivo: synthesis and biological applications. J Am Chem Soc 2002;124(21):6063–6076.

Agard DA, Hiraoka Y, Shaw P, Sedat JW. Fluorescence microscopy in three dimensions. Methods Cell Biol 1989;30:353–377.

Agronskaia AV, Valentijn JA, van Driel LF, Schneijdenberg CT, Humbel BM, van Bergen en Henegouwen PM, Verkleij AJ, Koster AJ, Gerritsen HC. Integrated fluorescence and transmission electron microscopy J Struct Biol 2008;164(2):183–9.

Al-Amoudi A, Chang JJ, Leforestier A, McDowall A, Salamin LM, Norlen LP, Richter K, Blanc NS, Studer D, Dubochet J. Cryo-electron microscopy of vitreous sections. EMBO J 2004;23(18):3583–3588.

Alroy J, Ucci AA. Skin biopsy: a useful tool in the diagnosis of lysosomal storage diseases. Ultrastruct Pathol 2006;30(6):489–503.

Andresen M, Schmitz-Salue R, Jakobs S. Short tetracysteine tags to beta-tubulin demonstrate the significance of small labels for live cell imaging. Mol Biol Cell 2004;15(12):5616–5622.

Baschong W, Stierhof YD. Preparation, use, and enlargement of ultrasmall gold particles in immunoelectron microscopy. Microsc Res Tech 1998;42(1):66–79.

Beck M, Forster F, Ecke M, Plitzko JM, Melchior F, Gerisch G, Baumeister W, Medalia O. Nuclear pore complex structure and dynamics revealed by cryoelectron tomography. Science 2004;306(5700):1387–1390.

Biel SS, Gelderblom HR. Diagnostic electron microscopy is still a timely and rewarding method. J Clin Virol 1999;13(1–2):105–119.

Biel SS, Kawaschinski K, Wittern KP, Hintze U, Wepf R. From tissue to cellular ultrastructure: closing the gap between micro- and nanostructural imaging. J Microsc 2003; 212(Pt 1):91–99.

Braet F, Wisse E, Bomans P, Frederik P, Geerts W, Koster A, Soon L, Ringer S. Contribution of high-resolution correlative imaging techniques in the study of the liver sieve in three-dimensions. Microsc Res Tech 2007;70(3):230–242.

Brock R, Jovin TM. Fluorescence correlation microscopy (FCM)-fluorescence correlation spectroscopy (FCS) taken into the cell. Cell Mol Biol 1998;44(5):847–856.

Bruchez MP. Turning all the lights on: quantum dots in cellular assays. Curr Opin Chem Biol 2005;9(5):533–537.

de Bruijn WC, Sorber CW, Gelsema ES, Beckers AL, Jongkind JF. Energy-filtering transmission electron microscopy of biological specimens. Scanning Microsc 1993;7(2):693–708, discussion 709.

Buckley IK. A simple technique for comparative light and electron microscopy of designated living cultured cells. Lab Invest 1971;25(4):295–301.

Cabantous S, Terwilliger TC, Waldo GS. Protein tagging and detection with engineered self-assembling fragments of green fluorescent protein. Nat Biotechnol 2005;23(1):102–107.

Capani F, Deerinck TJ, Ellisman MH, Bushong E, Bobik M, Martone ME. Phalloidin-eosin followed by photo-oxidation: a novel method for localizing F-actin at the light and electron microscopic levels. J Histochem Cytochem 2001;49(11):1351–1361.

Carlemalm E, Kellenberger E. The reproducible observation of unstained embedded cellular material in thin sections: visualisation of an integral membrane protein by a new mode of imaging for STEM. EMBO J 1982;1(1):63–67.

Carlen B, Stenram U. Primary ciliary dyskinesia: a review. Ultrastruct Pathol 2005;29(3–4):217–220.

Chalfie M, Tu Y, Euskirchen G, Ward WW, Prasher DC. Green fluorescent protein as a marker for gene expression. Science 1994;263(5148):802–805.

Chang E, Thekkek N, Yu WW, Colvin VL, Drezek R. Evaluation of quantum dot cytotoxicity based on intracellular uptake. Small 2006;2(12):1412–1417.

Chiu W, Baker ML, Almo SC. Structural biology of cellular machines. Trends Cell Biol 2006;16(3):144–150.

Cochilla AJ, Angleson JK, Betz WJ. Monitoring secretory membrane with FM1-43 fluorescence. Annu Rev Neurosci 1999;22:1–10.

Coleman RA, Liu J, Wade JB. Use of anti-fluorophore antibody to achieve high-sensitivity immunolocalizations of transporters and ion channels. J Histochem Cytochem 2006;54(7):817–827.

Corstjens PL, Li S, Zuiderwijk M, Kardos K, Abrams WR, Niedbala RS, Tanke HJ. Infrared up-converting phosphors for bioassays. IEEE Proc Nanobiotechnol 2005;152(2):64–72.

Costello MJ. Cryo-electron microscopy of biological samples. Ultrastruct Pathol 2006;30(5):361–371.

van Dam GJ, Bogitsh BJ, Fransen JA, Kornelis D, van Zeyl RJ, Deelder AM. Application of the FITC-anti-FITC-gold system to ultrastructural localization of antigens. J Histochem Cytochem 1991;39(12):1725–1728.

Darcy KJ, Staras K, Collinson LM, Goda Y. Constitutive sharing of recycling synaptic vesicles between presynaptic boutons. Nat Neurosci 2006;9(3):315–321.

van Driel LF, Knoops K, Koster AJ, Valentijn JA. Fluorescent labeling of resin-embedded sections for correlative electron microscopy using tomography-based contrast enhancement. J Struct Biol 2008;161(3):372–83.

Duan H, Nie S. Cell-penetrating quantum dots based on multivalent and endosome-disrupting surface coatings. J Am Chem Soc 2007;129:3333–3338.

Egner A, Hell SW. Fluorescence microscopy with super-resolved optical sections. Trends Cell Biol 2005;15(4):207–215.

Evans WH, Martin PE. Lighting up gap junction channels in a flash. Bioessays 2002;24(10):876–880.

Fairen A. Pioneering a golden age of cerebral microcircuits: the births of the combined Golgi-electron microscope methods. Neuroscience 2005;136(3):607–614.

Foster K, Markowitz GS, D'Agati VD. Pathology of thin basement membrane nephropathy. Semin Nephrol 2005;25(3):149–158.

Frischknecht F, Renaud O, Shorte SL. Imaging today's infectious animalcules. Curr Opin Microbiol 2006;9(3):297–306.

Gaietta G, Deerinck TJ, Adams SR, Bouwer J, Tour O, Laird DW, Sosinsky GE, Tsien RY, Ellisman MH. Multicolor and electron microscopic imaging of connexin trafficking. Science 2002;296(5567):503–507.

Gaietta GM, Giepmans BN, Deerinck TJ, Smith WB, Ngan L, Llopis J, Adams SR, Tsien RY, Ellisman MH. Golgi twins in late mitosis revealed by genetically encoded tags for live cell imaging and correlated electron microscopy. Proc Natl Acad Sci U S A 2006;103(47):17777–17782.

Genovesio A, Liedl T, Emiliani V, Parak WJ, Coppey-Moisan M, Olivo-Marin JC. Multiple particle tracking in 3-D+t microscopy: method and application to the tracking of endocytosed quantum dots. IEEE Trans Image Process 2006;15(5):1062–1070.

Geuze HJ. A future for electron microscopy in cell biology? Trends Cell Biol 1999;9(3):92–93.

Ghosh I, Hamilton AD, Regan L. Antiparallel leucine zipper-directed protein reassembly: application to the green fluorescent protein. J Am Chem Soc 2000;122(23):5658–5659.

Giddings TH. Freeze-substitution protocols for improved visualization of membranes in high-pressure frozen samples. J Microsc 2003;212(Pt 1):53–61.

Giepmans BN, Adams SR, Ellisman MH, Tsien RY. The fluorescent toolbox for assessing protein location and function. Science 2006;312(5771):217–224.

Giepmans BN, Deerinck TJ, Smarr BL, Jones YZ, Ellisman MH. Correlated light and electron microscopic imaging of multiple endogenous proteins using Quantum dots. Nat Methods 2005;2(10):743–749.

Grabenbauer M, Geerts WJ, Fernadez-Rodriguez J, Hoenger A, Koster AJ, Nilsson T. Correlative microscopy and electron tomography of GFP through photooxidation. Nat Methods 2005;2(11):857–862.

Groos S, Reale E, Luciano L. Re-evaluation of epoxy resin sections for light and electron microscopic immunostaining. J Histochem Cytochem 2001;49(3):397–406.

Grunewald K, Medalia O, Gross A, Steven AC, Baumeister W. Prospects of electron cryotomography to visualize macromolecular complexes inside cellular compartments: implications of crowding. Biophys Chem 2003;100(1–3):577–591.

Hanker JS. Osmiophilic reagents in electronmicroscopic histocytochemistry. Prog Histochem Cytochem 1979;12(1):1–85.

Hanson DA, Ziegler SF. Fusion of green fluorescent protein to the C-terminus of granulysin alters its intracellular localization in comparison to the native molecule. J Negat Results Biomed 2004;3(1):2.

Hardman R. A toxicologic review of quantum dots: toxicity depends on physicochemical and environmental factors. Environ Health Perspect 2006;114(2):165–172.

Hayat MA. *Correlative Microscopy in Biology: Instrumentation and Methods*. London: Academic Press, Inc.; 1987.

Hell SW, Schrader M, van der Voort HT. Far-field fluorescence microscopy with three-dimensional resolution in the 100-nm range. J Microsc 1997;187(Pt 1):1–7.

Henkel AW, Lubke J, Betz WJ. FM1-43 dye ultrastructural localization in and release from frog motor nerve terminals. Proc Natl Acad Sci U S A 1996;93(5):1918–1923.

Hollander H. The section embedding (SE) technique. A new method for the combined light microscopic and electron microscopic examination of central nervous tissue. Brain Res 1970;20(1):39–47.

Hoshino A, Fujioka K, Oku T, Nakamura S, Suga M, Yamaguchi Y, Suzuki K, Yasuhara M, Yamamoto K. Quantum dots targeted to the assigned organelle in living cells. Microbiol Immunol 2004;48(12):985–994.

Howell DN, Payne CM, Miller SE, Shelburne JD. Special techniques in diagnostic electron microscopy. Hum Pathol 1998;29(12):1339–1346.

Jaiswal JK, Simon SM. Potentials and pitfalls of fluorescent quantum dots for biological imaging. Trends Cell Biol 2004;14(9):497–504.

Jones S, Chapman SK, Crocker PR, Carson G, Levison DA. Combined light and electron microscope in routine histopathology. J Clin Pathol 1982;35(4):425–429.

Kandela IK, Albrecht RM. Fluorescence quenching by colloidal heavy metals nanoparticles: implications for correlative fluorescence and electron microscopy. Scanning 2007;29:152–161. [E-pub ahead of print].

Koster AJ, Grimm R, Typke D, Hegerl R, Stoschek A, Walz J, Baumeister W. Perspectives of molecular and cellular electron tomography. J Struct Biol 1997;120(3):276–308.

Koster AJ, Klumperman J. Electron microscopy in cell biology: integrating structure and function. Nat Rev Mol Cell Biol 2003;9 Suppl: SS6–SS10.

Larson DR, Zipfel WR, Williams RM, Clark SW, Bruchez MP, Wise FW, Webb WW. Water-soluble quantum dots for multiphoton fluorescence imaging in vivo. Science 2003;300(5624):1434–1436.

Leapman RD. Novel techniques in electron microscopy. Curr Opin Neurobiol 2004;14(5):591–598.

Leis A, Andrees L, Gruska M, Al-Amoudi A, Sartori A, Dubochet J, Baumeister W. Cryo-electron tomography and fluorescence microscopy of unicellular algae in vitreous cryosections. Microsc Microanal 2005;11 Suppl 2:330–331.

Liou W, Geuze HJ, Slot JW. Improving structural integrity of cryosections for immunogold labeling. Histochem Cell Biol 1996;106(1):41–58.

Liu J, Li H, Wang W, Xu H, Yang X, Liang J, He Z. Use of ester-terminated polyamidoamine dendrimers for stabilizing quantum dots in aqueous solutions. Small 2006;2(8–9):999–1002.

Lucic V, Forster F, Baumeister W. Structural studies by electron tomography: from cells to molecules. Annu Rev Biochem 2005;74:833–865.

Machleidt T, Robers M, Hanson GT. Protein labeling with FlAsH and ReAsH. Methods Mol Biol 2007;356:209–220.

Magliery TJ, Wilson CG, Pan W, Mishler D, Ghosh I, Hamilton AD, Regan L. Detecting protein-protein interactions with a green fluorescent protein fragment reassembly trap: scope and mechanism. J Am Chem Soc 2005;127(1):146–157.

Manfredi JJ, Parness J, Horwitz SB. Taxol binds to cellular microtubules. J Cell Biol 1982;94(3):688–696.

Maranto AR. Neuronal mapping: a photooxidation reaction makes Lucifer yellow useful for electron microscopy. Science 1982;217(4563):953–955.

Marko M, Hsieh C, Moberlychan W, Mannella CA, Frank J. Focused ion beam milling of vitreous water: prospects for an alternative to cryo-ultramicrotomy of frozen-hydrated biological samples. J Microsc 2006;222(Pt 1):42–47.

Marko M, Hsieh C, Schalek R, Frank J, Mannella C. Focused-ion-beam thinning of frozen-hydrated biological specimens for cryo-electron microscopy. Nat Methods 2007;4:215–217.

Marsh BJ. Lessons from tomographic studies of the mammalian Golgi. Biochim Biophys Acta 2005;1744(3):273–292.

Martin BR, Giepmans BN, Adams SR, Tsien RY. Mammalian cell-based optimization of the biarsenical-binding tetracysteine motif for improved fluorescence and affinity. Nat Biotechnol 2005;23(10):1308–1314.

McDonald KL, Auer M. High-pressure freezing, cellular tomography, and structural cell biology. Biotechniques 2006;41(2):137, 139, 141 passim.

McEwen BF, Heagle AB, Cassels GO, Buttle KF, Rieder CL. Kinetochore fiber maturation in PtK1 cells and its implications for the mechanisms of chromosome congression and anaphase onset. J Cell Biol 1997;137(7):1567–1580.

McEwen BF, Marko M. The emergence of electron tomography as an important tool for investigating cellular ultrastructure. J Histochem Cytochem 2001;49(5):553–564.

McIntosh JR. Electron microscopy of cells: a new beginning for a new century. J Cell Biol 2001;153(6):F25–F32.

McIntosh R, Nicastro D, Mastronarde D. New views of cells in 3D: an introduction to electron tomography. Trends Cell Biol 2005;15(1):43–51.

McNary WF Jr, Rosan RC, Kerrigan JA. Fluorescent microscopy of thin sections as an adjunct to electron microscopy. J Histochem Cytochem 1964;12:216–217.

Medalia O, Weber I, Frangakis AS, Nicastro D, Gerisch G, Baumeister W. Macromolecular architecture in eukaryotic cells visualized by cryoelectron tomography. Science 2002;298(5596):1209–1213.

Michalet X, Pinaud FF, Bentolila LA, Tsay JM, Doose S, Li JJ, Sundaresan G, Wu AM, Gambhir SS, Weiss S. Quantum dots for live cells, in vivo imaging, and diagnostics. Science 2005;307(5709):538–544.

Mironov A Jr, Latawiec D, Wille H, Bouzamondo-Bernstein E, Legname G, Williamson RA, Burton D, DeArmond SJ, Prusiner SB, Peters PJ. Cytosolic prion protein in neurons. J Neurosci 2003;23(18):7183–7193.

Mironov AA, Beznoussenko GV, Luini A, Polishchuk RS. Visualizing intracellular events in vivo by combined video fluorescence and 3-D electron microscopy. Methods Enzymol 2005;404:43–57.

Mironov AA, Polishchuk RS, Luini A. Visualizing membrane traffic in vivo by combined video fluorescence and 3D electron microscopy. Trends Cell Biol 2000;10(8):349–353.

Monosov EZ, Wenzel TJ, Luers GH, Heyman JA, Subramani S. Labeling of peroxisomes with green fluorescent protein in living P. pastoris cells. J Histochem Cytochem 1996;44(6):581–589.

Mori M, Ishikawa G, Takeshita T, Goto T, Robinson JM, Takizawa T. Ultrahigh-resolution immunofluorescence microscopy using ultrathin cryosections: subcellular distribution of caveolin-1alpha and CD31 in human placental endothelial cells. J Electron Microsc (Tokyo) 2006;55(2):107–112.

Morozov Y, Khalilov I, Ben-Ari Y, Represa A. Correlative fluorescence and electron microscopy of biocytin-filled neurons with a preservation of the postsynaptic ultrastructure. J Neurosci Methods 2002;117(1):81–85.

Murk JL, Posthuma G, Koster AJ, Geuze HJ, Verkleij AJ, KLeijmeer MJ, Humbel BM. Influence of aldehyde fixation on the morphology of endosomes and lysosomes: quantitative analysis and electron tomography. J Microsc 2003;212(Pt 1):81–90.

Muscariello L, Rosso F, Marino G, Giordano A, Barbarisi M, Cafiero G, Barbarisi A. A critical overview of ESEM applications in the biological field. J Cell Physiol 2005;205(3):328–334.

Najlah M, D'Emanuele A. Crossing cellular barriers using dendrimer nanotechnologies. Curr Opin Pharmacol 2006;6(5):522–527.

Nelson AC. Computer-aided microtomography with true 3-D display in electron microscopy. J Histochem Cytochem 1986;34(1):57–60.

Newman GR, Hobot JA. Resins for combined light and electron microscopy: a half century of development. Histochem J 1999;31(8):495–505.

Nickell S, Kofler C, Leis AP, Baumeister W. A visual approach to proteomics. Nat Rev Mol Cell Biol 2006;7(3):225–230.

Nickell S, Mihalache O, Beck F, Hegerl R, Korinek A, Baumeister W. Structural analysis of the 26S proteasome by cryoelectron tomography. Biochem Biophys Res Commun 2007;353(1):115–120.

Nikonenko I, Boda B, Alberi S, Muller D. Application of photoconversion technique for correlated confocal and ultrastructural studies in organotypic slice cultures. Microsc Res Tech 2005;68(2):90–96.

Nishikawa S, Sasaki F. Internalization of styryl dye FM1-43 in the hair cells of lateral line organs in Xenopus larvae. J Histochem Cytochem 1996;44(7):733–741.

Nisman R, Dellaire G, Ren Y, Li R, Bazett-Jones DP. Application of quantum dots as probes for correlative fluorescence, conventional, and energy-filtered transmission electron microscopy. J Histochem Cytochem 2004;52(1):13–18.

Nogales E, Grigorieff N. Molecular Machines: putting the pieces together. J Cell Biol 2001;152(1):F1–10.

Oorschot V, de Wit H, Annaert WG, Klumperman J. A novel flat-embedding method to prepare ultrathin cryosections from cultured cells in their in situ orientation. J Histochem Cytochem 2002;50(8):1067–1080.

Paddock SW. Further developments of the laser scanning confocal microscope in biomedical research. Proc Soc Exp Biol Med 1996;213(1):24–31.

Peters A. Examining neocortical circuits: some background and facts. J Neurocytol 2002;31(3–5):183–193.

Pfeiffer S, Beese M, Boettcher M, Kawaschinski K, Krupinska K. Combined use of confocal laser scanning microscopy and transmission electron microscopy for visualisation of identical cells processed by cryotechniques. Protoplasma 2003;222(3–4):129–137.

Pfeiffer S, Vielhaber G, Vietzke JP, Wittern KP, Hintze U, Wepf R. High-pressure freezing provides new information on human epidermis: simultaneous protein antigen and lamellar lipid structure preservation. Study on human epidermis by cryoimmobilization. J Invest Dermatol 2000;114(5):1030–1038.

Polishchuk RS, Polishchuk EV, Marra P, Alberti S, Buccione R, Luini A, Mironov AA. Correlative light-electron microscopy reveals the tubular-saccular ultrastructure of carriers operating between Golgi apparatus and plasma membrane. J Cell Biol 2000;148(1):45–58.

Polishchuk RS, San Pietro E, Di Pentima A, Tete S, Bonifacino JS. Ultrastructure of long-range transport carriers moving from the trans Golgi network to peripheral endosomes. Traffic 2006;7(8):1092–1103.

Porter KR, Claude A, Fullam EF. A study of tissue culture cells by electron microscopy: methods and preliminary observations. J Exp Med 1945;81(3):233–246.

Powell RD, Halsey CM, Hainfeld JF. Combined fluorescent and gold immunoprobes: reagents and methods for correlative light and electron microscopy. Microsc Res Tech 1998;42(1):2–12.

Prasher DC, Eckenrode VK, Ward WW, Prendergast FG, Cormier MJ. Primary structure of the Aequorea victoria green-fluorescent protein. Gene 1992;111(2):229–233.

Roberts JC, Adams YE, Tomalia D, Mercer-Smith JA, Lavallee DK. Using starburst dendrimers as linker molecules to radiolabel antibodies. Bioconjug Chem 1990;1(5):305–308.

Robinson JM, Takizawa T, Pombo A, Cook PR. Correlative fluorescence and electron microscopy on ultrathin cryosections: bridging the resolution gap. J Histochem Cytochem 2001;49(7):803–808.

Robinson JM, Vandre DD. Efficient immunocytochemical labeling of leukocyte microtubules with FluoroNanogold: an important tool for correlative microscopy. J Histochem Cytochem 1997;45(5):631–642.

Rudner L, Nydegger S, Coren LV, Nagashima K, Thali M, Ott DE. Dynamic fluorescent imaging of human immunodeficiency virus type 1 gag in live cells by biarsenical labeling. J Virol 2005;79(7):4055–4065.

Ryman-Rasmussen JP, Riviere JE, Monteiro-Riviere NA. Surface coatings determine cytotoxicity and irritation potential of quantum dot nanoparticles in epidermal keratinocytes. J Invest Dermatol 2007;127(1):143–153.

Salmon ED, Tran P. High-resolution video-enhanced differential interference contrast light microscopy. Methods Cell Biol 2003;72:289–318.

Sartori A, Gatz R, Beck F, Kossel A, Leis A, Baumeister W, Plitzko JM. Correlation microscopy: bridging the gap between light- and cryo-electron microscopy. Microsc Microanal 2005;11 Suppl 2:16–17.

Sawada H, Esaki M. A practical technique to postfix nanogold-immunolabeled specimens with osmium and to embed them in Epon for electron microscopy. J Histochem Cytochem 2000;48(4):493–498.

Schneckenburger H. Total internal reflection fluorescence microscopy: technical innovations and novel applications. Curr Opin Biotechnol 2005;16(1):13–18.

Seleverstov O, Zabirnyk O, Zscharnack M, Bulavina L, Nowicki M, Heinrich JM, Yezhelyev M, Emmrich F, O'Regan R, Bader A. Quantum dots for human mesenchymal stem cells labeling. A size-dependent autophagy activation. Nano Lett 2006;6(12):2826–2832.

Shimomura O. The discovery of aequorin and green fluorescent protein. J Microsc 2005;217(Pt 1):1–15.

Shiurba R. Freeze-substitution: origins and applications. Int Rev Cytol 2001;206:45–96.

Small J, Rottner K, Hahne P, Anderson KI. Visualising the actin cytoskeleton. Microsc Res Tech 1999;47(1):3–17.

Sosinsky GE, Gaietta GM, Hand G, Deerinck TJ, Han A, Mackey M, Adams SR, Bouwer J, Tsien RY, Ellisman MH. Tetracysteine genetic tags complexed with biarsenical ligands as a tool for investigating gap junction structure and dynamics. Cell Commun Adhes 2003;10(4–6):181–186.

Soto GE, Young SJ, Martone ME, Deerinck TJ, Lamont S, Carragher BO, Hama K, Ellisman MH. Serial section electron tomography: a method for three-dimensional reconstruction of large structures. Neuroimage 1994;1(3):230–243.

Spagnuolo CC, Vermeij RJ, Jares-Erijman EA. Improved photostable FRET-competent biarsenical-tetracysteine probes based on fluorinated fluoresceins. J Am Chem Soc 2006;128(37):12040–12041.

Sternberger LA. *Immunocytochemistry*. New York: John Wiley & Sons; 1986.

Steven AC, Aebi U. The next ice age: cryo-electron tomography of intact cells. Trends Cell Biol 2003;13(3):107–110.

Stewart WW. Lucifer dyes-highly fluorescent dyes for biological tracing. Nature 1981;292(5818):17–21.

Stirling JW. Immuno- and affinity probes for electron microscopy: a review of labeling and preparation techniques. J Histochem Cytochem 1990;38(2):145–157.

Stroffekova K, Proenza C, Beam KG. The protein-labeling reagent FLASH-EDT2 binds not only to CCXXCC motifs but also non-specifically to endogenous cysteine-rich proteins. Pflugers Arch 2001;442(6):859–866.

Sundara Rajan S, Vu TQ. Quantum dots monitor TrkA receptor dynamics in the interior of neural PC12 cells. Nano Lett 2006;6(9):2049–2059.

Suzuki Y, Yuen SR, Ashley R. Short, thin asbestos fibers contribute to the development of human malignant mesothelioma: pathological evidence. Int J Hyg Environ Health 2005;208(3):201–210.

Svitkina TM, Borisy GG. Correlative light and electron microscopy of the cytoskeleton of cultured cells. Methods Enzymol 1998;298:570–592.

Svitkina TM, Bulanova EA, Chaga OY, Vignjevic DM, Kojima S, Vasiliev JM, Borisy GG. Mechanism of filopodia initiation by reorganization of a dendritic network. J Cell Biol 2003;160(3):409–421.

Takizawa T, Robinson JM. Ultrathin cryosections: an important tool for immunofluorescence and correlative microscopy. J Histochem Cytochem 2003;51(6):707–714.

Timp W, Watson N, Sabban A, Zik O, Matsudaira P. Wet electron microscopy with quantum dots. Biotechniques 2006;41(3):295–298.

Tokuyasu KT. A technique for ultracryotomy of cell suspensions and tissues. J Cell Biol 1973;57(2):551–565.

Trucco A, Polishchuk RS, Martella O, Di Pentima A, Fusella A, Di Giandomenico D, San Pietro E, Beznoussenko GV, Polishchuk EV, Baldassarre M, Buccione R, Geerts WJ, Koster AJ, Burger KN, Mironov AA, Luini A. Secretory traffic triggers the formation of tubular continuities across Golgi sub-compartments. Nat Cell Biol 2004;6(11):1071–1081.

Tsien RY. Building and breeding molecules to spy on cells and tumors. FEBS Lett 2005;579(4):927–932.

Valentijn JA, van Daal JH, Jenks BG, van Abeelen JH. A method permitting precise trimming of resin-embedded tissue for ultrathin sectioning in pre-embedding immunoelectronmicroscopy. J Neurosci Methods 1989;30(1):55–58.

Verdijk P, Dijkman R, Plasmeijer EI, Mulder AA, Zoutman WH, Mommaas MA, Tensen CP. A lack of Birbeck granules in Langerhans cells is associated with a naturally occurring point mutation in the human Langerin gene. J Invest Dermatol 2005;124(4):714–717.

Vetter J. Toxins of Amanita phalloides. Toxicon 1998;36(1):13–24.

Walz J, Erdmann A, Kania M, Typke D, Koster AJ, Baumeister W. 26S proteasome structure revealed by three-dimensional electron microscopy. J Struct Biol 1998;121(1):19–29.

van der Wel NN, Fluitsma DM, Dascher CC, Brenner MB, Peters PJ. Subcellular localization of mycobacteria in tissues and detection of lipid antigens in organelles using cryo-techniques for light and electron microscopy. Curr Opin Microbiol 2005;8(3):323–330.

Westbroek W, Lambert J, Bahadoran P, Busca R, Herteleer MC, Smit N, Mommaas M, Ballotti R, Naeyaert JM. Interactions of human Myosin Va isoforms, endogenously expressed in human melanocytes, are tightly regulated by the tail domain. J Invest Dermatol 2003;120(3):465–475.

Wisher AC, Bronstein I, Chechik V. Thiolated PAMAM dendrimer-coated CdSe/ZnSe nanoparticles as protein transfection agents. Chem Commun (Camb) 2006;15:1637–1639.

Wouters CH, Koerten HK. Combined light microscope and scanning electron microscope, a new instrument for cell biology. Cell Biol Int Rep 1982;6(10):955–959.

Wulf E, Deboben A, Bautz FA, Faulstich H, Wieland T. Fluorescent phallotoxin, a tool for the visualization of cellular actin. Proc Natl Acad Sci U S A 1979;76(9):4498–4502.

Zeuschner D, Geerts WJ, van Donselaar E, Humbel BM, Slot JW, Koster AJ, Klumperman J. Immuno-electron tomography of ER exit sites reveals the existence of free COPII-coated transport carriers. Nat Cell Biol 2006;8(4):377–383.

Zhang S, Ma C, Chalfie M. Combinatorial marking of cells and organelles with reconstituted fluorescent proteins. Cell 2004;119(1):137–144.

7

TRACER IMAGING

RAINER HINZ
Wolfson Molecular Imaging Centre, University of Manchester, Manchester, UK

7.1 INTRODUCTION

The Nobel Prize in Chemistry 1943 was awarded to George de Hevesy for his work on the use of isotopes as tracers in the study of chemical processes. This was just 8 years after the first radioindicator study in life sciences with a manmade radionuclide was reported (Chievitz and Hevesy, 1935). Since then, the use of the tracer principle has provided a wealth of knowledge about the biochemical pathways in living organisms. In particular, combination with imaging, that is, the recording of spatial and temporal distributions of radiolabeled molecules within the body, has made it possible to quantitatively acquire parameters such as blood flow, rates of metabolism, or receptor binding to describe physiological processes.

In the first tracer studies, only crude spatial information about radioactive source distributions was available by positioning a single detector at various locations around the subject. In 1950, Benedict Cassen invented the rectilinear scanner. This device produced planar images by mechanically scanning a detector in a rasterlike pattern over the area of interest. However, because of the sequential nature of the scanning, this technique required very long imaging times.

By 1952, Hal Anger completed the first prototype of a pinhole camera with a photographic plate. In late 1956, he developed the design now seen in current "Anger camera" systems replacing the film and screen with a single sodium iodide (NaI) crystal and a Photomultiplier Tube (PMT) array (Anger, 1958). The first use of the Anger camera to produce tomographic images was reported by

Biomedical Imaging: Principles and Applications, First Edition. Edited by Reiner Salzer.

Kuhl and Edwards (1964). In conjunction with Allan M. Cormack and Godfrey N. Hounsfield's developments of computer-assisted tomography, for which they were awarded the 1979 Nobel Prize in Physiology or Medicine, the first tomographs were built. By acquiring views of the tracer distribution from a variety of angles, the three-dimensional tracer distribution within the body can be reconstructed. In contrast to conventional Computed Tomography (CT) where X-ray transmissions are used, in Single-Photon Emission Computed Tomography (SPECT) γ-rays and in Positron Emission Tomography (PET) positrons are the sources of image information.

Figure 7.1 demonstrates how, through imaging, molecular pathways and molecular interactions in human tissue are studied (Jones, 1996). It serves as an illustration for the challenge of a highly interdisciplinary field stretching from basic science disciplines such as physics, chemistry, biology, and mathematics through applied sciences such as engineering and computing to matters of quality assurance, compliance, and regulatory affairs.

The following sections provide a quick overview of SPECT and PET imaging, starting with isotope production and continuing through radiochemistry and radiopharmacy to a description of measurement techniques and applications.

7.2 INSTRUMENTATION

To perform tracer imaging studies, a comprehensive instrumentation set is required. In this chapter, a brief overview of the tracer imaging instrumentation is provided in four sections. The first section introduces the production of short-lived isotopes that are commonly used in imaging. The second section summarizes some of the main radiolabeling strategies. The last two sections of this chapter provide an introduction to the devices used for imaging as well as to peripheral detectors and bioanalysis systems required to perform quantitative imaging studies.

For more details on the instrumentation of molecular imaging, the reader is referred to monographs such as Phelps et al., (1986) or Valk et al., (2003).

7.2.1 Radioisotope Production

Radioisotopes for tracer imaging are either γ- or positron emitters. For most practical applications in imaging, they are produced in specially designed generators or with cyclotrons.

The most widely used SPECT isotope ^{99m}Tc is a fission product from the fission of uranium or plutonium in nuclear reactors. The vast majority of the ^{99m}Tc used in medical work is generated from ^{99}Mo, which is formed by the neutron activation of ^{98}Mo. ^{99}Mo has a half-life of 67 h, so short-lived ^{99m}Tc (half-life = 6 h), which results from its decay, is being constantly produced. The imaging unit then chemically extracts the technetium from the solution by using a technetium-99m generator, which is also known as a *technetium cow*.

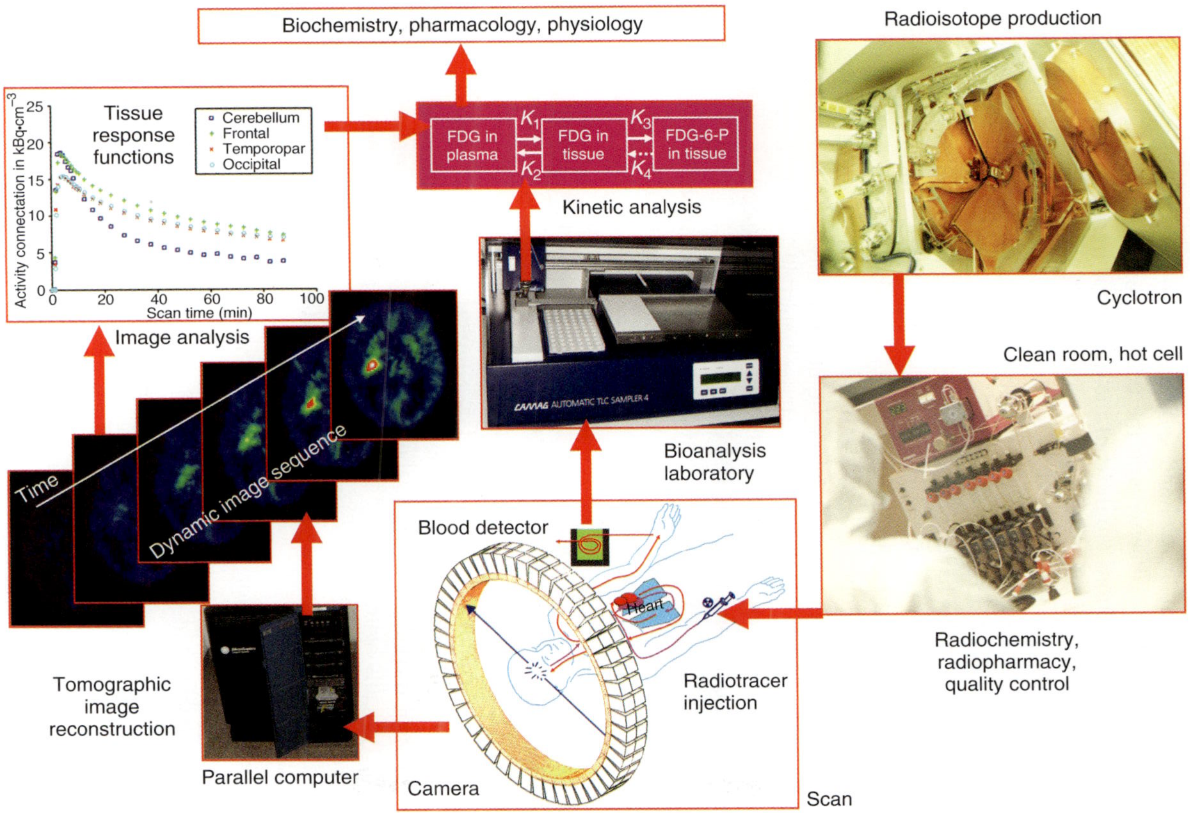

Figure 7.1. Tracer imaging science. The schematic illustrates the path of molecular imaging from the preparation of the radiotracer through the scanning session to the kinetic analysis of data that provides parameters that are meaningful in the fields of biochemistry, pharmacology, and physiology. With its superior sensitivity and specificity, tracer imaging is the means to bridge human molecular biology and molecular medicine.

Other single-photon emitters such as ^{201}Tl, ^{123}I, and ^{67} Ga and positron emitters (^{18}F, ^{15}O, ^{13}N, ^{11}C) are produced in cyclotrons using specific gas, solid, or liquid targets. The group of positron-emitting radionuclides can be produced by inducing energies in the order of a few to about 10 MeV in so-called PET cyclotrons that are small in size and self-shielded so that they can be installed directly in the imaging center without the need to build a costly shelter (vault). The most effective reactions are those of the (p, n) type implemented with highly enriched stable nuclides and protons accelerated in these small PET cyclotrons, for example,$^{14}N(p, \alpha)^{11}C$ and $^{18}O(p, n)^{18}F$. In such cases, the radionuclides obtained are not contaminated with any stable nuclide of the same element and are referred to as *No Carrier Added* (NCA) *substances*.

Liquid target systems have been developed for the production of nucleophilic [^{18}F]fluoride from the $^{18}O(p, n)^{18}F$ reaction using highly enriched [^{18}O]water targets. The volume of the liquid target is generally kept low in order to minimize the use of enriched isotopes. Target cooling is critical as hundreds of watts are usually imparted into less than 1 ml of liquid. The target pressure in a sealed system increases with the temperature of the liquid as it turns to vapor. This process allows the production of [^{18}F] fluoride with high specific activity within a few hours at quantities of about 100 GBq.

A gas target system is frequently used to produce electrophilic [^{18}F] fluorine gas from the $^{20}Ne(d, \alpha)^{18}F$ reaction by deuteron bombardment. This method, however, produces relatively low yields of [^{18}F] F_2 gas (less than 37 GBq) and a lower specific activity than with the $^{18}O(p, n)^{18}F$ reaction.

Oxygen-15 is one of the earliest radioisotopes used in PET and continues to be used for studies of blood flow and blood volume, using primarily [^{15}O]water and [^{15}O]CO. It has also been used directly in the form of [^{15}O]O_2 for tissue oxygen utilization measurements. The simplest reaction to produce ^{15}O is $^{14}N(d, n)^{15}O$, taking advantage of the high yields at low energy and the economical use of the natural isotopic abundance of the target material. Gas targets are used, typically with 99% N_2 gas and an admixture of an appropriate gas to form the required chemical product. In the case of [^{15}O]water, hydrogen is used as the mix gas. Similarly, replacing the hydrogen with oxygen produces [^{15}O]O_2.

Several routes exist for ^{11}C production, which can be performed with low energy particles and allow the recovery of ^{11}C from the target with automated systems. In contrast to the solid target technology of the $^{11}B(p, n)^{11}C$ reaction that requires subsequent extraction of ^{11}C from the target, the gas phase production with $^{14}N(p, \alpha)^{11}C$ has the advantage of greatly simplifying the subsequent chemistry, as the ^{11}C is produced in the form of carbon dioxide CO_2 or methane CH_4. The basic system is identical to that for ^{15}O production, in that the target gas is primarily natural nitrogen, with a small admixture of an appropriate balance gas to produce the desired product. In the case of [^{11}C]CO_2, the mix is $<1\%$ oxygen, while for methane, a higher mix of hydrogen is optimal, on the order of 10%.

7.2.2 Radiochemistry and Radiopharmacy

After the production of radioisotopes, a radiochemistry procedure is used to produce the radiolabeled compounds for the imaging study.

^{18}F can react as an electrophile (i.e., an electron-deficient species that seeks electron-rich reactants with high electron densities such as carbon) or as a nucleophile (i.e., an electron-rich species that seeks electron-deficient reactants).

The nucleophilic routes use high specific activity [^{18}F]fluoride and are substitution reactions of different types. The electrophilic reaction routes use [^{18}F]fluorine with lower specific activity and are direct fluorination of aromatic rings or regioselective demetallations.

For the production of ^{11}C-labeled compounds, methyl iodide [^{11}C]CH_3I is widely used as an alkylating agent for nucleophiles. It is produced either by conversion of carbon dioxide [^{11}C]CO_2 to [^{11}C]methoxide followed by reaction with hydroiodic acid or by a gas phase reaction of methane [^{11}C]CH_4 with iodine. Another widely used labeling agent for the production of amines, amides, and carboxylic acids is [^{11}C]cyanide, which can be obtained from carbon dioxide [^{11}C]CO_2 or from methane [^{11}C]CH_4.

The manufacturing of radiopharmaceutical products for administration to human subjects requires the manufacturer to hold a licence from the regulatory body. The licensing agency, for example, in the United Kingdom, the Medicines and Healthcare Products Regulatory Agency (MHRA), expects a quality assurance system in place to ensure that the procedures used are in accordance with the principles of Good Manufacturing Practice (GMP). This quality assurance system covers all activities from design, development, production, and installation to servicing and documentation (Långström and Hartvig, 2008).

In GMP, an important part is the documentation of every aspect of the process, activities, and operations involved in the manufacture of pharmaceuticals. This documentation must show how the product was made and tested. GMP requires that all manufacturing and testing equipment has been qualified as suitable for use, and that all operational methodologies and procedures such as manufacturing, cleaning, and analytical testing utilized in the pharmaceutical manufacturing process have been validated according to predetermined specifications, to demonstrate that they can perform their purported functions.

Quality Control (QC) is concerned with checking and testing the radiopharmaceuticals for release (Frier, 2000). QC is performed independently of the radiopharmaceutical production. Because the physical half-life of the radionuclides is short in relation to the time required for some of the QC tests, for instance, for sterility and for apyrogenicity, these tests are performed retrospectively. Most of the tests, however, are performed before the release of the radiopharmaceutical for administration. These are measurements of radionuclide purity, radiochemical purity, the specific activity and the amount of stable impurities, for instance, the precursor. For a ^{11}C-labeled product, these QC tests should not require more than 20 min (one isotope half-life) to release the product for injection.

For ^{99m}Tc technetium kits, the most likely radiochemical impurities are pertechnetates. Chromatographic methods that separate the components of a mixture by exploiting differences in the relative affinities for an adsorbent (stationary phase) and a developing solvent (mobile phase) are used to check the continued stability of the kit.

7.2.3 Imaging Devices

The basis of tracer imaging is the detection by external devices of the radiation emitted from the radiolabel attached to the tracer injected into humans or animals. In most cases, nuclear disintegration of the radiolabel is detected via registering photons, which are either uncorrelated (hence single-photon imaging) or which are paired as the result of positron annihilation. This imaging technique is then known as *coincidence imaging* or *positron imaging*. Other imaging modalities such as fluorescence imaging are not covered here; see Chapter 8 in this book.

The imaging devices described here are subdivided into cameras for planar imaging and tomographs. They can also be classified in terms of the way they are operated; they acquire either static images, which are snapshots of the tracer distribution not taking note of the changes over time, or dynamic sequences of images, which are series of consecutively acquired images reflecting not only the spatial but also the temporal distribution of the imaging probe.

In a simple planar imaging setup, for instance, for bone scans, the detector array is in a fixed position over the patient and all data are acquired from a single angle. The acquired image then closely resembles that of a radiological X-ray image.

If multiple planar images, each of which is the result of summing data over a short time interval, are acquired over time, then the kinetics of the tracer distribution in the organ is also captured. For example, kidney function is assessed by renal dynamic imaging with the agent ^{99m}Tc-diethylene triamine pentaacetic acid (^{99m}Tc-DTPA).

In contrast to planar imaging, multiple views of the tracer distribution are acquired from a variety of angles in tomographic imaging. This is achieved by rotating either one or multiple camera heads around the patient, a system design that is commonly found in SPECT. The other option that is usually employed in PET is to build a ring of detectors, thus acquiring entire sets of projections in planes perpendicular to the axis of the tomograph. Explanations on how the original activity distribution can be restored from the measurements of the projections follow later in the section on image reconstruction.

As in planar imaging, tomographic images can be acquired in the static mode or as a dynamic sequence of consecutive images. A special acquisition protocol is that of whole-body imaging, which is used in [^{18}F]Fluorodeoxyglucose ([^{18}F]FDG) PET to scan the entire body for metastatic disease. Here, the patient couch is moved through the scanner step by step, acquiring one image per bed position such that at the end of the acquisition a whole-body image can be assembled from this series of images.

After this general overview of the different acquisition modes in tracer imaging, a more detailed description of the physical processes underlying PET imaging are provided as an example highlighting various aspects specific to tracer imaging technology.

The positron emission occurs in proton-rich nuclei, the positron emitter, whereby in the nuclear field a proton **p** is converted into a neutron **n** emitting a positron $\mathbf{e}^+$ and an electron neutrino $\boldsymbol{\nu}_\mathbf{e}$. For example, the nuclear disintegration of ^{11}C via positron emission follows the reaction

$$^{11}\mathrm{C} \rightarrow {}^{11}\mathrm{B} + \mathrm{e}^+ + \nu_\mathrm{e}$$

Both the positron and the neutrino leave the nucleus. As the neutrino is without electric charge and has only a minuscule mass, it passes through matter almost undisturbed. The positron, however, interacts with the surrounding matter until it finally undergoes positron–electron annihilation. In the annihilation, the positron and electron are converted into two or three photons, with the cross section for the conversion into two photons being 372 times higher than the cross section for the conversion into three photons.

$$\mathrm{e}^+ + \mathrm{e}^- \rightarrow 2\gamma$$

These two photons each have an energy of 511 keV and travel on an almost collinear path in opposing directions. The detection of these two photons in coincidence by two detectors constitutes the principle of positron imaging and is illustrated in Figure 7.2.

The connection of the two points where the photons are detected is known as the *Line of Response* (LOR), illustrated in Figure 7.3a. As the photons interact with matter on their paths, they may be absorbed or scattered. As shown in Figure 7.3b where the photon γ_2 is deflected as the result of scatter, LORs are then incorrectly assigned. Two main strategies are used to compensate the errors arising from photon scattering. First, because the photon loses energy when it undergoes Compton scattering, the detectors register only the photons that fall in a preset energy window, for example, between 400 keV and 600 keV. This means that all photons with energy below the lower level of the energy window will not be passed on to form coincidence events. Second, the tomographic image reconstruction procedure contains special mathematical components to perform a scatter correction. With the help of a scatter model, the contribution of scattered photons within the energy window to the acquired projections is estimated from the distribution of the attenuation coefficients in the object and from an assumed positron emitter distribution. These estimated scattered events can then be subtracted from the measured coincidences, thus removing the impact of the scattered events from the data.

The coincidence processing unit pairs two single events into one coincidence if these two events fall within the coincidence time window, which is, depending on the timing resolution of the detectors, typically a few nanoseconds long. Photons

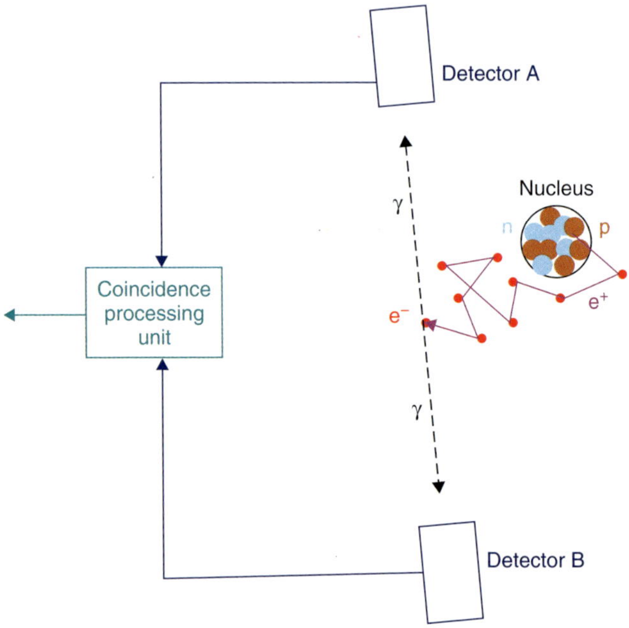

Figure 7.2. Principle of the positron detection. A pair of detectors A and B registers in coincidence the photon pair that has been produced by the annihilation of the positron e^+ with the electron e^-.

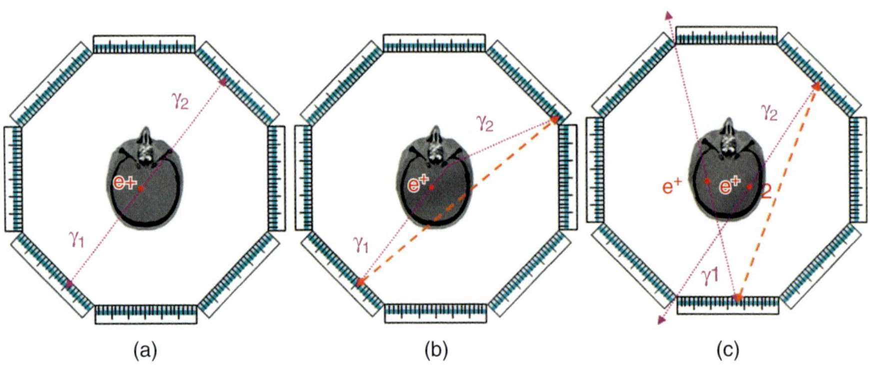

Figure 7.3. Coincidence types in PET. The PET scanner shown in the diagram consists of eight planar detector heads, a design that has been adopted for the High Resolution Research Tomograph (HRRT). (a) A true coincidence occurs when both detected photons γ_1 and γ_2 originate from the same positron annihilation. If at least one of the two photons is deflected as a result of being scattered in tissue, then a scattered coincidence (b) is recorded. If the two detected photons γ_1 and γ_2 are produced by two separate positron annihilations, then a random or accidental coincidence is recorded (c).

originating from two different positron annihilations may accidentally be detected as a coincidence event (Fig. 7.3c). However, because these two sources are not correlated, an estimate of random coincidences can be obtained from acquiring delayed coincidences, that is, the combination of two single events that occur in a delayed time window.

As the processing of an event in the radiation detector and the subsequent electronic circuitry requires a small, but finite, amount of time, two events following each other very shortly cannot always be identified as two separate events. This effect of the system being temporarily "blind" to events is characterized by a "dead time," which is the minimum time the system needs to again be able to process another event following an initial event. The fraction of events lost because of dead time increases with the activity of the radiation source, therefore making it important to apply a correction to SPECT and PET data. On the basis of the characterization of the count rate performance of a particular scanner, mathematical methods of dead time correction are implemented in the tomographic image reconstruction.

At present, all commercially produced PET systems use inorganic scintillator crystals, for instance, thallium-activated sodium iodide NaI(Tl), bismuth germanate BGO, lutetium oxyorthosilicate LSO, or gadolinium oxyorthosilicate GSO, for the detection of photons. These scintillators emit visible light that can be measured with a position-sensitive photo detector, such as PMTs or an array of avalanche photodiodes, from the interaction with the incident photons. The preference for these scintillators results from their good stopping power for 511 keV photons because of their high effective atomic number and density and their good energy resolution due to their light output. For small animal imaging, however, High Density Avalanche Chamber Positron Cameras (HIDACs) are also used because of their excellent spatial resolution. These devices are based on the principle of position-sensitive multiwire proportional chambers, although they have a poor detection efficiency for 511 keV photons and a very limited energy resolution.

Most commercially available PET systems record coincidence events only by the LOR where the photon pair was registered. However, some systems have, because of shorter coincidence time windows of less than 1 ns, the ability to measure in addition to the LOR the Time of Flight (TOF) of the photons. The tomographic image reconstruction process can then take not only the detected LOR into account but also a probability distribution for where along the LOR the annihilation occurred.

In order to be able to correct the emission images for the effects of photon attenuation and scatter in the object, the knowledge of the distribution of the attenuation coefficients in the object is required. For relatively simple objects such as the head, sometimes a calculated attenuation map is used, which is derived from a crude estimate of the contour of the skull from the acquired emission data. In most cases, an attenuation map of the object is generated from a CT scan in combined SPECT/CT or PET/CT systems, or from a transmission scan performed with rotating external rod or point sources. Figure 7.4 provides

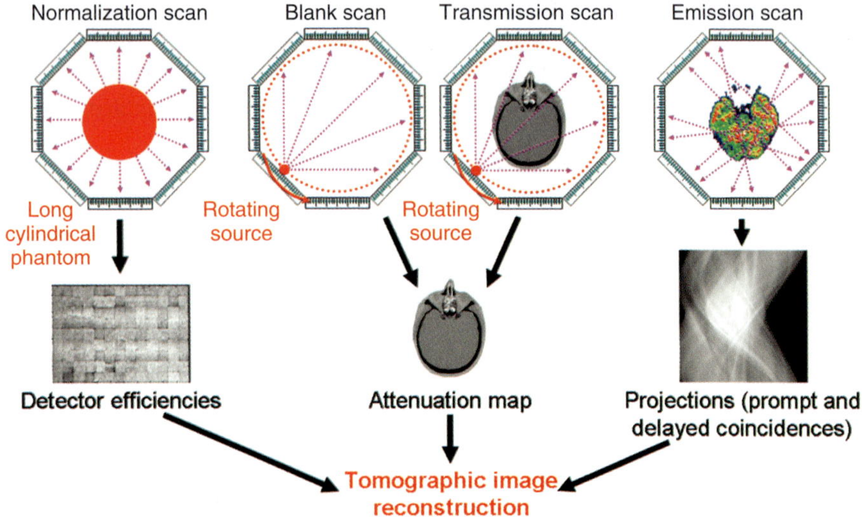

Figure 7.4. PET data acquisition. The diagram shows the set of scans that is required to quantitatively reconstruct the images of the emission scan. On combined PET/CT systems, a CT scan is performed to obtain the attenuation map, thus replacing both the blank scan and the transmission scan.

an overview of the scans that comprise the PET data acquisition. In contrast to the transmission scan that is required every time the object in the scanner is changed, the blank scan is acquired once per day or so, often in combination with the daily system stability tests. For the characterization of the detector efficiencies, an acquisition with good statistical quality, that is, a large enough number of counts per detector element, is required. This is the reason why these normalization scans, which can take up to 1 week on some scanners such as the High Resolution Research Tomograph (HHRT), are usually performed only after maintenance cycles or in case of replacement of scanner components.

Dual modality SPECT/CT and PET/CT systems have been hugely successful over the last decade as they provide anatomical data from the CT colocalized with functional data from the SPECT or PET investigation. This is a particular advantage outside the head where the simple rigid body coregistration of images normally is not satisfactory. Furthermore, it also reduces the time required for the transmission scan (typically between 5 and 15 min per bed position) to just a few seconds for a CT scan, thus substantially increasing the throughput in whole-body imaging studies with multiple bed positions.

First prototypes of combined PET and Magnetic Resonance Imaging (MRI) systems suitable for human imaging are being evaluated at the moment. Owing to the strong electromagnetic fields in and around an MR scanner, it is a bigger challenge to design the PET components for a PET/MR system than it is for the combined PET/CT systems, which were—and still are—basically a CT scanner and a PET scanner set up next to each other such that the patient bed can be used by both scanners.

All PET scanners available today operate in a three-dimensional (3D) mode. This means that there are no septa in the scanner to collimate the radiation, and that, in principle, LORs exist between any combination of two detector elements in the tomograph. Some scanners are still equipped with retractable septa that can be moved into the scanner for 2D acquisitions or to perform transmission scans with external sources using positron emitters such as ^{68}Ge. The scanner's sensitivity is significantly lower in the 2D mode than it is in the 3D mode, although the fraction of scattered events is also smaller because of the smaller solid angle in axial direction.

SPECT entirely relies on the use of collimators to generate images from single-photon emitters without the "electronic collimation" via the detection of coincidences between pairs of photons. Different designs of collimators are used to project the images onto the detector heads. Dependent on the imaging needs, pinhole, parallel-hole, converging-hole, or diverging-hole collimators are used. The trade-off in the choice of the best collimator is between efficiency and resolution. A collimator with longer septa and smaller holes provides a higher resolution as it defines better the direction of the photons but it lets fewer photons through to the detector. On the other hand, collimators with larger holes and shorter septa have a higher efficiency but provide a lower image resolution. For isotopes with higher photon energies (Table 7.1), collimators with thicker septa are needed to reduce the penetration of the septa by the γ-rays.

Many of the techniques described above for providing quantitative PET data are also used on SPECT and combined SPECT/CT systems. Nonetheless, the accuracy of the quantification in SPECT does not reach that of PET.

7.2.4 Peripheral Detectors and Bioanalysis

In addition to the imaging devices already described, an instrumentarium of peripheral devices is required to perform quantitative tracer imaging. The procedures for the production of radioactivity, radiosynthesis, and QC all require specialized equipment for measuring masses, activities, and other parameters.

Before human administration, the activity dispensed is usually measured in a dose calibrator, which is a shielded ion chamber specially designed to provide immediate readings of the activity in a vial or syringe. This measurement of the injected activity enables the calculation of a semiquantitative parameter of tracer uptake in tissue, the Standardized Uptake Value (SUV).

$$\mathrm{SUV} = \frac{\text{Tissue activity concentration}}{\text{Injected activity} \cdot \text{body weight} \cdot \text{tissue density}}$$

The SUV is a unitless entity, and normally the tissue density is assumed to be equal to that of water, and a value of 1 g cm^{-3} is used. Oncology applications often use the SUV as a measure to characterize the malignancy of lesions in [^{18}F]FDG PET studies, although the SUV has been described as being subject to many sources of variability not least due to the inhomogeneities in body composition. For example,

TABLE 7.1. Physical properties of radioisotopes most commonly used in SPECT and PET listed by half-life

SPECT			
Isotope	Half-Life	Principal Photon Energy (keV)	Number of Photons per 100 Disintegrations
^{99m}Tc (technetium)	6.01 h	140.5	88.5
^{123}I (iodine)	13.22 h	27.2	24.69
		27.5	45.98
		159.0	83.25
^{111}In (indium)	2.8049 d	171.28	90.61
		245.35	94.12
^{67}Ga (gallium)	3.2613 d	93.31	37.8
		184.58	20.9
		300.22	16.8

PET				
Isotope	Half-Life (min)	Maximum in Positron Energy (MeV)	Mean Positron Range in Water (mm)	Branching Fraction
^{15}O (oxygen)	2.041	1.7350	2.8	0.9989
^{13}N (nitrogen)	9.967	1.1985	1.6	0.9982
^{11}C (carbon)	20.37	0.9605	1.2	0.9975
^{18}F (fluorine)	109.7	0.6335	0.6	0.9686

Values are taken from Laboratoire National Henri Becquerel recommended data (http://www.nucleide.org/DDEP_WG/DDEPdata.htm)

a positive correlation with body weight is the consequence of a lower uptake of [^{18}F]FDG in adipose tissue in comparison with other types of tissue.

The absolute quantification of the radiotracer kinetics in the tomographic images normally requires an input function. This is the time course of the radiotracer in the supply stream that drives the tissue response, which is the time course of the concentration of the radiolabeled compound in arterial plasma. In contrast to the acquisition of the images that is performed by a single instrument, the SPECT or PET camera, the measurement of the plasma input function requires the combination of several laboratory devices.

Online blood detector devices are used to provide whole blood activity measurements of continuously withdrawn blood. These online blood counters provide data with excellent temporal resolution (typically about one activity reading per second), but because of the small counting volume, their sensitivity is inferior to counting discrete blood samples of a larger volume, that is, of a few milliliters. Because the tubing has to be directly connected to the subject, they have to be operated directly at the bedside, which exposes them to the radiation background originating from the injected activity in the patient and require bigger efforts for shielding.

A series of discrete blood samples is collected during the scan in syringes that are heparinized to prevent coagulation, that is, to stop the blood from clotting. By centrifuging the blood samples, blood plasma is separated from the erythrocytes and other blood cells, that is, thrombocytes (platelets) and leukocytes. The activities of whole blood and of plasma are measured in well counter devices. For PET, well counters are often custom made of big crystals in order to provide sufficient stopping power and counting efficiency for the 511-keV photons. For the commonly used SPECT isotopes, automated γ-counters are commercially distributed devices, in which racks with samples are automatically handled by a robotic system, placing one or multiple samples at the same time into a single well or a multiwell counter. Such systems achieve a high sample throughput; however, measurements often need to be corrected for cross talk between the wells.

For radiotracers that undergo metabolism in the body, quantitative assays of the plasma samples to determine the fraction of radioactivity that is due to unmetabolized parent compound may also be required to obtain the input function. The laboratory setup required for these investigations often involves Solid Phase Extraction (SPE) followed by High Performance Liquid Chromatography (HPLC) or Thin Layer Chromatography (TLC). Figure 7.5 shows an example chromatogram obtained from an HPLC analysis run.

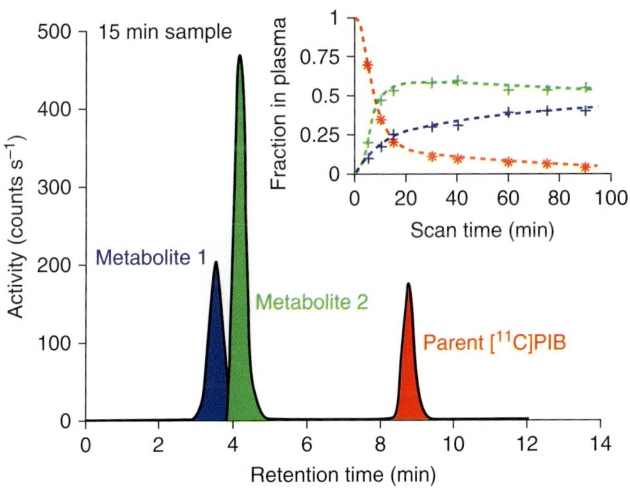

Figure 7.5. Analysis of radiolabeled metabolites in a plasma sample. The data are from the 15-min sample of a human subject injected with 370 MBq of Pittsburgh Compound-B or [^{11}C]PIB, a marker of amyloid deposition in brain. The large plot shows the HPLC trace with three identifiable peaks. The peak of the unmetabolized parent compound with about 9 min retention time follows two more hydrophylic metabolites that partly overlap. The figure inset shows the measurements of the fractions of radioactivity in plasma belonging to metabolite 1, metabolite 2, and [^{11}C]PIB. Eight plasma samples were analyzed for this 90-min PET scan. The plot illustrates that the parent [^{11}C]PIB (red line) is rapidly metabolized in humans.

Other ancillary measurement systems are used in conjunction with tracer imaging studies to improve the quality of the imaging data. For example, in cardiac studies, the signal from an electrocardiograph, which records the electrical activity of the heart over time, is used to gate the imaging data. By reconstructing images according to the phases of the cardiac cycle, the blurring of the heart in the images due to cardiac motion can be greatly reduced.

In brain imaging studies, infrared motion tracking systems are used to track involuntary movements of the head during the image acquisition. As head motion can been seen as rigid body motion, a resorting of the lines of response from the PET emission scan can be performed with the motion tracking information.

7.3 MEASUREMENT TECHNIQUES

This portion of the chapter on tracer imaging measurement techniques is subdivided into two sections. The first section provides a short introduction into tomographic image reconstruction, that is, the restoration of activity distribution in the object imaged. The second section on quantification method then takes us forward to the field of kinetic modeling, that is, the extraction of physiologically interpretable parameters from the imaging data.

7.3.1 Tomographic Image Reconstruction

In tomographic tracer imaging, sets of projections through the object of interest are acquired. The role of image reconstruction is to accurately restore the original distribution of the activity concentration in three-dimensional space. Using mathematical language, the imaging process can be described in terms of integral theory, and then methods of solving inverse problems can be applied to the measured data (Natterer and Wübbeling, 2001).

Two main strategies are used to reconstruct tomographic images, Filtered Back Projection (FBP) and iterative image reconstruction. FBP is an analytical reconstruction method and is widely used to reconstruct images from scanners with ring geometry and in modalities with a high signal to noise ratio, such as X-ray CT and MRI. FBP is computationally fast and has linear properties, which means the precision of the reconstructed images is independent of the location within the image and the intensity of the object. Data from 3D acquisitions normally need to be preprocessed in a Fourier rebinning step to estimate equivalent parallel projections before they can be reconstructed with FBP.

Iterative image reconstruction starts from an initial estimate of the source distribution, usually a constant activity value; predicts the response of the imaging system to this source distribution (this step is also called *forward projection*); and then derives from the comparison of the measured projections with the calculated projections a set of corrections to apply to each element of the image volume. This process of repeated updates of the image continues until the predicted projections have converged sufficiently close to the measured projections.

The Maximum Likelihood Expectation Maximization (ML-EM, Shepp and Vardi, 1982) algorithm forms the basis of the majority of the iterative image reconstruction techniques used in tracer imaging today. It is, however, very slow to converge. By grouping projection data into an ordered sequence of subsets and processing the data in these subsets within each iteration, an acceleration of the convergence by a factor proportional to the number of subsets can be achieved (Hudson and Larkin, 1994).

As iterative image reconstruction is a nonlinear process, the precision of the reconstructed voxel counts is dependent on the original intensity and also on the distribution of the activity across the reconstructed object. For example, the convergence of the iteratively reconstructed images is slower in areas of low activity (often referred to as *cold spots*, which could, for instance, be areas of an infarct in myocardial images) than in the surrounding areas of the image with higher activity. Voxels close to high intensity objects (this could be, e.g., the bladder for tracers with high renal excretion) are not as precisely reconstructed as in other parts of the image. These nonlinear properties make it particularly challenging to obtain quantitative images with iterative image reconstruction.

On the other hand, iterative image reconstruction provides the possibility to more accurately model the entire imaging process than FBP. For example, resolution effects can be included into the system matrix such that the EM algorithm gradually recovers the modeled resolution with each update (Reader et al., 2003). For data from tomographs with nonring geometry, which do not provide complete sets of projections and with spatially varying point spread functions, FBP cannot be used. High resolution tomographs inherently deal with a small number of counts per voxel such that the approximation of the Poisson distribution for the description of the probability of the nuclear disintegration by the Gaussian distribution is no longer accurate. Again, iterative image reconstruction offers the advantage over FBP that accurate models for the underlying statistical processes can be incorporated.

To visually appreciate the difference in image quality provided by FBP and Ordered Subset Expectation Maximization (OSEM), Figure 7.6 shows an example from a PET scan in the abdomen.

7.3.2 Quantification Methods

The genuine strength of imaging with radiolabeled tracers in comparison with many other imaging modalities is that estimates of parameters of biological function can be obtained. Quantification in the first instance applies to the physics of the imaging process, that is, the accurate restoration of the activity concentrations in the blood and the tissue. This quantitative tracer concentration signal acquired in a dynamic sequence then paves the way to quantifying the underlying physiological processes, for instance, blood flow, metabolic rates, or ligand binding to receptors. This link is established via a tracer kinetic model whose model parameters describe the exchange of the tracer between compartments. As examples, Figure 7.7 shows the configuration of three widely used compartmental models.

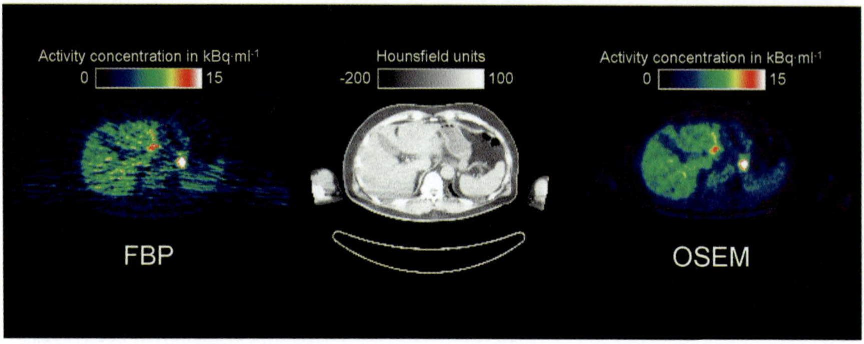

Figure 7.6. Tomographic image reconstruction. Displayed is a transaxial slice from a scan of the abdomen performed on a combined PET/CT system following the intravenous injection of an [^{18}F]FDG bolus. On the left hand side, the result from the reconstruction with filtered back projection (FBP) is shown. It has streak artefacts characteristic of FBP across the entire image, including the parts outside the body. On the right hand side is the result from iterative image reconstruction using the Ordered Subset Expectation Maximization (OSEM) method after 4 iterations with 16 subsets. It visually appears much smoother and has no image artefacts. The image reconstructed from the spiral CT scan is shown for comparison in the center. Because the trans axial field of measurement of the CT scanner is with 500 mm smaller than that of the PET scanner, the outer parts of the arms are cut. For patient comfort during the PET scan, the subject was positioned with the arms next to the body. In between the two arms, some artefacts due to beam hardening can be seen in the CT image.

7.3.2.1 ***The Flow Model.*** The blood flow model in Figure 7.7a has been introduced by Kety and Schmidt (1948). It was originally developed for quantitative Cerebral Blood Flow (CBF) studies with nitrous oxide N_2O but is now widely used with all freely diffusable tracers, for example, [^{15}O]water. In this one-tissue compartment model, the rate constant K_1 describes the transfer of the tracer from arterial blood plasma into the tissue and is—- under the assumption that the properties of this transfer, that is, the tracer extraction, are constant over the measurement duration—proportional to tissue perfusion. The ratio of K_1/k_2 is known as the *partition coefficient* and is equal to the distribution volume of the tracer in tissue.

7.3.2.2 ***The Irreversible Model for Deoxyglucose.*** The two-tissue compartment model shown in Figure 7.7b was developed by Sokoloff and coworkers for [^{14}C]deoxyglucose (Sokoloff et al., 1977) and was soon applied to human [^{18}F]fluorodeoxyglucose ([^{18}F]FDG) studies (Reivich et al., 1979). It is the basis for the measurement of the regional cerebral metabolic rate of glucose $rCMR_{glu}$ with [^{18}F]FDG in brain PET studies. The two rate constants, K_1 and k_2, in the model reflect the transport of FDG across the Blood–Brain Barrier (BBB). The rate constant k_3 represents the phosphorylation of FDG by hexokinase into FDG-6-phosphate, which—in contrast to glucose—does not undergo further

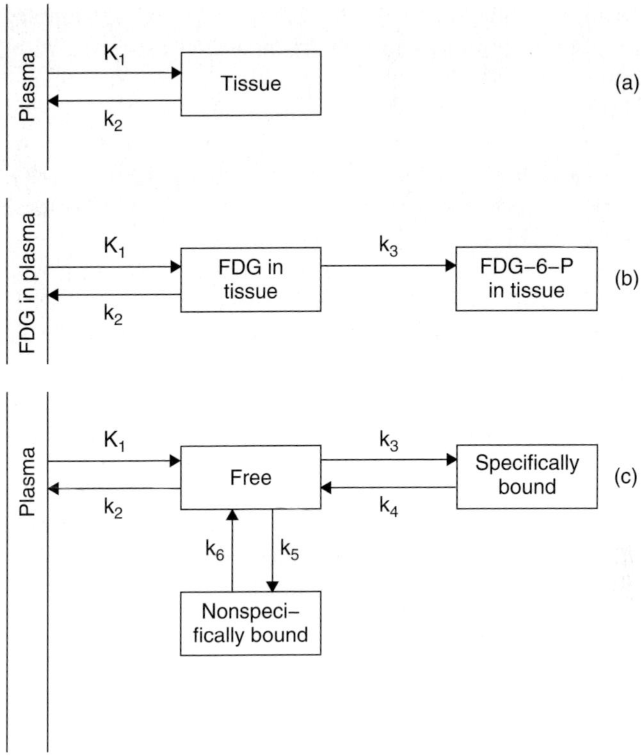

Figure 7.7. Examples of compartmental models. (a) the flow model (Kety and Schmidt, 1948), (b) the deoxyglucose model (Sokoloff et al., 1977), and (c) the neuroreceptor binding model (Mintun et al., 1984).

glycolysis. With estimates of these three rate constants, the combined forward rate constant K_I can be calculated, from which $\mathrm{rCMR}_{\mathrm{glu}}$ is obtained

$$rCMR_{\mathrm{glu}} = \frac{C_{\mathrm{glu}}}{\Lambda} \cdot K_I = \frac{C_{\mathrm{glu}}}{\Lambda} \cdot \frac{k_1 \cdot k_3}{k_2 + k_3}$$

The steady-state concentration of glucose C_{glu} in plasma has to be measured in conjunction with the PET scan. The so-called lumped constant Λ is required to convert the metabolic rate of FDG into the metabolic rate of glucose and accounts for differences in enzyme affinities and in the transport across the BBB between glucose and FDG.

Estimates of the model microparameters can be obtained by fitting the tissue time-activity curve using the measured input function, that is, the time course of radioactivity in plasma, and the equations describing the compartmental model. Bias-free parameter estimates are generally provided by weighted nonlinear least squares methods. However, these methods are time consuming, require initial parameter estimates as starting values for the optimization algorithm and may not converge to a unique solution. Therefore, linearized versions of the model equations are often used in order to obtain parameter estimates with linear least squares methods (Blomqvist, 1984). These rapid methods enabled the generation of parametric maps, that is, images representing the estimated values of parameters such as CBF or $rCMR_{glu}$. Figure 7.10 shows examples of parametric images generated with spectral analysis (Cunningham and Jones, 1993), which is based on the general properties of linear systems rather than assuming a specific compartmental model configuration.

An alternative method to obtain estimates of the combined forward rate constant K_I from graphical analysis has been published by Gjedde (1981) and Patlak et al. (1983). The idea of this graphical analysis of irreversible binding is to replace the measurement time t on the abscissa with a "virtual" or "stretched" time obtained by dividing the plasma integral with the plasma concentration. Furthermore, if the concentration in tissue on the ordinate is replaced by the ratio of the tissue concentration over the plasma concentration, then for any irreversible system, the obtained plot asymptotically approaches a straight line, whose slope is equal to K_I (Patlak and Blasberg, 1985). The result of the data transform of the Gjedde-Patlak plot is how the tissue time-activity curve would have looked if the input function had been a unit step function or, in terms of tracer imaging, if the concentration of radiotracer in plasma had been kept constant over time by continuous tracer infusion. In Figure 7.8, an example plot from a dynamic PET study with [^{18}F]FDG is shown.

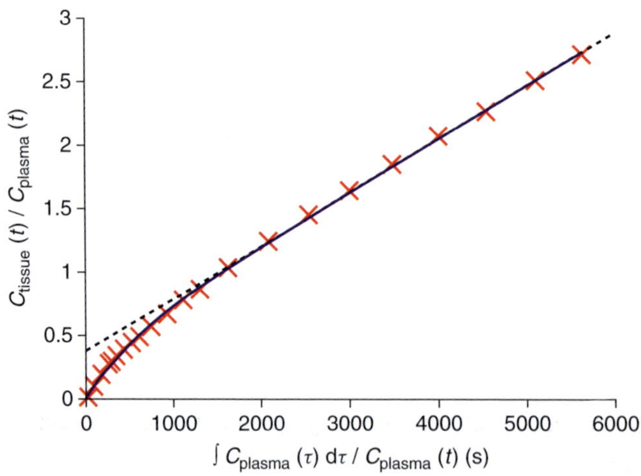

Figure 7.8. Example of graphical analysis of irreversible binding (Gjedde-Patlak plot). The 28 data points (red crosses) were acquired over 60 min in a dynamic [^{18}F]FDG PET study with simultaneous measurement of the plasma input function. The blue solid line depicts the fit obtained from a single exponential approaching a straight line. The dashed gray line is the estimated asymptote whose slope equals to the combined forward rate constant K_I.

7.3.2.3 The Neuroreceptor Binding Model. The standard model for the quantification of neuroreceptor binding in dynamic PET studies is shown in Figure 7.7c (Mintun et al., 1984). It has subsequently been adopted for dynamic SPECT neuroreceptor studies (Laruelle et al., 1994).

The most widely used outcome parameter of neuroreceptor imaging studies, the binding potential BP, was defined based on this model as

$$BP = \frac{k_3}{k_4} = \frac{B_{\text{max}}}{K_{\text{D}}}$$

The binding potential links the two rate constants k_3 and k_4 of the *in vivo* imaging model with the two parameters B_{max}, denoting the maximum concentration of receptors that are available for binding, and K_{D}, the radioligand equilibrium dissociation constant. This model, therefore, translates concepts established in traditional *in vitro* neuroreceptor binding assays to *in vivo* molecular imaging.

The model contains three separate tissue compartments for free radioligand in brain tissue, for nonspecifically bound radioligand, and for radioligand specifically bound to the binding sites of interest (Cunningham and Lammertsma, 1995). Specific binding refers to binding that is displaceable by the unlabeled ligand or other compounds that compete for the same binding site with the radioligand. On the other hand, the concept of nonspecific binding accounts for all binding that is not displaceable by an excess of unlabeled ligand and that usually occurs to lipids, proteins, cell membranes, and so on. It is assumed that the binding follows the classic kinetics of bimolecular association and unipolar dissociation. If the rate constants for these two reactions are k_{ON} and k_{OFF}, respectively, then the dissociation constant K_{D} equals to $k_{\text{OFF}}/k_{\text{ON}}$.

Radioligands may bind specifically to several targets, for instance, N-[^{11}C-Methyl]spiperone (NMSP) binds to dopamine D_2 receptors and serotonin 5-HT_2 receptors. This property is referred to as *nonselective binding* and needs particular consideration in the design and analysis of the imaging study. In the striatum, where the concentration of D_2 receptors is much higher than the concentration of 5-HT_2 receptors, NMSP was used to study binding to D_2 receptors (Wagner et al., 1983).

Changes of the binding potential BP determined in *in vivo* imaging studies cannot distinguish between changes in the concentration of the binding sites, changes in the apparent affinity, and changes due to the concentration of competitors to the same binding sites, for example, endogenous neurotransmitters. In order to examine these contributions to the binding potential, scanning protocols with multiple tracer injections with varying amounts of co-injected stable ligand have been developed (Delforge et al., 1990).

In most receptor imaging studies, the tracer is administered as a bolus that is the closest approximation of an impulse input function that is achievable. As it is usually assumed that the rate constants of the underlying model are constant over the period of the scan, from a bolus injection scan the estimates of the model microparameters can be obtained. Other studies aim at identifying changes of binding during the scan, for instance, due to a pharmacological challenge. Here, the radiotracer is administered as a bolus followed by a constant infusion to maximize the ability to detect changes of the specific binding of the radiotracer (Carson et al., 1997).

As with the Gjedde-Patlak plot for irreversibly binding tracers, graphical methods have been developed to estimate the total volume of distribution of a tracer with reversible binding. This Logan plot (Logan et al., 1990) allows the quantification of radioligand binding without the knowledge of a specific compartmental configuration. It does, however, suffer from a noise-induced bias (underestimation of the total volume of distribution) due to the transformation of the time-activity data into the new co-ordinates of the Logan plot.

7.4 APPLICATIONS

From the very beginning, PET applications were focused on the brain and the heart as the principle organs of interest (Phelps et al., 1986). This has dramatically changed over time, and today the vast majority of PET scans in the clinical field is performed with [^{18}F]FDG in oncological applications, and molecular imaging has become a major tool for research in oncology (Kim and Yang, 2000). In this chapter, short introductory summaries of the role of molecular imaging in neuroscience, cardiology, and oncology are given. Two brief sections on the use of tracer imaging for drug development and on small animal imaging conclude this chapter.

7.4.1 Neuroscience

In brain research, SPECT and PET are primarily used as tools for measuring cerebral physiologic function, such as blood flow and glucose metabolism, and neurochemical systems, for example, the synthesis, storage, release, receptor binding, and reuptake of neurotransmitters. In terms of disease areas, molecular imaging is used to study epilepsy, cerebrovascular disease, movement disorders, dementia, and a range of psychiatric disorders, for example, schizophrenia, depression, and substance abuse (Duncan, 1997; Herholz et al., 2004).

7.4.1.1 Cerebral Blood Flow. The most widely used techniques for the measurement of Regional Cerebral Blood Flow (rCBF) are [^{99m}Tc]HMPAO/SPECT and [^{15}O]water/PET. The use of these two tracers is based on different principles. [^{99m}Tc]HMPAO acts as a "chemical microsphere," that is, it is intravenously administered and completely extracted and retained in proportion to local flow. Radiolabeled water, on the other hand, is seen as an example of a freely diffusible tracer to which the reversible one-tissue compartment model (Fig. 7.7a) applies. Under the assumption of a complete extraction, the rate constant K_1 of the model represents tissue blood flow. However, the diffusion of water into tissue is limited, which results in an incomplete extraction of water. As a consequence of less tracer entering the tissue, the flow is underestimated by the flow model, an effect with increasing severity as the flow increases.

Another widespread application of rCBF measurements using [^{15}O]water PET but without full quantification is in functional brain mapping. The acquired PET images are interpreted in an autoradiographic way, that is, it is assumed that the acquired voxel counts are proportional to rCBF, thus avoiding the need for measuring the arterial input function. In a repeated scan design, automated [^{15}O]water generator systems produce a series of activity boli, which are highly reproducible in terms of the administration length and profile in comparison with manual injection of the activity from a syringe.

During a typical scanning session in an activation study, the subject repeats certain neurobehavioral tasks, normally one of which is used to characterize the "resting state" or "baseline" condition, while the others are motor or cognitive tasks. Active nerve cells consume oxygen carried by hemoglobin from the capillaries. The local response to oxygen utilization is an increase in rCBF to the areas of increased neural activity, occurring after a delay of a few seconds. This hemodynamic response is captured in the repeated measurements of rCBF with [^{15}O]water PET. Special statistical analysis software known as *Statistical Parametric Mapping* (SPM) has been developed to identify clusters of task-associated differences in rCBF (Frackowiak et al., 2004). This methodology of functional brain mapping has been very successfully adopted by Functional Magnetic Resonance Imaging (fMRI); however, [^{15}O]water PET is still the modality of choice for studies of subjects with implanted stimulators or other materials that are incompatible with strong magnetic fields. As an example, Figure 7.9 shows a typical output from an SPM analysis, highlighting the areas of the brain that were shown to be functionally involved in the task performance.

7.4.1.2 Neurotransmitter Systems. Owing to its superior sensitivity, molecular imaging is the principal tool for performing studies of the neurotransmitter systems in the living human brain. A wide spectrum of imaging probes has been developed for both the excitatory and the inhibitory systems (Table 7.2). γ-Aminobutyric Acid (GABA) is the main inhibitory neurotransmitter that hyperpolarizes the postsynaptic membranes at the inhibitory synapses. On the other hand, excitatory neurotransmitters, for example, dopamine, depolarize the postsynaptic membrane at the excitatory synapses.

For many steps of the neurochemistry chain of neurotransmitter systems, for example, neurotransmitter synthesis from precursor, neurotransmitter storage and release, the interaction of neurotransmitter with the receptors, and the reuptake of the neurotransmitter into the presynaptic terminal or the metabolic breakdown of the neurotransmitter, imaging biomarkers have been used. A field that has been particularly intensely studied with PET and SPECT is neuroreceptor imaging. One of the typically asked questions is whether there is a group difference in neuroreceptor binding, for example, between gender- and age-matched healthy control subjects and a cohort of patients.

Another application of tracer imaging is the *in vivo* measurement of brain receptor occupancy by drugs. For example, the central occupancy by

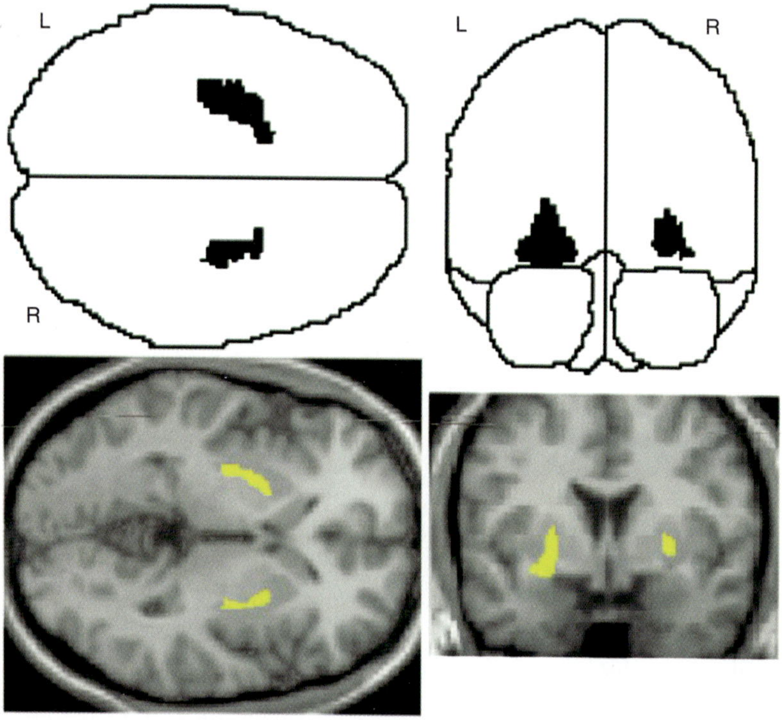

Figure 7.9. Example output from a statistical parametric mapping (SPM) analysis. Regions of the brain in which there was a statistically significant correlation between reduced [^{11}C]raclopride binding potential and task performance. The task in this study was playing a video game, which led to an increased release and binding of dopamine to its receptors. Top row, the transverse and coronal glass brain views show those voxels with a significant inverse correlation of [^{11}C]raclopride binding potential with the highest performance level reached. Bottom row, three-dimensional SPM projections superimposed on representative transaxial and coronal magnetic resonance image brain slices. *Source:* Figure adapted by permission from Macmillan Publishers Ltd: Koepp et al., 1998. This study published for the first time behavioral conditions under which dopamine is released in humans, illustrating the ability of PET to detect neurotransmitter fluxes *in vivo* during manipulations of behavior.

antipsychotic and antidepressant drugs has been studied in relationship to the administered dose, plasma concentration, and clinical response.

PET investigations demonstrated that the occupancy of dopamine D_2/D_3 receptors correlates better with the plasma concentration than with the doses of the antipsychotics. From analysis of the clinical effects, it was established that 60–70% dopamine receptor occupancy is required to effectively treat the positive symptoms of schizophrenia (Farde et al., 1988). Furthermore, extrapyramidal side effects were associated with higher occupancies of 80% or more. These findings subsequently led to an improvement of the treatment

TABLE 7.2. Brain neurotransmitter systems with example imaging markers

Neurotransmitter System with Target	Tracer
Dopaminergic System	
Dopamine synthesis	[^{18}F]6-Fluoro-L-DOPA [^{18}F]6-Fluoro-L-*m*-tyrosine
Dopamine transporter	[^{11}C]PE2I [^{99m}Tc]TRODAT-1 [^{123}I]FP-CIT [^{123}I]PE2I
Striatal dopamine D_2/D_3 receptors	[^{11}C]Raclopride [^{123}I]IBZM
Extrastriatal dopamine D_2/D_3 receptors	[^{11}C]FLB457 [^{123}I]Epidepride
Striatal and extrastriatal dopamine D_2/D_3 receptors	[^{11}C]Fallypride
D_1 receptors	[^{11}C]SCH23390 [^{11}C]NNC 112
Serotonergic System	
Serotonin transporter	[^{123}I]β-CIT [^{11}C](+)McN-5652 [^{11}C]DASB
Serotonin 5-HT_{1A} receptors	[^{11}C]WAY-100635 [^{18}F]MPPF
Serotonin 5-HT_{2A} receptors	[^{18}F]Setoperone [^{18}F]Altanserin [^{11}C]MDL 100,907 [^{123}I]5-I-R91150
Other Systems	
Opiod receptors (several subtypes)	[^{11}C]Carfentanil [^{11}C]Diprenorphine [^{18}F]Cyclofoxy
γ-Aminobutyric acid $GABA_A$ receptors	[^{11}C]Flumazenil [^{123}I]Iomazenil
Peripheral benzodiazepine binding site	[^{11}C]PK11195 [^{11}C]DPA-713
Neurokinin NK_1 receptors	[^{11}C]GR205171 [^{18}F]SPA-RQ
Histamine H_1 receptors	[^{11}C]Doxepine
Adenosine A_1 receptors	[^{18}F]CPFPX
Adenosine A_{2A} receptors	[^{11}C]SCH442416 [^{11}C]TMSX
Norepinephrine NET transporter	[^{11}C]MeNER
Muscarinic cholinergic receptors, M2 subtype	[^{18}F]FP-TZTP
Nicotinic acetylcholine receptors (nAChR0), $\alpha 4\beta 2$ subunit	[^{11}C]Nicotine 2-[^{18}F]F-A-85380 [^{123}I]5-IA-85380
Acetylcholinesterase activity	[^{11}C]PMP [^{11}C]MP4A
Monoamine oxidase type A (MAO-A)	[^{11}C]Clorgyline [^{11}C]-Deuterium-clorgyline
Monoamine oxidase type B (MAO-B)	[^{11}C]L-Deprenyl [^{11}C]L-Deuterium-deprenyl
Vesicular monoamine transporter 2 (VMAT2)	[^{11}C]DTBZ
N-methyl-D-aspartate (NMDA) receptor	[^{123}I]CNS-1261

[a]This list comprises mostly tracers that have been used in human clinical research

of patients with antipsychotics such as clozapine, haloperidol, risperidone, perphenazine, and olanzapine.

7.4.1.3 Metabolic and Other Processes. As the main energy substrate for the brain is glucose, a lot of effort has been spent on imaging studies of glucose metabolism, predominantly using [^{18}F]FDG. Virtually in all brain disorders, $rCMR_{glu}$ measurements have been performed over the last 30 years; a comprehensive review can be found in Herholz et al. (2004). As an example, the lower part of Figure 7.10 illustrates the characteristic pattern of glucose hypometabolism in the temporal and parietal cortex obtained in subjects with Alzheimer's Disease (AD) dementia.

Another enzymatic system that has been the subject of a number of quantitative tracer imaging studies not only in brain but also in peripheral organs such as the lungs is that of Monamine Oxidase MAO (Fowler et al., 1996). The enzyme MAO plays a major role in controlling the levels of neurotransmitters, amines, and drugs. There are two MAO subtypes, MAO-A and MAO-B, with different specificities for the endogenous amines, for which irreversible inhibitors have been radiolabeled with ^{11}C as imaging markers (Table 7.2). By substituting the hydrogen with deuterium in the carbon–hydrogen bond of [^{11}C]clorgyline and [^{11}C]L-deprenyl, the isotope effect was exploited to improve the properties of the radiotracer.

Two of the hallmark pathological features of AD are amyloid plaques and neurofibrillary tangles in the brain. Neuropathological dyes such as Congo red have been used for a long time for postmortem staining of human brain tissue samples. Attempts to develop radiolabeled *in vivo* imaging markers have been hampered by the poor brain penetration of most of these compounds. Just recently, a ^{11}C-labeled thioflavin T derivate called [^{11}C]6-OH-BTA-1, or more commonly [^{11}C]PIB for "Pittsburgh Compound-B," and a hydrophobic radiofluorinated derivative of 2-{1-[6-(dimethylamino)-2-naphthyl]ethylidene} malononitrile, named [^{18}F]FDDNP, brought the breakthrough to human imaging studies involving large subject cohorts and longitudinal follow-up of patients (Nordberg, 2004). The example data from [^{11}C]PIB scans of an elderly control subject and an AD patient, shown in the upper part of Figure 7.10, illustrate the huge qualitative difference, making the imaging agent a quasi binary marker of amyloid deposition with an "OFF" (low cortical gray matter signal) and an "ON" (high cortical gray matter signal) state. Ongoing studies investigate the usefulness of PET imaging for the early and potentially specific diagnosis of AD and the effects of treatment with antiamyloid agents (de Leon et al., 2007).

Imaging studies have been performed to study the function of efflux pump systems. Active efflux is a mechanism responsible for extrusion of toxic substances and antibiotics outside the cell. The transporter hypothesis states that the efflux pump systems contribute to the phenomenon of multidrug resistance, that is, the lack of effectiveness of drug treatment in diseases such as epilepsy and cancer in certain patients, which can be attributed to an overexpression of efflux transport systems in those individuals.

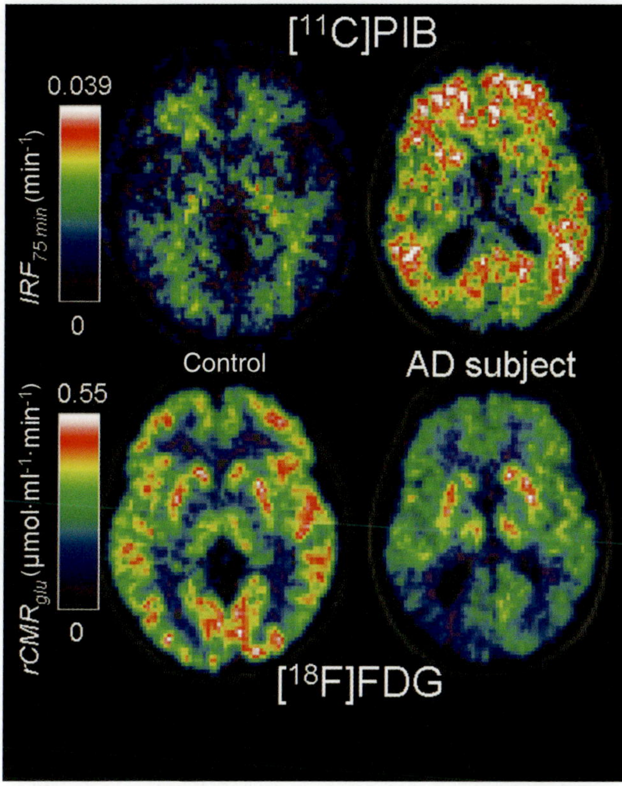

Figure 7.10. Dementia imaging with PET. Depicted are transaxial slices from an elderly healthy control subject (on the left) and a patient with Alzheimer's disease (AD) (on the right) superimposed onto a structural MR image in grayscale. The scans were performed with the Pittsburgh Compound-B or [^{11}C]PIB, a marker of the brain amyloid load, and with fluorodeoxyglucose or [^{18}F]FDG to measure $rCMR_{glu}$. The parametric images were generated with spectral analysis, a technique that calculates the values of the unit Impulse Response Function (IRF) voxel by voxel (Cunningham and Jones, 1993). The IRF at 75 min is a measure of [^{11}C]PIB retention in tissue, providing maximal discrimination between controls, with only some signal in white matter, and AD subjects, with high intensity signal throghout the cortical white matter (top row). A typical pattern of [^{18}F]FDG hypometabolism, in particular, in the temporoparietal cortex, distinguishes the AD subject from the control (bottom row).

P-glycoprotein (Pgp) is an efflux pump with broad substrate specificity that is extensively distributed and expressed in normal cells such as those lining the intestine, liver cells, and capillary endothelial cells comprising the BBB. Verapamil, a substatrate for Pgp, has been radiolabeled with ^{11}C and is used as an imaging agent for Pgp function.

7.4.2 Cardiology

The applications of molecular imaging in cardiology range over a wide spectrum from atherosclerosis over myocardial ischemia, myocardial viability, heart failure, and gene therapy, to stem cell transplantation (Wu et al., 2007). Here, only a few examples can be highlighted.

Measurements of Myocardial Blood Flow (MBF) are performed with $[^{15}O]H_2O$, $[^{13}N]NH_3$ or ^{82}Rb in PET or with $[^{99m}Tc]$sestamibi in SPECT. From the MBF measurements under two conditions, at rest and under stress, the coronary flow reserve is calculated.

The heart utilizes various sources for energy production, such as glucose, free fatty acids, lactate, and ketones. Under aerobic and fasting conditions, the heart primarily uses free fatty acids because their degradation yields an abundance of energy-rich phosphates. Ischemia causes a shift of myocardial metabolism from fatty acids to glucose. $[^{18}F]$FDG is widely used for imaging cardiac glucose metobolism. Several fatty acids have been labeled with the single-photon emitter ^{123}I, for example, β-methyl-p-$[^{123}I]$iodophenyl-pentadecanoic acid. But only straight-chain fatty acids that are labeled in the C-1 position accurately reflect physiologic oxidation, because all other carbons in the chain can undergo other metabolic fates. For quantitative measurements of metabolism with PET, fatty acids such as acetate and palmitate have been labeled with ^{11}C in this position.

One of the key applications of tracer imaging in cardiology are studies to distinguish viable from nonviable tissue in patients with ischemic cardiomyopathy. By measuring MBF and glucose metabolism in dysfunctional myocardium with PET, Tillisch et al., (1986) demonstrated that recovery of myocardial function after surgical revascularization coincided with either preserved perfusion/metabolism or reduced perfusion and preserved metabolism, as from the underlying pathophysiology these combinations reflect stunned and hibernating myocardium. On the other hand, the concordant reduction of perfusion and metabolism is indicative of scar tissue.

As in neuroscience, tracer imaging studies are also performed for evaluation of receptors in heart and lung tissue. In Table 7.3 a short list of tracers is given. As an example, Figure 7.11 shows images from a self-inhibition study with $[^{11}C]$GB67, a ligand for cardiac α1-adrenoceptors.

7.4.3 Oncology

Today, oncology is one of the major drivers behind the developments in molecular imaging. The complex molecular biology, biochemistry, immunology, pathology, and physiology of cancer demand a wide spectrum of imaging biomarkers that can only be briefly mentioned here. The following subsections go through the key processes targeted by molecular imaging probes.

7.4.3.1 Angiogenesis. The formation of new blood vessels via the proliferation of endothelial and muscle cells is known as *angiogenesis* and is an essential component of the metastatic pathway. Antiangiogenic drugs, for example, Vascular

TABLE 7.3. Imaging examples for the nervous system in the heart and the lung

Neurotransmitter System with Target	Tracer
Nonselective β-adrenoceptor	[^{11}C]CGP-12177, [^{11}C]CGP-12388, [^{18}F]CGP-12388, [^{18}F]fluorocarazolol
Cardiac α1-adrenoceptor	[^{11}C]GB67
Peripheral muscarinic receptors	[^{11}C]MQNB, [^{11}C]-VC002
Tracers for mapping cardiac sympathetic neurons	[^{123}I]MIBG, [^{11}C]HED

Endothelial Growth Factor (VEGF) inhibitors, are investigated for their therapeutic potential. Tracer imaging is used to provide quantitative measurements of tumor perfusion and vascular volume. Clinical feasibility of these techniques has been demonstrated in several studies with antiangiogenic and vascular disruptive agents (Laking et al., 2006).

7.4.3.2 Proliferation. The increase in cell number by division is also referred to as *cell proliferation*. By synthesizing DNA during the S phase of the cell cycle, proliferating cells differ from cells at resting state. Therefore, measuring cell proliferation is widely seen as a target for differentiating between benign tissue and malignant tissue, for measuring the aggressiveness of a tumor, and for trying to evaluate the early response in therapy.

To provide a method for measuring human tumor proliferation *in vivo*, a number of radiotracers have been developed, for example, 2-[^{11}C]thymidine, and compared with well-established immunohistochemical measures of tumor proliferation, such as the Ki-67 index. Among those candidates, [^{18}F]-fluoro-3′-deoxy-3′-L-fluorothymidine or [^{18}F]FLT appears the currently most widely used tracer to image cell proliferation (Been et al., 2004). However, care is required when interpreting [^{18}F]FLT data, as they do not always reflect the cell proliferation rate because [^{18}F]FLT is a substrate of Thymidine Kinase 1 (TK_1), and TK_1 activity and the S phase fraction of cells are not always correlated, in particular, after treatment with certain chemotherapeutic agents.

7.4.3.3 Hypoxia. Sensitivity of cells to conventional radiation is higher in the presence of oxygen, and even a small proportion of hypoxic cells within a tumor reduces the response to radiation therapy. Measurements of hypoxia are performed with oxygen electrodes, however, their invasiveness could be overcome with suitable imaging biomarkers (Padhani et al., 2007).

The hypoxic cell sensitizer misonidazole (MISO) has been radiolabeled with ^{18}F, ^{123}I, and ^{99m}Tc for the evaluation of tumor hypoxia. This compound is reduced enzymatically and trapped within hypoxic cells, but the uptake of FMISO in hypoxic tissues remains relatively low. Alternatively, [^{60}Cu] ATSM is assessed as a putative marker for delineating the extent of hypoxia within tumors with PET.

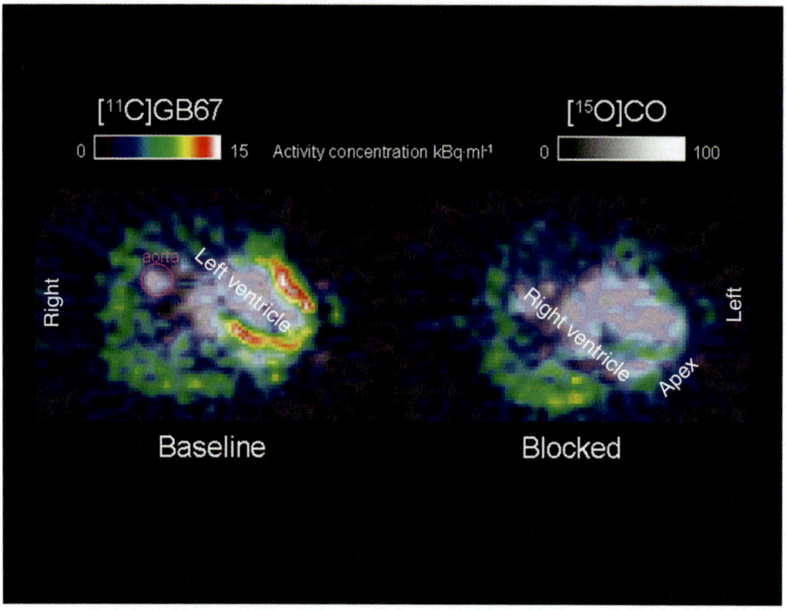

Figure 7.11. Cardiac receptor study. In an anesthetized pig, scans with [^{11}C]GB67, a ligand for cardiac α1-adrenoceptors, were performed after measuring the blood volume with [^{15}O]CO, which is shown in grayscale. The baseline scan was acquired with the tracer alone, the blocked scan started 20 min after the administration of 0.12 μmol$\cdot$kg^{-1} body weight of unlabeled GB67. This dose led to a significant reduction of [^{11}C]GB67 binding in the myocardial wall (on the image visible around the left ventricle). The mostly nonspecific binding of [^{11}C]GB67 in the lungs remained largely unaffected by predosing with the cold compound.

7.4.3.4 Apoptosis. Programmed cell death or apoptosis occurs during the treatment of tumors with radiation or anticancer drugs. Assessment of apoptosis is a useful tool for the evaluation of disease progression or regression during anticancer therapy. However, these assessments are currently done by immunohistochemical or flow cytometric analysis of tissue samples. For imaging apoptosis *in vivo*, annexin V, which binds to phosphatidylserine on the surface of apoptotic cells, has been labeled with ^{99m}Tc for SPECT and ^{124}I for PET and used in animal models (Keen et al., 2005).

7.4.3.5 Receptor Imaging. Many malignancies are characterized by an overexpression of receptors. It is hoped that receptor imaging in oncology provides more tumor-specific information than the measurement of the rates of glucose metabolism or protein synthesis. For example, most endocrinal tumors overexpress somatostatin-subtype receptors such that [^{68}Ga]DOTATOC and [^{111}In]DTPAOC have been used for imaging these tumors with PET and SPECT. Imaging of estrogen receptors with [^{18}F]fluoroestradiol has been performed in primary and metastatic breast cancer (Mintun et al., 1988). The overexpression of folate receptors on many cancer tissues can be exploited for PET imaging with folic acid derivative labeled with ^{18}F.

7.4.3.6 ***Imaging Gene Therapy.*** Different approaches for treating cancer by introducing genes into tumor cells are under investigation. For imaging therapeutic gene expression, "direct" and "indirect" imaging strategies are pursued. If the therapeutic protein substrate can be radiolabeled, then the specific expression of that protein can be directly imaged. In the indirect imaging approach, the therapeutic gene is coupled to a reporter gene, which is then tracked by SPECT or PET.

As an example, the herpes simplex virus type-1 thymidine kinase (HSV-1-*tk*) gene has been used as a reporter gene for which radiolabeled substrates exist. In PET, ^{124}I-labeled FIAU is such a specific substrate for HSV-1-*tk*, which has been used to noninvasively monitor patients with glioblastoma who underwent HSV-1-*tk* suicide gene therapy (Jacobs et al., 2001). It is expected that reporter gene imaging will contribute to the optimization of the various gene therapy approaches in humans.

7.4.4 Molecular Imaging for Research in Drug Development

Molecular imaging is increasingly used to advance drug development because of its ability to study molecular pathways and physiological function. Major pharmaceutical companies have launched imaging programmes and already either set up their own facilities to perform tracer imaging studies in animals and humans or established partnerships and collaborations with academic imaging research centers.

Three main application areas are most commonly named for accelerating drug discovery with molecular imaging:

1. Noninvasive measurements of downstream physiological and metabolic responses to drug action.
2. Binding and competition studies where a molecular imaging probe for the target of the drug is available. A classic example is dose-occupancy studies, which establish the relationship between plasma concentration of a drug and the occupancy at a binding site, for example, Farde et al. (1988).
3. Direct assessment of the biodistribution and pharmacokinetics of a drug, if the drug can be radiolabeled.

As the first two uses of molecular imaging have already been discussed in this chapter, only a few words on the third point are added. Tracer imaging is well suited to adopt the microdosing concept, which is the study of the behavior of investigational compounds *in vivo* at concentrations so low that they do not produce a pharmacological effect. Generic labeling techniques used in PET allow the radiolabeling of a whole range of organic compounds with positron emitters. In combination with the superior sensitivity of PET, drug distributions can be studied in humans without the need to perform a full toxicological assessment, which would otherwise be required to study the pharmacokinetics of a new compound in humans (Bergström et al., 2003).

For example, the injection of 480 MBq of a ^{11}C-labeled compound corresponds to 1.4 pmol or 0.5 ng, assuming a relative molecular mass of 350 g mol^{-1}. With only a very moderate specific activity of 40 GBq µmol^{-1}, the injected amount of stable compound would still be only 4.2 µg, hence a true microdose.

7.4.5 Small Animal Imaging

Over the past years, there has been a rapid growth in the field of *in vivo* tracer imaging in small laboratory animals such as mice and rats (Myers and Hume, 2002). Small animal scanners are now commercially available and are often multimodality devices, such as combined SPECT/CT, PET/CT, PET/SPECT/CT, or PET/MRI systems. As before, in human whole-body applications, this allows reliable colocalization between functional and anatomical images.

Animal models, in particular genetically modified mice, are often expensive; therefore, it is beneficial to avoid traditional autoradiographic techniques and use *in vivo* imaging approaches. Furthermore, it reduces variability because multiple time points are obtained from the same individual instead of from a set of animals. Frequently, animals are scanned several times (e.g., prior and after intervention) and with multiple modalities. A particular challenge for the quantitative analysis of small animal imaging data is to accurately obtain the input function from very small blood samples, which are often just of a volume of a few microliters.

ACKNOWLEDGEMENTS

The author gratefully acknowledges Dr Marie-Claude Asselin's help in the preparation of the Cardiology and Oncology sections. The author thanks all the volunteers who participated in the PET studies from which data presented in this chapter originate and all former colleagues at Hammersmith, without whose invaluable help it would have been impossible to prepare this chapter.

REFERENCES

Anger HO. Scintillation camera. Rev Sci Instrum 1958;29:27.

Been LB, Suurmeijer AJ, Cobben DC, Jager PL, Hoekstra HJ, Elsinga PH. [^{18}F]FLT-PET in oncology: current status and opportunities. Eur J Nucl Med Mol Imaging 2004;31:1659–1672.

Bergström M, Grahnén A, Långström B. Positron emission tomography microdosing: a new concept with application in tracer and early clinical drug development. Eur J Clin Pharmacol 2003;59:357–366.

Blomqvist G. On the construction of functional maps in positron emission tomography. J Cereb Blood Flow Metab 1984;4:629–632.

Carson RE, Breier A, Bartolomeis Ade, Saunders RC, Su TP, Schmall B, Der MG, Pickar D, Eckelman WC. Quantification of amphetamine-induced changes in [^{11}C]raclopride binding with continuous infusion. J Cereb Blood Flow Metab 1997;17:437–447.

Chievitz O, Hevesy G. Radioactive indicators in the study of phosphorus metabolism in rats. Nature 1935;136:754–755.

Cunningham VJ, Jones T. Spectral analysis of dynamic PET studies. J Cereb Blood Flow Metab 1993;13:15–23.

Cunningham VJ, Lammertsma AA. Radioligand studies in brain; kinetic analysis of PET data. Med Chem Res 1995;5:79–96.

Delforge J, Syrota A, Mazoyer BM. Identifiability analysis and parameter identification of an in vivo ligand-receptor model from PET data. IEEE Trans Biomed Eng 1990;37:653–661.

Duncan R, editor. *SPECT Imaging of the Brain*. Dordrecht: Kluwer Academic Publishers; 1997.

Farde L, Wiesel FA, Halldin C, Sedvall G. Central D2-dopamine receptor occupancy in schizophrenic patients treated with antipsychotic drugs. Arch Gen Psychiatry 1988;45:71–76.

Fowler JS, Volkow ND, Wang GJ, Pappas N, Logan J, MacGregor R, Alexoff D, Shea C, Schlyer D, Wolf AP, Warner D, Zezulkova I, Cilento R. Inhibition of monoamine oxidase B in the brains of smokers. Nature 1996;379:733–736.

Frackowiak RSJ, Friston KJ, Frith CD, Dolan RJ, Price CJ, Zeki S, Ashburner JT, Penny WD, editors. *Human Brain Function*. 2nd ed. San Diego (CA): Academic Press; 2004.

Frier M. Quality testing of radiopharmaceuticals. Hosp Pharm 2000;7:89–93.

Gjedde A. High- and low-affinity transport of D-glucose from blood to brain. J Neurochem 1981;36:1463–1471.

Herholz K, Heiss WD, Herscovitch P. *NeuroPET: PET in Neuroscience and Clinical Neurology*. Berlin, Heidelberg: Springer-Verlag; 2004.

Hudson HM, Larkin RS. Accelerated image reconstruction using ordered subsets of projection data. IEEE Trans Med Imaging 1994;13:601–609.

Jacobs A, Voges J, Reszka R, Lercher M, Gossmann A, Kracht L, Kaestle C, Wagner R, Wienhard K, Heiss WD. Positron-emission tomography of vector-mediated gene expression in gene therapy for gliomas. Lancet 2001;358:727–729.

Jones T. The imaging science of positron emission tomography. Eur J Nucl Med 1996;23:807–813.

Keen HG, Dekker BA, Disley L, Hastings D, Lyons S, Reader AJ, Ottewell P, Watson A, Zweit J. Imaging apoptosis in vivo using ^{124}I-annexin V and PET. Nucl Med Biol 2005;32:395–402.

Kety SS, Schmidt CF. The nitrous oxide method for the quantitative determination of cerebral blood flow in man: theory, procedure and normal values. J Clin Invest 1948;27:476–483.

Kim EE, Yang DJ, editors. *Targeted Molecular Imaging in Oncology*. New York: Springer-Verlag New York, Inc; 2000.

Koepp MJ, Gunn RN, Lawrence AD, Cunningham VJ, Dagher A, Jones T, Brooks DJ, Bench CJ, Grasby PM. Evidence for striatal dopamine release during a video game. Nature 1998;393:266–268.

Kuhl DE, Edwards RQ. Cylindrical and section radioisotope scanning of the liver and the brain. Radiology 1964;83:926–938.

Laking GR, West C, Buckley DL, Matthews J, Price PM. Imaging vascular physiology to monitor cancer treatment. Crit Rev Oncol Hematol 2006;58:95–113.

Långström B, Hartvig P. GMP-three letters with many interpretations: protection of patients or killing the clinical and research applications of PET? Eur J Nucl Med Mol Imaging 2008;35:693–694.

Laruelle M, van Dyck C, Abi-Dargham A, Zea-Ponce Y, Zoghbi SS, Charney DS, Baldwin RM, Hoffer PB, Kung HF, Innis RB. Compartmental modeling of iodine-123-iodobenzofuran binding to dopamine D2 receptors in healthy subjects. J Nucl Med 1994;35:743–754.

de Leon MJ, Mosconi L, Logan J. Seeing what Alzheimer saw. Nat Med 2007; 13:129–131.

Logan J, Fowler JS, Volkow ND, Wolf AP, Dewey SL, Schlyer DJ, MacGregor RR, Hitzemann R, Bendriem B, Gatley SJ, Christman DR. Graphical analysis of reversible radioligand binding from time-activity measurements applied to [N-^{11}C-methyl]-(-)-cocaine PET studies in human subjects. J Cereb Blood Flow Metab 1990;10:740–747.

Mintun MA, Raichle ME, Kilbourn MR, Wooten GF, Welch MJ. A quantitative model for the in vivo assessment of drug binding sites with positron emission tomography. Ann Neurol 1984;15:217–227.

Mintun MA, Welch MJ, Siegel BA, Mathias CJ, Brodack JW, McGuire AH, Katzenellenbogen JA. Breast cancer: PET imaging of estrogen receptors. Radiology 1988;169:45–48.

Myers R, Hume S. Small animal PET. Eur Neuropsychopharmacol 2002;12:545–555.

Natterer F, Wübbeling F. *Mathematical Methods in Image Reconstruction, Series: Monographs on Mathematical Modeling and Computation No. 5*. Philadelphia: Society for Industrial and Applied Mathematics (SIAM); 2001.

Nordberg A. PET imaging of amyloid in Alzheimer's disease. Lancet Neurol 2004;3:519–527.

Padhani AR, Krohn KA, Lewis JS, Alber M. Imaging oxygenation of human tumours. Eur Radiol 2007;17:861–872.

Patlak CS, Blasberg RG. Graphical evaluation of blood-to-brain transfer constants from multiple-time uptake data. Generalizations. J Cereb Blood Flow Metab 1985;5:584–590.

Patlak CS, Blasberg RG, Fenstermacher JD. Graphical evaluation of blood-to-brain transfer constants from multiple-time uptake data. J Cereb Blood Flow Metab 1983;3:1–7.

Phelps ME, Mazziotta J, Schelbert HR, editors. *Positron Emission Tomography and Autoradiography: Principles and Applications for the Brain and Heart*. New York: Raven Press; 1986.

Reader AJ, Julyan PJ, Williams H, Hastings DL, Zweit J. EM algorithm resolution modeling by image-space convolution for PET reconstruction. IEEE Trans Nucl Sci 2003;50:1392–1397.

Reivich M, Kuhl D, Wolf A, Greenberg J, Phelps M, Ido T, Casella V, Fowler J, Hoffman E, Alavi A, Som P, Sokoloff L. The [^{18}F]fluorodeoxyglucose method for the measurement of local cerebral glucose utilization in man. Circ Res 1979;44:127–137.

Shepp LA, Vardi Y. Maximum likelihood reconstruction for emission tomography. IEEE Trans Med Imaging 1982;1:113–121.

Sokoloff L, Reivich M, Kennedy C, Des Rosiers MH, Patlak CS, Pettigrew KD, Sakurada O, Shinohara M. The [^{14}C]deoxyglucose method for the measurement of local cerebral glucose utilization: theory, procedure, and normal values in the conscious and anesthetized albino rat. J Neurochem 1977;28:897–916.

Tillisch J, Brunken R, Marshall R, Schwaiger M, Mandelkern M, Phelps M, Schelbert H. Reversibility of cardiac wall-motion abnormalities predicted by positron tomography. N Engl J Med 1986;314:884–888.

Valk PE, Bailey DL, Townsend DW, Maisey MN, editors. *Positron Emission Tomography: Basic Science and Clinical Practice*. London: Springer-Verlag; 2003.

Wagner HN Jr, Burns HD, Dannals RF, Wong DF, Långström B, Duelfer T, Frost JJ, Ravert HT, Links JM, Rosenbloom SB, Lukas SE, Kramer AV, Kuhar MJ. Imaging dopamine receptors in the human brain by positron tomography. Science 1983;221(4617):1264–1266.

Wu JC, Bengel FM, Gambhir SS. Cardiovascular molecular imaging. Radiology 2007;244:337–355.

8

FLUORESCENCE IMAGING

NIKOLAOS C. DELIOLANIS
Institute for Biological and Medical Imaging (IBMI), Helmholtz Zentrum München and Technische Universität München, Munich, Germany

CHRISTIAN P. SCHULTZ
Siemens Medical and Center for Molecular Imaging Research, Massachusetts General Hospital, Charlestown, MA, USA

VASILIS NTZIACHRISTOS
Institute for Biological and Medical Imaging (IBMI), Helmholtz Zentrum München and Technische Universität München, Munich, Germany

8.1 INTRODUCTION

Fluorescence imaging is an emerging field of imaging sciences that encompasses a diverse arena of methods and techniques utilized in biomedical research and clinical application. Fluorescence methods attain widespread use in the biomedical laboratory because light is an easily manipulated modality and the corresponding measurements or image formation can reveal highly diverse anatomical, physiological, and molecular features of the structure studied. Additional applications are found in the fields of biotechnology, genomics, proteomics, and systems biology, and there is increasing use of fluorescence methods for *in vivo* imaging of development, disease, and drug discovery.

Fluorescence imaging can be generally classified according to (i) the physical size of the object imaged and (ii) the contrast mechanism utilized in image formation. *Microscopy* is the most common optical imaging method for imaging thin tissue slices up to about a millimeter of depth or thickness. The resolution

Biomedical Imaging: Principles and Applications, First Edition. Edited by Reiner Salzer.

typically achieved is diffraction limited for each corresponding wavelength. Imaging deeper in tissue is generally achieved with *macroscopic imaging*; however, typically the resolution then depends on the depth and the optical properties of the object studied. Typically, penetration of the order of several centimeters is possible, especially in the Near-Infrared (NIRs) (650–950 nm), because of the low light absorption by tissue in this spectral region. From a contrast perspective, fluorescence imaging can be classified into endogenous and exogenous contrast mechanisms. Natural endogenous tissue autofluorescence has often been considered for diagnosis as it carries information on key tissue structural elements or metabolites such as collagen or NADH. More commonly, however, fluorescence imaging is utilized with exogenous or induced expression of fluorochromes. Examples of exogenous fluorescence contrast are the injection of specific fluorescent dyes, fluorescent probes, or fluorescence-labeled antibodies, antibody fragments, and peptides. Induced fluorescence generally refers to the genetic manipulation of cells and organisms to express fluorescence proteins.

Fluorescence contrast is further affected by the tissue's natural optical properties, especially when imaging thick tissue specimens or *in vivo*. Tissue optical properties are primarily dependent on endogenous absorbers (primarily hemoglobin in the visible and NIR) and scattering due to index of refraction changes in the different cellular interfaces and cellular organelles. Correspondingly, the fluorescence field that propagates in tissues can undergo various phenomena, such as refraction, absorption, or scattering, that modify its spatial and temporal characteristics. In general, light–tissue interaction properties can be utilized as stand-alone methodologies to generate images of endogenous contrast, for example, in cellular imaging using Phase Contrast (PC) microscopy or tissue imaging using optical coherence tomography. The addition of exogenous fluorescence contrast, however, greatly increases the ability to study diverse processes and biomarkers that would be impossible to visualize with endogenous contrast, for example, the expression of a certain gene or the interaction of two proteins.

The first part of this chapter reviews the contrast mechanisms that are used in optical and fluorescence imaging. In particular, it briefly discusses the optical properties of biological tissue in the visible and NIR spectrum range and explains their role in light propagation and imaging. Subsequently, different reporter technologies used in fluorescence are presented, and a short explanation of an associated modality, that is, bioluminescence imaging is discussed. The second part of the chapter then presents current microscopic and macroscopic imaging methods for fluorescence imaging and expands on some applications of the methods described.

8.2 CONTRAST MECHANISMS

8.2.1 Endogenous Contrast

The propagation of light in bulk biological tissue is dominated by multiple scattering, since tissues are mostly consisted of closely packed cells and the size of the inhomogeneities in their structure is comparable to the wavelength of light. The optical properties of tissues are generally described by the refractive index η, the absorption coefficient μ_a, the scattering coefficient μ_s, and the probabilistic description of the scattering direction of a photon given a scattering event. For simplification in macroscopic observations, μ_s can be replaced with the reduced scattering coefficient $\mu_s' = \mu_s(1 - g)$, where g is a parameter accounting for the scattering anisotropy. The spectral dependence of the reduced scattering coefficient in the approximation of Mie scattering theory is

$$\mu_s'(\lambda) = a \times \lambda^b, \tag{8.1}$$

where a and b are parameters that are typically set heuristically (Alexandrakis et al., 2005). The various tissue chromophores provide the endogenous contrast for optical imaging, with the oxy- and deoxyhemoglobin molecules being the major contributors to the absorption of light. As seen in Figure 8.1, the absorption coefficient for both oxygenated (HbO) and deoxygenated (Hb) blood below 600 nm is considerably high. Therefore, the penetration depth in the visible region is limited to a few millimeters.

Tissue absorption imaging is generally used to reveal information on spatially varying hemoglobin concentration, which can be anatomical information (e.g., the presence of a blood vessel or a hemodynamic change) or information on disease (e.g., tumor contrast due to angiogenesis (Hielscher, 2005). Scattering contrast is associated with abnormally high tissue organelles, for example, those associated with highly packed cancer cells. Macroscopic scattering imaging is therefore occasionally used in the detection of abnormal tissue characteristics. In contrast, microscopic methods generally operate by "rejecting" scattering in

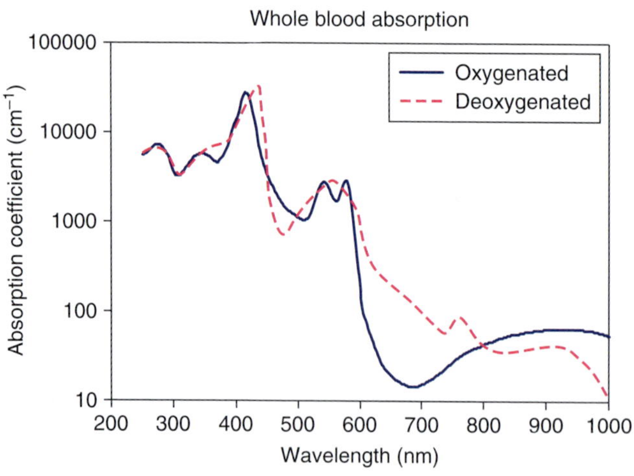

Figure 8.1. Absorption spectrum of oxygenated and deoxygenated whole blood in the 200-1000-nm range.

order to improve resolution, and therefore, scattering is not an important contrast mechanism in microscopy.

8.2.2 Exogenous Contrast

A long-standing practice in contrast enhancement in optical microscopy is tissue staining, where tissue is processed with specific tagging techniques, so that different types of cells and cellular structures can be identified. This paradigm further extends to *in vivo* staining methods to significantly improve the ability to visualize specific cells and subcellular moieties and processes *in vivo*. The different state-of-the-art *in vivo* staining methods go beyond contrast enhancement commonly available to clinical imaging methods, such as X-ray Computed Tomography (CT) or Magnetic Resonance Imaging (MRI), and include elaborate techniques to engineer fluorescent molecules or nanoparticles with particular accumulation properties or highly specific targeted characteristics.

8.3 DIRECT METHODS: FLUORESCENT PROBES

Fluorescent tagging techniques are widely used in microscopic and macroscopic imaging as well as in flow cytometry and are classified into *direct* and *indirect reporter technologies*. In the former, an engineered fluorescent probe is administered *in vivo* to target a specific moiety such as a receptor or an enzyme. Fluorescent probes can be further categorized as active or activatable. *Active probes* are fluorochromes attached to affinity ligands such as antibodies and peptides (Gurfinkel et al., 2003–2004; Ntziachristos, 2006) specific for a certain target, for example, tumors or molecular processes marking a disease. The active probes fluoresce even when they are not bound to the indented target and thus increase the background fluorescence. In consequence, a long circulation period should be allowed for the nonbound probe to clear out from the body and improve the signal to background ratio. *Activatable probes* use fluorochromes in close proximity to each other or to a quenching molecule, using appropriate peptides, so that their fluorescence is partially quenched. By utilizing peptide sequences that can be cleaved in the presence of a particular enzyme (Weissleder et al., 1999) or an acid (Licha et al., 1999), it is possible to activate the molecule's fluorescence by freeing the linked fluorochromes. Fluorescence probes typically consist of the active component, which interacts with the target (an affinity ligand or enzyme substrate), the reporting component (a fluorescent dye or a quantum dot), and possibly a delivery vehicle (e.g., a biocompatible polymer). Examples of identifying a series of proteases have been reported *in vivo* in tumors (Bremer et al., 2001; Mahmood and Weissleder, 2003; Weissleder et al., 1999), apoptosis (Bullok and Piwnica-Worms, 2005), myocardial infarction (Chen et al., 2005), and arthritis (Wunder et al., 2004).

8.4 INDIRECT METHODS: FLUORESCENT PROTEINS

Indirect imaging generally refers to genetic manipulations that can induce fluorescence contrast, by means of expressed fluorescence reporters. The most common practice is to introduce a gene into a cell that encodes for a Fluorescent Protein (FP). Protein expression can be constitutive or be in response to external stimuli, for example, a certain promoter. Fusing the FP-encoding gene to a gene of interest allows fluorescent tagging of the corresponding protein. The resulting fused protein generally maintains the functionality of the original protein but can be visualized either *in vitro* or *in vivo*.

The most commonly used protein is eGFP (Enhanced-Green Fluorescent Protein) derived from the wild type FP found in the jellyfish *Aequorea victoria*; different color proteins, such as Cyan Fluorescent Protein (CFP) and Yellow Fluorescent Protein (YFP) have been produced from mutations on the GFP gene. Recently, cloning of the Red Fluorescent Protein (RFP) has produced a number of important variants (Shaner et al., 2004; Tsien, 2005) that emit beyond the 600-nm barrier. This is of great importance since autofluorescence is reduced at the longer wavelengths (Muller et al., 2001) and, most significantly, light absorption in tissue is considerably decreased, enabling *in vivo* FP detection located deeply inside tissue and with higher sensitivity. FPs have been used in numerous applications such as cancer and stem cell research (Dewhirst et al., 2002; Hoffman, 2002; Paris and Sesboue, 2004; Shah et al., 2004; Wobus and Boheler, 2005), immunology (Griekspoor et al., 2005), drug discovery (Hoffman, 2002), and so on.

A powerful variation of the indirect reporter technologies is Fluorescence Resonant Energy Transfer (FRET), which is used to monitor protein–protein interactions. Two different proteins are labeled with a pair of FPs with, for example, CFP acting as a donor and YFP acting as an acceptor, since the latter can be excited and fluoresce because of energy transfer from the CFP molecule when the two are in close proximity to each other. Therefore, with the two proteins separated, CFP fluorescence is dominant when excited at its peak absorption wavelength, whereas there is little fluorescence from the YFP molecule. However, when the proteins interact and come into close proximity, the CFP emission pumps YFP fluorescence. By using spectrally separated measurements, it is possible to record the color change, representative of protein proximity and interaction. FRET is therefore employed to study protein behavior in live cells (Chamberlain et al., 2000; van Roessel and Brand, 2002).

An associated method is *bioluminescence imaging*, where, in a manner similar to the use of fluorescence proteins, genetic manipulation of the cell allows the expression of an enzyme that can catalyze the reaction between an exogenously administered substrate, oxygen, and ATP. This process produces endogenously generated light (Contag and Bachmann, 2002), such as the one produced by the common firefly. One of the great advantages of bioluminescent reporter technology is that light is intrinsically generated only where luciferase is present, while there is extremely low background emission, thus the signal to background ratio is excellent. Luciferase obtained from *Photinus pyralis* has a peak emission at 560 nm, which is inside the tissue absorption spectral region (Fig. 8.1); however, a significant portion of its emission spectrum extends beyond 600 nm, which makes it possible for photons to reach the surface from deeper regions. Luciferase mutants with spectrum shifted to the red have also been produced (Contag and Bachmann, 2002; Nakatsu et al., 2006; Shapiro et al., 2005). Bioluminescence imaging is widely used in several biomedical imaging applications, for example, to report on tumor growth and metastasis, gene delivery and expression, or cell tracking applications (Bhaumik and Gambhir, 2002; Contag and Bachmann, 2002; Thorne and Contag, 2005). The bioluminescence technology analogous to FRET is Bioluminescence Resonant Energy Transfer (BRET), where the donor is expressing luciferase, bypassing the problems of photobleaching, autofluorescence, and simultaneous emission of FPs in FRET (Pfleger and Eidne, 2006).

8.5 MICROSCOPY

Optical microscopy has a long history of evolution and achievement, and it is one of the most valuable tools of biomedical research and clinical diagnosis. Importantly, novel methodologies that improve resolution, penetration depth, and acquisition speed or innovate on the contrast mechanism employed are continuously emerging. Herein, we only briefly summarize the major developments in the field of microscopy in biomedical imaging and emphasize on tissue imaging.

8.5.1 Optical Microscopy

Wide-field optical microscopy (Fig. 8.3a) utilizes lenses to magnify the field of view visualized in order to observe objects and structures that are smaller than the eye's resolving capacity, that is, 20–30 microns. Cells are, however, relatively transparent structures that offer limited contrast for direct visualization. Correspondingly, phase contrast (PC) microscopy, introduced by Zernike (1942a, 1942b), and Differential Interference Contrast (DIC) microscopy (Allen et al., 1969) are two widely used techniques employed to visualize cellular structures with increased sensitivity. The principle of operation is the visualization of spatial-dependent changes in the phase of light as it propagates through the cell, due to changes in thickness or the index of refraction. The PC microscope visualizes phase changes by inserting a $\lambda/4$ phase retardation plate at the back focal plane of the objective lens, in order to add a small phase shift to specific spatial components of the emerging light field in such a way as to interfere with the components that carry the phase modulation information (Fig. 8.2a). The result is an image where the intensity pattern is correlated to the difference in the optical path transversed by the different components. In differential interference microscopy, the object is illuminated by two slightly laterally displaced light wavefronts that are orthogonally polarized (Fig. 8.2b). Each of them undergoes

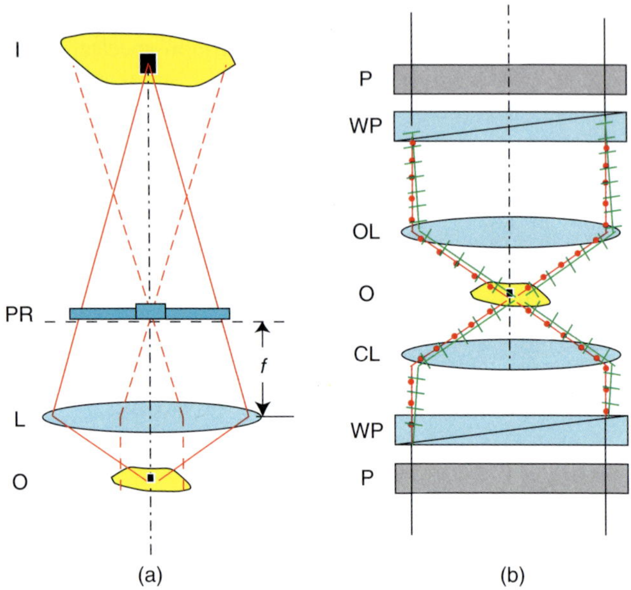

Figure 8.2. Phase detection techniques in microscopy. (a) PC microscope; O, object; L, objective lens; PR, phase retardation plate; I, image. The phase retarder is placed on the back focal (Fourier) plane to modulate the phase of the bulk component of the photon field. (b) P, polarizer; WP, modified Wolaston (Nomarsky) prism; CL, condenser lens; O, object; OL, objective lens. The modified Wolaston prism steers the two orthogonal polarizations to a slightly different direction that are focused on a slightly displaced position on the object. The two different beams pick up slightly different phase retardations due to the different optical paths through the sample. They are synthesized and interfere to convert the phase difference to intensity modulation.

a slightly different phase distortion, and they are appropriately synthesized in order to interfere. The resulting image encodes the gradient of the phase modulation of the object to intensity. In general, DIC microscopy exhibits superior characteristics in spatial and phase shift resolution compared to PC microscopy and can also handle a higher dynamic range of phase differences from the object. Although PC technologies have been developed for standard optical microscopy, they are also combined with fluorescence microscopes in multimodal systems.

8.5.2 Fluorescence Microscopy

As an exogenous contrast technique, *fluorescence microscopy*, has evolved into a widely used technology in biomedical imaging, which offers high levels of sensitivity, allowing even the detection of single molecules. In its basic form, it is a variation of the wide-field optical microscope, where light is filtered before forming the image by means of transmittance filters or dichroic mirrors. Figure 8.3a shows a schematic diagram of a wide-field epi-illumination microscope. The light

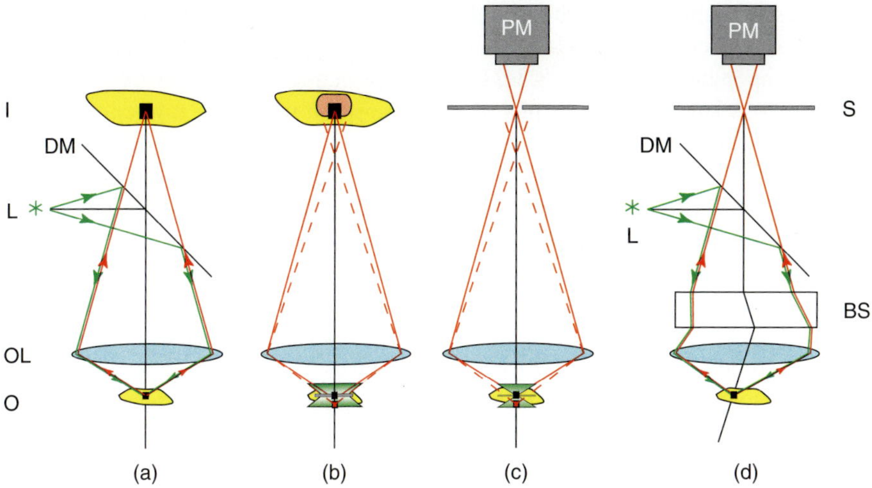

Figure 8.3. Fluorescence and confocal microscopy. O, object; OL, objective lens; L, light (laser) source; I, image; DM, dichroic mirror; S, screen; PM, photomultiplier tube; BS, beam scanning system; the green and red lines are the excitation and fluorescent emission rays, respectively. (a) Schematic diagram—principle of operation of an epi-illumination fluorescence microscope. Excitation and fluorescence light beams are filtered with a dichroic mirror. (b) Imaging characteristics of a wide-field microscope. Light from the point of interest (black square) is imaged sharply, while the rays from the deeper positioned red point (dashed lines) do not converge on the image plane and produce a blurred image. (c) Filtering in a confocal microscope. The illuminated field is reduced to a very narrow spot compared to a wide-field microscope. The pinhole on the screen located on the image plane allows only the light coming from the conjugate point in the object to reach the photomultiplier. (d) Schematic diagram of a confocal laser scanning microscope. The optomechanics in the white box steer the beam to scan the object, and the light returns back from the same optical path.

from the excitation source is directed on the object from the same path as the reflected light. The light in the excitation wavelength is reflected by the dichroic mirror, but it is transmitted in the fluorescent wavelength, and the rejection ratio of the system can be improved with the use of interference filters.

While standard microscopy is applied to imaging thin cellular or tissue layers (i.e., 5–10 μm), imaging thicker samples is complicated by photon scattering. In an aberration-free optical imaging system, each point on the image is generated only from light received from its conjugate point on the object plane. However, when imaging thick samples, light coming from different depths inside the tissue converges in different planes but remains unfocused on the imaging plane (Fig. 8.3b). The image formed is a superposition of a sharply focused plane and the unfocused projections of adjacent planes. In addition, in a wide-field imaging system, a wide area of the object is illuminated, and photons coming from adjacent points on the same plane might project on the same point on the imaging plane because of aberrations or scattering inside the tissue. Confocal imaging is a microscopy method in which the light collected and recorded in the image plane is spatially filtered by an aperture, to reject the undesired unfocused and scattered components. In Figure 8.3c, the basic principle of confocal microscopy is illustrated: A small pinhole is placed on the position where the rays coming from the point inside the object converge and most of the stray light is blocked. The volume of the object from which the rays are entering the pinhole depends on the shape of the illuminating beam (which is very sharply focused), the Numerical Aperture (NA) of the objective lens, and the optical characteristics of the tissue. The light from the aperture is collected, and its intensity is measured by a detector, typically a photomultiplier tube. Confocal Laser Scanning Microscopy (CLSM) is a technique developed to produce images, generated by scanning a laser beam onto the specimen of interest and measuring the corresponding signal at the pinhole over the entire volume scanned point by point. Images are formed by a posteriori synthesizing each individual measurement. While scanning, the point of interest should always be imaged on the aperture, and this can be implemented in three ways: (i) stage scanning, where the object is translated on the x-, y-, and z-axis; (ii) laser beam scanning (Fig. 8.3d), where the illuminating beam is usually steered by a set of two orthogonally placed galvanoactuated mirrors. The beam emerging from the point of interest returns from the same path and converges on the aperture; and (iii) use of spinning disks with multiple holes and microlenses (Nipkow disks). In Figure 8.4, an example of imaging HeLa cells with CLSM is presented, where the overexpression of parathymosin damages the nuclear structure.

Confocal microscopy can typically image at depths of up to 200 μm depending on the tissue optical properties. To allow *in vivo* visualization of deeper sitting structures, invasive approaches have been developed using implanted transparent windows (Helmchen and Denk, 2005; Jain et al., 2002) or surgical and endoscopic approaches (Molitoris and Sandoval, 2005). Endoscopically driven intravital microscopy allows microscopy for the first time to measure tissue and cell parameters directly within the surrounding environment before tissue resection for pathology may alter such conditions. The concept of optical biopsy has been suggested as a new tool for medical diagnostics, and endoscopy-based optical technologies may just support such future approaches in surgery. Although microscopic by nature, high resolution optical imaging through fibers may be combined with macroscopic guiding and positioning tools in order to provide targeted tissue diagnostics and potentially therapy monitoring. *In Vivo* applications of the technique include studies of tumor angiogenesis (Sipkins et al., 2005), pharmacological studies (Norman, 2005), neurological imaging (Kleinfeld et al., 1998), or the microdistribution of fluorescent probes (Bogdanov et al., 2002). One of the major disadvantages of fluorescent confocal microscopy is the use of very high light intensities to compensate for the light blocked by the pinhole filter, which results in the fast bleaching of the fluorescent dyes or proteins.

An alternative microscopic technique that enables imaging deeper than confocal microscopy is *two-photon* or *multiphoton microscopy*. This technique utilizes the multiphoton excitation phenomenon, where two or more photons are absorbed

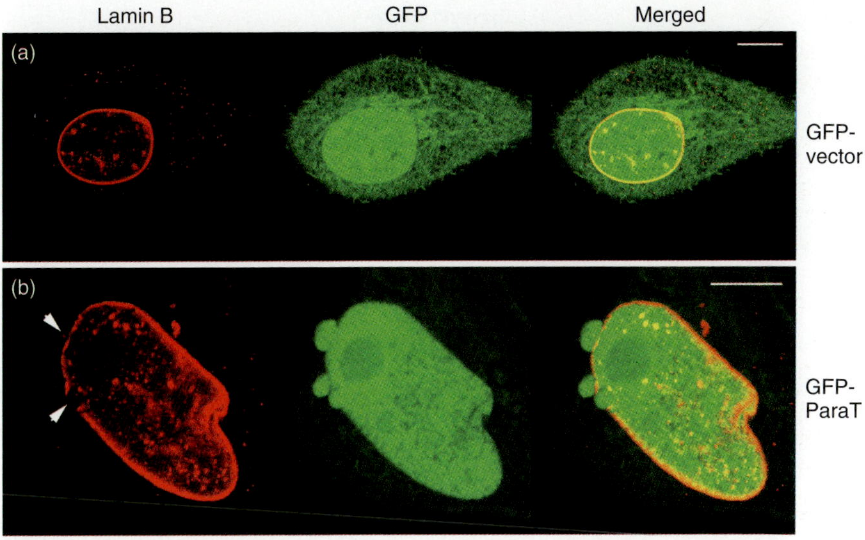

Figure 8.4. Overexpression of parathymosin (ParaT) in HeLa cells decondenses chromatin and damages nuclear sructure. (a) Lamin B-TRITC staining (left), GFP (middle), and the merge of both pictures (right) of HeLa cells expressing GFP. Lamin B (TRITC, excitation 532 nm and emission 580 nm) stains the nuclear envelope, and GFP (excitation 488 nm, emission 514 nm) can be found both in the nucleus and in the cytoplasm. (b) HeLa cells overexpressing GFP-tagged ParaT show distorted nuclear structure. Arrows indicate nuclear envelope irregularities. Bars: 10 μm (courtesy of Goran Martic, University of Ioannina).

almost simultaneously by a molecule. In this process, a molecule is excited to an intermediate state by the first photon, and consecutively, within 10^{-15} s, the second photon excites it to a state from which it can decay after fluorescence emission. The same stepwise excitation can also be achieved with more than two photons arriving within the same ultrafast time window. In this case, the combined energy of the two or more photons needs to be equal to the energy of the one-step excitation, as shown in Figure 8.5. Two- and multiphoton excitation is feasible only when there is a high density of photons in the tissue, and this can be achieved with the use of ultrafast light pulses (usually from a Ti:sapphire laser) and high NA objective lenses. In this geometry, the photon density is high enough to produce multiple excitations within the geometrical confinement of the focus of the beam, while there is no excitation outside the focal area, resulting in reduced photobleaching effects outside the laser beam focus. An additional advantage of two- and multiphoton microscopy over confocal microscopy is that the use of laser sources in the NIR (needed to excite FPs in the visible) allows penetration deeper in tissues (~500 μm) (Helmchen and Denk, 2005; Zipfel et al., 2003), although in principle resolution is decreased because of the longer wavelength utilized. Multiphoton laser scanning microscopy applications include visualization of vascularization (Kleinfeld et al., 1998), angiogenesis (Bird et al., 2005; Brown

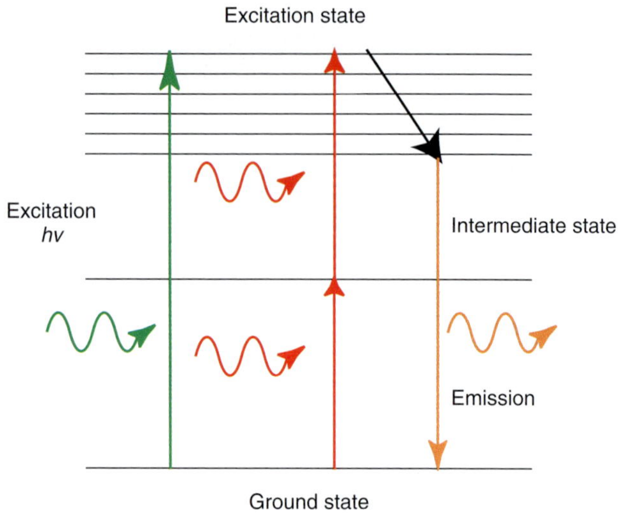

Figure 8.5. One- and two-photon excitation and fluorescent emission (green, red, and orange).

et al., 2001), metastasis (Voura et al., 2004; Wang et al., 2002), immunological studies (Germain et al., 2005; Runnels et al., 2006), kidney physiology (Dunn et al., 2002; Molitoris and Sandoval, 2005) and neurological research (Majewska et al., 2006; Mansfield et al., 2005).

Postacquisition image processing techniques can be further employed to enhance the contrast of the images or to reconstruct the three-dimensional structure of the object. Each image produced is a convolution of the actual image and the Point Spread Function (PSF) of the imaging system, that is, the blurring that occurs when the system images an ideal point. If the PSF is known, then it is possible to process the z-axis stack of images and produce an aberration-free and defocus-free 3D image of the object. This technique is called *deconvolution microscopy* (McNally et al., 1999), and the algorithms used can be classified as deblurring, in which the images are processed in a 2D basis and out-of-focus photons are just removed from a slice, and restoration, in which the whole z-stack is processed simultaneously and these photons are reassigned to their original position. These techniques can operate as a stand alone in regular wide-field or fluorescence microscopy or can be implemented as an add-on improvement on confocal techniques (Yaksi and Friedrich, 2006).

The microscopic methods described above operate with very thin specimens or by rejecting scattered light, whereas Total Internal Reflection Fluorescence Microscopy (TIRFM) is a method that achieves object illumination at very shallow depths (~100 nm) using evanescent fields. In this way, only very superficial fluorochromes are excited, which can reduce blurring effects since no fluorescence from deeper in the tissue is present on the resulting microscopic image. This technique is typically applied to imaging tagged cellular receptors or single molecules (Funatsu et al., 1995; Mashanov et al., 2003) and appropriately places the cell or medium of interest on a special glass plate in order to form a flat surface area over the field of view. The illuminating light is incident on the surface of the object at an angle larger than the internal reflection critical angle so that the entire light is reflected, but a shallow evanescent field component is established inside the object.

Currently there is significant progress with optical imaging beyond the diffraction limit. A recent development that achieves "nanoscopic" imaging is Stimulated Emission Depletion (STED) fluorescence microscopy. As in confocal and two-photon microscopy, a small area on the object is excited by a short pulse and its lateral size cannot be smaller than the diffraction limit. In STED, however, the size of the volume excited is reduced by sending a second pulse at the same wavelength as the fluorescent emission (Hell and Wichmann, 1994). The second pulse is formed has a donut-shaped profile, that is, of high intensity in the periphery and zero in the center; its wavelength is longer than the excitation pulse and is delivered at times that are much shorter compared to the fluorochrome's life time. The energy of the photons of the second pulse is tuned to stimulate the emission of the excited molecules but is not enough to excite new molecules. As a result, the ring around the spot is depleted, and only a fine spot of excited molecules remains in the center. The spontaneous fluorescence from the nondepleted molecules is collected by the detector. The resolution achieved combined with improved object illumination system can reach 50–100 nm, which is a threefold to fivefold improvement over conventional confocal microscopes (Hell, 2003). Early applications in biology include subdiffraction imaging of GFP-labeled retrovirus particles and epithelial cells (Willig et al., 2006).

An alternative subdiffraction limit fluorescence imaging method developed recently, reported as *stochastic optical reconstruction microscopy* (Rust et al., 2006) or *photoactivated localization microscopy* (Betzig et al., 2006), enables fluorescence imaging down to the molecular scale. An object tagged with a fluorescent molecule or protein is illuminated with a very low intensity using the TIRFM technique. To compensate for the very low intensity, the image acquisition process has to be repeated over thousands of cycles. In each cycle, only a few of the fluorescent single molecules are excited because of the low intensity, and the image captured from the fluorescent emission of each single molecule is blurred because of the diffraction limit. The advantage lies in the fact that the density of the excited single molecule in each cycle is low because of the low excitation intensity; thus, their blurred images are generally not overlapping. By postprocessing each one of the acquired images, the center of the PSF of each emitting source can be localized with an accuracy of 20 nm, and superimposing the processed stack of images from all the cycles yields the ultrahigh resolution. One of the disadvantages of the method is the very long acquisition time, about 2–12 h.

8.6 MACROSCOPIC IMAGING/TOMOGRAPHY

Macroscopic biomedical imaging operates at depths beyond the ones achieved by microscopic techniques. To achieve this, the technique utilizes photons that have scattered multiple times and therefore exchanges resolution for penetration depth. Macroscopic imaging is increasingly used for *in vivo* imaging of entire tissues and animals and in select clinical applications. Macroscopic imaging can be generally classified into planar qualitative techniques and quantitative tomographic methods. Analogous to microscopy, they can be further characterized in relation to the contrast mechanism used.

8.7 PLANAR IMAGING

Planar imaging is technologically and methodologically a simple technique, in which the photon field emerging from the object is recorded using a photographic system with high sensitivity (typically a Charge-Coupled Device (CCD) camera with a lens and appropriate filters). There are many alternative configurations depending on the geometry of illumination and the contrast mechanism used. From the geometrical standpoint, a spatially expanded light wavefront can either be incident from the same side of the camera detector (epi-illumination or reflectance imaging) or from the opposite side of the camera detector (transillumination), as shown in Figure 8.6.

When operating in the fluorescence mode, the excitation light field propagates into the object, excites the fluorochromes (which serve as secondary sources),

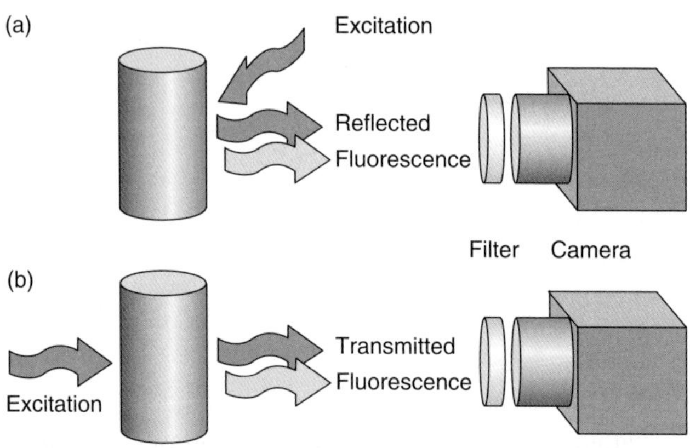

Figure 8.6. The two alternative configurations for optical planar imaging. (a) Epi-illumination (or reflectance configuration), where the illumination source and the camera are on the same side of the object. (b) Transilluminescence, where the illumination source and the camera are placed on opposite sides of the object.

and the emitted field is acquired with the use of bandpass filters to isolate the emission wavelength and reject the excitation. Fluorescence Reflectance Imaging (FRI) (Fig. 8.6a) performs better when the fluorescent source is located near surface areas, as, for example, when performing in vivo studies of fluorescent probe uptake in superficial tumors (Bugaj et al., 2001; Ke et al., 2003; Mahmood et al., 1999) or osteoblastic activity (Zaheer et al., 2001). Fluorescence Transillumination Imaging (FTI) (Fig. 8.6b) is more suitable for deeply located sources, because in FRI, signal from deep-seated activity is strongly attenuated compared to the signal coming from superficial activity, and when both deep-seated and superficial activities exist, contrast from deeper lesions is significantly reduced. In FTI, there is more symmetric attenuation of superficial and deep-seated signals since the combined path of propagation of excitation and emission light is the same, independent of the depth of the fluorochrome. Planar fluorescence images can be significantly improved by a simple normalization technique (Ntziachristos et al., 2005; Zacharakis et al., 2006). Absorption inhomogeneities inside the tissue result in unequal absorption of the fluorescent signal, which deteriorates image quality and quantification and can lead to erroneous conclusions. Dividing the fluorescent image with an image recorded at the excitation wavelength compensates for the uneven illumination and improves image quality. Figure 8.7 shows transillumination images obtained *in vivo* from FP-expressing cells stereotactically impanted in the brain of nu/nu mice and the superior imaging accuracy imparted by normalized images. *In vivo* planar imaging of bioluminescence can be similarly obtained; in this case, no illumination is required but only the use of highly sensitive CCD cameras. However, the method is similarly prone to spatial variation of the bioluminescence signal collected due to background optical attenuation heterogeneity, which may result in inaccurate observations, especially from deep-seated activity.

In many applications, multiple fluorescent probes or proteins can be used simultaneously to tag different cell types or cellular structures. It is possible that some spectral overlap may be present in the resulting images (e.g.,when one excitation wavelength excites two or more fluorochromes or when their emission spectra have an overlap). In these cases, spectral unmixing techniques are required to determine the contribution of each emitter, in analogy to methods used in microscopy (Zimmermann et al., 2003). Another aspect that requires attention in fluorescence imaging is the effects of autofluorescence or background fluorescence on the resulting images. Tissue autofluorescence, that is, fluorescence due to endogenous fluorochromes, is a broadband emission that is higher in the blue-green visible part of the spectrum and that significantly reduces in the NIR (Georgakoudi et al., 2002). Depending on the spectral region where imaging is performed, autofluorescence may reduce the contrast from fluorochromes of interest. Spectral unmixing techniques or careful filter selection can be used to reject background fluorescence and improve contrast and detection sensitivity (Mansfield et al., 2005; Troy et al., 2004).

Modern Liquid Crystal Tunable Filter (LCTF) devices provide new technology and the means to differentiating signal content beyond simple physical resolution

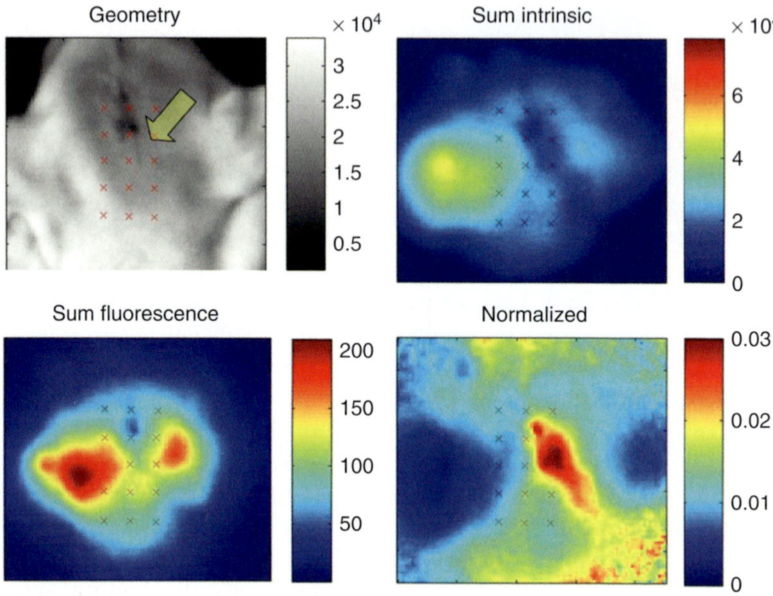

Figure 8.7. Transillumination imaging of brain tumor. One-half million glioma cells expressing tdTomato FP were stereotactically injected into the brain in the right cranial side and imaged 4 days later. The images are planar reflectance of the cranium, sum of the intrinsic signals for all the sources, sum of the fluorescence, and the fluorescence normalized with the intrinsic signal. The red crosses indicate the location of the laser sources projected on the ventral side of the head, and the arrow indicates the location of the implanted cells.

of optical information. Creating stacks of images at different frequencies allows the generation of complex spectral information that can then be processed with focus on background subtraction and multiple fluorescent probes separation with significant spectral overlap (Mansfield et al., 2005).

One important aspect of current development in planar imaging is the design of flexible, small, and versatile Handheld Devices (HHDs) (Fig. 8.8) (Kirsch et al., 2007). The area of focus of such technology development is the creation of new surgical tools, providing physicians with devices for direct tissue guidance. Targeted optical fluorescent probes connected to tissues that are subject to resection during procedures would fluoresce if illuminated and be made visible through HHDs. In contrast to common practice, surgeons would be able to see the tissue material that requires removal. Such devices are currently developed through many different initiatives and tested in animal models.

8.8 TOMOGRAPHY

The quantification and penetration limitations of planar imaging have led to the development of optical tomography. Optical tomography employs theoretical

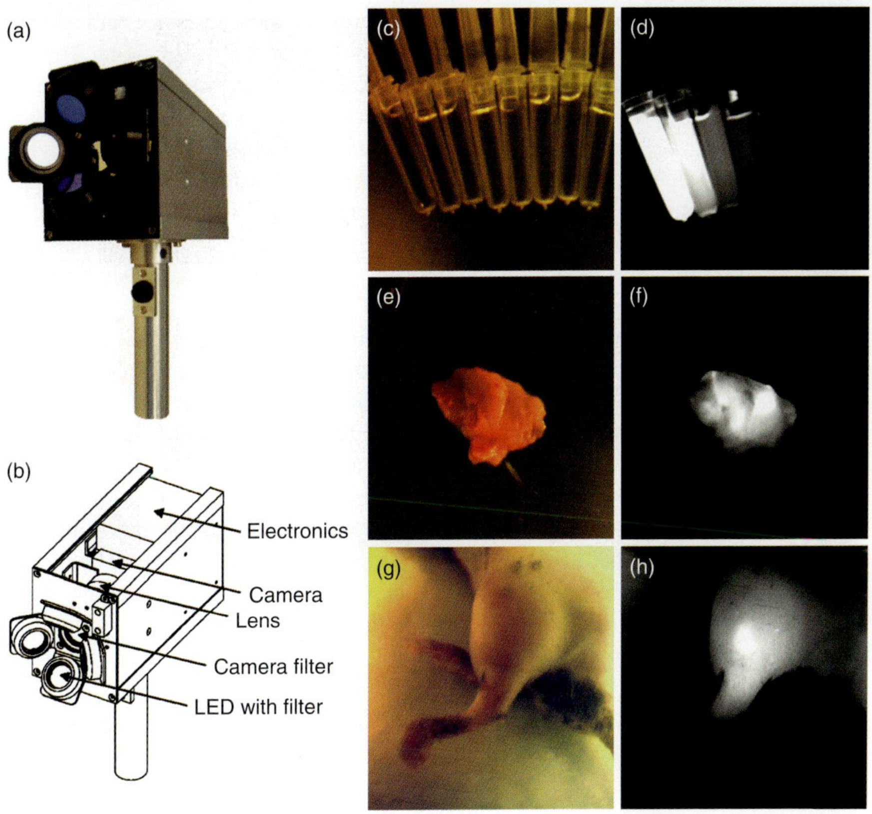

Figure 8.8. Handheld device prototype for interventional optical fluorescence imaging. (a) Front view of the device showing the four-angled laser diode mounts, the center objective, the electronic case, front mounted distance sensor, and LED trigger. (b) Schematic drawing of the handheld device. (c) Visible image of the dilution series of AngioSense 750 (VisEn Medical, MA, USA) for fluorescence response calibration of the handheld device (left to right: 2000, 1000, 500, 250, 125, 62.5, 31.25, and 15.625 pM). (d) Simultaneously measured fluorescence image. (e) Visible image of excised tumor tissue. (f) Simultaneously measured fluorescence image of the tumor tissue showing the heterogeneous distribution of tumor cells labeled with ProSense 750 (VisEn Medical). (g) Visible image of a laboratory mouse with a growing tumor before surgical tumor resection. (h) Simultaneously measured fluorescence image of the mouse showing the glowing tumor tissue labeled with ProSense 750 (VisEn Medical) through the surrounding healthy tissue of the mouse leg. (The handheld device developments are part of a strategic effort in molecular imaging between Siemens Medical Solution and the Center for Molecular Imaging Research).

models of photon propagation, coupled to multi-illumination approaches to provide three-dimensional information of optical contrast. Fluorescence tomography utilizes the general theoretical mainframe developed for Diffuse Optical Tomography (DOT). The resolution achieved is of the order of 1 mm in small animals and of the order of centimeters for large structures such as the human breast. However, these methods can reveal cellular and subcellular information when coupled to fluorochromes with specificity to certain tissue biomarkers. A particular tomographic approach developed, Fluorescence Molecular Tomography (FMT), makes use of such fluorescent probes while utilizing a particular normalization scheme that is appropriate for *in vivo* imaging, as it significantly minimizes the dependence of spatially varying attenuation.

There are various geometrical implementations for DOT and FMT. A common approach utilizes a cylindrical chamber that is used to bring fibers in contact with the tissue of investigation either by utilizing matching fluids or by mechanically moving the fibers onto the tissue (Brooksby et al., 2004; Ntziachristos and Weissleder, 2002b; Xu et al., 2001) (Fig. 8.9). Another common geometry is the slab, where the object is placed inside a rectangular chamber. This implementation offers only limited angle illumination, analogous to X-ray tomosynthesis, but allows for simpler hardware requirements. Similar to the cylindrical chamber approach, fibers that are brought in contact with the tissue or matching fluids have been utilized for optimal photon coupling between the optical system and the tissue under interrogation (Choe et al., 2005; Graves et al., 2003; Patwardhan et al., 2005; Turchin et al., 2006).

More recently, the appearance of noncontact systems has simplified experimental procedures and the quality and size of the data set collected. Noncontact

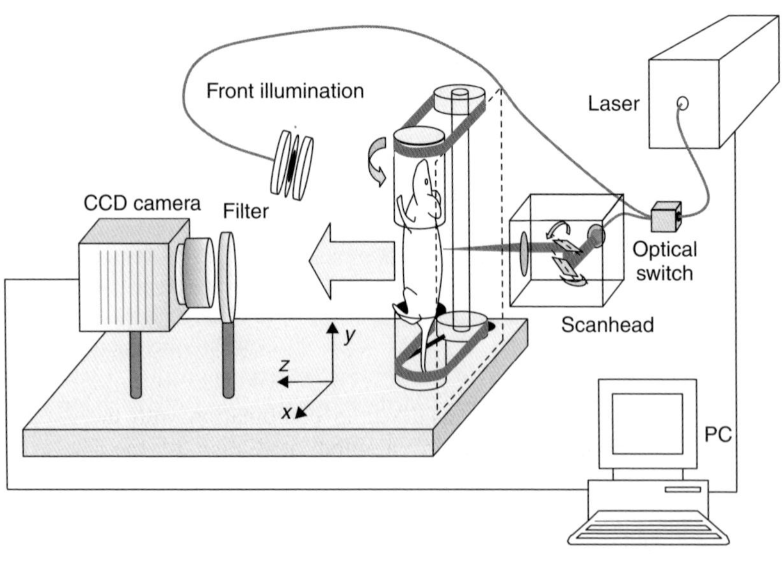

Figure 8.9. Schematic of the experimental setup for free-space full-projection FMT.

systems do not generally utilize fibers to guide light, but employ direct imaging of the free surface using a CCD camera or other detectors. Illumination is similarly achieved by scanning a laser beam on the surface of an animal. When operating in the free-space mode, these approaches also avoid the use of matching fluids, that is, the object is suspended in free space (Chaudhari et al., 2005; Deliolanis et al., 2007; Hielscher et al., 2002; Schulz et al., 2004; Schulz et al., 2006). In these systems, the object is not compressed, but keeps its natural shape; thus, for reconstruction it is necessary to capture the geometry of the surface of the body as well. Finally, there are reflection tomographic geometries in which the sources and detectors are on the same side of the object (Bluestone et al., 2001; Meyer, 2007). These geometries are more suitable for reconstruction of volumes located near the surface.

Regarding the illumination and detection technique used, optical tomographic imaging systems can be divided into three categories: Continuous Wave (CW), Time Domain (TD), and Frequency Domain (FD) systems systems. The CW systems use constant intensity light sources and regular CCD cameras or light detectors, combining simple low-cost implementation with high detection sensitivity and signal to noise ratio. They are suitable for fluorescent tomography; however, they cannot distinguish between absorption and scattering and therefore do not offer optimal implementations for imaging endogenous nonfluorescence contrast. In *time domain* systems, short-pulse lasers (typically <10 ps) are used with detection techniques based on time-gated or time-resolved imaging, which are able to record the intensity of light as a function of time, with resolutions on the order of picoseconds to hundreds of picoseconds. TD systems have the capability to disentangle scattering and absorption coefficients and to image fluorescence lifetime. The main disadvantage of TD systems compared to CW systems is the lower signal to noise ratio achieved because of the low duty cycles employed due to pulsing. In *frequency domain* systems, the intensity of the illuminating light is modulated typically in the 100-1000-MHz range. The recorded signal is demodulated, and the amplitude A and the phase retardation ϕ are measured at a single or multiple modulation frequency. The main advantage of the FD technique over TD methods is the high rejection ratio of the nonmodulated noise components such as ambient light and potentially the improved signal to noise ratio of operation.

Optical tomography is generally a computationally intensive method (Chapter 2). Typically, implementations discretize the volume of interest in a 3D mesh, and the problem can be solved in two steps: First, the light propagation inside the object imaged is described with a mathematical model known as the *forward problem*. Then, in the inverse problem, a solution of internal distribution is reached when (considered in combination with the theoretically calculated forward model) it yields a good prediction of the data collected experimentally. Optical tomography problems are typically ill-posed because of the high light diffusion present (Kak and Slaney, 1999). This implies that the solutions are sensitive to noise and can be reached only after regularization. Photon propagation is theoretically modeled utilizing an approximate solution to the radiation transport equation (Ishimaru, 1997). A common simplification, however, is to utilize the diffusion approximation that models light propagation as a diffusion process. Consequently, simple solutions that facilitate practical inversion schemes can be reached.

8.8.1 Diffuse Optical Tomography

In DOT, the unknown distribution of the scattering and absorption coefficients (μ_s' and μ_a, respectively) is reconstructed, assuming that the refractive index η is known. As described earlier, the reconstructed optical properties μ_s' and μ_a are associated with different physiological and disease states, in particular, organelle density represented by μ_s' and oxy- and deoxyhemoglobin (and to a certain extent water and lipids) represented byμ_a. By performing tomography in multiple wavelengths, the concentrations of oxy- and deoxyhemoglobin can be derived and spatially resolved. DOT has been used in various *in vivo* applications, such as brain functional studies, stroke monitoring, joint imaging, and breast cancer imaging (for a comprehensive description, see references Brooksby et al., 2006; Choe et al., 2005; Hielscher et al., 2002 and references therein). Approaches that improve image reconstruction consider the use of a priori information, as derived from another high resolution modality (Brooksby et al., 2005) or using multispectral information (Corlu et al., 2003, Corlu et al., 2005; Srinivasan et al., 2006; Xu et al., 2004) to improve the ill-posed nature of the inverse problem.

8.8.2 Fluorescence Tomography

Forward problems utilized in fluorescence tomography typically need to solve two separate problems, one that solves for the propagation of the excitation light and one that solves for the propagation of the emitted light (Jiang, 1998; O'Leary et al., 1996; Paithankar et al., 1997). A relatively more simple approach increasingly used for *in vivo* imaging is the use of the normalized Born approximation (Ntziachristos and Weissleder, 2001). In this case, similar to the normalization methods developed for planar imaging, fluorescence measurements are divided with corresponding measurements at the excitation wavelength. The ratio of the fluorescent over the excitation photon field that reach the boundary of the object is then given by

$$\frac{\Phi_{\mathrm{fl}}(r_{\mathrm{d}}, r_{\mathrm{s}}, \omega)}{\Phi_{\mathrm{exl}}(r_{\mathrm{d}}, r_{\mathrm{s}}, \omega)} = \frac{\Theta}{\Phi(r_{\mathrm{d}}, r_{\mathrm{s}}, \omega)} \int g_{\mathrm{em}}(r_{\mathrm{d}}, r, \omega) O_{\mathrm{fl}}(r, \omega) \Phi(r, r_{\mathrm{s}}, \omega)\, \mathrm{d}r, \qquad (8.2)$$

where r_s, and r_d are the position vectors of the source and detector, respectively; $\Phi(r, r_s, \omega)$ is the field reaching a point inside the object; g_{em} is the Green's function solution of a delta function at the position r; $O_{fl}(r, \omega)$ is the emission yield, which is proportional to the fluorophore concentration; and Θ is a factor accounting for various gain factors such as filter transmittance and camera sensitivity for the different wavelengths. The advantages of the normalized Born approximation are that the division performs corrections for spatially dependent gain factors between different sources and detectors and significantly reduces the sensitivity to the background optical heterogeneity, thus offering a method appropriate for *in vivo* imaging (Soubret et al., 2005).

FMT implemented in the noncontact slab geometry has been employed in resolving protease and receptor upregulation, chemotherapeutic responses, or fluorochrome accumulation *in vivo* (Ntziachristos et al., 2002a; Ntziachristos et al., 2004; Patwardhan et al., 2005) as well as in FP expression in small animals (Zacharakis et al., 2005). Recently, the first demonstration of free space, noncontact FMT, in the 360° implementation mode has been achieved using a CW domain prototype. The system is shown in Figure 8.9.

Animals are scanned by a laser beam that is focused on their surface and translated in the *xy* plane using two orthogonally placed galvanometer-actuated mirrors. The transmitted and fluorescent emitted photon field is collected in transillumination using a high sensitivity low noise CCD camera, through a photographic lens and appropriate bandpass filters tuned at the wavelengths of the excitation and fluorescent emission of the fluorophore of interest. The animals in this implementation are placed in a vertical rotation stage and imaged in free space over multiple projections. *In vivo* imaging of a mouse model of lung cancer is shown in Figure 8.10. The mouse shown was implanted with 1×10^6 Lewis Lung Carcinoma (LLC) cells administered intercostally into the right lung parenchyma. Twelve days after implantation, the mouse received 2 nmol of Angioscence750 (Visen Medical) via the tail vein and was imaged 36 h later. During the experiment, the mouse was anesthetized with ketamine and xylazine. The images demonstrate protease imaging in 360° free-space FMT mode and coregistered X-ray CT images acquired before FMT imaging, showing virtually identical mouse placement. The FMT images highlight areas of increased fluorescence concentration congruent with the location of tumor seen on the X-ray CT images.

8.9 CONCLUSION

Optical and fluorescent imaging technology is an emerging field in biomedical research. Chemically and genetically engineered optical reporter technologies that enable visualization of a large number of tissue biomarkers have been introduced. In parallel, significant developments in imaging technology now allow visualization from the level of protein and DNA to entire animals and human organs. The high implementation flexibility combined with relatively low cost makes optical imaging a highly disseminated technology in the biomedical laboratory. Various optical imaging systems, including advanced macroscopic methods and optical tomographic imaging, are becoming increasingly available for biomedical research and drug discovery. Overall, therefore, the use of optical contrast, and in particular fluorescence, offers an increasingly useful readout for basic research, preclinical imaging, and potential clinical translation as well.

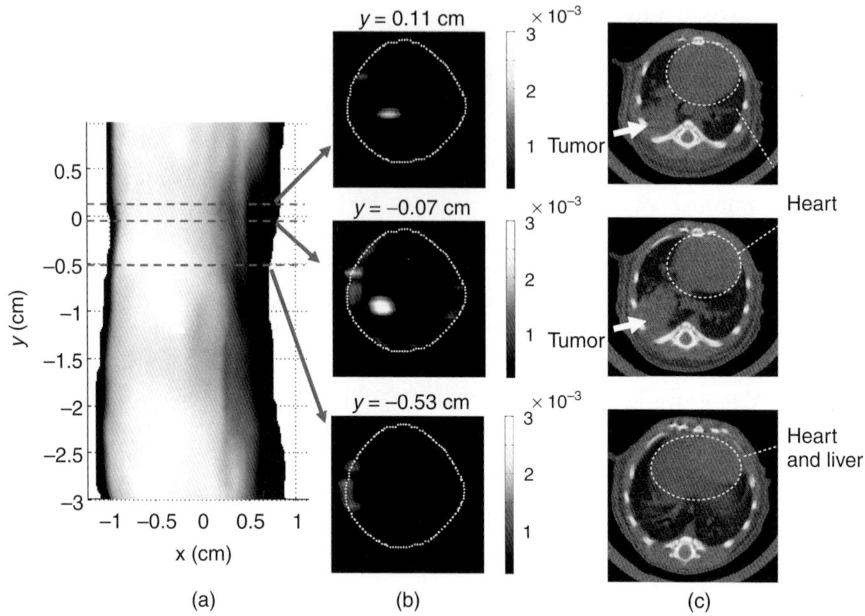

Figure 8.10. Free-space multiprojection FMT imaging lung tumor in a mouse *in vivo*. (a) Planar reflectance image of the torso of the mouse. (b) FMT axial slices of the reconstructed fluorescence concentration at different heights; the dotted line is the animal surface. Experimental details: 36 different projections with 21 sources and 132 detectors per projection arranged in a rectangular grid. Reconstructed fluorescence was calculated in a rectangular mesh consisting of 7932 points 15 min on a Pentium 4 on 3.32 GHz and 3 Gb of RAM. (c) Corresponding X-ray CT images, showing the location of the heart, liver, tumor (appearing gray), and lung (black).

ACKNOWLEDGMENTS

The authors thank Goran Martic for providing the microscopy image and gratefully acknowledge the financial support from the National Institutes of Health grants NIH NIBIB R01 EB006432 and NIH NIBIB RO1 EB00750.

REFERENCES

Alexandrakis G, Rannou FR, Chatziioannou AF. Tomographic bioluminescence imaging by use of a combined optical-PET (OPET) system: a computer simulation feasibility study. Phys Med Biol 2005;50(17):4225–4241.

Allen R, David G, Nomarski G. The Zeiss-Nomarski differential interference equipment for transmitted-light microscopy. Z Wiss Mikrosk Mikrosk Tech 1969;69(4):193–221.

Betzig E, Patterson GH, Sougrat R, Lindwasser OW, Olenych S, Bonifacino JS, Davidson MW, Lippincott-Schwartz J, Hess HF. Imaging intracellular fluorescent proteins at nanometer resolution. Science 2006;313(5793):1642–1645.

Bhaumik S, Gambhir SS. Optical imaging of Renilla luciferase reporter gene expression in living mice. Proc Natl Acad Sci U S A 2002;99(1):377–382.

Bird DK, Yan L, Vrotsos KM, Eliceiri KW, Vaughan EM, Keely PJ, White JG, Ramanujam N. Metabolic mapping of MCF10A human breast cells via multiphoton fluorescence lifetime imaging of the coenzyme NADH. Cancer Res 2005;65(19):8766–8773.

Bluestone AY, Abdoulaev G, Schmitz CH, Barbour RL, Hielscher AH. Three-dimensional optical tomography of hemodynamics in the human head. Opt Express 2001;9(6):272–286.

Bogdanov AA, Lin CP, Simonova M, Matuszewski L, Weissleder R. Cellular activation of the self-quenched fluorescent reporter probe in tumor microenvironment. Neoplasia 2002;4(3):228–236.

Bremer C, Tung CH, Weissleder R. *In vivo* molecular target assessment of matrix metalloproteinase inhibition. Nat Med 2001;7(6):743–748.

Brooksby B, Jiang SD, Dehghani H, Pogue BW, Paulsen KD, Kogel C, Doyley M, Weaver JB, Poplack SP. Magnetic resonance-guided near-infrared tomography of the breast. Rev Sci Instrum 2004;75(12):5262–5270.

Brooksby B, Pogue BW, Jiang SD, Dehghani H, Srinivasan S, Kogel C, Tosteson TD, Weaver J, Poplack SP, Paulsen KD. Imaging breast adipose and fibroglandular tissue molecular signatures by using hybrid MRI-guided near-infrared spectral tomography. Proc Natl Acad Sci U S A 2006;103(23):8828–8833.

Brooksby B, Srinivasan S, Jiang SD, Dehghani H, Pogue BW, Paulsen KD, Weaver J, Kogel C, Poplack SP. Spectral priors improve near-infrared diffuse tomography more than spatial priors. Opt Lett 2005;30(15):1968–1970.

Brown EB, Campbell RB, Tsuzuki Y, Xu L, Carmeliet P, Fukumura D, Jain RK. *In vivo* measurement of gene expression, angiogenesis and physiological function in tumors using multiphoton laser scanning microscopy (Erratum in: Nat Med 2001;7(9):1069). Nat Med 2001;7(7):864–868.

Bugaj JE, Achilefu S, Dorshow RB, Rajagopalan R. Novel fluorescent contrast agents for optical imaging of *in vivo* tumors based on a receptor-targeted dye-peptide conjugate platform. J Biomed Opt 2001;6(2):122–133.

Bullok K, Piwnica-Worms D. Synthesis and characterization of a small, membrane-permeant, caspase-activatable far-red fluorescent peptide for imaging apoptosis. J Med Chem 2005;48(17):5404–5407.

Chamberlain C, Hahn KM. Watching proteins in the wild: Fluorescence methods to study protein dynamics in living cells. Traffic 2000;1(10):755–762.

Chaudhari AJ, Darvas F, Bading JR, Moats RA, Conti PS, Smith DJ, Cherry SR, Leahy RM. Hyperspectral and multispectral bioluminescence optical tomography for small animal imaging. Phys Med Biol 2005;50(23):5421–5441.

Chen JQ, Tung CH, Allport JR, Chen S, Weissleder R, Huang PL. Near-infrared fluorescent imaging of matrix metalloproteinase activity after myocardial infarction. Circulation 2005;111(14):1800–1805.

Choe R, Corlu A, Lee K, Durduran T, Konecky SD, Grosicka-Koptyra M, Arridge SR, Czerniecki BJ, Fraker DL, DeMichele A, Chance B, Rosen MA, Yodh AG. Diffuse optical tomography of breast cancer during neoadjuvant chemotherapy: a case study with comparison to MRI. Med Phys 2005;32(4):1128–1139.

Contag CH, Bachmann MH. Advances *in vivo* bioluminescence imaging of gene expression. Annu Rev Biomed Eng 2002;4 235–260.

Corlu A, Choe R, Durduran T, Lee K, Schweiger M, Arridge SR, Hillman EMC, Yodh AG. Diffuse optical tomography with spectral constraints and wavelength optimization. Appl Opt 2005;44(11):2082–2093.

Corlu A, Durduran T, Choe R, Schweiger M, Hillman EMC, Arridge SR, Yodh AG. Uniqueness and wavelength optimization in continuous-wave multispectral diffuse optical tomography. Opt Lett 2003;28(23):2339–2341.

Deliolanis NC, Lasser T, Hyde D, Soubret A, Ripoll J, Ntziachristos V. Free-space fluorescence molecular tomography utilizing 360° geometry projections. Opt Lett 2007;32(4):382–384.

Dewhirst MW, Shan S, Cao YT, Moeller B, Yuan F, Li CY. Intravital fluorescence facilitates measurement of multiple physiologic functions and gene expression in tumors of live animals. Dis Markers 2002;18(5-6):293–311.

Dunn KW, Sandoval RM, Kelly KJ, Dagher PC, Tanner GA, Atkinson SJ, Bacallao RL, Molitoris BA. Functional studies of the kidney of living animals using multicolor two-photon microscopy. Am J Physiol-Cell Physiol 2002;283(3): C905–C916.

Funatsu T, Harada Y, Tokunaga M, Saito K, Yanagida T. Imaging of single fluorescent molecules and individual ATP turnovers by single myosin molecules in aqueous-solution. Nature 1995;374(6522):555–559.

Georgakoudi I, Muller MG, Feld MS. Intrinsic fluorescence spectroscopy of biological tissue. In: Mycek MA, Pogue B, editors. *Fluorescence in Biomedicine*. New York: Marcel Decker; 2002. pp. 109–142.

Germain RN, Castellino F, Chieppa MC, Egen JG, Huang AYC, Koo LY, Hai Q. An extended vision for dynamic high-resolution intravital immune imaging. Semin Immunol 2005;17(6):431–441.

Graves EE, Ripoll J, Weissleder R, Ntziachristos V. A submillimeter resolution fluorescence molecular imaging system for small animal imaging. Med Phys 2003;30(5): 901–911.

Griekspoor A, Zwart W, Neefjes J. Presenting antigen presentation in living cells using biophysical techniques. Curr Opin Microbiol 2005;8(3):338–343.

Gurfinkel M, Ke S, Wen XX, Li C, Sevick-Muraca EM. Near-infrared fluorescence optical imaging and tomography. Dis Markers 2003–2004;19(2–3):107–121.

Hell SW. Toward fluorescence nanoscopy. Nat Biotechnol 2003;21(11):1347–1355.

Hell SW, Wichmann J. Breaking the diffraction resolution limit by stimulated-emission-stimulated-emission-depletion fluorescence microscopy. Opt Lett 1994;19(11): 780–782.

Helmchen F, Denk W. Deep tissue two-photon microscopy (Erratum: 2006;3:235). Nat Methods 2005;2(12):932–940.

Hielscher AH. Optical tomographic imaging of small animals. Curr Opin Biotechnol 2005;16(1):79–88.

Hielscher AH, Bluestone AY, Abdoulaev GS, Klose AD, Lasker J, Stewart M, Netz U, Beuthan J. Near-infrared diffuse optical tomography. Dis Markers 2002;18(5-6): 313–337.

Hoffman RM. Green fluorescent protein imaging of tumour growth, metastasis, and angiogenesis in mouse models. Lancet Oncol 2002;3(9):546–556.

Ishimaru A. *Wave Propagation and Scattering in Random Media*. New York: IEEE Press; 1997.

Jain RK, Munn LL, Fukumura D. Dissecting tumour pathophysiology using intravital microscopy. Nat Rev Cancer 2002;2(4):266–276.

Jiang HB. Frequency-domain fluorescent diffusion tomography: a finite-element-based algorithm and simulations. Appl Opt 1998;37(22):5337–5343.

Kak AC, Slaney M. *Principles of Computerized Tomographic Imaging*. New York: IEEE Press; 1999.

Ke S, Wen XX, Gurfinkel M, Charnsangavej C, Wallace S, Sevick-Muraca EM, Li C. Near-infrared optical imaging of epidermal growth factor receptor in breast cancer xenografts. Cancer Res 2003;63(22):7870–7875.

Kirsch DG, Dinulescu DM, Miller JB, Grimm J, Santiago PM, Young NP, Nielsen GP, Quade BJ, Chaber CJ, Schultz CP, Takeuchi O, Bronson RT, Crowley D, Korsmeyer SJ, Yoon SS, Hornicek FJ, Weissleder R, Jacks T. A Spatially and temporally restricted mouse model of soft tissue sarcoma. Nat Med 2007;13(8):992–997.

Kleinfeld D, Mitra PP, Helmchen F, Denk W. Fluctuations and stimulus-induced changes in blood flow observed in individual capillaries in layers 2 through 4 of rat neocortex (Erratum: 1999;96:8307). Proc Natl Acad Sci U S A 1998;95(26):15741–15746.

Licha K, Becker A, Kratz F, Semmler W. New contrast agents for optical imaging: acid-cleavable conjugates of cyanine dyes with biomolecules. Proc SPIE 1999;3600 29–35.

Mahmood U, Tung CH, Bogdanov A, Weissleder R. Near-infrared optical imaging of protease activity for tumor detection. Radiology 1999;213(3):866–870.

Mahmood U, Weissleder R. Near-infrared optical imaging of proteases in cancer. Mol Cancer Ther 2003;2(5):489–496.

Majewska AK, Newton JR, Sur M. Remodeling of synaptic structure in sensory cortical areas *in vivo*. J Neurosci 2006;26(11):3021–3029.

Mansfield JR, Gossage KW, Hoyt CC, Levenson RM. Autofluorescence removal, multiplexing, and automated analysis methods for *in vivo* fluorescence imaging. J. Biomed Opt 2005;10, 041207.

Mashanov GI, Tacon D, Knight AE, Peckham M, Molloy JE. Visualizing single molecules inside living cells using total internal reflection fluorescence microscopy. Methods 2003;29(2):142–152.

McNally JG, Karpova T, Cooper J, Conchello JA. Three-dimensional imaging by deconvolution microscopy. Methods 1999;19(3):373–385.

Meyer H, Garofalakis A, Zacharakis G, Psycharakis S, Mamalaki C, Kioussis D, Economou EN, Ntziachristos V, Ripoll J. Non-contact optical imaging in mice with full angular coverage and automatic surface extraction. Applied Optics 2007;46(17):3617–3627.

Molitoris BA, Sandoval RM. Intravital multiphoton microscopy of dynamic renal processes. Am J Physiol Renal Physiol 2005;288(6): F1084–F1089.

Muller MG, Georgakoudi I, Zhang QG, Wu J, Feld MS. Intrinsic fluorescence spectroscopy in turbid media: disentangling effects of scattering and absorption. Appl Opt 2001;40(25):4633–4646.

Nakatsu T, Ichiyama S, Hiratake J, Saldanha A, Kobashi N, Sakata K, Kato H. Structural basis for the spectral difference in luciferase bioluminescence. Nature 2006;440(7082):372–376.

Norman K. Techniques: intravital microscopy-a method for investigating disseminated intravascular coagulation? Trends Pharmacol Sci 2005;26(6):327–332.

Ntziachristos V. Fluorescence molecular imaging. Annu Rev Biomed Eng 2006;8:1–33.

Ntziachristos V, Schellenberger EA, Ripoll J, Yessayan D, Graves E, Bogdanov A, Josephson L, Weissleder R. Visualization of antitumor treatment by means of fluorescence molecular tomography with an annexin V-Cy5.5 conjugate. Proc Natl Acad Sci U S A 2004;101(33):12294–12299.

Ntziachristos V, Tung CH, Bremer C, Weissleder R. Fluorescence molecular tomography resolves protease activity *in vivo*. Nat Med 2002a;8(7):756–760.

Ntziachristos V, Weissleder R. Charge-coupled-device based scanner for tomography of fluorescent near-infrared probes in turbid media. Med Phys 2002b;29(5):803–809.

Ntziachristos V, Turner G, Dunham J, Windsor S, Soubret A, Ripoll J, Shih HA. Planar fluorescence imaging using normalized data. J. Biomed Opt 2005;10, 064007.

Ntziachristos V, Weissleder R. Experimental three-dimensional fluorescence reconstruction of diffuse media by use of a normalized Born approximation. Opt Lett 2001;26(12):893–895.

O'Leary MA, Boas DA, Li XD, Chance B, Yodh AG. Fluorescence lifetime imaging in turbid media. Opt Lett 1996;21(2):158–160.

Paithankar DY, Chen AU, Pogue BW, Patterson MS, SevickMuraca EM. Imaging of fluorescent yield and lifetime from multiply scattered light reemitted from random media. Appl Opt 1997;36(10):2260–2272.

Paris S, Sesboue R. Metastasis models: the green fluorescent revolution? Carcinogenesis 2004;25(12):2285–2292.

Patwardhan SV, Bloch SR, Achilefu S, Culver JP. Time-dependent whole-body fluorescence tomography of probe bio-distributions in mice. Opt Express 2005;13(7): 2564–2577.

Pfleger KDG, Eidne KA. Illuminating insights into protein-protein interactions using bioluminescence resonance energy transfer (BRET). Nat Methods 2006;3(3):165–174.

van Roessel P, Brand AH. Imaging into the future: visualizing gene expression and protein interactions with fluorescent proteins. Nat Cell Biol 2002;4(1): E15–E20.

Runnels JM, Zamiri P, Spencer JA, Veilleux I, Wei XB, Bogdanov A, Lin CP. Imaging molecular expression on vascular endothelial cells by *in vivo* immunofluorescence microscopy. Mol Imaging 2006;5(1):31–40.

Rust MJ, Bates M, Zhuang XW. Sub-diffraction-limit imaging by stochastic optical reconstruction microscopy (STORM). Nat Methods 2006;3(10):793–795.

Schulz RB, Peter J, Semmler W, D'Andrea C, Valentini G, Cubeddu R. Comparison of noncontact and fiber-based fluorescence-mediated tomography. Opt Lett 2006;31(6): 769–771.

Schulz RB, Ripoll J, Ntziachristos V. Experimental fluorescence tomography of tissues with noncontact measurements. IEEE Trans Med Imaging 2004;23(4):492–500.

Shah K, Jacobs A, Breakefield XO, Weissleder R. Molecular imaging of gene therapy for cancer. Gene Ther 2004;11(15):1175–1187.

Shaner NC, Campbell RE, Steinbach PA, Giepmans BNG, Palmer AE, Tsien RY. Improved monomeric red, orange and yellow fluorescent proteins derived from Discosoma sp red fluorescent protein. Nat Biotechnol 2004;22(12):1567–1572.

Shapiro E, Lu C, Baneyx F. A set of multicolored Photinus pyralis luciferase mutants for *in vivo* bioluminescence applications. Protein Eng Des Sel 2005;18(12):581–587.

Sipkins DA, Wei XB, Wu JW, Runnels JM, Cote D, Means TK, Luster AD, Scadden DT, Lin CP. *In vivo* imaging of specialized bone marrow endothelial microdomains for tumour engraftment. Nature 2005;435(7044):969–973.

Soubret A, Ripoll J, Ntziachristos V. Accuracy of fluorescent tomography in the presence of heterogeneities: study of the normalized born ratio. IEEE Trans Med Imaging 2005;24(10):1377–1386.

Srinivasan S, Pogue BW, Dehghani H, Leblond F, Intes X. Data subset algorithm for computationally efficient reconstruction of 3-D spectral imaging in diffuse optical tomography. Opt Express 2006;14(12):5394–5410.

Thorne SH, Contag CH. Using *in vivo* bioluminescence imaging to shed light on cancer biology. Proc IEEE 2005;93(4):750–762.

Troy T, Jekic-McMullen D, Sambucetti L, Rice B. Quantitative comparison of the sensitivity of detection of fluorescent and bioluminescent reporters in animal models. Mol Imaging 2004;3(1):9–23.

Tsien RY. Building and breeding molecules to spy on cells and tumors. FEBS Lett 2005;579(4):927–932.

Turchin IV, Balalaeva IV, Vasil'ev RB, Zlomanov V, Plehanol V, Orlova AG, Zagaynova EV, Kamensky VA, Kleshnin MS, Shirmanova MV, Dorofeev SG, Dirin DM. Imaging of QDs-labeled tumors in small animals by fluorescence diffuse tomography. Laser Phys Lett 2006;3(4):208–211.

Voura EB, Jaiswal JK, Mattoussi H, Simon SM. Tracking metastatic tumor cell extravasation with quantum dot nanocrystals and fluorescence emission-scanning microscopy. Nat Med 2004;10(9):993–998.

Wang WG, Wyckoff JB, Frohlich VC, Oleynikov Y, Huttelmaier S, Zavadil J, Cermak L, Bottinger EP, Singer RH, White JG, Segall JE, Condeelis JS. Single cell behavior in metastatic primary mammary tumors correlated with gene expression patterns revealed by molecular profiling (Erratum in: Cancer Res 2002;62(23):7132). Cancer Res 2002;62(21):6278–6288.

Weissleder R, Tung CH, Mahmood U, Bogdanov A. *In vivo* imaging of tumors with protease-activated near-infrared fluorescent probes. Nat Biotechnol 1999;17(4): 375–378.

Willig KI, Kellner RR, Medda R, Hein B, Jakobs S, Hell SW. Nanoscale resolution in GFP-based microscopy. Nat Methods 2006;3(9):721–723.

Wobus AM, Boheler KR. Embryonic stem cells: Prospects for developmental biology and cell therapy. Physiol Rev 2005;85(2):635–678.

Wunder A, Tung CH, Muller-Ladner U, Weissleder R, Mahmood U. *In vivo* imaging of protease activity in arthritis-A novel approach for monitoring treatment response. Arthritis Rheumatism 2004;50(8):2459–2465.

Xu Y, Iftimia N, Jiang HB, Key LL, Bolster MB. Imaging of in vitro and in vivo bones and joints with continuous-wave diffuse optical tomography. Opt Express 2001;8(7):447–451.

Xu H, Pogue BW, Dehghani H, Paulsen KD, Springett R, Dunn JF. Absorption and scattering imaging of tissue with steady-state second-differential spectral-analysis tomography. Opt Lett 2004;29(17):2043–2045.

Yaksi E, Friedrich RW. Reconstruction of firing rate changes across neuronal populations by temporally deconvolved Ca2+ imaging. Nat Methods 2006;3(5):377–383.

Zacharakis G, Kambara H, Shih H, Ripoll J, Grimm J, Saeki Y, Weissleder R, Ntziachristos V. Volumetric tomography of fluorescent proteins through small animals *in vivo*. Proc Natl Acad Sci U S A 2005;102(51):18252–18257.

Zacharakis G, Shih H, Ripoll J, Weissleder R, Ntziachristos V. Normalized transillumination of fluorescent proteins in small animals. Mol Imaging 2006;5(3):153–159.

Zaheer A, Lenkinski RE, Mahmood A, Jones AG, Cantley LC, Frangioni JV. *In vivo* near-infrared fluorescence imaging of osteoblastic activity. Nat Biotechnol 2001; 19(12):1148–1154.

Zernike F. Phase contrast, a new method for the microscopic observation of transparent objects Part II. Physica 1942a;9:974–986.

Zernike F. Phase contrast, a new method for the microsopic observation of transparent objects. Physica 1942b;9:686–698.

Zimmermann T, Rietdorf J, Pepperkok R. Spectral imaging and its applications in live cell microscopy. FEBS Lett 2003;546(1):87–92.

Zipfel WR, Williams RM, Webb WW. Nonlinear magic: multiphoton microscopy in the biosciences. Nat Biotechnol 2003;21(11):1368–1376.

9

INFRARED AND RAMAN SPECTROSCOPIC IMAGING

Gerald Steiner
Clinical Sensoring and Monitoring, Faculty of Medicine Carl Gustav Carus, Dresden University of Technology, Dresden, Germany.

9.1 INTRODUCTION

Infrared and Raman spectroscopic imaging are relatively new techniques that reveal the biochemical composition of cells, tissue, and even organs. Advances in instrumentation have made these imaging modalities a tool of choice for an increasing number of medical applications. The greatest benefit of these techniques lies in their high molecular sensitivity combined with a spatial resolution of less than 1 μm. Another advantage is their ability to probe samples under *in situ* conditions, which allows new insights into living cells without the need for fixation, stains, or markers.

Both infrared and Raman spectroscopy probe vibrations of the atoms within a molecule; hence, infrared and Raman spectra are summarized as vibrational spectra. The infrared spectral region is divided into three subregions, the sort-wavelength Near-Infrared (NIR) region, the Mid-Infrared (MIR or simply IR) region, and the Far-Infrared (FIR) region. The last region recently attracted some interest under the new name terahertz (THz) region. By far, the most important region is the IR region. NIR spectroscopy has also become an interesting tool in clinical medicine. NIR spectra result from overtones and combinations of fundamental vibrations occurring in the IR spectral range. Raman spectra of biomolecules are usually excited in the visible or the NIR spectral regions. The following chapter describes the new imaging techniques based on vibrational

Biomedical Imaging: Principles and Applications, First Edition. Edited by Reiner Salzer.

spectroscopy that have a clear potential in medical diagnostic when rapid and objective detection of complex samples is required.

Vibrational spectroscopy is commonly used to obtain the molecular fingerprint of the sample under investigation. IR and Raman spectroscopy are complementary, whereby IR spectroscopy is more sensitive to vibrations of polar species and Raman spectroscopy is more sensitive to vibrations of nonpolar species. Molecular details are obtained by monitoring spectral frequencies, intensities, and bandwidth parameters of spectral bands. All three parameters together reflect a sample's molecular structure like a fingerprint. Raman spectroscopy has two advantages over IR spectroscopy for the analysis of biological samples: it is less sensitive to water that is present in tissue, and no sample preparation is necessary. On the other hand, Raman spectroscopy needs a laser, which can destroy the tissue. Moreover, the measurement time is often longer than in IR spectroscopy. In addition, IR spectroscopy provides quantitative information from the application of Beer's law. Both IR and Raman spectroscopy exhibit very high sensitivity toward molecular structure and permit the acquisition of spectra from samples as small as 10 pg.

IR as well as Raman spectroscopy is used to investigate living systems since the late 1980s. A milestone in the application to biological samples was the development of high sensitive array detectors with a large number of small detector elements. Each detector element is capable of simultaneously collecting data and recording a two-dimensional spectroscopic image. The resulting image is recorded at a spatial resolution that is diffraction limited. This allows the characterization of objects as small as a fraction of single cells to monitor processes in cells and to reveal information about distribution of cellular components. Thus, spectroscopic images show a distribution of chemical information and give the chances of identifying molecular indicators of pathological processes and diseases. IR and Raman imaging are highly complementary. Both permit a more complete examination of the tissue in question and contribute substantially to an objective histopathological diagnosis of tissue sections. The high spatial resolution in combination with the high degree of biochemical information provides an exceptional capability of performing *in situ* tissue diagnosis. One of the most promising applications is the use for guidance during surgical intervention and treatment.

Each molecule has its own characteristic IR and Raman spectrum. The IR spectrum, for example, from brain tissue, contains information from all molecules in the investigated sample (Fig. 9.1). All observed absorption bands can be assigned to groups of biochemical compounds. Some of the most prominent bands are labeled in Figure 9.1. From the spectral position and intensity of the characteristic absorption bands, it is possible to identify the class of biochemical species, their abundance, and how they are related to other molecules. Because of different intensities, some vibrational bands are better seen in IR spectra, others in Raman spectra. A short overview about the most important characteristic IR absorption bands of biomolecules is given in Table 9.1. Important Raman bands are summarized in Table 9.2.

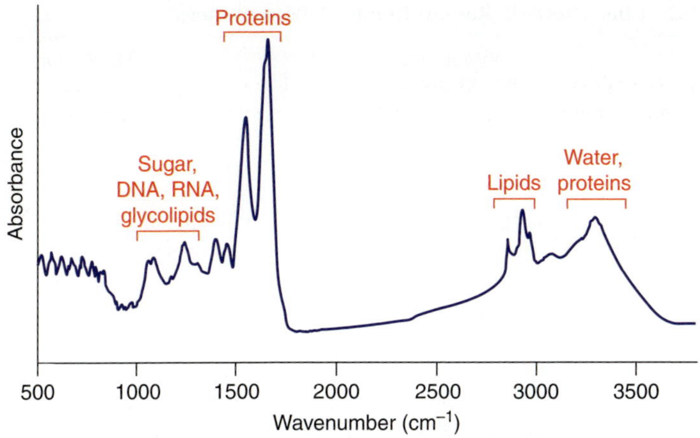

Figure 9.1. Typical IR transmission spectrum of a thin section prepared from extirpated human brain tumor tissue. The most prominent absorption bands arise from proteins. Other strong bands are related to carbohydrates and nuclei acids. Lipids appear relatively weak in the IR spectrum.

TABLE 9.1. Characteristic IR Absorption Bands of Biomolecules[a]

Spectral Range (cm^{-1})	Vibrational Mode	Molecular Origin
1090–1080	$\nu(PO_2)$, ν(C—O)	RNA, DNA
1120–1160	ν(C—O)	RNA, DNA, carbohydrates
1200–1245	ν(P—O)	RNA, DNA
1235–1260	ν(P=O)	Lipids, phosphate esters
1330–1200	Amide III	Proteins
1420–1440	$\delta(CH_2)$	Lipids
1550–1530	δ(N—H) amide II	Proteins
1610	ν(C=C)	DNA, RNA
1640	δ(OH)	Water
1700–1620	ν(C=O) amide I	Proteins
1760–1720	ν(C=O)	Lipids, amino acids, carboxyl acids
3000–2800	$\nu(CH_2, CH_3)$	Lipids
3800–3200	ν(O—H)	Water

[a] ν indicates stretching vibrations, δ indicates deformation vibrations.

Two technical approaches are employed to obtain IR and Raman spectroscopic images: mapping with a single detector and imaging with a multielement (so-called Focal-Plane Array (FPA)) detector.

Mapping is a point-by-point rastering across a sample. This single-detector-based technique uses an aperture window, which determines the spatial resolution. It is an inherently slow method.

TABLE 9.2. Characteristic Raman Bands of Biomolecules[a]

Spectral Range (cm^{-1})	Vibrational Mode	Molecular Origin
540	S—S	Disulfide bridges
853–870	ν(C—C) ring breathing, ν(O—P—O)	Proteins, tyrosine, DNA
935–975	ν(C—C), α-helix	Proteins, glycogen
1080–1100	ν(C—C), $\nu(PO_2)$, ν (C—O)	Lipids, nucleic acids, proteins, carbohydrates
1300–1310	$\delta(CH_2)$, $\delta(CH_3CH_2)$	Adenine, cytosine, collagen, lipids
1445	$\delta(CH_2)$	Lipids carbohydrates, proteins
1746	ν(C=O)	Lipids
1640–1660	ν(C=O) of 0061 mide I, α-helix	Proteins
2020–2090	ν(C≡C)	Lipids, fatty acids, hormones

[a] ν indicates stretching vibrations, δ indicates deformation vibrations

Imaging is based on array detectors, which enable the simultaneous collection of all spectra across the image. Imaging is faster than mapping.

The mapping technique is preferred in Raman spectroscopy. Imaging is more frequently used in IR spectroscopy.

Different types of detectors are used in Raman mapping and IR spectroscopic imaging. Raman spectroscopy and Raman mapping are often used in the visible and NIR spectral range so that high sensitive Si charge-coupled-device (Si-CCD) detectors are used. IR FPA detectors are fabricated from material that is sensitive in the spectral range from approximately 1 to 10 μm (10.000–1.000 cm^{-1}). These IR FPAs, originally developed for military applications, have become available for research and civic applications in the 1990s. Today, there are several types of FPA detectors available. For spectroscopic measurement in the NIR range, indium antimonite (InSb) FPA detectors with typically 128×128 up to 512×512 elements are available. Mercury Cadmium Telluride (MCT) FPA detectors are used for IR imaging and range from 64×64 up to 512×512 elements. Other types such as lead-salt-based array detectors and bolometers are used in spectroscopic imaging as well but are currently of less importance in medical imaging. Table 9.3 summarizes array detectors that are used in IR spectroscopic imaging.

9.2 INSTRUMENTATION

9.2.1 Infrared Imaging

An infrared imaging instrument consists of an FPA detector coupled to a common IR spectrometer. A microspectroscopic imaging instrument in addition needs an IR microscope attached to the spectrometer. Most imaging spectrometers use a Michelson-type interferometer. The FPA collects the data

TABLE 9.3. Array Detectors Used In Ir Spectroscopic Imaging

Detector Material	D* (cm Hz$^{1/2}$ W^{-1})[a]	Typical Array Dimensions (pixels)	Operating Temperature	Wavelength Range (μm)
InSb	1×10^{11}	128 × 128, 256 × 256, 512 × 512	<80 K	0.4–5
HgCdTe (MCT)	1×10^{11}	64 × 64, 128 × 128, 256 × 256	<80 K	2–10
PbS, PbSe	$8 \times 10^9 - 6 \times 10^{10}$	1 × 256, 1 × 512	Room temperature	0.4–4
GaAlAs (quantum well)	2×10^9	640 × 512	<70 K	2–12
Microbolometer	10^9	320 × 240	Room temperature	7–20

[a]The symbol D* is a quality feature of the detector called *detectivity*, which is equal to the reciprocal of the noise equivalent power, normalized to unit area and unit bandwidth.

once the moving mirror in the interferometers stops. After the data from all FPA elements are read out, the mirror is advanced to the next position. Step by step, the interferogram is built up for the detector array; hence, the method is called *step scan*. In the case of the more recent continuous-scan interferometers, the mirror movement does not stop. The FPA rate of data acquisition and readout is now sufficiently high, and stops of the mirror movement are not required.

The general configuration of an IR imaging instrument is shown in Figure 9.2. Most IR imaging instruments today provide measurements both in the micro and macro modes.

The beam path in the microscope for the often preferred transmission mode is sketched in Figure 9.2a. The infrared light passes the interferometer, where it is spectrally encoded. The infrared light is then guided through the microscope, passes the sample on the *xy* stage, and is finally collected by the FPA detector. Visible light can be coupled to the IR beam path in order to observe the sample area visually. In modern instruments, the IR and visible lights are separated by dichromatic mirrors, which ensure that exactly the same sample area is observed by the visible light and by the FPA detector. Samples that are not transparent in the IR spectral range have to be investigated in the reflection mode (Fig. 9.2b). In this case, substrates with reflectivity have to be used in order to ensure a high intensity of the reflected IR light. Using a typical Cassegrainian objective with an aperture of 0.4, the image size captured by a single shot with a 64 × 64 FPA is 270 × 270 μm, both in transmission and reflection modes. Larger sample areas can be investigated in the so-called macrochamber (Fig. 9.2c). If the same FPA array is used as before, the sample size captured in one shot is approximately 4 × 4 mm, and the spatial resolution is approximately 65 μm.

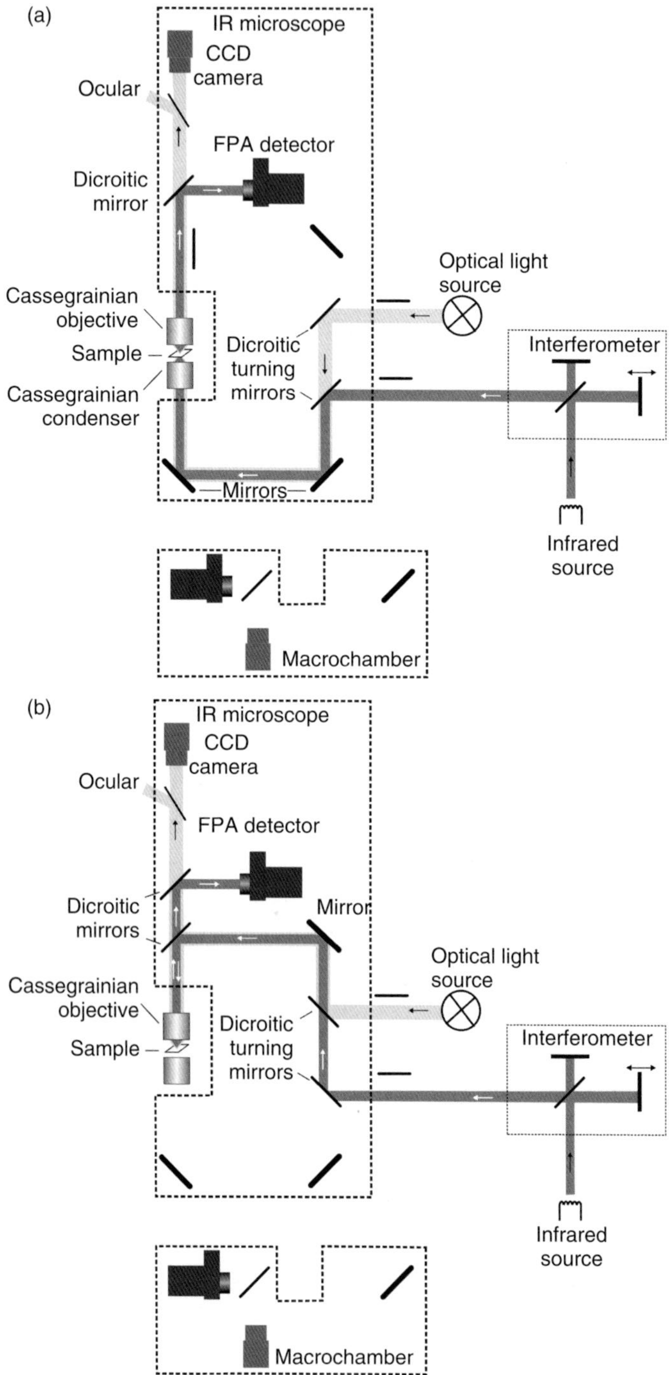

Figure 9.2. Optical diagram of an IR imaging instrument showing the path from the source via the interferometer to microscope. (a) Microscopic transmission mode, (b) microscopic reflection mode, and (c) transmission macromode. The visible optical light is used to control the sample position either by a CCD camera or by an ocular camera.

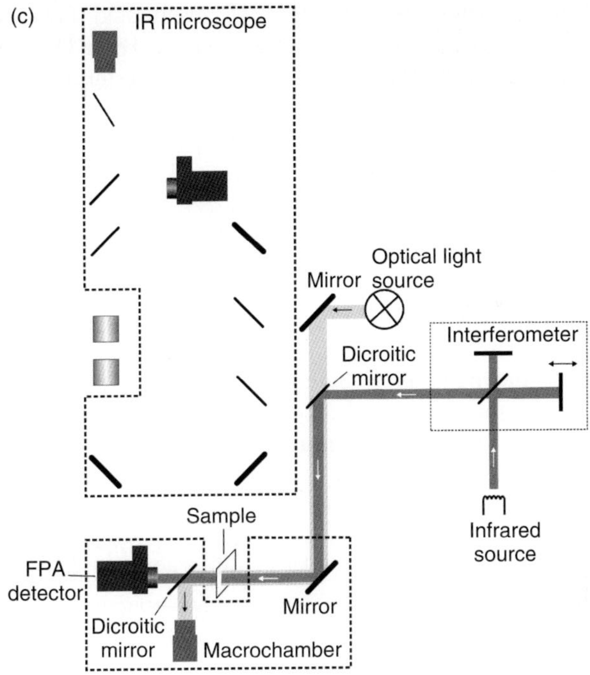

Figure 9.2. (*Continued*)

9.2.2 Near-Infrared Imaging

NIR spectroscopy is accomplished by measuring light between 700 and 2500 nm wavelength of the electromagnetic spectrum. The interaction of NIR light with cells and tissue is governed by both absorption and scattering processes. Absorption of light is similar to IR imaging, but in the NIR imaging, it is based on overtone and combination of O—H, N—H, and C—H vibrations and to some extent of C=O vibrations. Scattering of light is dictated by the morphology of the tissue such as size and shape of cells or particles as well as boundaries and interfaces between several types of tissue. Compared to IR and Raman spectra, NIR spectra have the highest signal to noise ratio for spectra recorded in equal time.

Among the optical spectroscopic methods, NIR spectroscopy usually provides the highest penetration depth into tissue. The penetration of NIR light is mainly limited by scattering and by absorption of water. The presence of some characteristic biomolecules may already be evident from the raw spectra. Chemometric approaches allow a more detailed evaluation and/or quantitative analysis. Technological developments in data communication in the early 1990s have driven NIR spectroscopic applications to noninvasive or minimally invasive medical diagnosis. In recent years, NIR spectroscopy has become a powerful tool in a number of different ways. NIR spectroscopy has been used in lipid analysis to determine saturation of unsaturated fatty acid esters, to examine lipids *in vitro* and *in vivo*, and to analyze High Density Lipoprotein (HDL), Low Density Lipoprotein (LDL), and cholesterol in blood vessels. Analytes include glucose, lactate, proteins, hemoglobin, and deoxyhemoglobin in blood. The large-format NIR FPA detectors (1024 × 1024 pixels) provide high image fidelity for small and large samples. NIR spectroscopic imaging can be performed in transmission and reflection modes. Most commercially available NIR spectral imaging systems are spectrally extended IR imaging systems.

9.3 RAMAN IMAGING

Raman spectroscopic imaging is based on conventional Raman spectroscopy, similar IR spectroscopic imaging. Raman scattering is excited by a laser. Sometimes the laser light is coupled into an optical fiber in order to illuminate the sample conveniently. Raman scattering from the sample is collected by an objective. Figure 9.3 illustrates the so-called 180° geometry, as the angle at the sample between the incoming and the excited light is 180°. Alternative geometries are 90° and 0°. Rayleigh scattering, excited together with Raman scattering, has a much higher intensity than Raman scattering but contains no chemical information; hence, it is blocked by a holographic filter. The radiation that passes the holographic filter is spectrally analyzed either by a monochromator or by a polychromator (Fig. 9.3a). Typical excitation wavelengths range from the green (532 nm) to the NIR (830 nm) region, so that the Raman spectrum can finally be measured by a Si detector (single detector or CCD array). Fluorescence, which occurs in nearly all biological samples, can be a problem when green light is used for illumination. For this reason, biological samples are often excited by NIR radiation, where usually much less fluorescence is observed. Unfortunately, detector sensitivities are mostly distinctly lower in the NIR region.

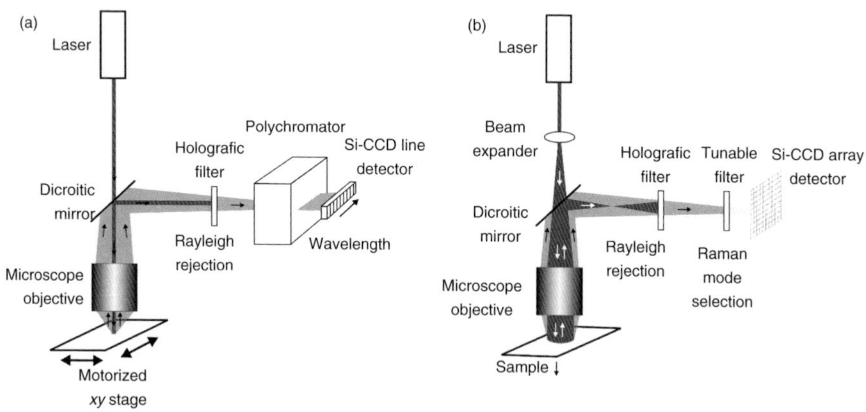

Figure 9.3. Schematic diagram of (a) a Raman mapping instrument and (b) a Raman imaging instrument.

The common technique to measure Raman images is the mapping technique (Section 9.1). Point mapping is the sequential registration of a series of single Raman spectra at different positions of the sample, followed by the reconstruction of the spectroscopic map (Fig. 9.3a). The achievable spatial resolution depends on both the accuracy of the motorized *xy* stage and on the optical resolution of the Raman microscope. The "true" Raman imaging technique is similar to the IR spectroscopic imaging technique, where the spectroscopic image is captured with an array detector. The optical layout of a Raman imaging device is depicted in Figure 9.3b. The illuminated area on the surface determines the measured sample size and the intensity of the Raman signals. The size of the illuminated area can be adjusted by using a beam expander. The figure of merit of tunable filters improved in recent years; hence, this technique gains in practical importance.

Raman microscope turrets incorporate 5×, 20×, and 50× objectives, which can be employed to give sampled areas from 40 × 40 μm to 480 × 480 μm. A spatial resolution below 1 μm can be achieved. Raman images are often measured with confocal optics so that a particular depth of the sample can be chosen, from which the image is measured. Table 9.4 summarizes important parameters of NIR and IR as well as of Raman imaging spectrometers.

9.4 SAMPLING TECHNIQUES

Appropriate sample preparation is essential and often has to be chosen as a compromise between the different requirements of sample, the method, and the aim of the investigation. Generally, each sample preparation technique is intended for use with specific types of cells and tissue and has its own strengths and weaknesses. The first step is to select the spectroscopic imaging method.

Several sampling techniques are available for NIR and IR spectroscopic imaging. Water exhibits very intense, broad absorption bands in its NIR and IR spectrum. These strong bands overlay the relatively weak absorption bands of cells. Layers of single cells, thin films, and tissue sections up to a thickness of 50 μm on IR transparent substrates can be imaged. These samples can also be investigated in the reflection mode when the sample is placed on a substrate surface of high reflectivity (e.g., gold). In this case, the optical path through the sample is twice as long as in the transmission technique (back and forth). This leads to higher sensitivity for weak absorbing samples but to nonlinearity in absorbance for strong absorbing samples. The reflection technique is used for thicker samples (thickness over 50 μm). Attenuated Total Reflection (ATR) imaging has a potential for thick samples without any sample preparation. ATR imaging spectroscopy requires a special accessory that either mounts in the sample compartment of the spectrometer or equips with the microscope. The heart of an ATR system is an IR transparent optical crystal. A schematic diagram of an ATR accessory is shown in Figure 9.4.

A typical ATR crystal has the form of an inverted prism (Fig. 9.4). On reflection of the IR light at the prism surface an evanescent field is generated. A sample

TABLE 9.4. Characteristics of NIR, IR, and Raman Spectroscopic Imaging Instruments

Description	NIR, IR Imaging	Raman Imaging
Detector	FPA MCT 64 × 64; 128 × 128 pixel	Si-based CCD line, Si-based CCD array,Ge, InGaAs
Detector sensitivity	Excellent	Si-CCD is detector of choice; Ge, InGaAs are poor
Operating modes	Transmission, reflection, total reflection, optical fibers (NIR)	Reflection
Extended experimental conditions	Microscopes, transmission, reflection and ATR accessory, optical fibers (NIR)	Microscopes, optical fibers, microprobes
Sample preparation	Cells, not required or minimal; tissue, thin tissue sections for transmission, not required for reflection and ATR modes	Tissue and cells, not required or minimal
Effects on the sample	Nondestructive harmless	Usually nondestructive, laser radiation can heat the sample
Sensitive against	Polar groups	Nonpolar groups
Sensitivity	High (<0.01 wt%) for IR, moderate (1 wt%) for NIR	Moderate (0.1–1 wt%) for cells and tissue
Noise limitation	Detector noise limited	Signal shot noise limited
Biofluids	In IR difficult, strong absorption of water, NIR possible	No problem
Solid samples	No problem	No problem except dark samples (intense thermal emission possible)
Good for	Tissue sections, single cells	Thick native tissue samples, tissue sections, single cells
Typical applications	*Ex vivo* (IR), *in vivo* (NIR)	*In vivo*
Spatial resolution	5–10 μm (IR), 2–5 μm (NIR)	<1 μm
Spectral range	4 000–900 cm^{-1} (IR), 10,000–4 000 cm^{-1} (NIR)	4 000–100 cm^{-1}
Spectral resolution	Typically 4–8 cm^{-1}, up to 2 cm^{-1}	
Fluorescence	No problem	Fluorescence may occur upon excitation by visible radiation, good suppression for NIR excitation wavelengths
Illumination, excitation	IR source (globar, halogen lamp)	Diode lasers, Nd-YAG laser, gas lasers
Costs for instrumentation	>$200,000	>$150,000

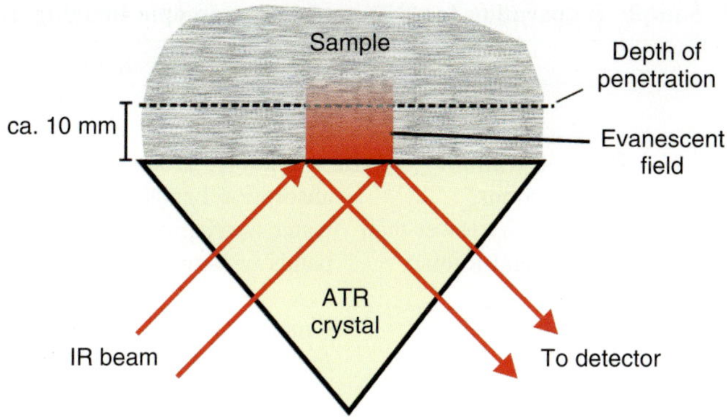

Figure 9.4. Illustration of the IR ATR technique.

brought in contact with the crystal can interact with the evanescent field. The penetration depth of the evanescent wave is dependent on the refractive indexes of the prism and the sample, the wavelength of the IR light, and the angle of incidence. IR ATR spectroscopic imaging has two important advantages: the sample can be kept under native conditions, and the lateral resolution is improved, because of the high refractive index of the prism. Even hard samples such as bone can be investigated when the sample is pressed onto the crystal. With the improved lateral resolution, individual cells can be imaged by ATR. Although the ATR technique is versatile in the types of samples that can be characterized, a large problem is the contact between the sample and the prism. Often it is difficult to achieve good optical contact. Another problem in terms of native tissue is a liquid film that develops between the tissue and the prism. The thickness of this aqueous film may be minimized by applying a tolerable force while maintaining the native condition of the tissue.

Raman spectroscopy usually does not require sample preparation. It might be preferred when a thick or very wet sample is to be imaged. IR spectroscopy usually requires sample preparation. Solid samples—for example, tissue and thin sections—are usually investigated by the 180° collection geometry, whereas the 90° collection geometry is often used for liquid samples. Raman imaging with a confocal microscope allows deep-resolved spectroscopic information of solid samples with a depth resolution of 2 μm and a lateral resolution of less than 1 μm. Table 9.5 summarizes different sampling techniques.

9.5 DATA ANALYSIS AND IMAGE EVALUATION

A common feature of most biological samples is the small spectral variance between the objects. In order to display such small variances in a spectral image and to render the underlying molecular information, techniques for data and image evaluation have to be used (Chapter 1, (1)). Chemometric imaging is the

TABLE 9.5. Sample Preparation for Different Spectroscopic Imaging Techniques

	Spectroscopic Imaging Technique		
Sample	NIR	IR	Raman
Native tissue, *in vivo*	Possible with no restrictions, sensitivity lower than in IR and Raman	Less suitable, strong absorption bands of water overlap many bands of biomolecules	Suitable with restrictions, laser can heat or burn the tissue, precise focusing required
Native tissue, *ex vivo*	See native tissue *in vivo*	See native tissue *in vivo*, ATR imaging also possible	See native tissue *in vivo*
Single living cells, *in vivo*	NIR not suitable	IR not suitable	Raman suitable, laser can heat or burn cells
Single living cells, *ex vivo*	NIR not recommended, low sensitivity	ATR possible when cells are adherent on optical crystal surface	Raman well suitable
Single cells (dried), *ex vivo*	NIR not recommended, low sensitivity	IR well suitable	Raman suitable, precise focusing required
Thin tissue section	NIR not recommended, low sensitivity	IR well suitable	Raman suitable, precise focusing required
Soft tissue blocks	NIR suitable, transmission or reflection mode	ATR or external reflection suitable	Raman well suitable
Hard tissue blocks	Reflection mode suitable	ATR or external reflection mode suitable	Raman well suitable, when focus adjusted to the surface
Hemodynamic and other dynamic processes, *in vivo*	NIR suitable	IR not suitable	Raman not suitable

term that encompasses a wide range of mathematical techniques for classifying data, pattern recognition, and generating false color images. In general, data and image evaluation is a multistage process. A long list of different methods or of combinations of different methods can be compiled. The best strategy for data and image evaluation is dependent on a variety of different factors, for example, on the sample, the experimental and environmental conditions, and the information required. Four main steps can be discerned between raw spectra and medical diagnosis.

1. Data preprocessing
2. Feature selection

3. Spectral classification
4. Image processing including pattern recognition

9.5.1 Data Preprocessing

Raw spectra obtained from a spectroscopic imaging system are subject to variations in sensitivity and linearity between detectors or between individual elements of array detectors. In addition, various physical properties of the sample, experimental conditions, and the environment itself may have an impact on the raw data. Data preprocessing aims at the removal such influences, which may even obscure the desirable information from the sample. Data preprocessing is therefore crucial for obtaining "correct" spectra. Moreover, data preprocessing can also help to reduce the large number of less important spectral features. This should make the covered information more accessible, but information from the sample may easily be removed together with the unwanted variations.

There is a long list of mathematical correction methods that can be applied to spectroscopic data. The strategy for preprocessing is strongly dependent on the quality of the data set. Few general points should be highlighted:

(i) Offset correction is generally recommended since physical properties of the sample and influences from the experimental conditions will be removed.
(ii) Smoothing, often used in conventional (nonimaging) spectroscopy to reduce the noise level, is not recommended in imaging spectroscopy. The noise signal has statistical character. Owing to a larger number of spectra in imaging data sets, the noise can be isolated from the chemical information by using statistical methods.
(iii) Changes in sample thickness lead to different intensities of absorption bands in IR spectroscopy, which should be compensated by normalization. In Raman spectroscopy, normalization eliminates variances in physical properties (e.g., different density of cells) within the sample or in experimental conditions (e.g., laser power) that are often much higher than different spectral features of complex biological samples.

Whenever preprocessing is performed, it is absolutely important to understand the features appearing in the spectra and to know how the mathematical methods affect spectroscopic data. Steady evaluation of the results of the preprocessing steps is strongly recommended.

9.5.2 Feature Selection

Detailed information about different methods for classification and pattern recognition are given in Chapter 1. This section summarizes important techniques of chemometric imaging, which are often used in IR and Raman biospectroscopy.

The fundamental function of feature selection is to find a set of features that will represent the wanted molecular information in a most optimal way at high specificity. Information that is either redundant or irrelevant to the following classification task is removed from the data set. When performing analysis of complex data, one of the major problems is based on the number of variables involved. The dimension of the selected spectral feature is usually much smaller than the dimension of the origin data set so that the computation time and the memory requirements are greatly reduced. Feature selection can also be used as a tool to test the discriminatory potential of the chosen features. Finally, feature selection can also be used to reduce the noise level. Common approaches for feature selection involve Principal Components Analysis (PCA) (2), Partial Least Squares (PLS) analysis (3), and wavelets (4, 5).

PCA is a mathematical transformation, which transforms spectral data to a new coordinate system such that the greatest variance by any projection of the data comes to lie on the first coordinate, which is called the *first principal component*, the second greatest variance on the second coordinate, and so on. Retaining those characteristics of the spectra that contribute most to its variance by keeping the corresponding principal components reduces the dimension of the data set. Usually, lower order principal components contain the most important aspects, whereas higher order ones represent the basic characteristics.

PLS calculates a linear model describing some predicted variables in terms of other observable variables. It is often used to find the fundamental relationships between two matrices (e.g., spectral regions X and Y). A PLS model will try to find the multidimensional direction in one spectral region that explains the maximum multidimensional variance direction in the Y direction, which leads to a reduction of the data set

Wavelets and wavelet transformation represent a set of spectra in terms of a fast decaying oscillating waveform. This waveform is scaled and translated to match the original spectrum. Wavelet transformation is related to the subject of harmonic analysis. The projection of a spectrum on a single wavelet or of a series of wavelets reduces the dimension of the data set. Wavelet transforms are broadly divided into three classes, the continuous wavelet transform, the discrete wavelet transform, and multiresolution-based wavelet transforms. In the continuous wavelet transform, every frequency band is considered. By integration over all obtained frequency components one can reconstruct the original spectrum. In the discredited wavelet transform, a discrete subset of wavelets is used to reconstruct a signal from the corresponding wavelet coefficients. The advantage is reduced computing time. The multiresolution-based wavelet considers only a finite number of wavelet coefficients. This avoids numerical complexity and further speeds up the computation.

9.5.3 Spectral Classification

Spectral classification is a procedure in which individual spectra are placed into groups based on quantitative spectral information. The algorithms can be subdivided into supervised and unsupervised classification. Supervised classification is based on a training set of spectra of known assignment, for example, tumor or normal tissue. In unsupervised classification, there is no prior information about the origin of the spectra required. Examples of classification algorithms often used in spectroscopic image analysis are Linear Discriminant Analysis (LDA), Cluster Analysis (CA), Artificial Neural Network (ANN), and Factor Analysis (FA) (6).

LDA is used to find the linear combination of spectral features that optimally separate two or more classes. LDA is closely related to the analysis of variance and regression analysis, which also attempt to express one dependent variable as a linear combination of other features or measurements and PCA. An example of LDA is illustrated in Figure 9.5. Two different types of samples, normal tissue of a maxilla and epithelial odontogenic tumor tissue of the maxilla, were characterized by IR spectroscopic imaging. Inputs to the LDA are sets of spectra from normal tissue and from tumor tissue together with the histological assignment. The red dots in Figure 9.5 indicate tumor tissue, and blue dots belong to normal tissue. The calculated linear function discriminates the two types of tissue so that subsequent unknown samples will be assigned either to the red field (tumor tissue) or to the blue field (normal tissue).

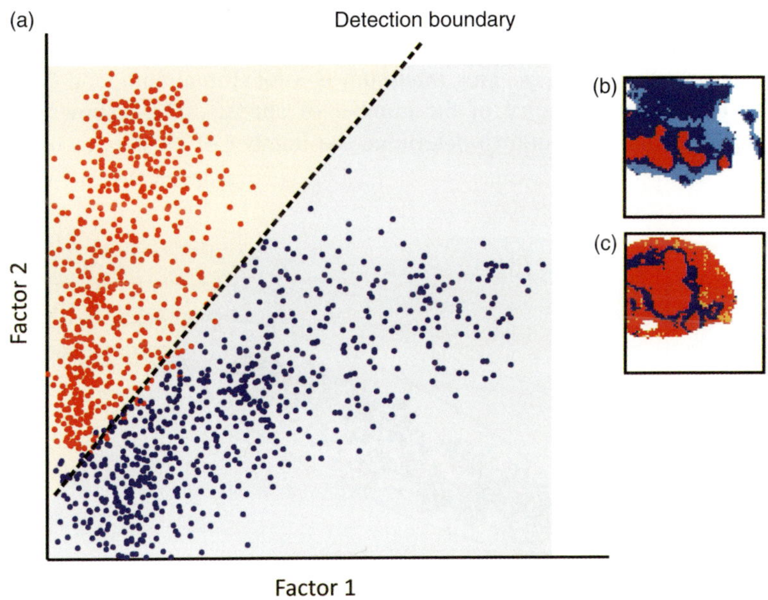

Figure 9.5. Linear discriminant analysis of IR spectra obtained from epithelial odontogenic tumor tissue of the maxilla (red dots) and from normal tissue of the same maxilla (blue dots). The figures on the right side show the Fourier Transform Infrared (FTIR) spectroscopic images of (b) expected normal tissue and (c) tumor tissue. Bright blue and orange pixels indicate spectra that are closer to the other group (located close to the dashed line in (a). Image (b) reveals that tumor cells have already infiltrated the expected normal tissue.

CA classifies spectra into different groups, or more precisely, partitions a data set into subsets (clusters), so that the spectra in each subset ideally share some common trait—often proximity according to some defined distance measure. There are several methods for CA:

Hierarchical clustering builds a hierarchy of clusters. The traditional representation of this hierarchy is a tree, called *dendrogram*, with individual elements at one end and a single cluster containing its elements at the other. Cutting the tree at a given height will result in a clustering at a selected precision. The k-means CA assigns each spectrum to the cluster whose center, also called *centroid*, is nearest. The centroid spectrum is the average of all the spectra in the cluster. The goal of the k-means CA is a large distance between neighboring centroid spectra and at the same time a small spread of the clusters. The number of clusters has to be estimated a priori. Each spectrum belongs to just one cluster, whereas in fuzzy c-means CA, each spectrum has a degree of belonging to clusters, as in fuzzy logic. Spectra on the edge of a cluster may have a smaller membership value than spectra in the center of the cluster. With fuzzy c-means CA, the centroid spectrum of a cluster is the mean of all spectra, weighted by their membership value. Figure 9.6 shows the results of the fuzzy c-means CA for spectra from normal tissue of a maxilla and epithelial odontogenic tumor tissue of the same maxilla. Both types of tissue are now more clearly separated into two clusters.

CA algorithms maximize the distance between the centroid spectra and minimize intracluster variances. This minimum is a local minimum, and the results depend on the initial choice of the number of clusters. The "elbow criterion" is a common rule of thumb to determine the number of clusters to be chosen.

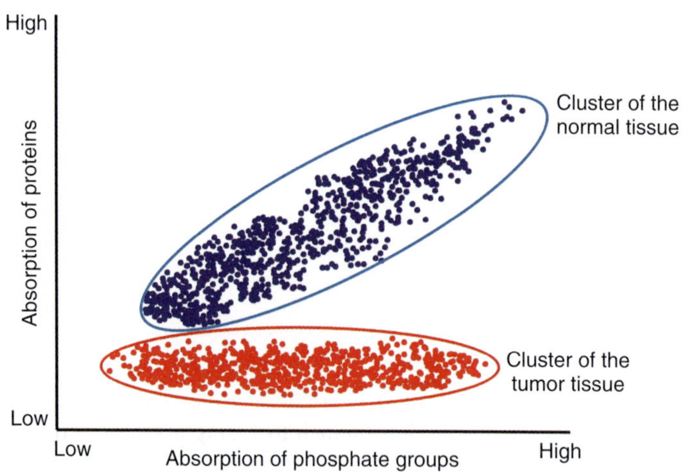

Figure 9.6. Illustration of k-means cluster analysis. Spectra of the data set shown in Figure 9.5 were separated into two clusters. Each spectrum is assigned to exactly one cluster representing normal or tumor tissue.

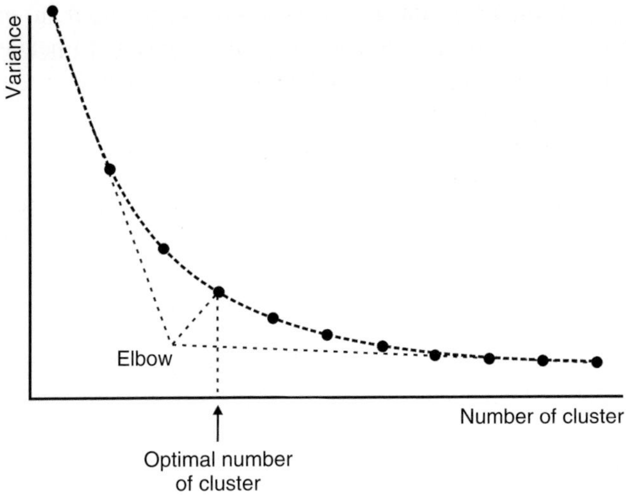

Figure 9.7. Elbow criterion to determine the optimal number of clusters for image segmentation.

Figure 9.7 shows the variance against the number of clusters. The elbow is indicated by an arrow. In this example, the number of clusters chosen should be five. In summary, CA is recommended when similarities of spectra should be highlighted. One advantage of CA is its relatively good robustness against artifacts and noise. CA is also recommended as the initial step when spectra exhibit a poor signal to noise ratio.

An ANN is an interconnected group of artificial neurons that uses a mathematical model or computational model for information processing based on a connectionist approach to computation. In most cases, an ANN is an adaptive system that changes its structure based on external or internal information that flows through the network. ANN is a very sophisticated method and should be used for a well-characterized training set. ANN can be very sensitive to slight spectral variations and to artifacts and distortions. Therefore, ANN is recommended for very good spectra without artifacts and with a high signal to noise ratio.

FA is a technique used to explain variability within a number of spectra in terms of fewer unobserved variables called *factors*. The spectra are modeled as linear combinations of the factors and an error term. FA is often used in combination with PCA, since the abstract principal components are transformed into an initial set of factors, which describe either species or certain biochemical characteristics. FA has several advantages, such as (i) the reduction in the number of absorbance values by combining them into a single factor and (ii) the identification of relevant spectral regions and the definition of relationships between variables (spectral regions). The interpretation of FA is almost based on heuristic approaches. Thus, more than one interpretation can be obtained from the same data factored the same way, and FA cannot be used to identify causalities.

Although multivariate methods are more commonly used in spectroscopic imaging analysis, univariate techniques are also used, in particular, when the statistical relationship of one variable to another is concerned.

9.5.4 Image Processing Including Pattern Recognition

Image processing aims at visualizing the classified spectra based on either a priori knowledge or on information extracted from the pattern. The simplest way of image processing is to assign different colors to the classified spectra and to create a false color image. In many cases, it is necessary and helpful to consider the distribution of the classified spectra and to highlight areas either with similar or different features. Rendering is used to eliminate the "noise" in the distribution. Pattern recognition techniques are also used to visualize the extracted features. Finally, the combination of spectroscopic images with other imaging systems can help to increase the specificity of the extracted features.

9.6 APPLICATIONS

9.6.1 Single Cells

Single Cells were characterized by IR and Raman spectroscopic imaging (7–9). The high spatial resolution of Raman imaging of less than 1 μm allows the examination of cell compartments, for example, the cell core or mitochondria. A Raman image also shows the distribution of lipids, nucleic acids, and protein in an individual cell (10). Images of cancer cells before, during, and after drug treatment provide keys to the drug mechanism and cell apoptosis. Cell stress and different stages of cell development can be imaged as well. Another example of Raman imaging is the characterization of drug distribution and other biochemical complexes in living cells (11–14). IR spectroscopic images reveal the biochemical characteristic of complete individual cells. Figure 9.8 shows the results of spectral classification of cells of the human glioma cell lines U343, T1115, and T508. The first row shows the microscopic image of the cell culture in the visible range. The rectangle indicates the sample area chosen for the IR spectroscopic investigation. Images in the lower panel summarize the results of the classification. Blue pixels indicate cells of the U343 cell line; yellow pixels, cells of T1115; and red pixels, cells of T508. The results demonstrate the potential of IR spectroscopic imaging to identify cells with only a few misclassifications.

9.6.2 Tissue Sections

Identification of tumor tissue was among the first biomedical applications of IR spectroscopic imaging (16–19). The approach provides within few seconds a classification of the tissue without staining or biochemical labeling. Striking chemical differences are observed between tumor and nontumor tissue. The photograph of a Hematoxylin–Eosin (HE)-stained tissue section of tumor in a

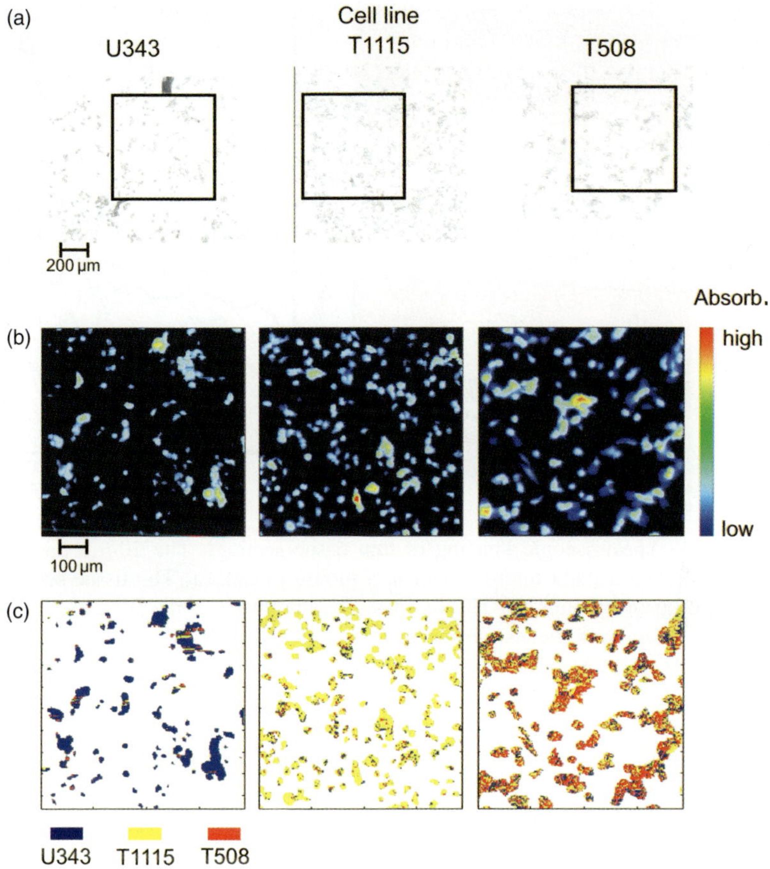

Figure 9.8. IR spectroscopic classification of human glioma cells of the cell lines U343, T1115, and T508. (a) Microscopic images in the visible range of the unstained cell populations. Differentiation between the cell lines is not possible. (b) IR spectroscopic images of the investigated sample. The images show total IR absorption by the cell samples (color coded according to the bar at right). Differentiation between the cell lines is not possible. (c) Cell classification of the spectral data of (b) by LDA. The assignment of the individual cells to corresponding cell lines is given by the color bar below. *Source:* Reproduced with permission from Reference 15.

mouse model for different types of tissue is shown in Figure 9.9a. The IR spectroscopic image in Figure 9.9b, evaluated by fuzzy k-means CA, reveals the same structure as the parallel HE-stained thin section. The tumor tissue (red, orange, and yellow clusters) is clearly discriminated. The segmentation in the spectroscopic image is based on several spectral features (Fig. 9.9c). Tumor tissue has a slightly lower absorbance in the spectral range between 1000 and 1100 cm^{-1}, indicating lower concentrations of gangliosides. Moreover, changes in amide I region (around 1640 cm^{-1}) indicate changes in the composition of

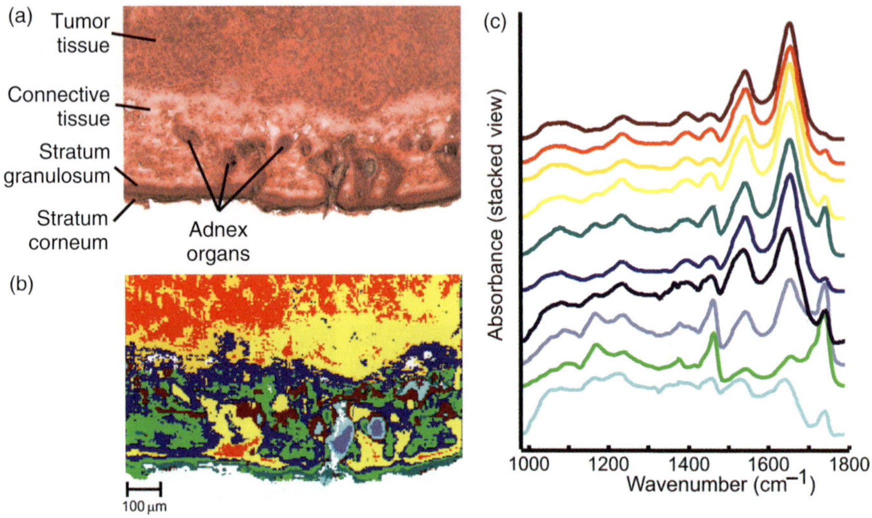

Figure 9.9. IR spectroscopic imaging of thin tissue sections. The 20-μm thick sample was obtained from a Fadu tumor grown in a mouse model. (a) The tissue section after hematoxylin–eosin staining. (b) The IR spectroscopic image of the adjacent thin section after segmentation by k-means cluster analysis. (c) The centroid spectra of the cluster shown in (b). The colors of the spectra traces are identical to the clusters in (b).

proteins. In contrast to that of the tumor and connective tissue, spectra of adnex organs exhibit elevated absorbance at 1740 cm^{-1}, 1460 cm^{-1} and between 1100 and 1200 cm^{-1}. The higher concentration of fatty acids is responsible for this elevated absorbance, whereas the absorption bands for proteins (amid I and amid II between 1480 and 1720 cm^{-1}) are reduced here. The following sections give a short overview of spectroscopic imaging analysis of different types of tissue.

9.6.2.1 Brain Tissue. Cancerous brain tissue can be well distinguished from normal brain tissue by their IR and Raman spectra (20, 21). The degree of malignancy can even be discriminated from one another when grades form a histological continuum and the histological assignment is known to be difficult. An example is the four tumor grades of increasing malignancy: pilocytic astrocytoma, low grade astrocytoma, anaplastic astrocytoma, and glioblastoma. Figure 9.10 shows IR images of normal tissue, astrocytoma degree 2, astrocytoma degree 3, and the most aggressive type glioblastoma. Grading the tumors based on IR spectroscopic classification is practically consistent with conventional histopathology; the IR spectroscopic classifications generally show no confusion between tumor and normal tissues.

Another example concerns the identification of brain metastases with unknown primary tumor. The management of metastases involves a combination of neurosurgery and therapies by radiation treatment and chemotherapy. The effective

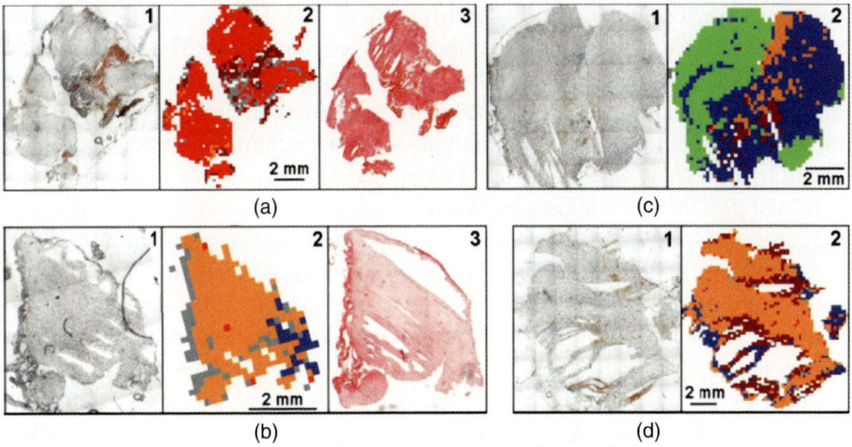

Figure 9.10. IR spectroscopic imaging of tissue section of various brain tumors: multifocal glioblastoma (a,b) and astrocytoma degree 3 (c,d). The spectral classification was obtained by LDA. Color codes: green, normal brain tissue; blue, astrocytoma degree 2; orange, astrocytoma degree 3; red, glioblastoma; brown, hemorrhage; and gray, leptomeninges.

(a) (1) Unstained cryosection, (2) IR spectroscopic image indicating glioblastoma, and (3) HE-stained parallel tissue section diagnosed as glioblastoma.

(b) (1) Unstained cryosection, (2) IR spectroscopic image indicating astrocytoma degree 3, and (3) HE-stained parallel tissue section diagnosed as astrocytoma degree 3.

(c) Unstained cryosection and (2) IR spectroscopic image indicating transition from normal tissue to astrocytoma degree 2 and a low fraction of astrocytoma°°3.

(d) (1) Unstained cryosection and (2) IR spectroscopic image indicating a high fraction of astrocytoma degree 3. *Source:* Reproduced with permission from Reference 22.

management is related to the origin of the metastasis. Thus, localization of the primary tumor is in the forefront for the management of metastases. Metastases exhibit a molecular fingerprint from the primary tumor. IR and Raman spectroscopy permit the rapid determination of spatial extension of metastases and of the type of the primary tumor.

9.6.2.2 Skin Tissue. Human skin consists of different layers of various functional structures. This structural organization can be characterized by spectroscopic methods, in particular, with deep-resolved Raman imaging (23). The stratum corneum, epidermis, and dermis are clearly visible in the images because of their content of lipids and specific proteins. For example, the upper stratum corneum exhibits larger areas with a high content of lipids and aggregated corneocytes.

Identification and more important demarcation of tumor from surrounding normal tissue as well as diagnosis of the growing state can be determined by spectroscopic imaging methods. Several studies have demonstrated the potential of IR spectroscopic imaging to identify benign skin lesions and to distinguish benign tumors associated with thyroid gland carcinoma (24). The distribution of exogene molecules, components of sun creams, and triglycerides in the different skin layers has also been measured with spectroscopic imaging. Figure 9.11 shows the IR spectroscopic determination of the permeation of Dimethylsulfoxide (DMSO) through skin. A series of visible and IR images was recorded from a section of porcine skin cut perpendicular to the surface. The visible micrograph of each section is shown in the right-hand panel. The spatial distribution of amino acids, protein, lipids constituents, and DMSO were derived from the intensity of the representative bands. The penetration enhancer DMSO is used in several treatment plans for skin diseases. Knowledge of permeation pathways provides a basis for a better understanding of the situation and processes in the skin.

Stitching of individual maps provides a cross section of skin. Figure 9.12 demonstrates the ability of Raman microimaging to reveal different layers of skin. The importance of these investigations lies in the fact that protein structures may be changed irreversibly because of outer influences or as a consequence of certain diseases of the organism.

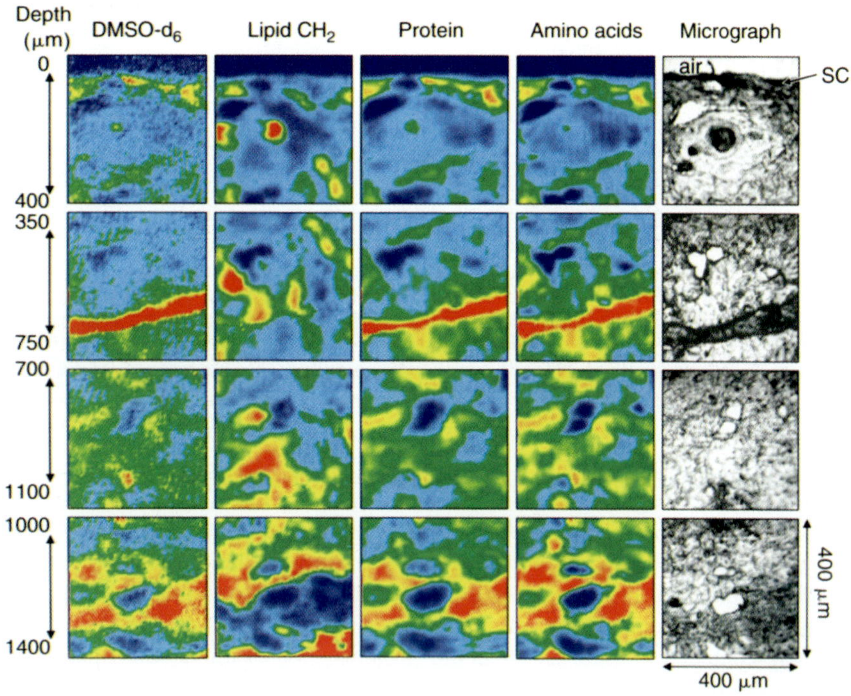

Figure 9.11. Permeation of the penetration enhancer DMSO-d_6 through the skin. The last column on the right shows the micrographs. The color-coded IR images represent various components. In the first column, DMSO-d_6 is determined by the evaluation of CD_3 vibrations. *Source:* Reproduced with permission from Reference 25.

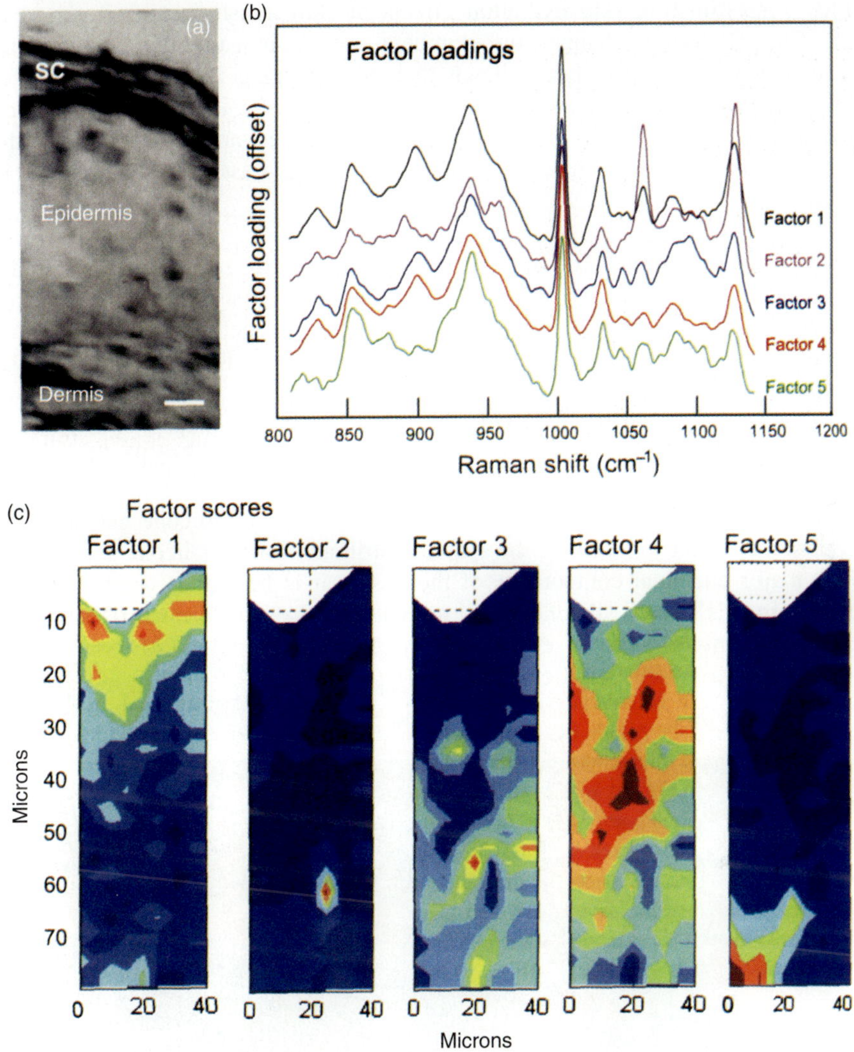

Figure 9.12. Confocal Raman spectroscopic images of pigskin. (a) Optical micrograph of a 5-μm thick section. (b) Five distinct factor loadings generated by a special segregation algorithm. (c) Spatial distribution of factor scores for each loading. Factor 1 represents the stratum corneum, factor 4 corresponds to the viable epidermis, and factor 5 corresponds to the dermis. The two remaining factors, 2 and 3, represent particular features of the skin. *Source:* Reproduced with permission from Reference 26.

NIR imaging for measuring skin hydration has been applied in a clinical study for estimating skin hydration effects of skin moisturizers and cleansers (27, 28). Hydration changes on treatment with a moisturizing cream could be detected. It has also been shown that NIR imaging is more sensitive for discriminating between treatments and control. Moreover, it is rapid, noncontact, and noninvasive, and has the additional important advantage of showing the degree of hydration as a function of location, for rapid assessment of change in hydration.

9.6.2.3 Breast Tissue. One of first applications of IR spectroscopic imaging of tissue was the characterization of breast implants consisting of silicone elastomers, filled with saline or silicone gel (29). The silicone gel may leak, leading to complications such as calcification, connective tissue disorders, and capsular contracture. For an optimized therapy, it is necessary to confirm the presence of silicone gel within the breast tissue. In spectroscopic images, silicone elastomers can be clearly found by the Si—CH_3 vibrations. Small silicone gel inclusions could also be found in samples in which microscopic contrast was poor. Figure 9.13 shows an NIR spectroscopic image of silicone gel inclusion in tissue. In order to visualize the spatial distribution of the silicone gel together with major chemical components of the tissue, it is helpful to create an RGB image. In this image, silicone gel is assigned to the red channel, tissue which consists mainly of type III collagen is in blue, and green shows tissue with a high correlation with type I collagen.

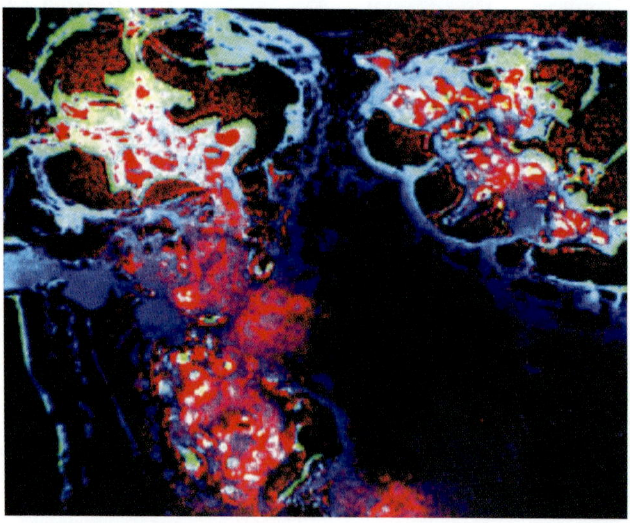

Figure 9.13. NIR spectroscopic image of silicone gel inclusion within tissue. The spectral information of silicone gel is transferred to an RGB image. Red indicates silicon, blue shows mainly type III collagen, and green is assigned to type I collagen. *Source:* Reproduced with permission from Reference 30.

Breast tumor tissue could be identified by evaluation of intensities at 1084 cm^{-1}, which is ascribed to RNA and DNA. The study also reported a detection of micro areas of breast tumors, which could not be found by common microscopy. Although several studies demonstrated recognition of capabilities of IR spectroscopic imaging in the management of breast tumors, there are no reports on extensive clinical spectroscopic measurements.

9.6.2.4 Bone Tissue. IR and Raman spectroscopic imaging has been used to characterize mineralized structures in bone tissue. The images exhibit spatial variances of hydroxylapatite and other minerals, lipids, and proteins. For example, human iliac crest biopsies were monitored to correlate biochemical data with morphologic structures. The results show that a mineralization process increased from the middle of the osteon toward the outside. In addition, the distribution of proteins, by evaluation of the amide I band, showed a corresponding gradient. Several studies have demonstrated that IR and Raman spectroscopic imaging are very good methods to highlight the mineralization of bones (31, 32) or micro-damages in bone tissue (33). The distribution of phosphates, carbonates, proteins, and lipids of bone tissue is shown in Figure 9.14. The ratio of phosphate bands

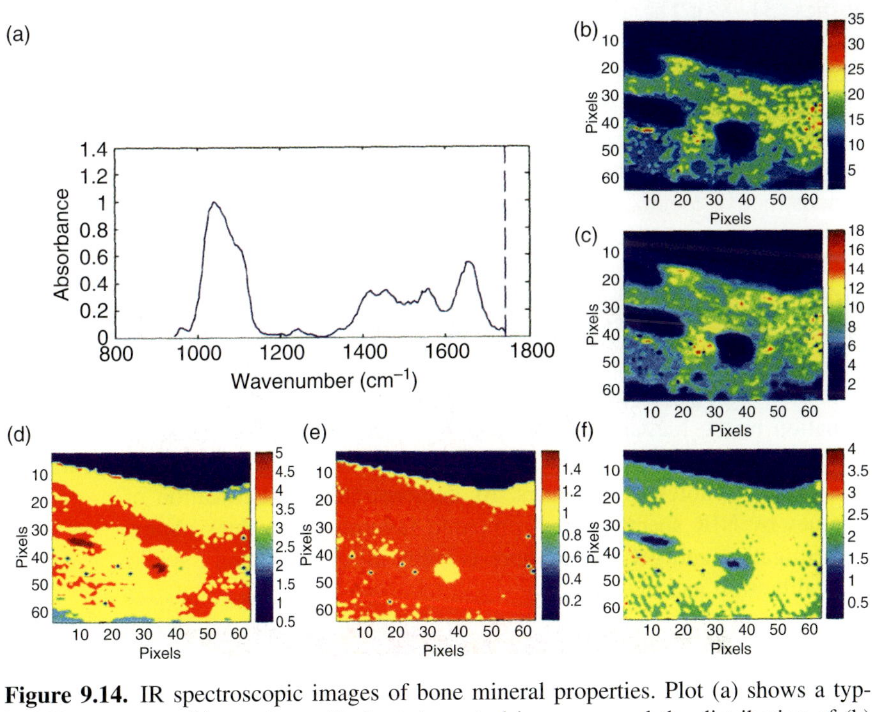

Figure 9.14. IR spectroscopic images of bone mineral properties. Plot (a) shows a typical IR spectrum of bone tissue. Evaluated spectral images reveal the distribution of (b) mineral, (c) matrix, (d) carbonate, (e) mineral to matrix and (f) crystallinity. *Source:* Reproduced with permission from Reference 31.

(900–1200 cm^{-1}) to amide I vibration (1580–1720 cm^{-1}) of proteins is directly related to mineral content. Spectroscopic investigations allow the characterization of the development of physiologically mineralized tissue and of the mineral content in cells.

IR spectroscopic imaging becomes useful for the diagnosis of bones. Changes in the chemical composition of bones are often a significant indicator for diseases such as osteogenesis imperfecta or osteoporosis.

Interaction between bone tissue and Poly(Methylmethacrylate) (PMMA), used as compartment in bone cements, could be monitored. Osteon centers were found to contain fewer minerals than peripheral areas. The investigation of osteoporotic ilica crest biopsies and normal tissue sections shows that the averaged mineral content in the osteoporotic samples were considerably reduced. The spectra revealed that, in the diseased state, the crystal size was substantially enhanced. Similar studies were performed to characterize the effects of estrogen therapy on fracture healing in rat femurs.

9.6.3 Diagnosis of Hemodynamics

NIR spectroscopic imaging is being increasingly applied in hemodynamic diagnostics (34–37). The ability of NIR spectroscopy to characterize oxyhemoglobin and deoxyhemoglobin under in situ conditions makes it extremely useful for monitoring blood perfusion and dysfunction of perfusion. For example, absolute measurements of Hb, Mb, HbO_2, and MbO_2 are possible, and NIR imaging can be also used to monitor cerebral oxygenation. More recently, NIR imaging has moved to the events preceding ischemic injury. Another large field is the nondestructive localization and quantitative determination of cholesterol, which may serve as an *in vivo* marker for atherosclerotic plaques. Several studies have demonstrated that IR and Raman imaging appear to be ideally suited for measuring the size, distribution, and chemical composition of lipid inclusions or particles. Accurate measurement of lipoprotein cholesterol in all its forms is a critical first step in intervention in the diseases of atherosclerosis. For example, NIR imaging of lipid and protein in primate brain tissue and noninvasive determination in the human body have been described. NIR imaging has also been used in human stroke patients to locate atherosclerotic plaques by identifying and locating cholesterol plaques. As demonstrated, quantification of proteins in plaques by NIR spectroscopy compared favorably to values obtained by ultracentrifugation and gel electrophoresis when these separation methods were used for calibration and validation.

In many cases, such as in neurosurgery ongoing in the brain, intraoperative monitoring and imaging of blood flow of the vessel is required. The concentrations of deoxyhemoglobin, oxhemoglobin, and water, which are the major NIR absorbers in tissues, can be imaged by NIR spectroscopy. Such an imaging system measures the regional blood volume and oxygen saturation and can assist surgeons.

Another application based on the measurement of blood is the treatment of burns. An important question is whether the tissue is viable or damaged. This is, in particular, of interest in the case of second-degree, or partial-thickness, burns. Whether second-degree burns heal on their own depends on the damage done to blood vessels in the skin's dermal layer. If blood is not oxygenated in the burned skin, it is not going to start the healing process at the burn site.

REFERENCES

1. Clark D, Sasic S. Chemical images: technical approaches and issues. Cytometry 2006;69A(8):815–824.
2. Kohler A, Bertrand D, Martens H, Hannesson K, Kirschner C, Ofstad R. Multivariate image analysis of a set of FTIR microspectroscopy images of aged bovine muscle tissue combining image and design information. Anal Bioanal Chem 2007;389(4):1143–1153.
3. Burger J, Geladi P. Hyperspectral NIR imaging for calibration and prediction: a comparison between image and spectrometer data for studying organic and biological samples. Analyst 2006;131(10):1152–1160.
4. Jetter K, Depczynski U, Molt K, Niemoller A. Principles and applications of wavelet transformation to chemometrics. Anal Chim Acta 2000;420(2):169–180.
5. Ehrentreich F. Wavelet transform applications in analytical chemistry. Anal Bioanal Chem 2002;372(1):115–121.
6. Wood BR, Bambery KR, Evans CJ, Quinn MA, McNaughton D. A three-dimensional multivariate image processing technique for the analysis of FTIR spectroscopic images of multiple tissue sections. BMC Med Imaging 2006;6:12.
7. Kalasinsky KS, Hadfield T, Shea AA, Kalasinsky VF, Nelson MP, Neiss J, Drauch AJ, Vanni GSt, Treado PJ. Raman chemical imaging spectroscopy reagentless detection and identification of pathogens: signature development and evaluation. Anal Chem 2007;79(7):2658–2673.
8. Diem M, Romeo M, Boydston-White S, Milijkovic M, Matthaeus C. A decade of vibrational microspectroscopy of human cells and tissue (1994–2004). Analyst 2004;129(10):880–885.
9. Lasch P, Pacifico A, Diem M. Spatially resolved IR microspectroscopy of single cells. Biopolymers 2002;67(4–5):335–338.
10. Krafft C, Knetschke T, Funk RHW, Salzer R. Studies on stress-induced changes at the subcellular level by Raman microspectroscopic mapping. Anal Chem 2006;78(13):4424–4429.
11. Florence D, Pierre J, Abdelilah B, Ali T, Nicolas F, Michel M, Josep S-S, Ganesh S. Raman spectral imaging of single living cancer cells: a preliminary study. Analyst 2009;134(3):542–548.
12. Hamada K, Fujita K, Smith NI, Kobayashi M, Inouye Y, Kawata S. Raman microscopy for dynamic molecular imaging of living cells. J Biomed Opt 2008;13(4): 044027.
13. Feofanov AV, Grichine AI, Shitova LA, Karmakova TA, Yakubovskaya RI, Egret-Charlier M, Vigny P. Confocal Raman microspectroscopy and imaging study of theraphthal in living cancer cells. Biophys J 2000;78(1):499–512.

14. Meister K, Niesel J, Schatzschneider U, Metzler-Nolte N, Schmidt DA, Havenith M. Label-free imaging of metal-carbonyl complexes in live cells by Raman microspectroscopy. Angew Chem Int Ed 2010;49(19):3310–3312.

15. Steiner G, Küchler S, Hermann A, Koch E, Salzer R, Schackert G, Kirsch M. Rapid and label-free classification of human glioma cells by infrared spectroscopic imaging. Cytometry 2008;73A(12):1158–1164.

16. Bhargava R. Towards a practical Fourier transform infrared chemical imaging protocol for cancer histopathology. Anal Bioanal Chem 2007;389(4):1155–1169.

17. Ferandez DC, Bhargava R, Hewitt StM, Levin IW. Infrared spectroscopic imaging for histopathologic recognition. Nat Biotechnol 2005;23(4):469–474.

18. Petibois C, Dèlèris G. Chemical mapping of tumor progression by FT-IR imaging: towards molecular histopathology. Trends Biotechnol 2006;24(10):455–461.

19. Steiner G, Shaw A, Choo-Smith L-P, Abuid MH, Schackert G, Sobottka S, Steller W, Salzer R, Mantsch HH. Distinguishing and grading human gliomas by IR spectroscopy. Biospectrosc Biopolym 2003;72:464–471.

20. Krafft C, Sobottka SB, Schackert G, Salzer R. Analysis of human brain tissue, brain tumors and tumor cells by infrared spectroscopic mapping. Analyst 2004;129(10):921–925.

21. Beleites C, Steiner G, Sowa MG, Baumgartner R, Sobottka S, Schackert G, Salzer R. Classification of human gliomas by infrared imaging spectroscopy and chemometric image processing. Vib Spectrosc 2005;38(1–2):143–149.

22. Krafft C, Thümmler K, Sobottka SB, Schackert G, Salzer R. Classification of malignant gliomas by infrared spectroscopy and linear discriminant analysis. Biopolymers 2006;82(4):301–305.

23. Xiao C, Flach C, Marcott C, Mendelsohn R. Uncertainties in depth determination and comparison of multivariate with univariate analysis in confocal Raman studies of a laminated polymer and skin. Appl Spectrosc 2004;58(4):382–389.

24. Tfayli A, Piot O, Durlach A, Bernard P, Manfait M. Discriminating nevus and melanoma on paraffin-embedded skin biopsies using FTIR microspectroscopy. Biochim Biophys Acta 2005;1724(5):262–269.

25. Mendelsohn R, Boskey AL, Camacho NP. Infrared microscopy and imaging of hard and soft tissue. In: Bhargava R, Levin IraW, editors. *Spectrochemical Analysis Using Infrared Multichannel Detectors*. Oxford: Blackwell publishing; 2005.

26. Zhang G, Moore DJ, Flach CR, Mendelsohn R. Vibrational microscopy and imaging of skin: from single cells to intact tissue. Anal Bioanal Chem 2007;387(8):1591–1599.

27. Zhang SL, Meyers CL, Subramanyan K, Hancewicz TM. Near infrared imaging for measuring and visualizing skin hydration. A comparison with visual assessment and electrical methods. J Biomed Opt 2005;10(3): 031107.

28. Attas EM, Sowa MG, Posthumus TB, Schattka BJ, Mantsch HH, Zhang S. Near-IR spectroscopic imaging for skin hydration: the long and the short of it. Biopolymers 2002;67(2):96–106.

29. Kidder LH, Kalasinsky VF, Luke JL, Levin IW, Lewis NE. Visualization of silicone gel in human breast tissue using new infrared imaging spectroscopy. Nat Med 1997;3(2):235–237.

30. Lee E, Kidder LH, Kalasinsky VF, Schoppelrei JW, Lewis EN. Forensic visualization of foreign matter in human tissue by near-infrared spectral imaging: methodology and data mining strategies. Cytometry 2006;69A(8):888–869.

31. Boskey AL, Mendelsohn R. Infrared spectrosocpic characterization of mineralized tissue. Vib Spectrosc 2005;38(1–2):107–114.

32. Faibish D, Gomes A, Boivin G, Binderman I, Boskey A. Infrared imaging of calcified tissue in bone biopsoes from adults with osteomalacia. Bone 2005;36(1):6–12.

33. Timlin JA, Garden A, Morris MD, David RM, Kohn H. Raman spectroscopic imaging markers for fatigue-related microdamage in bovine bone. Anal Chem 2000;72(10):2229–2236.

34. Piao D, Wogue PB. Rapid near-infrared diffuse tomography for hemodynamic imaging using a low-coherence wideband light source. J Biomed Opt 2007;12(1): 014016.

35. Abookasis D, Lay CC, Mathews MS, Linskey ME, Frostig RD, Tromberg BJ. Imaging cortical absorption, scattering, and hemodynamic response during ischemic stroke using spatially modulated near-infrared illumination. J Biomed Opt 2009;14(2): 024033.

36. Kohno S, Miyai I, Seiyama A, Oda I, Ishikawa A, Tsuneishi S, Amita T, Shimizu K. Removal of the skin blood flow artifact in functional near-infrared spectroscopic imaging data through independent component analysis. J Biomed Opt 2007;12(6): 062111.

37. Huppert TJ, Diamond SG, Franceschini MA, Boas DA. HomER: a review of time-series analysis methods for near-infrared spectroscopy of the brain. Appl Opt 2009;48(10): D280–D298.

10

COHERENT ANTI-STOKES RAMAN SCATTERING MICROSCOPY

ANNIKA ENEJDER
Department of Chemical and Biological Engineering, Chalmers University of Technology, Göteborg, Sweden

CHRISTOPH HEINRICH
Department für Physiologie und Medizinische Physik, Medizinische Universität Innsbruck, Innsbruck, Austria

CHRISTIAN BRACKMANN
Department of Chemical and Biological Engineering, Chalmers University of Technology, Göteborg, Sweden

STEFAN BERNET AND MONIKA RITSCH-MARTE
Department für Physiologie und Medizinische Physik, Medizinische Universität Innsbruck, Innsbruck, Austria

10.1 BASICS

10.1.1 Introduction

Generations of bioscientists have obtained microscopic images based on the light absorption, scattering, polarization, and fluorescence properties of their samples, providing information on different aspects of the fascinating world of the cell. In our quest to understand normal as well as disease conditions for the benefit of human health, the requirements of resolution and contrast have changed radically during the last decade. We want more than the morphological information

Biomedical Imaging: Principles and Applications, First Edition. Edited by Reiner Salzer.

typically provided; we now wish to follow changes in structural and physiological molecular properties as well as dynamic biochemical *processes* at the *molecular* level in *living* cells and in *real time*. This stimulates the development of a series of sophisticated microscopic methods based on multiphoton (nonlinear) interaction processes. Here, conventional light sources are replaced by short-pulsed laser systems generating the high peak intensities required. In the interaction process with the sample, the generated light signal is frequency shifted relative to the excitation light and can selectively be detected by means of filters or dispersive elements in front of a sensitive detector.

Molecular vibrations . . .

- are Raman active if the polarizability varies with the vibration
- are usually given in the unit of wavenumbers (cm^{-1}), a reciprocal wavelength defined as $10{,}000/\lambda$(λ in μm)
- of low weight atoms occur at higher frequencies: for example, carbon–hydrogen bonds (C—H) vibrate in the frequency range 2845–2950 cm^{-1}, while their corresponding deuterated forms (C—D bonds) vibrate at a lower frequency ~2100 cm^{-1}
- of stronger bonds occur at higher frequencies: for example the double bond C=C has a resonance at ~1650 cm^{-1} while that of the single bond C—C can be found at 1000–1100 cm^{-1}

One of these novel microscopic techniques is Coherent Anti-Stokes Raman Scattering (CARS) microscopy. Here, image contrast is given by the vibrational properties of molecules, highly dependent on the participating atoms, the character of the bond, the physical state of the molecule, and its environment. (see Factbox and Chapter 9). This allows for true chemical imaging. Although the first published experiments involving this particular third-order nonlinear effect were carried out at a company selling cars, the Ford Motor Company (Maker and Terhune, 1965), then studying imaging on a macroscopic scale in benzene derivatives, the acronym CARS was not coined only 9 years later (Begley et al., 1974). In the past 40 years, it has found numerous applications for qualitative and quantitative analysis of gas-phase and plasma systems, particularly within combustion diagnostics (for reviews see Druet and Taran, 1981; Zheltikov, 2000).

The exploration of the CARS process for microscopic imaging was, however, fairly recently initiated. In 1982, CARS was for the first time introduced in a microscope and employed for the visualization of deuterated water in onion skin cells, although with an image quality severely limited by available technology and strong background generation (Duncan et al., 1982). It required almost two decades of further laser system development, until CARS microscopy was taken up again for three-dimensional visualization of biological molecules in living cells

(Zumbusch et al., 1999). Today, it is on the verge of becoming a widespread and easy-to-use tool complementing other microscopic methods.

10.2 THEORY

In CARS microscopy, the characteristic vibrational properties of molecules in the sample are mapped to an image. This is achieved by tuning the frequency difference of two excitation laser beams, the pump (frequency ω_P) and Stokes (frequency ω_S) beams, to form a beating field with a frequency that matches the resonance frequency Ω of the target molecule, as illustrated in Figure 10.1. Ensembles of molecules in the high intensity region of the focal volume are set into a *coherent* vibration by the beating excitation field (Fig. 10.1a). They are then probed by another beam, a so-called probe beam (Fig. 10.1b), which is inelastically scattered with a positive frequency shift (anti-Stokes) corresponding to the molecular vibration (Fig. 10.1c). These coherently anti-Stokes Raman scattered (CARS) photons oscillate in phase and are all emitted in a specific direction set by the wave-matching (or phase-matching) condition, as explained below. The resulting CARS signal, I_{CARS}, is emitted as a laserlike beam at a wavelength (higher frequency ω_{aS}) shorter than the excitation beams I_P (used as both pump and probe beam) and I_S (Stokes beam), and can be clearly separated from the redshifted fluorescence background of the sample (Fig. 10.2).

This phenomenon is theoretically described in the literature of nonlinear optics and spectroscopy (Eesley, 1981; Shen, 1984). An analytical expression

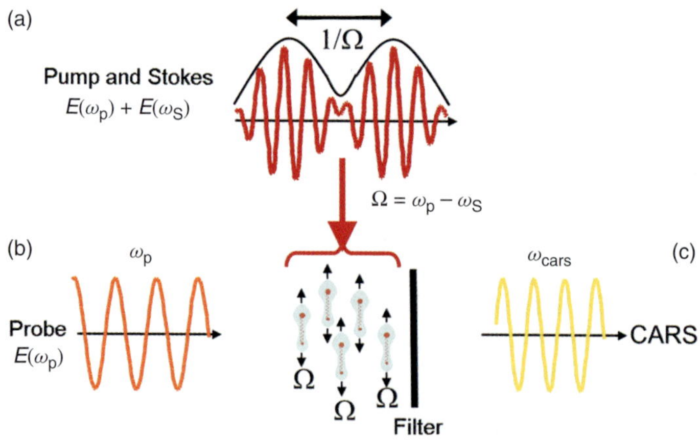

Figure 10.1. The classic picture of the CARS process: The pump and the Stokes beams form a beating field (a), which sets the target molecular groups in vibration when the beat frequency matches the resonance frequency Ω. The probe beam is inelastically scattered by the coherently vibrating cluster of molecules (b), resulting in a positive frequency shift. This coherent anti-Stokes Raman scattered light can then be separated from the excitation light by efficient optical filters before detection (c).

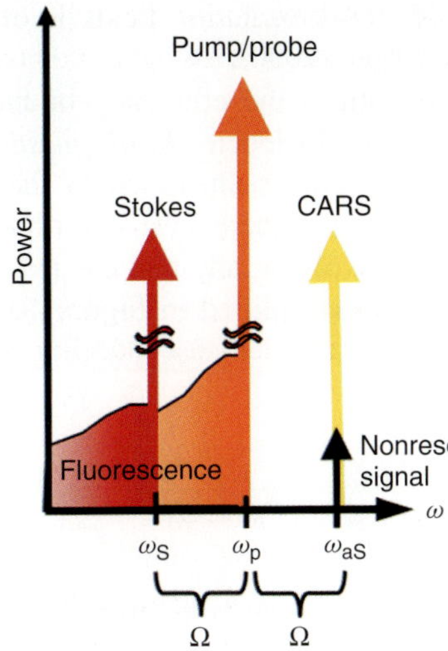

Figure 10.2. A schematic diagram illustrating the spectral separation of the CARS signal from the excitation beams and the resulting intrinsic fluorescence background.

for the emitted intensity at the resonance frequency ω_{aS} can be formulated for a nonabsorbing medium under the assumption of interaction between plane electromagnetic waves:

$$I(\omega_{\mathrm{aS}}) \propto \left| \sum_m N_m \chi_m^{(3)}(\omega_{\mathrm{aS}}) \right|^2 I_{\mathrm{P}}^2 I_{\mathrm{S}} \left(\frac{\sin\left(|\Delta\vec{k}|\,\frac{L}{2}\right)}{|\Delta\vec{k}|\,\frac{L}{2}} \right)^2 \tag{10.1}$$

where N_m is the number of molecules of type m in the probe volume and $\chi_m^{(3)}$ is the corresponding third-order susceptibility. $\Delta\vec{k} = \vec{k}_{\mathrm{aS}} - 2\vec{k}_{\mathrm{P}} + \vec{k}_{\mathrm{S}}$ is the wave-vector mismatch between the interacting electromagnetic fields, and L denotes the interaction length. The fundamental properties of the CARS process can be seen in Eq. (10.1), for example, the emitted intensity increases quadratically with the intensity I_{P} of the degenerate pump/probe beam and linearly with the intensity I_{S} of the Stokes beam. For quantitative microscopy, it is important to note the quadratic relationship between the output intensity and the number of molecules probed. Finally, the last factor, the *sinc* function, indicates the importance of the phase-matching condition $|\Delta\vec{k}| \approx 0$ of the interacting fields.

However, in the tight focus formed by an objective used for scanning CARS microscopy, a large spread in momentum is achieved, offering many possibilities for the photons to satisfy the wave-matching condition, $|\Delta\vec{k}| \approx 0$. In addition, phase matching becomes less critical within a small interaction length such as the size of the focal volume, which is on the order of the excitation wavelengths. For a more profound characterization of the CARS signal in CARS microscopy, the special case of tightly focused excitation fields is of particular importance (Cheng et al., 2002a; Potma et al., 2000).

The susceptibility $\chi_m^{(3)}$ quantifies the efficiency of the nonlinear four-wave mixing processes. It includes the efficiencies of *all possible* third-order resonant processes, vibrational and electronic, as illustrated by the energy level diagrams in Figure 10.3a and b. In addition, there is a contribution from nonresonant interaction processes, $\chi_{nr}^{(3)}$, not involving any real electronic or vibrational levels apart from the ground state, as exemplified in Figure 10.3c. This results in the following expression for the third-order susceptibility when probing a single vibration (Lotem et al., 1976):

$$\chi_m^{(3)}(\omega_{aS}) = \frac{A_R}{\Omega - (\omega_p - \omega_s) - i\Gamma_R} + \frac{A_e}{\omega_e} - 2\omega_p - i\Gamma_e + \chi_{nr}^{(3)}. \qquad (10.2)$$

This expression contains contributions from resonant vibrational and electronic excitations (first two terms), as well as a nonresonant background (last term). Ω and ω_e are the resonant vibrational and electronic frequencies, respectively. Γ_R and Γ_e are the corresponding half width at half maximum linewidths. The constants A_R and A_e are related to the cross sections for Raman scattering and two-photon excitation, respectively. For biological molecules and Infrared (IR) excitation, the second term involving two-photon excitation to an electronic level can typically be neglected, because this level is too far detuned for the low energy Near-Infrared (NIR) or IR photons. The expression for the susceptibility then reduces to

$$\chi_m^{(3)}(\omega_{aS}) = \chi_r^{(3)}(\omega_{aS}) + \chi_{nr}^{(3)}. \qquad (10.3)$$

The first term of Eq. (10.3) is responsible for the desired chemically selective image contrast in CARS microscopy, whereas the last term is essentially a real,

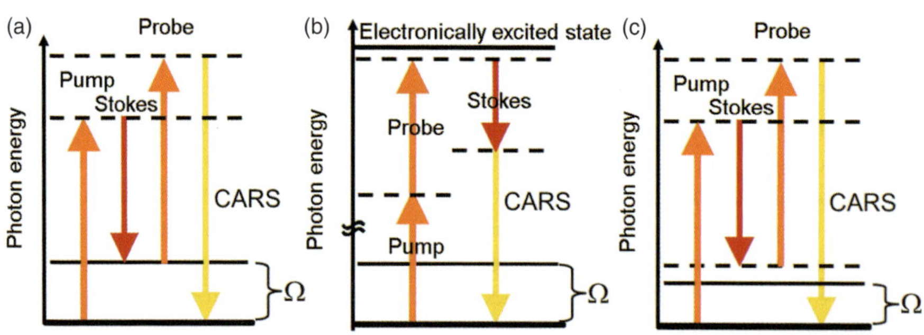

Figure 10.3. Energy level diagrams of all resonant third-order processes that are possible: (a) CARS process involving a vibrational energy level and (b) resonant electronic process involving an excited electronic state. (c) In condensed matter, such as biological samples, the nonresonant process is of particular importance.

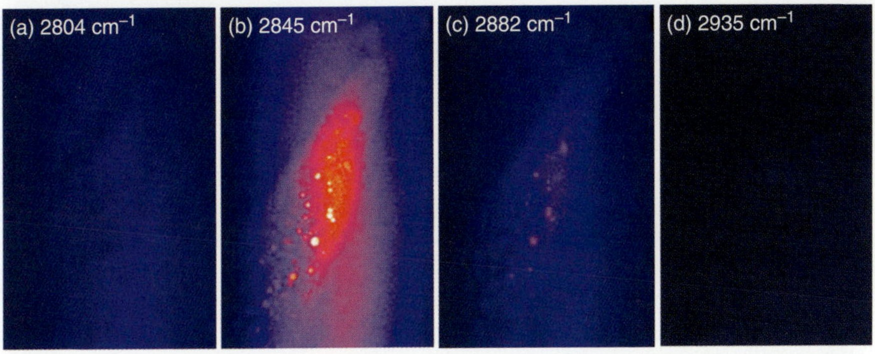

Figure 10.4. A series of CARS microscopic images of the lipid stores in a living *Caenorhabditis elegans* nematode collected at different vibrations in the region of C—H resonance, illustrating the chemical selectivity of CARS microscopy.

frequency-independent constant, not carrying any information on the molecular composition of the sample. Considering the wealth of different molecular species in the probe volume generating only nonresonant background, this part may contribute significantly to the CARS signal. Thus, experimental strategies are being developed in order to reduce and even remove the nonresonant background, resulting in improved sensitivity (Burkacky et al., 2006; Cheng et al., 2001a; Ganikhanov et al., 2006a; Potma et al., 2006; Volkmer et al., 2002; von Vacano et al., 2006). This is further elucidated in the Section "Measurement Techniques."

The primary feature of CARS microscopy is the ability to image with chemical specificity by tuning the frequency difference of the excitation fields to match the resonant vibration of the target molecule. This is illustrated by the series of CARS microscopic images shown in Figure 10.4, obtained by probing different frequencies in the range of the resonance of the C—H bond 2830–2930 cm^{-1}. The CARS images are collected (30 s integration time, 14 + 24 mW excitation power, $52.8 \times 82.1\ \mu m^2$) on the posterior end (tail) of a living nematode *C. elegans*. Four representative images are shown: (a) the nonresonant signal at 2804 cm^{-1}, (b) the symmetric CH_2-stretch vibration at 2845 cm^{-1}, (c) the antisymmetric CH_2 vibration at 2882 cm^{-1}, and (d) the symmetric CH_3 vibration at 2935 cm^{-1}. No lipid stores can be observed in the nonresonant images, whereas they can clearly be distinguished as bright spots in the C—H resonant images (b) and (c).

10.3 CARS MICROSCOPY IN PRACTICE

With present technology, CARS microscopic images are typically collected at average excitation powers in the order of 10 mW during tens of seconds up to 1 min. For NIR excitation light this is far from energy doses causing photodamage in biological materials (Chapter 9), and it is quite tolerable for living cells (Rajadhyaksha et al., 1999).

The sensitivity limit of conventional CARS microscopy is presently in the order of 10^6 vibrating modes per focal volume (Potma et al., 2006), which allows the imaging of single lipid bilayers and single cellular membranes by probing the symmetric CH_2 stretching mode (Potma and Xie, 2003). Bilayers separated by a distance smaller than the diffraction limit can clearly be distinguished, which indicates that ultrahigh resolution is possible in CARS microscopy. Polystyrene beads with a diameter of 0.2 μm have been visualized with a lateral resolution of 0.28 μm (Full Width at Half Maximum (FWHM)) and an axial resolution of 0.78 μm (Cheng and Xie, 2004). Images can be recorded at depths of 100 μm in living tissue, exemplified by the visualization of adipocytes in the subcutaneous layer of a mouse ear (Evans et al., 2005).

These data demonstrate that CARS microscopy has several unique and important virtues as follows:

1. No need for exogenous labeling molecules as the intrinsic vibrational properties are probed
2. Imaging with high three-dimensional resolution
3. Low average excitation powers
4. Efficient fluorescence background discrimination
5. Deep penetration into thick samples with NIR excitation

Thus, CARS microscopy takes molecular imaging beyond the limitations associated with fluorescence (perturbations to the function of the target molecule induced by labeling; Chapter 8), Raman scattering (long integration times and an overwhelming fluorescence background; Chapter 9), and FTIR (limited spatial resolution and absorption of the IR probe light by water; Chapter 9) microscopy. It allows functional imaging of micrometer-sized structures containing only picograms of the targeted substance at high three-dimensional resolution without labeling, which gives CARS microscopy a strong potential to become an important tool within the biosciences.

10.4 INSTRUMENTATION

To date, nearly all CARS microscopy setups utilize the frequency-degenerate excitation scheme, where two of the three incident photons originate from the same laser source, which makes the experimental setup less complicated. Figure 10.5 gives a schematic outline of the essential components of a CARS microscope: the laser system, the detection arrangement, and the actual microscope. The latter can fairly easily be adapted to CARS microscopy by the use of high Numerical Aperture (NA), large back aperture objectives, and NIR-transmitting optics in general. In addition, the optical paths must be optimized for efficient in-coupling of excitation light and detection. The microscope has a history of several hundred years of development to become such a flexible and almost perfect optical instrument enabling CARS microscopy, whereas the

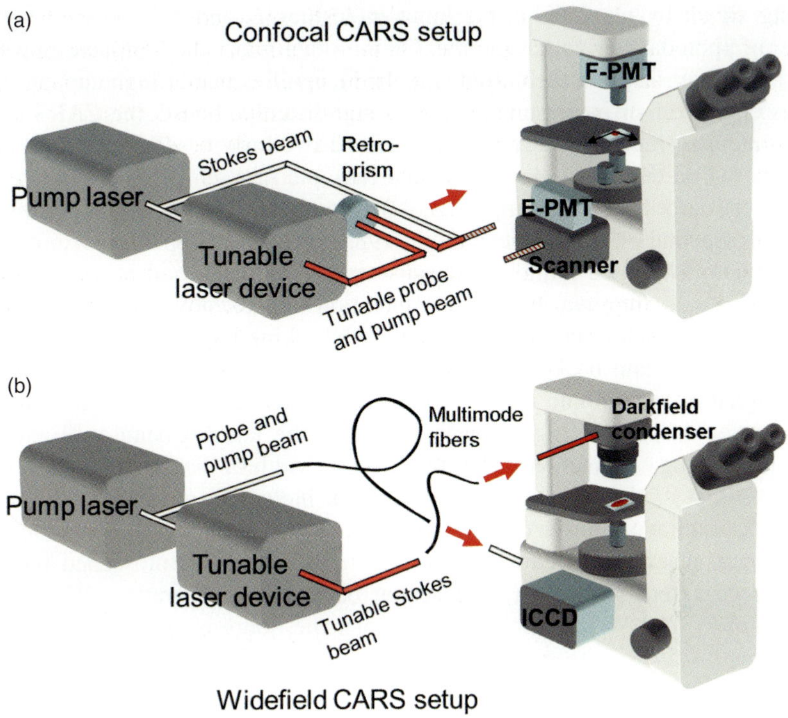

Figure 10.5. Schematic outline of the two principal categories of experimental setups for CARS microscopy: (a) scanning CARS microscope with forward and epidetection and (b) nonscanning wide-field CARS microscope.

development of the laser (Maiman, 1960) and highly sensitive detectors is far more recent and, consequently, in a more expansive phase.

Thus, the advancement of CARS microscopy is highly dependent on the continuing progress of laser and detector technology. An illustrative example of this is the revival of CARS microscopy in 1999 (Zumbusch et al., 1999), made possible by the development in high power short-pulsed lasers during the 1990s. The central role of laser and detector systems for CARS microscopy has been further exemplified.

10.5 LASER SOURCES

Three of the most central characteristics of the laser source for CARS microscopy are its spectral and temporal properties, as well as the peak power generated. The importance of the output power for the generation of the CARS process can be understood from Eq. 10.1, which indicates that the nonlinear response of the medium to the excitation beams is quantified by the third-order susceptibility tensor ($\chi_m^{(3)}$). Owing to weak susceptibilities one can only induce a sufficiently strong signal by maximizing the input intensities I_p and I_S, however, without causing photodamage to the sample. On the other hand, the nonlinear impact of the input intensities on the output (Eq. 10.1) signifies that at high enough intensities only a minor increase is needed to significantly "boost" the CARS signal. This intensity regime is successfully attained by short-pulsed excitation beams. Depending on the approach, nanosecond (ns), picosecond (ps), and femtosecond (fs) laser sources are being employed. After the first attempt at CARS microscopy with picosecond pulses (Duncan et al., 1982), there was hope that excitation by two transform-limited femtosecond pulse trains, allowing highest possible peak powers, would improve the signal generation and thereby enhance the image quality (Zumbusch et al., 1999). However, by taking the accompanying generation of nonresonant background also into account, it was soon realized that the best signal to background ratio is achieved for picosecond rather than femtosecond pulses despite the higher peak powers of the latter (Cheng et al., 2001b). The underlying explanation is that the spectral width of picosecond pulses better matches that of the vibrational resonances in biological matter (10–30 cm^{-1}). Thus the excitation power of picosecond pulses is efficiently used to induce the resonance, whereas the power of the spectrally broader femtosecond pulses is to a large extent wasted on nonresonant background generation. With a peak power of ~3750 W incident on the sample, the nonresonant contribution is in the order of 5% of the resonant signal in the C—H stretch vibrational region for femtosecond pulses (Zumbusch et al., 1999). For picosecond pulses a similar signal to background ratio is obtained, only requiring a peak power of 75 W (Enejder et al., unpublished data). To date, picosecond-pulsed laser sources are therefore primarily utilized for CARS microscopy. The exception is wide-field CARS microscopy, requiring larger energy densities to be distributed over the entire sample area, as offered by nanosecond lasers (Heinrich et al., 2004, 2006).

With the use of short-pulsed laser sources, it is crucial that the intensities of the pump/probe and Stokes beams are delivered simultaneously for efficient CARS generation. Thus the pulses must overlap not only in space in the probe volume but also in time. Time jittering between pulses causes variations in the CARS signal, deteriorating the true image contrast given by the spatial variations in vibrational properties. In the pioneering work of Duncan et al. (1982), two dye lasers were pumped by a single mode-locked argon ion laser in order to synchronize the picosecond excitation pulses. Xie and coworkers (Zumbusch et al., 1999) employed an Optical Parametric Amplifier (OPA) system, pumped by a femtosecond Ti:sapphire regenerative amplifier, also offering inherent pulse synchronization. Various synchronization schemes have been implemented for the use of two different picosecond Ti:sapphire lasers as pump/probe and Stokes sources (Cheng et al., 2001b; Jones et al., 2002; Potma et al., 2002). More recently, a passively mode-locked picosecond Nd:YVO_4 laser has been used with great success to pump one (Evans et al., 2005) and even two intracavity-doubled Optical Parametric Oscillators (OPOs) (Burkacky et al., 2006). A portion of the output from the pump laser serves as the Stokes beam, while the OPO output is used as the pump/probe beam. A new version of the OPO, pumped by a frequency-doubled Nd:YVO_4 laser, has been developed, where the signal and idler are used as pump/probe and Stokes beams (Ganikhanov et al., 2006b).

The evolution of laser systems for CARS microscopy has to a large extent also been driven by the desire for highly tunable laser sources, in order to probe molecular vibrations at free choice or at least over a wide frequency range. In addition, the operation in the NIR range has been shown to be advantageous as it reduces one- and two-photon electronic interactions, resulting in a lower nonresonant contribution, minimal risk of photodamage, and an improved probe depth for tissue imaging. The restricted tuneability of the dye lasers used in first attempts (Duncan et al., 1982) merely allowed imaging in a limited frequency range, not including any vibrations of natural biological molecules. In addition, excitation in the visible wavelength region resulted in a significant nonresonant background. The availability of femtosecond Ti:sapphire lasers (center wavelength at 855 nm) in the 1990s in combination with a widely tunable OPA (1.1–1.2 μm) resulted in improved image quality due to reduced generation of background originating from electronic transitions.

In addition, it gave access to molecular vibrations, for organic molecules, in the interesting region 2600–3300 cm^{-1} (Zumbusch et al., 1999). However, excitation in the wavelength region of 1.1–1.2 μm was found to be less suitable for CARS microscopy of biological cells, as the light absorption of water starts to become significant at approximately 1.15 μm. In addition, the broad spectral bandwidth of the transform-limited femtosecond laser pulses limited the spectral selectivity of the CARS signal. Numerous efforts have been made to overcome this problem by coherent control techniques (Oron et al., 2002, 2003) and spectral focusing (Hellerer et al., 2004), and today, a spectral resolution on the order of $\sim$5 cm^{-1} can be achieved with femtosecond laser systems.

The development of a picosecond dual-Ti:sapphire laser system with the aforementioned synchronization unit has also positively contributed to the spectral resolution of CARS microscopy (Cheng et al., 2001b; Jones et al., 2002; Potma et al., 2002). The lasers deliver pulses with a typical duration of 5 ps, corresponding to a spectral width of 3.6 cm^{-1}. Furthermore, they can be individually tuned in the optical window of biological matter, 700–1000 nm, giving access to most molecular vibrations of interest (100–3400 cm^{-1}) at favorable signal to background ratio levels due to the picosecond pulses. Unfortunately, the time jittering between the pulses was found to degrade the image quality significantly, despite the synchronization systems. The wish for a widely tunable picosecond laser system in the NIR range with inherent pulse synchronization prompted the development of the Nd:YVO_4 laser/OPO system (HighQ Laser Production GmbH 6830 Rankweil, Austria) emitting a highly stable 7-ps pulse train (spectral width: 3.5 cm^{-1}) through mode-locking using a semiconductor saturable absorber mirror in the pump laser. The combination of a Stokes beam fixed at 1064 nm and a tunable pump/probe beam in the range 780–930 nm gives access to a wide range of molecular vibrations (1350–3400 cm^{-1}) (Evans et al., 2005). With the use of two OPOs simultaneously pumped by a single Nd:YVO_4 laser, an even broader range of vibrations (0–3400 cm^{-1}) can be targeted (Burkacky et al.,

2006). A broad range (100–3700 cm^{-1}) is also accessible by the use of both signal and idler of a single OPO (Ganikhanov et al., 2006b).

Excellent spectral resolution of the CARS signal can be achieved in non-scanning CARS microscopy (Heinrich et al., 2004, 2006), further explained in "Measurement Techniques," which uses a nanosecond laser system. A Nd:YAG laser simultaneously emits three different beams at 1064 nm, 532 nm, and 355 nm, with a pulse duration of 3 ns. The 355-nm beam pumps an OPO, the output of which is continuously tunable between 410 and 2600 nm and serves as the Stokes beam in the CARS process. The second harmonic of the pump laser is used as the pump/probe beam. In contrast to other CARS microscope setups, the range of molecular vibrations accessible is not limited by the tuning range of the OPO but by the fulfillment of the wave-matching condition. This is a result of the excitation geometry employed (see later). The nanosecond-pulsed CARS microscopic system offers the widest spectral range to be probed (0–8000 cm^{-1}), with the disadvantage of a relatively low repetition rate (10 Hz) with the present laser system.

More laser lines are necessary if one wishes to probe not only one molecular vibration but two vibrations simultaneously, as, for instance, in dual-CARS microscopy (Burkacky et al., 2006). With broadband laser sources, even multiplex CARS microscopy (Cheng et al., 2002c; Müller et al., 2002) is possible within a limited vibrational region. This is done by synchronizing two tunable mode-locked Ti:Sapphire lasers: one narrow bandwidth laser (10 ps, bandwidth $\sim$1.5 cm^{-1}) acting as a pump/probe beam at a fixed wavelength and one broad bandwidth laser (80 fs, bandwidth $\sim$184 cm^{-1}), the Stokes beam, tunable from 700 to 1000 nm. This tunability allows access to a vibrational frequency range of 0–4000 cm^{-1}. The narrow-band laser sets the spectral resolution, while the broadband laser determines the spectral width of the generated CARS spectrum. Multiplex CARS microscopy is also possible by the use of a nonlinear fiber instead of a broadband laser system. Cicerone and coworkers (Kee and Cicerone, 2004) have realized a cost-efficient laser source on the basis of a single mode-locked femtosecond Ti:sapphire laser system combined with a nonlinear fiber. In short, a femtosecond pulse train is spectrally dispersed and split into two beams, one narrow bandwidth pulse train ($\sim$13 cm^{-1}) acting as the pump beam and one generating a broadband continuum inside a tapered nonlinear fiber. The long-wavelength part of the continuum forms the Stokes beam. With this approach, broadband multiplex CARS microscopy is possible over a vibrational range covering 2500 cm^{-1}, with a spectral resolution of 13 cm^{-1}.

10.6 DATA ACQUISITION

The generated CARS signal is typically detected by means of a Photomultiplier Tube (PMT) (Cheng et al., 2002b) or an avalanche photodiode (Duncan et al., 1982), depending on whether speed or sensitivity is an issue. Spectral measurements, as in multiplex CARS microscopy, require a Charge-Coupled Device

(CCD) camera attached to a spectrometer (Cheng et al., 2002c; Müller et al., 2002). The detector is mounted on the microscope such that either the transmitted (forward detection) or the back-scattered CARS light (epidetection) is collected, as outlined in Figure 10.5a. In order to prevent the excitation light, background light, and possible sum and mixing terms from being recorded, several optical filters are placed in front of the detector. For the generation of two-dimensional images, the sample is usually scanned by the excitation beams, which can be done in two ways; either the sample is physically translated with a piezo-driven stage (Duncan et al., 1982) or the position of the laser beam is scanned over the sample fixed on the microscope table with a pair of galvanometric mirrors (Cheng et al., 2002b). Mirror scanning in combination with a PMT detection system represents the fastest possibility for obtaining a CARS image with a confocal setup, enabling video-rate CARS microscopy with an acquisition of 20 frames per second (0.16 μs per pixel) (Evans et al., 2005). In addition, by either moving the sample or the microscope objective in the axial direction (z-direction), a series of two-dimensional CARS images can be collected, forming a three-dimensional image of the object.

Scanning can, however, be avoided by means of wide-field CARS microscopy (Heinrich et al., 2004, 2006) This nonscanning technique allows excellent time resolution, down to nanoseconds. Full-frame images can be collected instantaneously by means of an intensified, gated CCD imaging system mounted on one of the detection ports of the microscope, as illustrated in Figure 10.5b. Such wide-field, “snap-shot” CARS microscopic images, obtained by a single set of excitation pulses (pump/probe + Stokes), are shown in Figure 10.6. The upper row presents images of a test sample consisting of a 7-μm polystyrene bead at resonance (middle) and off-resonance (right). Detuning the pump frequency by 20 cm^{-1} results in a complete loss of the CARS signal, an indication of high spectral resolution and weak background signal from water. The left image shows the sample imaged with dark-field illumination. In the lower row of Figure 10.6, corresponding single-pulse pictures are shown for a biological sample, a water–olive oil emulsion. A strong resonant CARS signal is visible when tuning to the symmetric $C—H_2$ stretching vibration at 2850 cm^{-1} (middle). By detuning to 3100 cm^{-1}, the CARS signal again vanishes completely.

The CARS signal can also be collected by scanning an optical fiber probe (Schaller et al., 2002) or a silver coated silicon cantilever tip (Ichimura et al., 2004) over the sample. This near-field scanning approach allows spatial resolution far beyond the diffraction limit of light. For the subwavelength (50 nm) aperture fiber probe, only the locally emitted CARS photons have a chance to transmit into and tunnel through the fiber. This results in a spatial resolution of ~128 nm at the cost of the optical signal. For the metallic probe, an enhancement of the CARS polarization is achieved at the proximity of the tip and the signal is collected in the epi-mode by a high NA objective. The resolution is estimated to a few tens of nanometers.

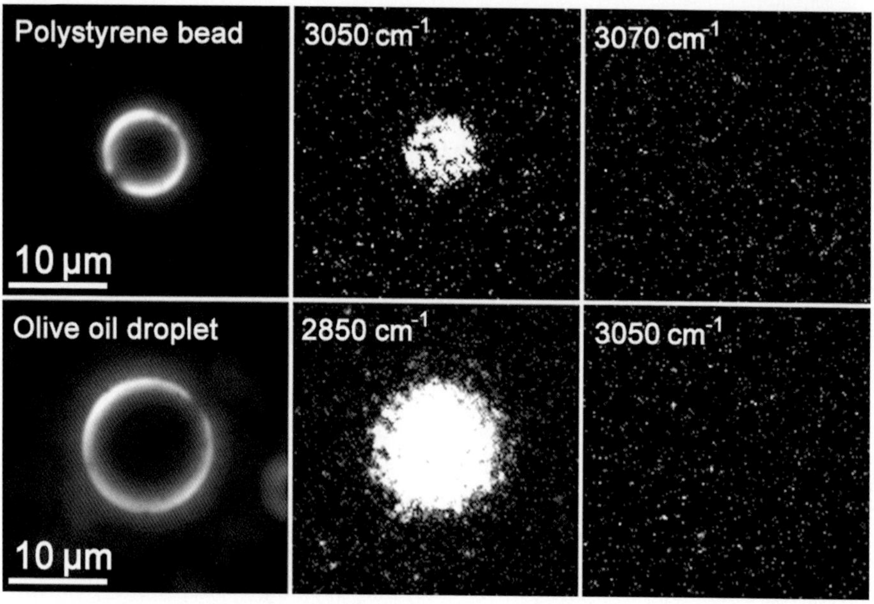

Figure 10.6. Snap-shot images of a polystyrene bead and an oil droplet recorded with *single* nanosecond pulses in nonscanning CARS microscopy. Left, dark-field images; middle, resonant CARS images by exciting the antisymmetric C—H stretching vibration at 3050 cm^{-1} or symmetric C—H_2 stretching vibration at 2850 cm^{-1}; right, nonresonant background by detuning the Stokes beam by 20 cm^{-1} or 200 cm^{-1} from the CARS resonance.

10.7 MEASUREMENT TECHNIQUES

Despite the short history of CARS microscopy, several different experimental protocols have been investigated in order to improve the resolution and sensitivity, many of which are inspired by macroscopic CARS spectroscopy (Eesley, 1981). There are numerous experimental parameters to vary, the most common of which are covered here: the excitation geometry, detection geometry, time-resolved detection, phase-sensitive detection, and amplitude-modulated detection.

10.7.1 Excitation Geometry

The formation of a beating excitation field in the probe volume at the vibrational resonance requires not only that the frequency is matched ($\omega_{aS} = 2\omega_p$-ω_S) but also that the excitation beam geometry is such that their wavevectors fulfill the phase-matching condition ($\overline{\Delta k} = \overline{k}_{aS} - 2\overline{k}_P + \overline{k}_S = 0$. The importance of this can be noted in Eq. 10.1, which tells us that the argument of the *sinc* function, $\overline{\Delta k}L$, must be minimized in order to boost the CARS signal. The most straightforward excitation geometry that satisfies the wave-matching condition for a nondispersive sample is the collinear beam geometry. Thus, it is not so surprising that this was the excitation geometry used in the very first CARS microscope (Duncan et al., 1982). A strong CARS signal was obtained; however, the long interaction length in the axial direction led to poor axial resolution and an overwhelming nonresonant background. In 1999, Zumbusch et al. circumvented this problem by means of a *confocal* CARS setup, similar to that shown in Figure 10.5a, employing tightly focussed beams of NIR laser pulses and oil-immersion objectives of high NA (NA = 1.4) (Zumbusch et al., 1999). Tight focusing in space leads to a narrow interaction length L and consequently "relaxes" the phase-matching condition, as it ascertains that the argument of the *sinc* function is small. Furthermore, the tight focussing assures a distribution of wavevectors, resulting in many combinations that fulfill the wave-matching condition. The confocal setup additionally enhances the axial resolution. In addition, as the generation of the CARS signal is limited to the high intensity, central part of the focal volume because of the nonlinear dependence on the excitation intensities, it offers three-dimensional sectioning. Owing to the many advantages, this confocal excitation geometry is most frequently used, although the so-called folded BOXCARS geometry has also been explored (Müller et al., 2000).

Wide-field CARS microscopy, a nonscanning variant of CARS microscopy as illustrated in Figure 10.5b, requires the use of a noncollinear beam geometry (Heinrich et al., 2004, 2006). The intensities of nanosecond excitation beams are distributed homogeneously over the whole sample region of interest. A complete CARS image from the entire region of interest can thus be obtained using a set of single laser pulses. Special noncollinear beam geometry (extremely folded BOXCARS) is implemented, which utilizes an ultradark-field condenser to deliver a cone of light at the frequency ω_p from earlier, while the Stokes beam is coupled through the objective of the inverted microscope from below. This gives rise to an anti-Stokes beam that counterpropagates relative to the Stokes beam and can conveniently be collected by the microscope objective. This kind of beam arrangement gives rise to a narrow interaction zone where all beams overlap, thus improving the axial resolution compared to collinear beam geometry. Extremely folded BOXCARS excitation also allows for optical sectioning, as demonstrated in Figure 10.7. The sample depicted contains 2-and 5-μm polystyrene beads. They were imaged by means of a Stokes beam at 1064 nm and pump/probe beam at 803.2 nm, exciting the vibrational resonance at 3052 cm^{-1} corresponding to the antisymmetric C—H stretching vibration. The axial resolution can be estimated from the fact that the two smaller beads in the center of the image can be axially resolved and illuminated *separately* by displacing the objective lens by 2 μm. Note that the axial resolution also strongly depends on the position of the dark-field condenser (NA = 1.3), which confines the generation of the CARS signal in the axial direction to a region only a few micrometers wide. The lateral resolution is determined to correspond to the diffraction limit, as in a conventional light microscope.

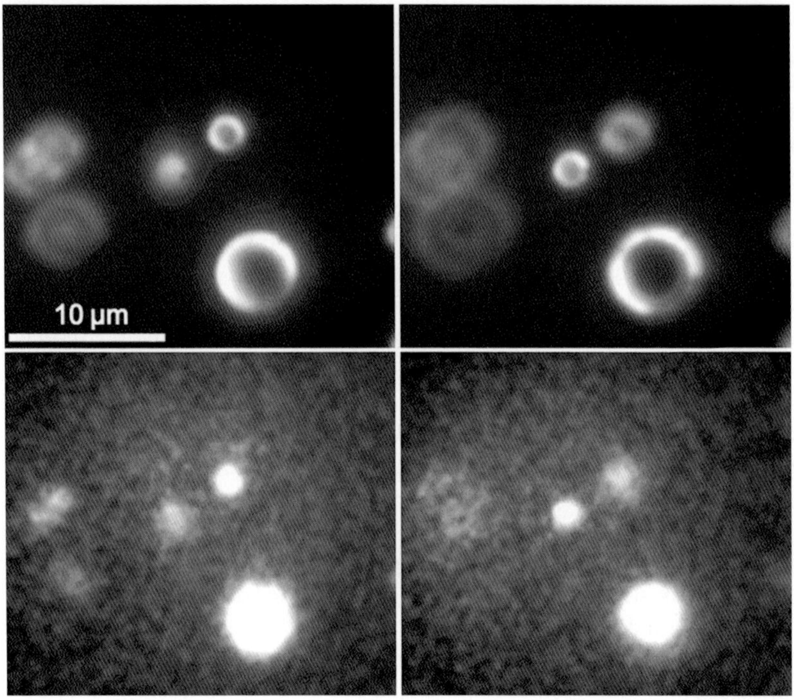

Figure 10.7. Experimental demonstration of optical sectioning in wide-field CARS microscopy for 2- and 5-μm polystyrene beads.

10.7.2 Detection Geometry

The major difficulty in CARS microscopy of condensed samples is that the resonant signal is accompanied by a significant inherent, nonresonant background, which negatively influences the signal to noise ratio and consequently the sensitivity. Thus, it is crucial to optimize the detection geometry of the CARS microscope such that the contribution from the nonresonant background is suppressed. This can be accomplished by detecting the CARS signal in the backward direction relative to the excitation beams, so-called epidetection. It delivers high contrast, particularly for scatterers smaller than the excitation wavelengths (Cheng et al., 2001b; Volkmer et al., 2001). For a monolayer of dipoles in a plane orthogonal to the propagation of the excitation fields, the emitted radiation shows a symmetrical pattern in the axial direction. Coherent addition of the radiation fields from a multilayer of dipoles lined up in axial direction, however, results in the generation of a large signal in the forward direction and a weak signal in the backward direction because of constructive and destructive interference. Thus, small objects emit as much CARS signal (both resonant and nonresonant) in the backward as in the forward direction, whereas the signal from larger objects is primarily forward directed. Using detection in the backward direction, the signal from small objects can be detected selectively without the impact of the large, forward-going nonresonant signal from the surrounding medium. The epidetection geometry has been shown to significantly improve the sensitivity of CARS microscopy for objects smaller than or in the order of the wavelength (Cheng et al., 2001b; Volkmer et al., 2001).

10.7.3 Time-Resolved Detection

Volkmer et al. have investigated the possibility of suppressing the nonresonant background in the time domain by means of pulsed-sequenced excitation (Volkmer et al., 2002). In this approach, three incident femtosecond pulse trains are required, of which one (the probe beam) interacts with the sample at a certain time delay τ relative to the other two, the pump and Stokes, beams. By varying the time delay, the time-dependence of the molecular vibration can be recorded, termed the *Raman Free Induction Decay* (RFID). As the nonresonant contribution is instantaneous, it can be separated from the resonant CARS signal by detection at a time delay of a few hundreds of femtosecond after excitation. Unfortunately, the improved signal to background ratio is accompanied by a significant reduction of the resonant CARS signal.

10.7.4 Phase-Sensitive Detection

Another possibility of improving the sensitivity of CARS microscopy is to utilize the fact that resonant objects induce a phase shift in the emitted CARS signal, whereas the nonresonant part is not associated with any shifts in phase. This results in a polarization difference between the resonant and nonresonant CARS fields (Cheng et al., 2001a). It is quantified by the depolarization ratio of the resonant object relative to the nonresonant solvent, which typically is 1/3. By excitation with linearly polarized pump/probe and Stokes fields having a relative difference in polarization direction of $\Phi = 71.6^\circ$, optimal separation of the nonresonant component from the resonant signal is achieved (Cheng et al., 2001a) by rotating an analyser positioned in front of the detector orthogonally with respect to the direction of the nonresonant polarization. Unfortunately, the resonant CARS signal is also reduced, which prevents the detection of weak Raman resonances using this approach.

The difficulty in imaging weak resonant signals overwhelmed by a strong nonresonant part can be circumvented by the interference with an intense nonresonant field that acts as a local oscillator: heterodyne CARS microscopy (Potma et al., 2006). In short, the pump and Stokes beams are collinearly combined and sent into a Mach-Zehnder-type interferometer. In one arm a strong nonresonant signal at the anti-Stokes frequency is generated in a reference sample. Alternatively, it can be generated in a photonic crystal fiber (Andresen et al., 2006). A phase modulation is applied at 10 MHz to this local oscillator beam, which is then recombined with the pump and Stokes beams by means of a dichroic mirror and collinearly sent into the microscope. The CARS signal, consisting of both nonresonant and resonant parts, generated in the sample is mixed with the co-propagating local oscillator field and finally detected by means of lock-in detection in order to isolate the heterodyne signal. This interferometric detection scheme allows the recovery of both the real and the imaginary parts of the third-order nonlinear susceptibility, resulting in imaging free of nonresonant background and a signal that is linearly dependent on the concentration of vibrational modes (Evans et al., 2004; Potma et al., 2006).

10.7.5 Amplitude-Modulated Detection

The separation of the nonresonant background from the CARS signal can also be accomplished by fast switching (>500 kHz) between resonant and pure nonresonant excitation. This results in an amplitude-modulated CARS signal. In practice, it can be achieved by alternately coupling two pump beams with two different wavelengths together with a common Stokes beam into the CARS microscope (Ganikhanov et al., 2006a). One pair excites the target molecules resonantly, while the second pair, slightly detuned, generates a pure nonresonant CARS signal. The constant nonresonant and the tuning-dependent resonant parts can then be separated with lock-in detection, improving the CARS signal detection sensitivity. This can also be achieved by means of dual-CARS microscopy, where the two pump/probe beams are jointly coupled into the microscope together with the Stokes beam. A resonant vibration and the nonresonant background can then be probed simultaneously using a dual-channel detector system (Burkacky et al., 2006).

10.8 APPLICATIONS

CARS microscopy has the ability to selectively visualize chemical species based on differences in their characteristic vibrational properties, allowing qualitative and quantitative mapping without the need to introduce artificial labels. Thus, this novel microscopic technique enables chemical imaging of living matter under close to natural conditions and is therefore considered to have a strong potential within the field of biological imaging. Time-resolved imaging of normal and malign biochemical processes, of dynamic changes in intra- and intercellular distributions of a target molecule, and of changes in molecular structure is foreseen. With improved sensitivity this should be possible for a broad range of molecular species. Thus, CARS microscopy is anticipated to take a complementary and just as important a role as that fluorescence microscopy presently plays within the biosciences. This expectation is supported by the growing number of applied studies emerging in well-recognized scientific journals, providing unique insights into a wide range of relevant biological and medical topics: composition and function of biological membranes, functional nutrients, cellular lipid dynamics and metabolism, cell hydrodynamics, growth of tumor cells, and tissue imaging of axonal myelin and skin.

10.8.1 Imaging of Biological Membranes

Despite its simple basic structure, namely, a phospholipid bilayer, the biological membrane is a complex organelle with multiple important tasks. It does not merely act as a passive barrier between cells or cellular subcompartments but regulates inter- and intracellular signal transduction and molecule transport in a subtle manner by local variations in the lipid composition (Simons et al., 2000). In order to study membrane microheterogeneity in detail and to elucidate possible molecular mechanisms behind membrane function, atomic force microscopy, single-particle tracking, and various high sensitivity fluorescence microscopic techniques are employed, all restricted to either *in vitro* studies or labeled molecules. As the intrinsic properties of lipids, such as their mobility and thermodynamic state, are altered *in vitro* and are severely influenced by labeling molecules, there is a profound need for new methods to study the function of lipid domains in biological membranes. CARS microscopy may serve as an important alternative, particularly multiplex CARS microscopy, as shown by several recent studies. It provides detailed spectral information over a vibrational region of ~400 cm^{-1}. By comparing trans- and gauche characteristic C—C skeletal stretching modes of the lipid acyl chains in the range 1000–1200 cm^{-1}, the thermodynamic state of the lipids (gel or liquid crystalline phase) in membranes can be characterized and visualized (Müller et al., 2002). This is also possible by relating the CH_2 and CH_3 stretching modes in the spectral range of 2800–3000 cm^{-1} (Cheng et al., 2002c; Rinia et al., 2007; Wurpel et al., 2004). The lipid density can be quantified, and even the orientation of the CH bonds in the lipid chains can be visualized by polarization sensitive imaging of the CH_2 stretch vibration (Potma and Xie, 2003; Wurpel et al., 2005).

10.8.2 Studies of Functional Nutrients

The ability of chemical imaging offered by CARS microscopy presents tempting opportunities for unique studies within nutrient research and industry. By simultaneously collecting images of the C=C (1660 cm^{-1}) and CH_2 (2845 cm^{-1}) stretch vibrations of lipids, a ratio can be formed, reflecting the relative contents of unsaturated fatty acids (Enejder et al., 2007). This is a highly relevant parameter, as it has been shown that dietary supplementation of Polyunsaturated Fatty Acids (PUFAs) such as in omega-3 has a positive health effect by repressing lipid synthesis and increasing lipid oxidation in adipose tissue (Sampath et al., 2004). Figure 10.8 a dual-CARS image, representing CH_2 and C=C vibrations, shows a glycerol tripalmitate crystal composed of a saturated fatty acid found to large extent in mammalian lipids (e.g., cream, milk, meat). The crystal is surrounded by omega-3 oil extracted from fish, with high contents of PUFAs. The crystal generates a strong resonant CARS signal at the general lipid vibration of CH_2, whereas merely nonresonant background light can be observed at the C=C vibration, typical for unsaturated lipids. In contrast, the omega-3 oil generates a resonant signal not only at the general lipid vibration but also at the C=C vibration because of the presence of PUFAs. This allows visual separation of lipids at

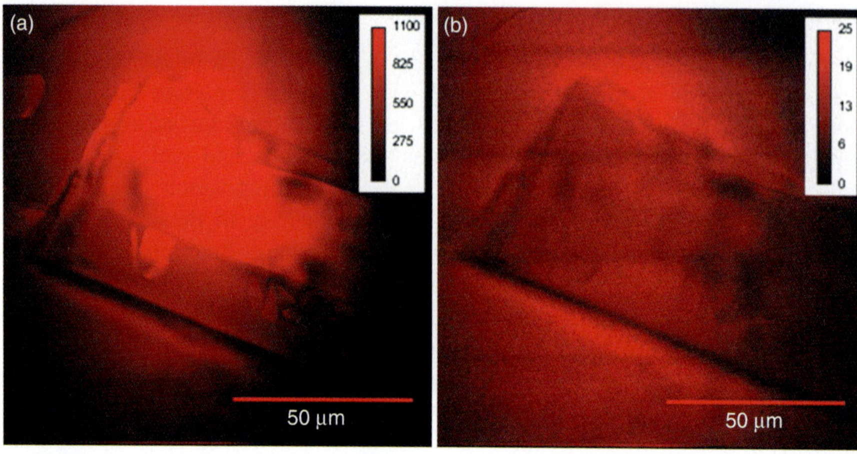

Figure 10.8. A dual-CARS microscopic image probing (a) the CH_2 vibration (2845 cm^{-1}) and (b) the C═C vibration (1660 cm^{-1}) for chemical imaging of the proportion of saturated and unsaturated lipids. A glycerol tripalmitate crystal is shown, composed of saturated fatty acids typically found in mammalian lipids, as, for instance, in cream. It generates a strong resonant CARS signal at the CH_2 vibrational frequency in (a) and merely a nonresonant background at the C═C vibration in (b). The crystal is surrounded by omega-3 oil from fish, with high contents of unsaturated fatty acids that generates a resonant signal at both vibrations. Excitation powers were 40 mW (pump/probe beam at 817 nm, CH_2), 38 mW (pump/probe beam at 907 nm, C═C), and 28 mW (Stokes beam at 1064 nm) with an integration time of 20 s.

a microscopic level with respect to their degree of saturation, and possibly also dynamic changes thereof.

10.8.3 Lipid Dynamics and Metabolism in Living Cells and Organisms

One of the strongest Raman scatterers in biological matter is the C—H bond with its different symmetric and antisymmetric stretch vibrations in the range of 2845–2950 cm^{-1}. All organic molecules contain C—H bonds, but lipids have a dominating fraction. Thus, in living matter, lipids are the most likely molecules to fulfill the minimum requirements to generate a coherent signal larger than the nonresonant background. By tuning the wavelengths of the excitation beams to match the C—H stretch vibrations, the principle organelle observed in most living cells are consequently the lipid droplet, primarily consisting of densely packed triacylglycerols (Zweytick et al., 2000). They can vary in number and size, from several micrometer-sized droplets typically observed in yeast cells (Fig. 10.9a) to a 100-μm-large reservoir filling the entire cell, as in the case of the mammalian fat-storing cell, the adipocyte (Fig. 10.9b).

Owing to the urgent need for better understanding of mammalian lipid storage and metabolism regulation, in order to explain the mechanisms behind metabolic

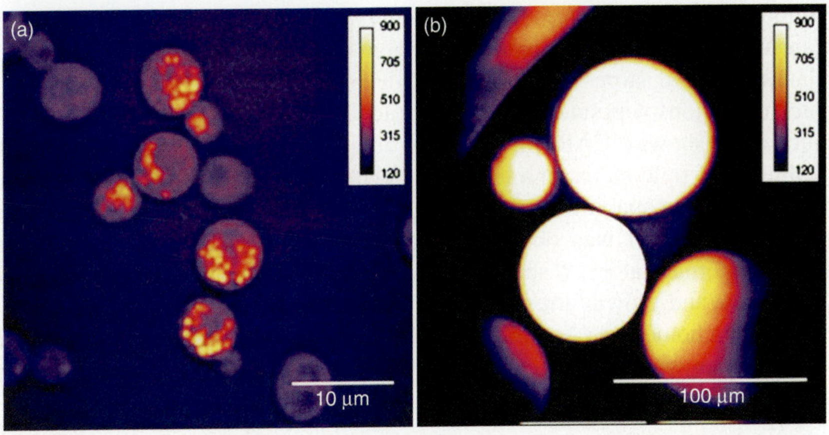

Figure 10.9. CARS microscopic images of lipid stores with (a) a size less than 1μm in yeast cells and (b) completely filling the entire cell in human adipocytes (diameters of 30–80 μm). The CH_2 vibration (2845 cm^{-1}) was probed with a pump/probe beam at 817 nm accompanied by a Stokes beam at 1064 nm. Excitation powers were 40 mW for the pump/probe beam and 28 mW for the Stokes beam, with an integration time of 20 s.

diseases, this has been the focus of several applied CARS microscopic studies. Nan et al., monitored the accumulation of lipid stores in 3T3-L1 cells during their differentiation into an adipocyte phenotype with many of the morphological, biochemical, and insulin-responsive features of the normal rodent adipocyte (Nan et al., 2003). The authors report that the lipid stores are newly synthesized during the differentiation process, following a clearance of the initially accumulated lipid deposits. The same group has studied the trafficking of lipid stores in mouse adrenal cortical cells and concludes that it occurs primarily in a subdiffusive manner in general (Nan et al., 2006). However, in conjunction with the production of steroid hormones, an active transport of the lipid deposits along the microtubules was observed for interaction with mitochondria. The accumulation of lipid stores has also been monitored in human hepatoma cells exposed to a drug for treatment of hepatitis C, altering the number and size of peroxisomes (Rakic et al., 2006).

Recently, wide-field CARS microscopy has been employed to distinguish cultivated mouse pre-adipocytes that were fed different diets (linoleic acid vs arachidonic acid), using the ratio between the strong —C—H CARS signal at 2850 cm^{-1} and the =C—H vibration around 3015 cm^{-1} for distinction (Heinrich et al., 2008). The quantitative comparison is challenging, since the =C—H resonance is weak, but it was possible to quantitatively assess differences on the order of only 5% in the concentration of polyunsaturated fatty lipids, which was checked against control measurements by High Performance Liquid Chromatography (HPLC). This nicely demonstrates that CARS microscopy can investigate lipid metabolism at the level of *individual* cells, which is clearly not possible in chromatography.

Lipid metabolism is regulated not only at a cellular level but also at an organism-wide level by the endocrine system and environmental cues. The accumulation of lipid stores during normal development as well as during stress-related conditions was studied in the nematode *C. elegans* (Hellerer et al., 2007). Figure 10.10 shows a CARS microscopic volume image of the three-dimensional distribution of lipid stores in a living *C. elegans* nematode, illustrating the excellent 3D-imaging capabilities of scanning CARS microscopy. A low energy status at the cellular level was observed to trigger the mobilization of lipid stores, whereas external caloric restriction and other environmental stresses promoted lipid storage and growth arrest. As the lipid regulatory genes of *C. elegans* have many human homologs (Ashrafi et al., 2003), these observations may contain relevant information with respect to the worldwide search for the causes of obesity.

10.8.4 Cell Hydrodynamics

The largest Raman cross section in biological matter is that of the O—H stretch mode in a broad range of 3000–3800 cm^{-1}, characteristic of liquid water. Water plays a principal and versatile role in cell and molecular biology. It influences protein and nucleic acid structure and function, as well as overall cellular activity. Thus, a method by which hydrodynamical phenomena can be observed at a cellular level is likely to provide unique insight into the tasks and properties of the most abundant molecule in living matter. The potential of CARS microscopy

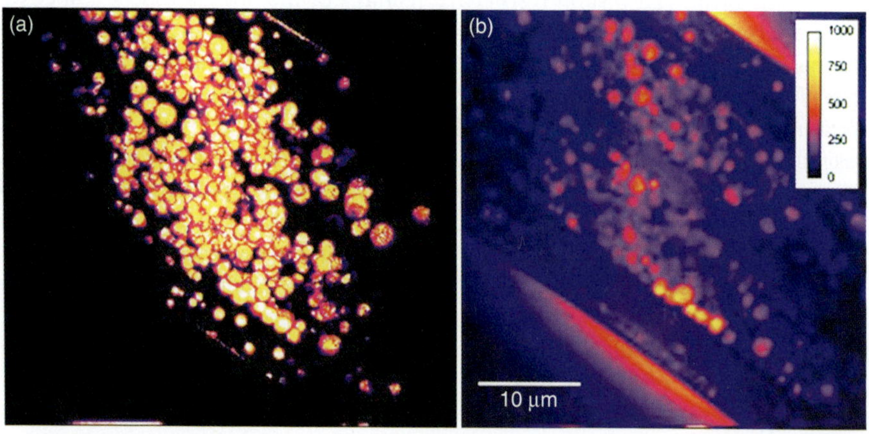

Figure 10.10. A normalized CARS volume image (a) showing the three-dimensional distribution of lipid stores in a living *C. elegans* nematode *(daf-2* mutant, L3). The volume image was reconstructed from a z-stack of 67 slides (40 × 40 μm) covering a depth of 20.1 μm, each with an integration time of 20 s. One of the central image planes is shown in (b), where the number of CARS photons registered is color coded according to the color bar. The CH_2 vibration at 2845 cm^{-1} was probed with the excitation powers 7.5 mW (1064 nm) and 15 mW (817 nm). This nicely illustrates the superior three-dimensional imaging capabilities of CARS microscopy.

for this has been illustrated by monitoring the plasma membrane permeability of water for the amoebae *Dictyostelium discoideum* (Potma et al., 2001). By flushing the cells with D_2O as a contrast agent while probing the O—H vibration, line scans of the CARS signal were collected versus time, indicating the presence of a region in the vicinity of the membrane where the mobility of water is reduced. By probing the O—H stretch mode of interlamellar water molecules in concentric phospholipid bilayers in combination with the CH_2 stretch mode of lipid hydrocarbon chains, an ordering of water molecules was observed (Cheng et al., 2003). It was shown that the water molecules align with their symmetry axis along the direction normal to the bilayer. Thus, this suggests that not only the distribution but also the orientation of specific molecules can be visualized by means of CARS microscopy.

10.8.5 Tumor Cells

The unique ability of CARS microscopy for imaging with high resolution in three dimensions was utilized for the monitoring of growth and invasion of the brain tumor *glioblastoma multiforme* (Kaufman et al., 2005). By varying the properties of the model tissue matrix, consisting of a three-dimensional collagen matrix, it was shown that the density of collagen fibers determines the tumor growth pattern.

10.8.6 Tissue Imaging

Owing to the low absorption and scattering properties of biological matter for the NIR excitation light typically used for CARS microscopy, images of cells in tissue can also be collected. The ordering degree of lipids in the axonal myelin sheath was visualized in spinal cord white matter samples from guinea pigs, showing that the lipids are in the liquid ordered phase (Haifeng et al., 2005). In addition, water molecules residing between adjacent bilayers of the myelin sheath were shown to be ordered with their symmetry axis perpendicular to that of the CH_2 groups of the lipids. A useful probe depth in spinal cord tissue, still allowing clear contrast of parallel axons, was estimated to be approximately 250 μm. This shows the potential for the use of CARS microscopy for studies of spinal cord injuries as well as the important category of demyelinating diseases.

Video-rate CARS microscopy shows the potential for imaging dynamic phenomena in living tissue in real time. This was exemplified in the skin of a mouse *in vivo*, clearly depicting the sebaceous glands, corneocytes, and adipocytes at a probe depth of up to 100 μm (Evans et al., 2005). However, the probe depth was limited by the working distance of the microscope objective. The diffusion of externally applied mineral oil was monitored; it penetrated the stratum corneum, although it did not reach the dermis.

The development of fiber-based CARS microscopy promises imaging of tissue in living organisms, even of deeper lying organs (Legare et al., 2006).

10.8.7 Imaging of Proteins and DNA

The Raman cross sections of DNA and protein are significantly lower than that of lipids. Thus, few studies of these relevant macromolecules have been conducted so far, as it requires the development of techniques that allow an improvement of the sensitivity by at least an order of magnitude. Large efforts are presently made to reduce the impact of the nonresonant background (Burkacky et al., 2006; Cheng et al., 2001a; Ganikhanov et al., 2006a; Potma et al., 2006; Volkmer et al., 2002; von Vacano et al., 2006;) and to enhance the signal by means of surface-enhanced Raman scattering (Koo et al., 2005) and thereby enable the visualization of weak Raman scatterers.

However, CARS images of proteins in yeast cells and epithelial cells have been reported (Cheng et al., 2001a; Hashimoto et al., 2000), and the chromosomes in an NIH3T3 cell were visualized during the metaphase by tuning to the DNA backbone vibrational band, the PO_2^- symmetric stretching vibration at 1090 cm^{-1} (Cheng and Xie, 2004). Clusters and networks of DNA have been depicted by scanning a silver tip over the sample and thus generating a locally enhanced CARS signal (Ichimura et al., 2004). Owing to an excitation volume limited to the end of the tip, a spatial resolution far beyond the diffraction limit of light was obtained.

10.9 CONCLUSIONS

CARS microscopy has many distinctive characteristics that facilitate functional imaging of complex and heterogeneous samples with high molecular specificity. As no exogenous labeling is required, samples and processes can be studied under close to natural conditions in a way not possible with present microscopic techniques. Thus, CARS microscopy has the potential to generate new and quite unique insights into the fascinating worlds of bio-, materials- and nanosciences. With major efforts being made to improve the sensitivity of the technique in order to lower the detection limit and to make the instrumentation more user-friendly and compact, it is anticipated that CARS microscopy will soon become an important tool within a broad range of disciplines.

ACKNOWLEDGEMENTS

The continuous support by the Swedish Research Council is gratefully acknowledged by A. Enejder. C. Brackmann is financially supported by the Trygger Foundation. The authors thank Madeleine Åkeson for her assistance in collecting many of the images shown. Samples were provided by Professors Marc Pilon, Lena Gustafsson, Joakim Norbeck, Malin Lönn, and Ann-Sofie Sandberg at Chalmers University of Technology and Göteborg University, Sweden. Part of the presented research was supported by the Austrian Science Fund FWF (grant P16658_N02).

REFERENCES

Andresen ER, Keiding SR, Potma EO. Picosecond anti-Stokes generation in a photonic-crystal fiber for interferometric CARS microscopy. Opt Express 2006;14:7246–7251.

Ashrafi K, Chang FY, Watts JL, Fraser AG, Kamath RS, Ahringer J, Ruvkun G. Genome-wide RNAi analysis of Caenorhabditis elegans fat regulatory genes. Nature 2003;421:268–272.

Begley RF, Harvey AB, Byer RL. Coherent anti-Stokes Raman spectroscopy. Appl Phys Lett 1974;25:387–390.

Burkacky O, Zumbusch A, Brackmann C, Enejder A. Dual-pump coherent anti-Stokes-Raman scattering microscopy. Opt Lett 2006;31:3656–3658.

Cheng JX, Book LD, Xie XS. Polarization coherent anti-Stokes Raman scattering microscopy. Opt Lett 2001a;26:1341–1343.

Cheng JX, Pautot S, Weitz DA, Xie XS. Ordering of water molecules between phospholipid bilayers visualized by coherent anti-Stokes Raman scattering microscopy. Proc Natl Acad Sci U S A 2003;100:9826–9830.

Cheng JX, Volkmer A, Book LD, Xie XS. An epi-detected coherent anti-Stokes Raman scattering (E-CARS) microscope with high spectral resolution and high sensitivity. J Phys Chem B 2001b;105:1277–1280.

Cheng JX, Volkmer A, Xie XS. Theoretical and experimental characterization of coherent anti-Stokes Raman scattering microscopy. J Opt Soc Am B 2002a;19:1363–1375.

Cheng JX, Jia YK, Zheng G, Xie XS. Laser-scanning coherent anti-Stokes Raman scattering microscopy and applications to cell biology. Biophys J 2002b;83:502–509.

Cheng JX, Volkmer A, Book LD, Xie XS. Multiplex coherent anti-Stokes Raman scattering microspectroscopy and study of lipid vesicles. J Phys Chem B 2002c; 106:8493–8498.

Cheng JX, Xie XS. Coherent anti-Stokes Raman scattering microscopy: instrumentation, theory, and applications. J Phys Chem B 2004;108:827–840.

Druet SAJ, Taran JPE. CARS spectroscopy. Prog Quantum Electron 1981;7(1):1–72.

Duncan M, Reintjes J, Manuccia T. Scanning coherent anti-Stokes Raman microscope. Opt Lett 1982;7:350–352.

Eesley GL. *Coherent Raman Spectroscopy*. New York: Pergamon Press; 1981.

Enejder A, Brackmann C, Burkacky O, Åkeson M. Dual CARS-CARS microscopy. In: Periasamy A, So PTC, editors. *Multiphoton Microscopy in the Biomedical Sciences*. Proceedings of the International Society for Optical Engineering; 2007. p. 6442.

Evans CL, Potma EO, Puoris'haag M, Côté D, Lin CP, Xie XS. Chemical imaging of tissue *in vivo* with video-rate coherent anti-Stokes Raman scattering microscopy. Proc Natl Acad Sci U S A 2005;102(46):16807–16812.

Evans CL, Potma EO, Xie XS. Coherent anti-Stokes Raman scattering spectral interferometry: determination of the real and imaginary components of nonlinear susceptibility chi(3) for vibrational microscopy. Opt Lett 2004;29:2923–2925.

Ganikhanov F, Carrasco S, Xie SX, Katz M, Seitz W, Kopf D. Broadly tunable dual-wavelength light source for coherent anti-Stokes Raman scattering microscopy. Opt Lett 2006b;31(9):1292–1294.

Ganikhanov F, Evans CL, Saar BG, Xie XS. High-sensitivity vibrational imaging with frequency modulation coherent anti-Stokes Raman scattering (FM CARS) microscopy. Opt Lett 2006a;31(12):1872–1874.

Haifeng W, Fu Y, Zickmund P, Shi R, Cheng JX. Coherent anti-Stokes Raman scattering imaging of axonal myelin in live spinal tissues. Biophys J 2005;89:581–591.

Hashimoto M, Araki T, Kawata S. Molecular vibration imaging in the fingerprint region by use of coherent anti-Stokes Raman scattering microscopy with a collinear configuration. Opt Lett 2000;25:1768–1770.

Heinrich C, Bernet S, Ritsch-Marte M. Wide-field coherent anti-Stokes Raman scattering microscopy. Appl Phys Lett 2004;84:816–818.

Heinrich C, Bernet S, Ritsch-Marte M. Nanosecond microscopy with spectroscopic resolution. New J Phys 2006;8:36–43.

Heinrich C, Hofer A, Ritsch A, Ciardi C, Bernet S, Ritsch-Marte M. Selective imaging of saturated and unsaturated lipids by wide-field CARS-microscopy. Opt Express 2008;16:2597–2708.

Hellerer T, Axäng C, Brackmann C, Hillertz P, Pilon M, Enejder A. Monitoring of lipid storage in *C. elegans* using CARS microscopy. Proc Natl Acad Sci U S A 2007;104:14658–14663.

Hellerer T, Enejder AMK, Zumbusch A. Spectral focusing: high spectral resolution spectroscopy with broad-bandwidth laser pulses. Appl Phys Lett 2004;85:25–27.

Ichimura T, Hayazawa N, Hashimoto M, Inouye Y, Kawata S. Tip-enhanced coherent anti-Stokes Raman scattering for vibrational nanoimaging. Phys Rev Lett 2004;92(22):220801.

Jones DJ, Potma EO, Cheng JX, Burfeindt B, Pang Y, Ye J, Xie XS. Synchronization of two passively mode-locked, picosecond lasers within 20 fs for coherent anti-Stokes Raman scattering microscopy. Rev Sci Instrum 2002;73(8):2843–2848.

Kaufman LJ, Brangwynne CP, Kasza KE, Filippidi E, Gordon VD, Deisboeck TS, Weitz DA. Glioma expansion in collagen I matrices: analyzing collagen concentration-dependent growth and motility patterns. Biophys J 2005;89:635–650.

Kee TW, Cicerone MT. Simple approach to one-laser, broadband coherent anti-Stokes Raman scattering microscopy. Opt Lett 2004;29(23):2701–2703.

Koo TW, Chan S, Berlin AA. Single-molecule detection of biomolecules by surface-enhanced coherent anti-Stokes Raman scattering. Opt Lett 2005;30(9):1024–1026.

Legare F, Evans CL, Ganikhanov F, Xie XS. Towards CARS endoscopy. Opt Express 2006;14(10):4427–4432.

Lotem H, Lynch RT Jr, Bloembergen N. Interference between Raman resonances in four-wave difference mixing. Phys Rev A 1976;14:1748–1755.

Maiman TH. Stimulated optical radiation in Ruby. Nature 1960;187:493–494.

Maker P, Terhune R. Study of optical effects due to an induced polarization third order in the electric field strength. Phys Rev A 1965;137:801–818.

Müller M, Schins JM. Imaging the thermodynamic state of lipid membranes with multiplex CARS microscopy. J Phys Chem B 2002;106(14):3715–3723.

Müller M, Squier J, De Lange CA, Brakenhoff GJ. CARS microscopy with folded Box-CARS phasematching. J Microsc 2000;197:150–158.

Nan XL, Cheng JX, Xie XS. Vibrational imaging of lipid droplets in live fibroblast cells with coherent anti-Stokes Raman scattering microscopy. J Lipid Res 2003;44:2202–2208.

Nan XL, Potma EO, Xie XS. Nonperturbative chemical imaging of organelle transport in living cells with coherent anti-Stokes Raman scattering microscopy. Biophys J 2006;91(2):728–735.

Oron D, Dudovich N, Silberberg Y. Single-pulse phase-contrast nonlinear Raman spectroscopy. Phys Rev Lett 2002;89:273001.

Oron D, Dudovich N, Silberberg Y. Femtosecond phase-and-polarization control for background-free coherent anti-Stokes Raman spectroscopy. Phys Rev Lett 2003;90: 213902.

Potma EO, de Boeij WP, van Haastert PJ, Wiersma DA. Real-time visualization of intracellular hydrodynamics in single living cells. Proc Natl Acad Sci USA 2001;98:1577–1582.

Potma EO, de Boeij WP, Wiersma DA. Nonlinear coherent four-wave mixing in optical microscopy. J Opt Soc Am B 2000;17:1678–1684.

Potma EO, Evans CL, Xie XS. Heterodyne coherent anti-Stokes Raman scattering (CARS) imaging. Opt Lett 2006;31(2):241–243.

Potma EO, Jones DJ, Cheng JX, Xie XS, Ye J. High-sensitivity coherent anti-Stokes Raman scattering microscopy with two tightly synchronized picosecond lasers. Opt Lett 2002;27:1168–1170.

Potma EO, Xie XS. Detection of single lipid bilayers with coherent anti-Stokes Raman scattering (CARS) microscopy. J Raman Spectrosc 2003;34:642–650.

Rajadhyaksha M, Anderson RR, Webb RH. Video-rate confocal scanning laser microscope for imaging human tissues *in vivo*. Appl Opt 1999;38:2105–2115.

Rakic B, Sagan MS, Noestheden M, Bélanger S, Nan X, Evans CL, Xie XS, Pezacki JP. Peroxisome proliferator-activated receptor alpha antagonism inhibits hepatitis C virus replication. Chem Biol 2006;13(1):23–30.

Rinia HA, Bonn M, Müller M, Vartiainen EM. Quantitative CARS spectroscopy using the maximum entropy method: the main lipid phase transition. ChemPhys Chem 2007;8(2):279–287.

Sampath H, Ntambi JM. Polyunsaturated fatty acid regulation of gene expression. Nutr Rev 2004;62(9):333–339.

Schaller RD, Ziegelbauer J, Lee LF, Haber LH, Saykaylly RJ. Chemically selective imaging of subcellular structure in human hepatocytes with coherent anti-Stokes Raman scattering (CARS) near-field scanning optical microscopy (NSOM). J Phys Chem B 2002;106:8489–8492.

Shen YR *The Principles of Nonlinear Optics*. New York: John Wiley & Sons; 1984.

Simons K, Toomre D. Lipid rafts and signal transduction. Nat Rev Mol Cell Biol 2000;1:31–39.

Volkmer A, Book LD, Xie XS. Time-resolved coherent anti-Stokes Raman scattering microscopy: imaging based on Raman free induction decay. Appl Phys Lett 2002;80(9):1505–1507.

Volkmer A, Cheng JX, Xie XS. Vibrational imaging with high sensitivity via epidetected coherent anti-Stokes Raman scattering microscopy. Phys Rev Lett 2001;87(2): 023901.

von Vacano B, Buckup T, Motzkus M. Highly sensitive single-beam heterodyne coherent anti-Stokes Raman scattering. Opt Lett 2006;31(16):2495–2497.

Wurpel GW, Rinia HA, Müller M. Imaging orientational order and lipid density in multilamellar vesicles with multiplex CARS microscopy. J Microsc 2005;218(Part 1):37–45.

Wurpel GWH, Schins JM, Müller M. Direct measurement of chain order in single phospholipid mono- and bilayers with multiplex CARS. J Phys Chem B 2004;108(11):3400–3403.

Zheltikov AM. Coherent anti-Stokes Raman scattering: from proof-of-the-principle experiments to femtosecond CARS and higher order wave-mixing generalizations. J Raman Spectrosc 2000;31(8–9):653–667.

Zumbusch A, Holtom GR, Xie XS. Three-dimensional vibrational imaging by coherent anti-Stokes Raman scattering. Phys Rev Lett 1999;82:4142–4145.

Zweytick D, Athenstaedt K, Daum G. Intracellular lipid particles of eukaryotic cells. Biochim Biophys Acta 2000;1469:101–120.

11

BIOMEDICAL SONOGRAPHY

GEORG SCHMITZ
Department for Electrical Engineering and Information Technology, Chair for Medical Engineering, Ruhr-University, Bochum, Germany

11.1 BASIC PRINCIPLES

11.1.1 Introduction

Ultrasound imaging was first introduced in 1950 by (Wild 1950) together with Reid. Since then, it developed to one of the most important diagnostic imaging modalities. With today's scanners, two-dimensional cross-sectional images of the body can be produced in real time with a spatial resolution below 1 mm. Ultrasound imaging relies on the propagation of mechanical waves with frequencies beyond the audible range into the body, the reflection and scattering of sound by tissue structures, and the registration of the echoes. Similar to sonar and radar, it is a pulse-echo ranging technique. Using the acoustical Doppler effect, the quantitative measurement of blood flow is possible, and flow velocity and direction can be presented in real time as colored overlays. To enhance the echoes from blood, ultrasound contrast media were developed. They show nonlinear behavior that can be used for their specific and sensitive detection. With the introduction of nonlinear imaging modes for contrast media also, nonlinear imaging of tissue became of interest and showed a significant improvement in many imaging situations. Recently, the higher integration of electronics and the increasing computer power led to the realization of real-time three-dimensional imaging, which is of special interest in cardiological applications.

After more than 50 years of development, ultrasound imaging is still enabling new applications, for example, by imaging of molecular markers with targeted

Biomedical Imaging: Principles and Applications, First Edition. Edited by Reiner Salzer.

contrast media or by the combination of imaging and therapy with local drug delivery.

11.1.2 Ultrasonic Wave Propagation in Biological Tissues

Ultrasound is a mechanical wave characterized by small pressure variations $p(\vec{r}, t)$ and a material displacement $\vec{x}(\vec{r}, t)$ propagating at the speed of sound c at frequencies beyond the hearing range. In biomedical sonography, typically frequencies in the range from 1 to 20 MHz are used for human examinations. In special applications such as imaging in dermatology, ophthalmology, or for small-animal imaging, higher frequencies up to 100 MHz are also common.

Soft tissues can be modeled as liquids in the respect that only longitudinal waves with the direction of displacement equal to the direction of propagation exist. The material can be described by its density ρ and compressibility κ. The propagating wave is characterized by its pressure $p(\vec{r}, t)$ and the particle velocity

$$\vec{v} = \frac{\partial \vec{x}}{\partial t}. \tag{11.1}$$

Often it is more convenient to use the velocity potential ϕ:

$$\vec{v} = -\nabla \phi \tag{11.2}$$

For small pressure variations, the wave equation can be linearized and holds in similar form for the pressure, the components of the displacement velocity, as well as for the velocity potential:

$$\nabla^2 \phi - \frac{1}{c^2} \frac{\partial^2 \phi}{\partial t^2} = 0 \tag{11.3}$$

where the speed of sound

$$c = \frac{1}{\sqrt{\rho \kappa}}. \tag{11.4}$$

The most important solutions to this equation are forward and backward traveling plane waves

$$\phi = \phi_{\mathrm{F}}(\omega t - \vec{k} \cdot \vec{r}) + \phi_{\mathrm{B}}(\omega t + \vec{k} \cdot \vec{r}). \tag{11.5}$$

In this, the wave vector $\vec{k}$ determines the direction of propagation

$$|\vec{k}| = \frac{2\pi}{\lambda} = \frac{\omega}{c} \tag{11.6}$$

where λ is the wavelength, the angular frequency $\omega = 2\pi f$, and f is the frequency of the ultrasound wave f. Wavelengths in water are in the range from 0.1 to 1 mm for the clinically used frequency range of 1.5 to 15 MHz. Pressure and particle velocity of the forward traveling plane wave have a fixed ratio, the acoustic impedance of the material

$$Z = \frac{p_F}{|\vec{v}_F|} = \sqrt{\frac{\rho}{\kappa}} = \rho c. \tag{11.7}$$

The acoustic impedance determines the reflection coefficient at a boundary between two media. For a wave traveling from a material with Z_1 to a material with Z_2 the amplitude reflection factor is

$$\Gamma = \frac{p_{1B}}{p_{1F}} = \frac{Z_2 - Z_1}{Z_2 + Z_1} \tag{11.8}$$

where p_{1B} and p_{1F} are the pressure amplitudes of the backward and forward traveling wave in material 1, respectively.

Ultrasonic imaging is based on the fact that soft tissues show only small variations in their acoustic impedance. Therefore, only a small amount of energy is reflected, which allows most of the wave's energy to propagate further into tissue. Table 11.1 shows average values of speed of sound and acoustic impedance for some tissues. A comprehensive overview of acoustical tissue parameters is given by Duck (1990). The soft tissue average is considered to be 1540 m s^{-1} and is used by most ultrasound scanners to calculate echo range from the time of echo arrival. Note that the large compressibility of air leads to an acoustic impedance close to zero. Thus, tissue–air boundaries will reflect sound totally.

11.1.3 Diffraction and Radiation of Sound

The sound field emitted from a vibrating surface can be derived by Huygen's principle: each point on the transducer aperture emits a spherical wave into the

TABLE 11.1. Speed of Sound and Acoustic Impedance for Tissues (Duck, 1990)

Material	Speed of Sound (m s^{-1})	Acoustical Impedance in MRayls = 10^6 kg m^{-2} s^{-1}
Air	330	0.0004
Water (20°C)	1480	1.48
Fat	1450	1.38
Liver	1570	1.65
Muscle	1580	1.70
Bone	3500	7.80
Soft tissue average	1540	1.63

medium, and the resulting pressure field is the superposition of the infinitesimal contributions of all source points. The mathematical formulation of this principle is the Rayleigh-Sommerfeld integral. For a sound-emitting aperture in a rigid baffle, it integrates over all source points on the transducer surface S to calculate the complex amplitude of the pressure for harmonic excitation at frequency ω (Morse and Ingard, 1968):

$$p_\omega(\vec{r}) = -j\omega\rho \iint\limits_S v_\omega(\vec{r}_0)\frac{\mathrm{e}^{jk|\vec{r}-\vec{r}_0|}}{2\pi|\vec{r}-\vec{r}_0|}\mathrm{d}\vec{r}_0. \tag{11.9}$$

Here, $v_\omega(\vec{r}_0)$ is the distribution of the complex amplitude of the velocity component normal to the emitting surface. The time varying pressure is related to the complex amplitude by

$$p(t,\vec{r}) = \mathrm{Re}\, p_\omega(\vec{r})\mathrm{e}^{j\omega t}. \tag{11.10}$$

This superposition results in field patterns that often can be calculated only by numerically solving Eq. (11.9). For example, the simulation software Field II developed by Jensen (1991) for MATLAB was used to produce the sound field simulations in the figures of this chapter.

In many situations, it is useful to analyze far field properties for which the Fraunhofer approximation holds. The far field distance is

$$d_{\mathrm{far}} = \frac{A}{\lambda}, \tag{11.11}$$

where A is the transducer area and λ is the wavelength. When the transducer is placed in the origin of a spherical coordinate system, the field distribution on a sphere with radius much greater than d_{far} will be the Fourier-transform of the aperture velocity distribution:

$$p_\omega(\vec{r}) \approx -j\omega\rho_0\frac{\mathrm{e}^{jk|\vec{r}|}}{2\pi|\vec{r}|}\iint\limits_A v_\omega(\vec{r}_0)\mathrm{e}^{-j\vec{k}\cdot\vec{r}_0}\mathrm{d}\vec{r}_0. \tag{11.12}$$

The apertures used for ultrasonic imaging are usually rectangular elements within an array of transducers. Thus, in the far field, the pressure distribution is a sinc function when all active array elements are pulsed with the same voltage, that is, energy is transmitted also in the side lobes. The side lobes in the diffraction pattern can be seen in Figure 11.1. Here, the maximum pressure of the sound field in front of a rectangular aperture built by 128 array elements with half-wavelength spacing and a total width of 28.1 mm is shown. In Figure 11.1a, the array elements are excited with identical pulses with a center frequency of 3.5 MHz. The pulses are time delayed to arrive at the focus at 40 mm at the same time. Clearly, side lobes can be seen behind the focus of the sound beam. In contrast, Figure 11.1b shows no side lobes. Here, the pulse amplitudes of the

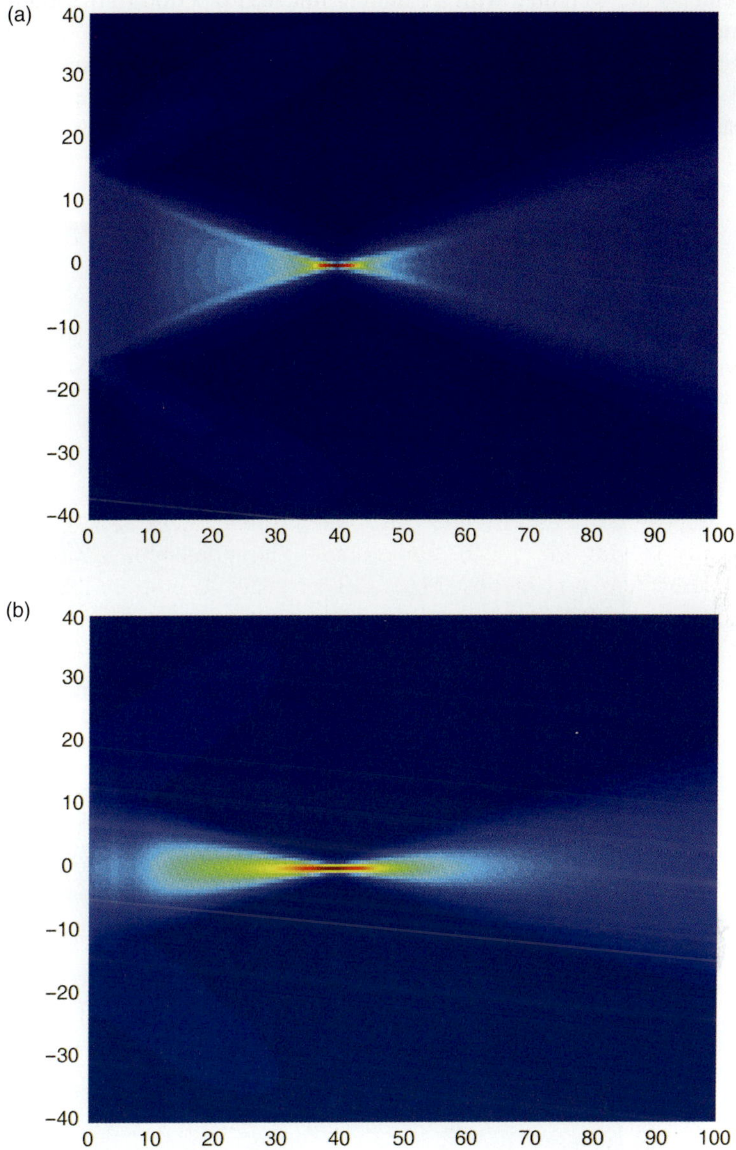

Figure 11.1. Sound field of a group of 128 rectangular array elements with half-wavelength spacing pulsed with a center frequency of 3.5 MHz. In (a), all elements are pulsed with the same amplitudes and are delayed for a focus in 40 mm distance. In (b), the focusing is identical, but the element amplitudes are varied with a Hanning window function over the length of the array. This leads not only to fewer side lobes but also to increased main lobe width and thus reduced spatial resolution in the lateral direction. Scales are in millimeters.

128 elements are weighted with a Hanning function (apodization). However, the focusing is weaker because of apodization.

In Figure 11.2, the effect of element spacing of a transducer array is demonstrated. While an element spacing of one wavelength as in Figure 11.2a is still acceptable for linear array imaging, arrays with larger element spacing such as 1.5

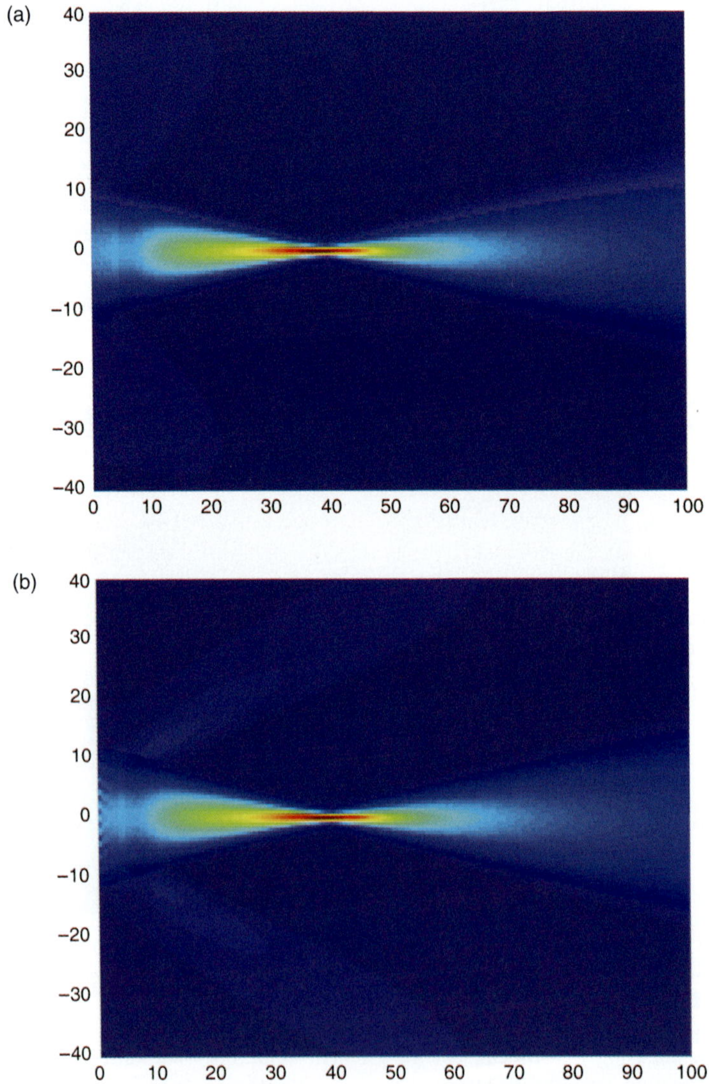

Figure 11.2. Effect of the variation of element spacing in a transducer array. Total transducer size and pulsing is kept identical to Figure 11.1(b), but element spacing is (a) one wavelength with 64 elements and (b) 1.5 wavelengths with 43 elements. Clearly, increasing grating lobes are visible.

wavelengths in Figure 11.2b show strong grating lobes, which can be explained by Eq. (11.12) in the far field as the Fourier transform of the periodic element structure. In imaging, grating lobes and side lobes will decrease imaging contrast because the system is sensitive to scatterers that lie off the main focusing direction. Usually, imaging arrays of high end systems have less than one wavelength spacing. The examples show that the design of transducer arrays and the pulsing schemes are crucial for the focusing of the sound beam and thus for image resolution.

11.1.4 Acoustic Scattering

Early ultrasonic imaging devices had a limited dynamic range and could only show reflections from tissue boundaries. However, also small fluctuations of density and compressibility at spatial dimensions at the scale of the wavelength or below scatter the sound waves. Modern ultrasound scanners have enough dynamic range to measure and display these backscattered signals. In fact, scattering from tissue provides most of the image information. Objects much larger than the wavelength show specular reflection. If the length scale of density and compressibility changes is in the range of the wavelength, resonances and complicated backscatter behavior arise. This can be seen for the example of a spherical solid elastic scatterer in water, one of the few geometrical objects for which an analytical expression of the scattered field was derived (Hickling, 1962). When scattering structures become much smaller than the wavelength of the incident wave, Rayleigh scattering is observed. Biological tissues are multiscale structures that show all of the different scattering domains simultaneously. So far, a general model for the acoustic description of biological tissue is not available. An appropriate model for the Rayleigh scattering in biological tissues can be given by modeling tissue as random fluctuations of the relative acoustic impedance (Schmitz, 2002)

$$\gamma(\vec{r}) = \frac{\Delta Z(\vec{r})}{Z_0} \tag{11.13}$$

described by its zero mean value and its autocovariance function

$$c_{\gamma\gamma}(\vec{u}) = E\gamma(\vec{r} + \vec{u})\gamma(\vec{r}) \tag{11.14}$$

where E denotes statistical expectation. The backscattering strength of the random medium is described by its backscattering coefficient (Schmitz, 2002), which can be calculated from the autocovariance function by Fourier-transformation:

$$\eta(\omega) = \frac{k^4}{16\pi^2} \int_V c_{\gamma\gamma}(\vec{u}) \mathrm{e}^{-j2\vec{k}\cdot\vec{u}} \mathrm{d}\vec{u}. \tag{11.15}$$

Its unit is per meter, and when integrated over a scattering volume, it gives the differential scattering cross section, which gives the ratio of scattered power per steradian to the incident intensity and has units of square meters. It can also be seen that the case of an ideal point scatterer can be considered by

$$c_{\gamma\gamma}(\vec{u}) = \gamma_0^2 \delta(\vec{u}) \tag{11.16}$$

and results in a constant integral and in the backscatter coefficient increasing with k^4, as known for Rayleigh scattering.

Although scattering is the cause of most of the signal power received by ultrasound scanners, it is difficult to quantify it absolutely for the purpose of tissue characterization. This is because of the unknown attenuation of intervening tissue and the dependency on the imaging system's transfer function. There have been many research efforts to analyze backscatter and its frequency dependence quantitatively to detect, for example, malignant tumors of the breast, the prostate, or the parotid gland.

11.1.5 Acoustic Losses

The wave equation, Eq. (11.3), does not include losses. In biological tissues, the relative attenuation per wavelength is small. Therefore, the attenuation can be accounted for by an additional exponential decay term for the wave amplitude. In the case of a wave propagating in the z-direction, the amplitude depends on the distance z according to

$$p(z) = p(0) \cdot \mathrm{e}^{-\alpha(f)z} = p(0) \cdot 10^{-\frac{a(f)}{20}z}. \tag{11.17}$$

Here, $\alpha(f)$ is the frequency-dependent attenuation in Nepers per centimeter. Often, attenuation is given in dB cm^{-1} as defined by $a(f)$. The frequency dependence of biological tissues can be described most correctly by a power law

$$a(f) = a_{p0} + a_p |f|^y \tag{11.18}$$

with exponents y close to one, different from the attenuation in water with $y = 2$. Ultrasound scanners typically use a limited frequency range, in which the attenuation can be approximated well to be linear with frequency

$$a(f) = a_0 + a_1 f \tag{11.19}$$

The linear attenuation coefficient is in the order of $0.5\,\mathrm{dB\,MHz^{-1}cm^{-1}}$ for soft tissues. For a typical frequency of 4 MHz and a penetration depth of 5 cm, to which sound has to travel and return, a total attenuation of $0.5\,\mathrm{dB\,MHz^{-1}cm^{-1}} \cdot 4\,\mathrm{MHz} \cdot 2 \cdot 5\,\mathrm{cm} = 20\,\mathrm{dB}$, that is, a tenth in amplitude, is expected. Considering the small reflection and backscatter coefficients in tissue, ultrasound receivers have to be very sensitive, because the maximum transmit amplitudes are limited by the onset of possible bioeffects. The total attenuation is caused by absorption and scattering, the latter accounting only for less than 15% (Bamber, 1998; Shung and Thieme, 1993).

11.1.6 Doppler Effect

When sound is transmitted and reflected or scattered by an object moving with speed v, the received sound wave is shifted in frequency. If the transmitter and receiver are in the same position and the speed of the scattering object is small compared to the speed of sound c, the frequency shift is

$$\Delta f = 2\frac{v}{c} f \cos\theta \tag{11.20}$$

where θ is the angle θ between the direction of sound propagation and the direction of the object movement. This effect can be used to measure blood flow by detecting the frequency shifts of ultrasound waves scattered back by red blood cells or ultrasound contrast media. For quantitative measurements, the angle between blood flow and sound propagation has to be measured interactively by the user. For physiological blood flow velocities (up to 3 ms^{-1} in the ascending aorta) the Doppler shifts are in the audible frequency range and can be listened to on most ultrasound imaging systems with Doppler capability.

Since blood flow velocity varies over the cross section of a blood vessel, a distribution of different velocities will be observed as a distribution of Doppler frequency shifts. Thus, a spectral decomposition of the Doppler signal allows measuring the velocity distribution within a vessel. Different Doppler measurement techniques are realized in diagnostic scanners and are discussed in more detail later.

11.1.7 Nonlinear Wave Propagation

The linear wave equation holds only for small sound pressures when it can be assumed that the material's density is proportional to the pressure. Modern diagnostic ultrasound scanners can reach local peak values of the intensity exceeding 100 W cm^{-2}, and the assumption of linearity is no longer valid. In this case, the transmitted waveform is deformed by a nonlinear transformation, leading to the generation of harmonic frequencies. In Figure 11.3, the effect on a sine-burst pulse with a center frequency of 1 MHz transmitted through 40 cm of water and measured by a hydrophone is demonstrated. The generation of higher harmonic frequencies by nonlinear propagation in tissue is used in Tissue Harmonic Imaging (THI) and often gives clearer images with higher resolution and better delineation of tissue boundaries.

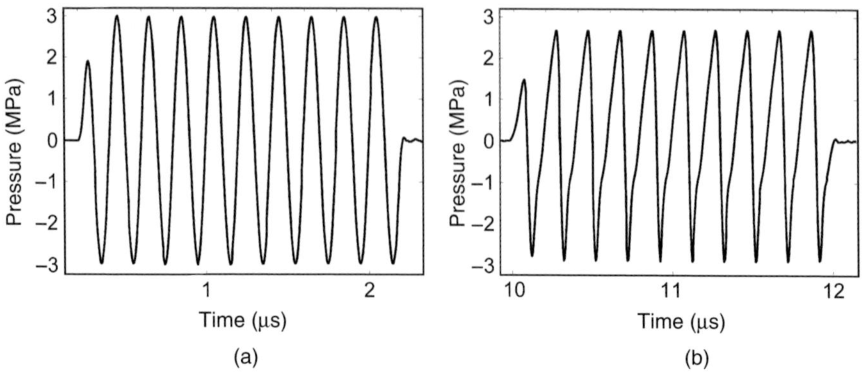

Figure 11.3. Simulation of the nonlinear wave propagation in water from an unfocused piston transducer excited with a 10-cycle sine burst. The waveform in (a) is observed at a distance of 0.3 mm to the transducer and shows a maximum peak pressure of 3 MPa. The waveform in (b) is measured at a distance of 15 mm and clearly shows the deviation from the sinusoidal waveform due to nonlinear propagation.

11.1.8 Biological Effects of Ultrasound

11.1.8.1 Thermal Effects. The absorption of ultrasound in tissue leads to a temperature increase that depends on the average intensity of the sound field. To give an indication of the temperature rise that can be expected in tissue, diagnostic ultrasonic scanners have to present a Thermal Index (TI) on the screen as part of the Output Display Standard (ODS). The TI is the ratio of the actual system power to the power needed to raise the temperature in the hottest spot of a model medium by 1°. If the TI is smaller than 0.4, it does not have to be displayed. Different TI calculations exist for soft tissue (TIS), bone (TIB), and cranial applications (TIC) in scanned and nonscanned modes. They all assume specific models that represent worst case scenarios and might not be the same as the actual scanning situation. Thus, the TI gives no measurement of the actual temperature increase but an indication of a possible risk of such an increase.

11.1.8.2 Cavitation Effects. A second effect that can be hazardous to tissue is the creation of cavitation. Cavitation may occur in the rarefactional phase of the pressure wave. It is more likely to occur if cavitation nuclei, for example, gas microbubbles, are present in the tissue. It has been shown that tissue tolerates negative pressures better at higher frequencies, and the Mechanical Index (MI) was introduced to give an indication of cavitation risk:

$$MI = \frac{p_{-,\max}}{\sqrt{f_c}} \frac{\sqrt{\text{MHz}}}{\text{MPa}} \qquad (11.21)$$

where $p_{-\max}$ is the maximum rarefactional pressure in megapascals and f_c is the center frequency in megahertz. The MI is dimensionless and takes the value of one for a maximum rarefactional pressure of 1 MPa at a frequency of 1 MHz. The MI is limited at 1.9 by the Us Food and Drug Administration (FDA), and values smaller than 0.4 do not have to be displayed. For ultrasound contrast media that consist of gas microbubbles, cavitation and additional effects such as cell membrane opening can occur and are still under investigation.

11.2 INSTRUMENTATION OF REAL-TIME ULTRASOUND IMAGING

11.2.1 Pulse-Echo Imaging Principle

Ultrasound imaging is based on the pulse-echo principle: a short sound pulse is transmitted into tissue from a focused transducer. The pulse propagates in the tissue with the speed of sound and is reflected and scattered at inhomogeneities of the acoustic material parameters. The echoes travel back to the transducer that has been switched to receive mode after transmitting the pulse. The focusing of the transducer restricts the energy of the propagating sound wave to approximately a line in a certain range around the focal depth. Current piezoelectric transducers emit short sine wave bursts with approximately a Gaussian envelope. The depth of the echo origin z can be calculated from the travel time t by

$$z = \frac{1}{2}ct \tag{11.22}$$

using the average speed of sound in tissue of 1540 m s^{-1}. A single scan line of echoes from a tissue is shown in Figure 11.4. Early medical ultrasound equipment showed such scan lines on an oscilloscope for inspection by the clinician, for example, to detect a midline shift in the brain. This representation of echo data

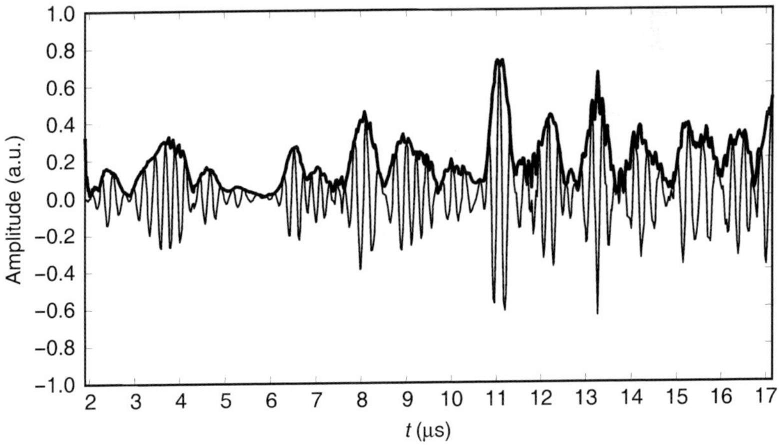

Figure 11.4. A-scan line of echoes from tissue and envelope signal without high frequency carrier signal.

is called an *A-line* or *A-scan* because the amplitude of the signal is shown. Owing to attenuation, the amplitude of the signal decays over increasing depth. Ultrasound scanners counteract with increasing the gain of the receive amplifiers with time. This Time-Gain Compensation (TGC) or Depth-Gain Compensation (DGC) is performed before analog signals are sampled and digitized to increase the dynamic range of the scanning equipment. However, in modern high end scanners, the TGC available as a setting to the clinical user is only an additional postprocessing method working on digitized data.

The information about echo strength is only contained in the envelope of the A-scan data, which can be calculated by envelope detection. The envelope of one A-scan line represents the echo strengths of objects along one line in the tissue. By moving the transducer, this line can be scanned, and a cross-sectional image of tissue is formed, in which the brightness represents the echo strength of image points. Therefore, this cross-sectional image is called a *B-scan* for *brightness scan*. The movement of the scan line can be realized by a mechanical translation or rotation of a single element transducer, as it was common in the first B-scan equipment. In today's clinical scanners, the transducer movement is realized by electronic switching of active elements of an array of small transducers as well as electronic beam forming and beam steering discussed in Section "Beamforming".

11.2.2 Ultrasonic Transducers

Currently, diagnostic ultrasound scanners use only piezoelectric transducers to generate sound waves. The scanhead of a diagnostic ultrasound scanner contains up to a few hundred transducer elements in linear arrays and up to thousands of elements in 2D arrays. The elements are driven with pulses with different time delays to influence the characteristics and directions of the sound beams interrogating the object of interest.

One transducer element consists of a piezoelectric ceramic, a typical material being lead zirconium titanate (PZT). The transducer is connected by metal electrodes on both sides as shown in Figure 11.5. The thickness of the transducer

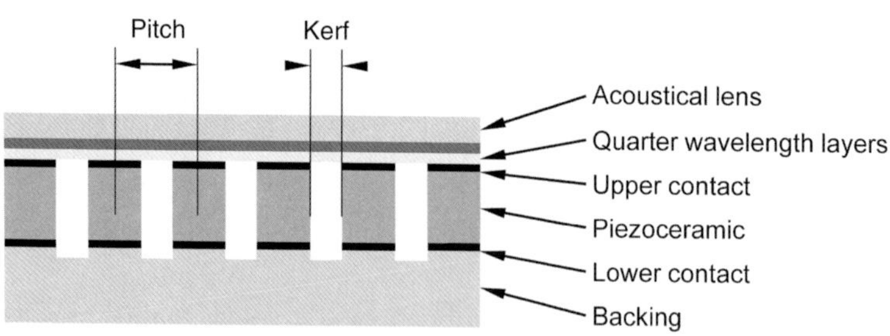

Figure 11.5. Part of a linear transducer array showing six piezoelectric transducer elements. The distance between element centers is the array pitch, and the element separation is the kerf. Sound is transmitted through quarter wavelength matching layers and an acoustical lens that focuses in the elevation direction perpendicular to the imaging plane. The backing attenuates sound transmitted to the back of the transducer.

element is half the wavelength of sound in the ceramic material for the center frequency. This makes the transducer resonant at the center frequency. The better the quality of the resonance, the more sensitive the transducer is. However, in this case, it transmits only long ringing pulses, rendering pulse-echo measurements with high resolution impossible.

Acoustic losses are introduced by the sound wave radiated into the medium at the front and even more by the backing material (Fig. 11.5). Owing to this, the resonance is less pronounced. This gives the transducer a larger bandwidth and enables it to emit short pulses. Thus, transducer design is a compromise between the sensitivity of the transducer and its bandwidth. Actual transducers reach bandwidths of up to 100% of the center frequency. Often, the band limits of a transducer array can be deduced from its name, but no standard naming convention is used: for instance, a Philips L8-4 transducer is a linear array transducer with a bandwidth from 4 to 8 MHz.

The quality of an imaging array is also characterized by the size and spacing of the elements. The element pitch is the distance between element centers, and the kerf is the space between elements. As discussed earlier, element pitch should typically be less than the wavelength in water at the center frequency.

A severe problem of piezoelectric transducers is the strong mismatch of acoustic impedances between the transducer material (ca. $Z_P = 34$ MRayls) and tissue (ca. $Z_W = 1.5$ MRayls). Owing to this, most of the acoustic energy would be reflected at the transducer surface. Therefore, quarter wavelength matching layers are used. If one-quarter wavelength layer is used, its acoustic impedance is chosen as $Z_M = \sqrt{Z_P Z_W}$, and no reflections are observed at the frequency for which the layer has quarter wavelength. For broadband pulses as used in ultrasound imaging, the matching is not perfect for frequencies away from the matching frequency, and the matching layer will limit the bandwidth of the transducer.

With higher electronic integration and increasing computer power, fully connected two-dimensional arrays also become available. This trend in increasing element counts and the need for the integration of electronics with the elements boosts development of novel transducer technology that is based on Microelectromechanical Systems (MEMS).

The most prominent new transducer design is the Capacitive Micromachined Ultrasound Transducer (CMUT), in which a thin metalized membrane covers a small gap to a second electrode as shown in Figure 11.6. If a voltage is supplied to the electrodes they will be attracted to each other by electrostatic forces, irrespective of the poling of the voltage. This nonlinear behavior is overcome by a bias DC voltage that brings the membrane into a working point and a small high frequency excitation around this point. If the DC voltage rises over a certain threshold where attractive electrostatic forces grow faster than the elastic forces pulling the membrane back, the membrane will collapse and touch the bottom of the transducer. Then, it can be released only when the voltage is lowered far beyond the collapse voltage. Theoretically, such transducers can reach very high coupling factors when driven close to the collapse point. However, parasitic capacitances limit the coupling factor in practice.

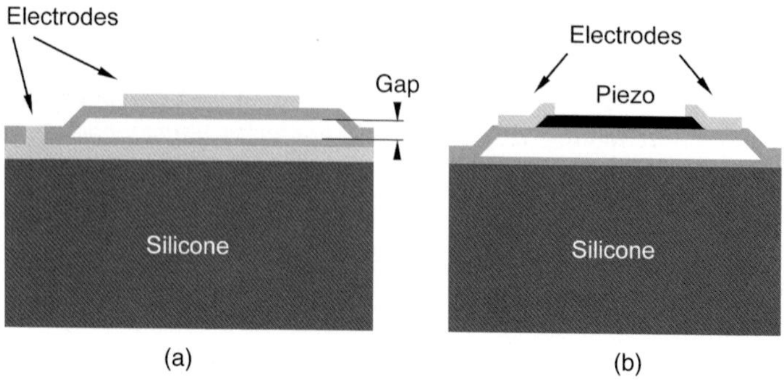

Figure 11.6. Micromachined transducers: principle of (a) capacitive micromachined ultrasound transducers (CMUT) and (b) piezoelectric micromachined ultrasound transducers (PMUT).

A different principle under investigation is the Piezoelectric Micromachined Ultrasound Transducer (PMUT), in which a piezoelectric thin film layer bends an elastic membrane (Fig. 11.6b). This principle has the advantage that it does not need a DC bias voltage and is more compatible with current scanner electronics.

Both technologies have the advantage that they use membranes with very low mechanical impedances that do not need any match to the tissue. Therefore, these transducers have a much larger bandwidth than conventional piezoelectric transducers. However, sensitivity and reliability are still an issue for both MUT principles. At the moment, manufacturers of diagnostic ultrasound equipment are still evaluating these technologies for the use in commercial equipment.

11.2.3 Beamforming

*11.2.3.1 **Beamforming Electronics.*** To focus sound beams and to direct them along different lines into tissue, the spatial distribution of the amplitude and phase of the emitting transducer excitation has to be controlled with respect to amplitude and phase. This is realized by the use of array transducers that consist of numerous small transducer elements. Several neighboring transducer elements of the array transducers build the active aperture. The transducer elements of such a group are driven all individually with different phases (delays) and amplitudes. In receive mode, the signals are also measured for each single element of the active aperture.

For this reason, current ultrasound scanners have about 64–256 parallel transmit and receive channels in the case of two-dimensional imaging with one-dimensional arrays. For three-dimensional imaging with two-dimensional arrays, even more channels are necessary, but because of cost, compromises are often made in 3D imaging. Transmitters are typically able to excite only rectangular pulses of positive and negative transmit voltages that will be bandlimited by the transducer transfer function. In high end systems, the transmit voltages can be adjusted for individual elements. The delay of the pulses to the elements is controlled digitally. In the receive mode, the echoes are amplified using TGC to account for tissue attenuation and digitized. The receive beamforming is then realized by digital signal processing of the individual echoes.

11.2.3.2 Array Beamforming. In array beamforming, the transducer elements are pulsed with individual delays, in such a way that the waves from the single elements reach the focal point F simultaneously (Fig. 11.7). Around this focal point, the sound wave propagation is nearly restricted to a line. The transmit focal point is fixed for one transmit/receive cycle. Often, more than one transmit focus is used in several transmit/receive cycles to combine the resulting images focused to different depths.

In the receive case, the echoes from a field point P will reach the transducer element with known differences in arrival times. The receiver is focused on point P by delaying the echoes in such a way that they are aligned in time and then summing the signals. In receive beamforming, the delays, and thus point P, can be adapted dynamically to the origin of echoes. Knowing the average speed of sound in tissue, the origin of echoes can be calculated by the time the transmit

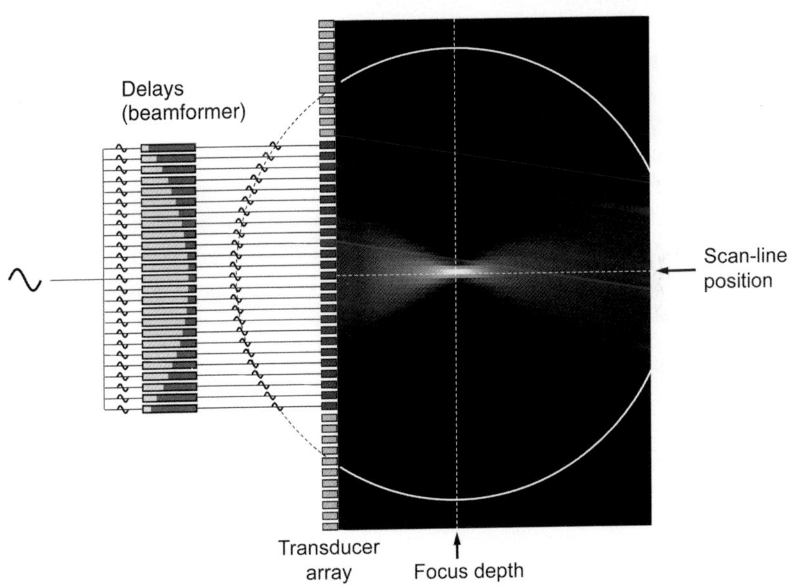

Figure 11.7. Linear array beamforming in transmit mode: a subgroup of the transducer array is active and focused to a fixed depth by the pulse delays realized in the beamformer. At the focus, waves of all elements arrive at the same time. The scan-line position can be moved by electronically switching to another subgroup of elements. The focus can be adapted by the choice of beamformer delays. In the background, a simulation of the maximum sound pressure is shown.

pulse needs to reach P and return to the transducer. Together with dynamic receive focusing, some scanners also enlarge the active aperture (dynamic aperture) for increasing depth to keep the focal point size constant.

With one-dimensional arrays, focusing perpendicular to the imaging plane (often named elevational focusing) cannot be realized electronically. Therefore, an acoustic lens with a fixed focus is used. With two-dimensional arrays, the elevational focus can also be realized by electronic beamforming, even if only a few elements (e.g., 5) in the second dimension are used. Such arrays are called *1.5D arrays*, in contrast to full two-dimensional arrays with equal element numbers and sizes in both dimensions as used for 3D imaging.

After recording one scan line, the position of the scan line has to be changed to gather image information along more lines. Two different principles exist to change the scan-line position: linear array scanning and phased array scanning. In linear array scanning, a subgroup of elements of a long array is active, and after recording one scan line, the active group is moved electronically along the array. By this, parallel scan lines are acquired (Fig. 11.8a). In some array designs, the elements are arranged on an arc to give a convex scan (Fig. 11.8b). However, the scan principle is the same. In phased array scanning, the focal points in transmit and receive are not on a line perpendicular to the transducer surface, but they are on a line steered under a steering angle ϕ. After one scan line is recorded, the steering angle is changed. Thus, a sector geometry with scan lines originating from one point on the transducer is generated (Fig. 11.8c). Which scan geometry is preferred depends on the application and the access to the organ of interest.

The phased array scan can also be used to sample volumes when a two-dimensional array is used to create a pyramid volume of scan lines originating in the transducer center. However, even for only 64 elements in one direction, a fully connected array would need 4096 individual channels. Therefore, first real-time 3D scanners used sparse random arrays in which only a random pattern of elements with a well-defined distribution is connected. With this, first real-time 3D images were realized at the cost of lower image quality. Now, fully connected 2D arrays use highly integrated electronics in the scan head to reduce connections to the system.

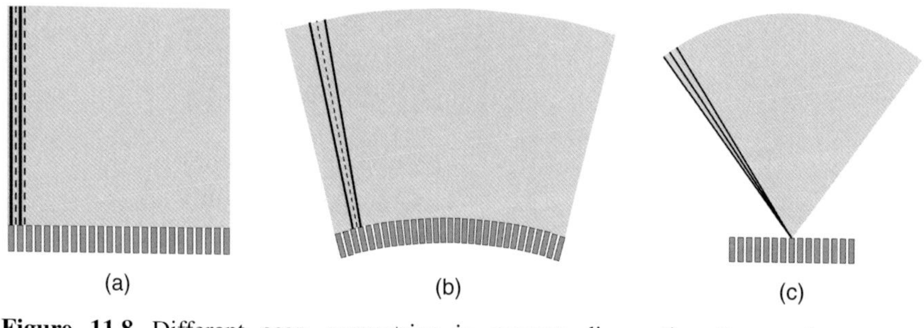

Figure 11.8. Different scan geometries in current diagnostic ultrasound scanners: (a) linear scan, (b) convex scan, and (c) phased array sector scan.

Apart from these technological problems, real-time volume scanning is also limited by the speed of sound, which determines the acquisition time of a single scan line. For an image depth of 75 mm, sound has to travel 150 mm through tissue at a speed of approximately 1.5 mm μs^{-1}, resulting in 100 μs per scan line. Two-dimensional images often have hundreds of scan lines, volume data can easily use 10,000 scan lines, demanding 1-s scan time, which is too slow for real-time imaging of the beating heart. For this reason, volumetric scan concepts often reduce transmit focusing and record several scan lines at the same time with parallel receive beamformers, again at the cost of image quality.

11.3 MEASUREMENT TECHNIQUES OF REAL-TIME ULTRASOUND IMAGING

11.3.1 Doppler Measurement Techniques

11.3.1.1 Continuous Wave Doppler. Continuous Wave Doppler (cw-Doppler) is a nonimaging method to detect blood flow using the Doppler shift caused by moving scatterers such as red blood cells. In cw-Doppler, one group of elements of the transducer array transmits a continuous sine wave signal into tissue while a second group of transducer elements records the echoes. If the received signal is mixed with a sinusoidal signal of the transmit frequency, the result contains one component with the sum of transmitted and received frequencies and a second component with their difference frequency. The first component can be suppressed by a low pass filter; the second component has the Doppler shift frequency. As mentioned earlier, the Doppler shift frequencies are in the audible range and can be listened to when supplied to a loudspeaker. B-mode images can be used to direct the interrogating beam to a vessel of interest.

With the processing described so far, only the absolute Doppler shift can be measured; the information if the frequency difference is positive (flow in the direction of the transducer) or negative (flow away from the transducer) is missing. This information can be extracted by using quadrature demodulation, also known as *IQ demodulation*. For this purpose, the received signal is mixed with the reference signal, resulting as above in the so-called I component (in-phase component). In addition, the signal is mixed with a 90° phase-shifted version of the reference signal, as shown in Figure 11.9. This results in the Q component. The Q component has a 90° phase shift with respect to the I component. The direction of this phase shift allows determination of the sign of the Doppler shift as illustrated in Figure 11.10. Both I and Q channels are shifted again by 90° and summed, resulting in the forward and backward flow signals that can be made audible on the two channels of stereo equipment. To remove the components of slow moving or stationary objects, a highpass filter is used, which is usually referred to as the *wall filter* because primarily vessel wall movements are suppressed.

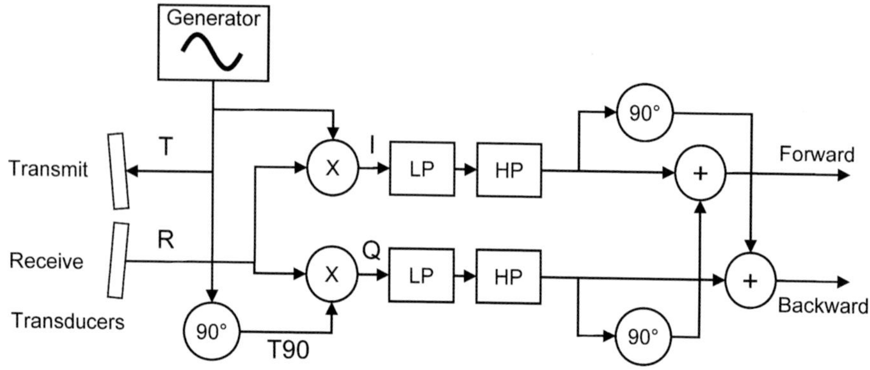

Figure 11.9. Block diagram of continuous wave Doppler processing. I and Q components are generated by mixing with a reference signal and its 90° phase-shifted version. Signals pass through a lowpass (LP) filter and a highpass (HP) wall filter. Adding original and 90° shifted I and Q signals as shown results in the forward and backward signals, which can also be connected to stereo speakers. Alternatively, I and Q components can be complex Fourier transformed for spectral Doppler analysis.

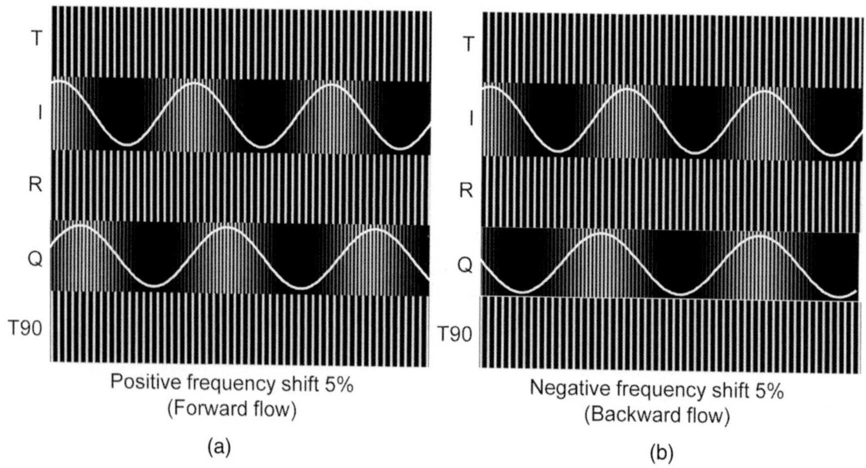

Figure 11.10. Demodulated I and Q signals for two received Doppler signals R shifted 5% up (a) and 5% down (b) in frequency by forward and backward flow, respectively. The overlaid sine shows the low frequency component, which is the demodulated Doppler signal after lowpass filtering. The phase shift of the Q component with respect to the I component is +90° for the forward flow and −90° for the backward flow. Signal names correspond to the figure above.

In practice, the Doppler signal of a blood vessel is not shifted to a single frequency but is a mixture of frequency shifts because blood flow varies over the cross section of the vessel. In addition, blood flow varies with the heart cycle. To determine the strength of the different frequency components, the Doppler signals are Fourier transformed in real time over short time intervals. The time varying frequency spectrum of the Doppler signal can be presented to the user as a brightness-coded image, as shown for pulsed Doppler measurements in Figure 11.12.

11.3.1.2 Pulsed Wave Doppler. The disadvantage of cw-Doppler is the range ambiguity of the method: all vessels intersecting the interrogating beam contribute to the Doppler signal. To restrict the Doppler measurement to a certain depth, a gated measurement technique that uses pulsed sine bursts was introduced (Baker, 1970; Wells, 1969). For easier detection of the Doppler shift, pulses are longer than the imaging pulses and are sent interleaved with the image acquisition. However, Doppler shifts cannot be measured by the frequency shift of the spectrum of a single pulse: the pulse duration determines the frequency resolution of the Fourier transform of the pulse. Even with a long sine burst of 10 cycles at 1 MHz, the pulse duration is 10 μs and the achievable frequency resolution is the reciprocal, that is, 100 kHz. This is obviously insufficient to measure typical Doppler shifts of less than 15 kHz. Therefore, the pulse measurement has to be repeated several times with a fixed phase relation of the sine-burst pulses as depicted in Figure 11.11.

The received signal is sampled at the time that corresponds to the desired measurement depth. Echoes from stationary objects will remain identical with

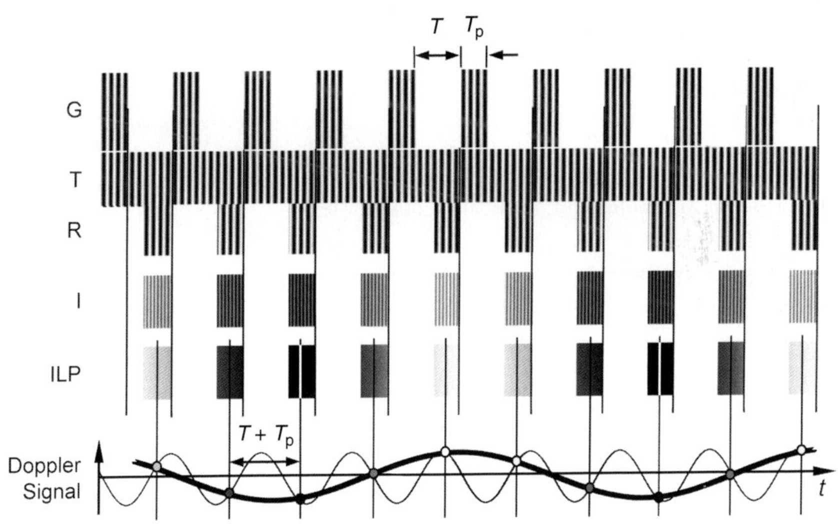

Figure 11.11. Pulse Doppler measurement: sine bursts G are sent with a fixed repetition time $T + T_p$, and the received echoes R are sampled after a fixed time delay corresponding to the measurement depth. The I signal is thus also gated, and after the lowpass filter, only a sampled version of the Doppler signal (thick line) is measured. Note that the second Doppler signal with a much higher frequency (thin line) has the same sample points, leading to velocity ambiguity if the repetition frequency is too low, that is, smaller than the double of the Doppler frequency.

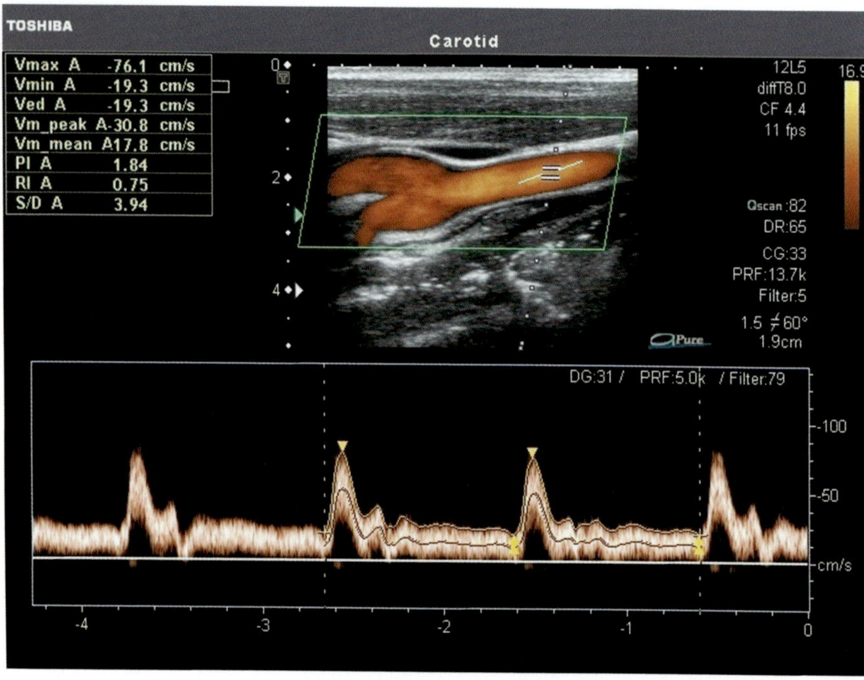

Figure 11.12. Pw-Doppler measurement and spectral Doppler representation. Blood flow is measured in the carotid close to the bifurcation. The red color overlay in the image is the color Doppler mode presentation. The direction of the measurement beam is represented by the dotted line in the image. The measurement window is marked by the two horizontal bars along the dotted line. In the vessel, angle direction measured by the user is presented by a further line. This allows presenting the data with the correct blood flow velocity. In the lower section, spectral Doppler measurements are overlaid with maximum and mean flow curves. Image courtesy of Toshiba Medical Systems.

each sampling, resulting in a constant signal. For a moving object, the phase of the returning sine wave will change. Ignoring propagation effects on the transmitted signal s, the received signal r from depth d will be (Jensen, 1996)

$$r(t) = s\left(\left[1 - 2\frac{v}{c}\cos\theta\right]t - \frac{2d}{c}\right) \tag{11.23}$$

which is a time-scaled version of the transmit pulse. In addition, the time delay τ between echo pulses is scaled relative to the time delay T_{PRF} between transmit pulses according to

$$\tau = \frac{2d}{c} = 2T_{\mathrm{PRF}}\frac{v}{c}\cos\theta. \tag{11.24}$$

This leads to a sampled signal slowly varying at the Doppler shift frequency. Again, as with cw-Doppler, quadrature demodulation can be used to detect the direction of flow. However, with Pulsed Wave Doppler (pw-Doppler), it is not realized by mixing with a phase-shifted reference signal but by sampling the echo signals a second time with a time delay corresponding to a 90° phase shift of the sine-burst frequency. For a detailed analysis of pw-Doppler, refer to the book by Jensen (1996).

In this technique, each pulse results only in a single sample point of the Doppler signal. Therefore, pw-Doppler is a sampling measurement of the Doppler signal that has to fulfill the sampling theorem: the sampling frequency, which is identical to the pulse repetition frequency, has to be twice as high as the frequency of the Doppler signal.

However, none of the two frequencies can be set freely by the user: The pulse repetition frequency depends on the depth of measurement. The closer the blood flow is to the transducer, the higher is the sampling frequency. Equation (11.20) shows the possibilities to lower the Doppler frequency shift for a given blood flow velocity: only the transmit frequency of the sine bursts can be lowered by the user. This is the reason why cardiac transducers use a lower frequency around 2 MHz at the cost of image resolution. However, the Doppler frequency shift may exceed half the pulse repetition rate, leading to aliasing and to the measurement of wrong Doppler shift frequencies and corresponding blood flow velocities. These situations have to be recognized by the clinical user.

11.3.1.3 Color Doppler Imaging and Power Doppler Imaging. Pw-Doppler measurements offer an exact assessment of blood flow velocity distributions over time in a single measurement window. However, often it is desired to get an overview of blood flow in a larger area such as in vessel bifurcations or in the heart. Unfortunately, it is not possible to quickly scan a pulsed Doppler measurement over an area of interest because pw-Doppler needs pulsing in the order of 100 times at one spot to calculate a Fourier transform. Scanning such a measurement would take too long and pose the risk of tissue heating. Therefore, by color Doppler imaging, only the average flow velocity is determined with fewer pulses and overlaid as a color-coded velocity image.

For this, similar to pw-Doppler, the echo signals are sampled at intervals T_{PRF} for the in-phase component I_n and with a time shift of 90° of the transmit frequency for the quadrature Q_n component. The most robust estimator (Evans, 1993) for the mean Doppler shift frequency can be calculated for N samples by the autocorrelator (Kasai et al., 1983):

$$\overline{f}_{\mathrm{D}} = \frac{1}{2\pi T_{\mathrm{PRF}}} \arctan\left[\frac{\sum_{n=1}^{N}(I_n Q_{n-1} - Q_n I_{n-1})}{\sum_{n=1}^{N}(I_n I_{n-1} + Q_n Q_{n-1})}\right] \tag{11.25}$$

The direction and mean frequency are color coded, typically in a red/blue color table. Some systems additionally calculate the variance of the velocity distribution and add a green color component to the color table if an increased variance is

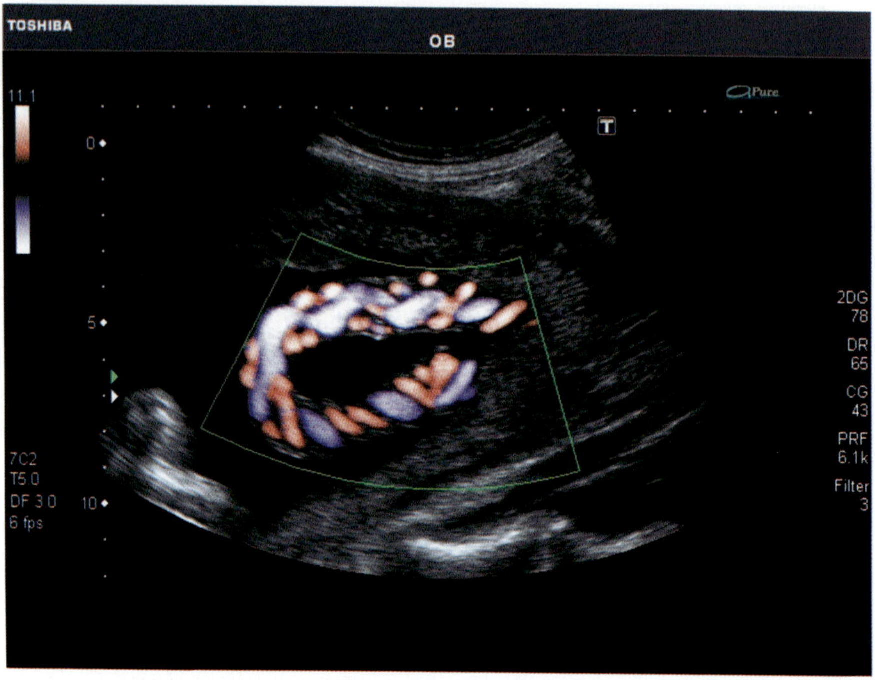

Figure 11.13. Example of color flow imaging in the fetal umbilical cord. The two smaller arteries and the larger single vein can be seen clearly with their opposing blood flow direction. Note the missing signal for any blood flow directed orthogonal to the insonifying beam. Image courtesy of Toshiba Medical Systems.

observed. This feature can be helpful in identifying turbulences in blood flow, which show large variances.

Color flow imaging also uses sampling of the Doppler signal and can show aliasing if the sampling frequency is too low for the measured flow velocities. Aliasing will show as a switch over from the end of the color scale to the beginning (e.g., from red to blue) and has to be differentiated from local turbulence that might also lead to a reversal of flow. Figure 11.13 shows an example of color flow imaging of the fetal umbilical cord.

Another variant of color Doppler imaging is power Doppler imaging (Rubin et al., 1994), in which only the average power of the sampled Doppler signal is presented, typically in a temperature color scale from red to yellow. It can also be calculated from the IQ components by

$$P = \sum_{n=1}^{N} (I_n^2 + Q_n^2). \tag{11.26}$$

Although the signal is sampled, no aliasing problems occur because the power of the signal is calculated correctly even in the case of aliasing: total power is

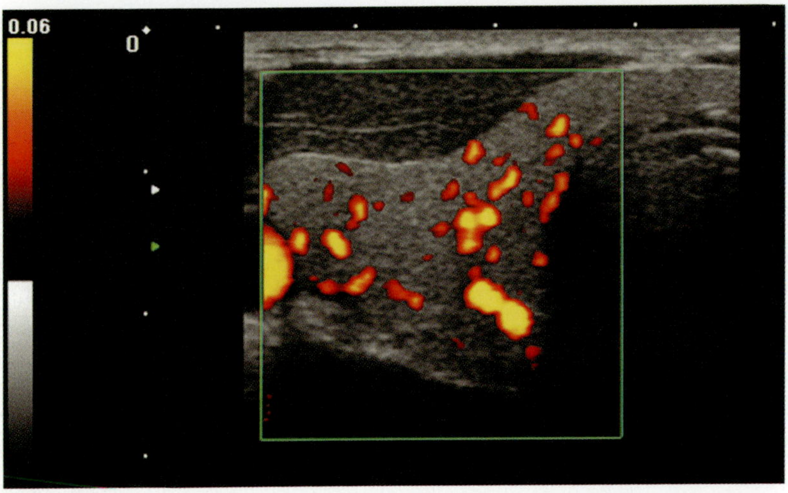

Figure 11.14. Power Doppler imaging of the thyroid. Very small vessels that cannot be visualized by color Doppler can be found by power Doppler. However, only the presence of blood flow is visualized, neither the flow velocity nor its direction can be determined from the image. Image courtesy of Toshiba Medical Systems.

calculated by integration over the frequency spectrum of the signal. Owing to aliasing, signal components may be misplaced in the frequency domain, but the integral is not affected by this. Power Doppler shows neither the direction nor the velocity but only the existence of flow. Signals do not get stronger because of higher flow rates but because of stronger scattering of the flowing medium. Power Doppler is more sensitive than color Doppler and is used to show the presence of blood flow even in small vessels (Fig. 11.14).

11.3.2 Ultrasound Contrast Agents and Nonlinear Imaging

11.3.2.1 Ultrasound Contrast Media. Scattering from blood is low compared to other tissues and makes blood flow difficult to image in small vessels. Gramiak and Shah (1968) were the first to use small gas bubbles to increase the echoes from blood. This led to the design of specific contrast agents consisting of gas microbubbles stabilized by a shell. It is obvious from the very low acoustic impedance of gases that microbubbles represent strong scatterers, and de Jong (1993) calculated that their scattering cross section is greater by a factor of 10^8 than that of an iron sphere of the same radius. In addition, gas microbubbles exhibit resonant and nonlinear properties that make them even stronger scatterers that can be sensitively detected by their nonlinear response.

Table 11.2 lists some contrast agents. First-generation microbubbles (Albunex, Levovist) were air-filled and were filtered out quickly by the lung. Second-generation contrast agents (Definity, Sonovue, Optison) are filled with low solubility gases and are stable for several minutes. They are administered

TABLE 11.2. Examples of Ultrasound Contrast Agents and Their Composition

Agent	Shell material	Gas	Ø (μm)	Manufacturer
Albunex	Albumin	Air	4.3	Molecular Biosystems Inc.
Levovist®	Lipid/galactose	Air	2–3	Schering AG
Sonovist®	Cyanoacrylate	Air	1–2	Schering AG
Definity®	Lipid/surfactant	C_3F_8	1.1–3.3	Lantheus Medical Imaging
Optison ™	Albumin	C_3F_8	2.0–4.5	GE Healthcare
SonoVue®	Lipid	SF_6	2.5	Bracco Diagnostics Inc.
CARDIOsphere®	Polyactide	N_2	4.0	POINT Biomedical Corp.

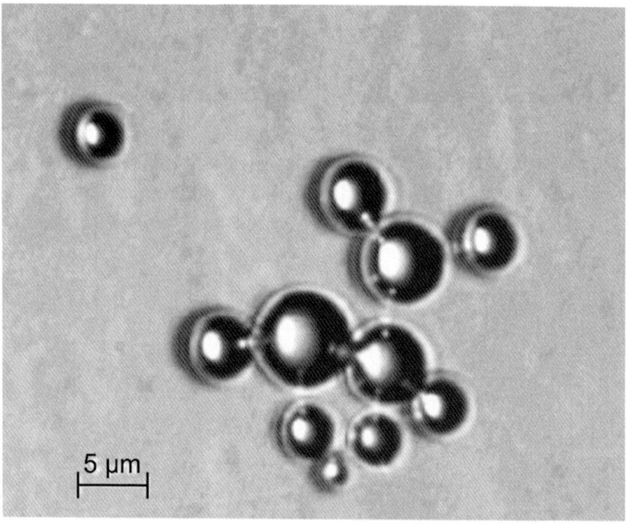

Figure 11.15. Contrast microbubbles containing sulfur hexafluoride with a phospholipid shell (optical microscopy, experimental microbubbles from the author's laboratory).

intravenously and can pass the lung. Polymer-shelled microbubbles such as Sonovist can live even longer and can be phagocytosed by the reticuloendothelial system and thus accumulate in the liver and spleen where they can last for several hours. Third-generation contrast agents (e.g., CARDIOSphere) aim at well-defined and reproducible bubble properties, such as constant shell thickness and a narrow radius distribution. Figure 11.15 shows a microscopic image of self-fabricated microbubbles with 5 μm average diameter with lipid shells filled with SF_6.

The oscillation of microbubbles in an ultrasound field is nonlinear; in the rarefaction phase the bubble expands and can reach several times its resting radius. However, in the compression phase, the bubble cannot be compressed as far. The motion equations for contrast media are nonlinear differential equations, such as the equation of Rayleigh, Plesset, Neppiras, Noltingk, and Poritsky (RPNNP

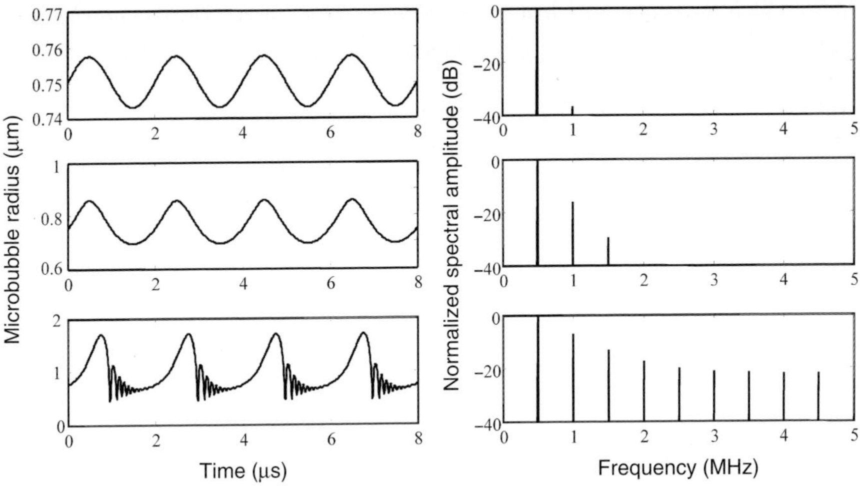

Figure 11.16. Simulated response of a microbubble with 0.75-μm resting radius and excitation at 500 kHz. For the panels on the left, the pressure increases from top to bottom, resulting in higher harmonics in the frequency representation in the panels on the right.

equation) modified for the stiffness of the shell or a modified Herring equation (Doinikov and Dayton, 2006). Figure 11.16 shows the simulated radius change for a free gas bubble for different driving pressures. For low pressures, also called *low MI imaging* because of the low mechanical index, the bubble behaves like a linear resonator. For increasing pressures, the bubble behavior becomes more and more nonlinear. This leads to increasing deviations from the sinusoidal form of the driving pressure and generates harmonic frequencies in the spectrum of the scattered signal of the bubble (Schrope and Newhouse, 1993). This can be used for the sensitive detection of bubbles as discussed below. In this so-called medium MI range, the bubble shows stable nonlinear oscillation. Apart from the generation of harmonics, microbubbles can generate subharmonics and ultraharmonics (Shi et al., 1999, 2001), an effect typical for nonlinear dynamic systems close to chaotic behavior.

The strong mechanical activity of microbubbles can lead to tissue damage such as capillary rupture (Miller and Quddus, 2000). Therefore, guidelines for the safe use of contrast media have been issued (Albrecht et al., 2004).

Increasing the driving pressure even further to the high MI range leads to bubble destruction (Chomas et al., 2001; de Jong et al., 2002). Destruction takes place during the very fast compression of the bubble and typically fragments the bubble into smaller bubbles that dissolve (Chomas et al., 2001; Postema et al., 2004). This effect is used in imaging protocols for destruction of contrast agents and the quantification of subsequent replenishment to assess tissue perfusion. When collapsing, the microbubbles emit a broadband signal that can be detected and is known as *Stimulated Acoustic Emission* (SAE). The disappearance of the microbubble leads also to a loss of correlation and thus to a strong short Doppler signal (Tiemann et al., 2000), which can also be used for microbubble detection.

11.3.2.2 Harmonic Imaging Techniques. The first method to detect the harmonic response from microbubbles was to use bandpass filters for the second harmonic (Schrope and Newhouse, 1993). This technique has several disadvantages: the broadband spectrum of an imaging pulse shows considerable overlap with the second harmonic and the pulse spectrum as well as the second harmonic must fit in the limited bandwidth of transducers. To better understand the generation of harmonics, the nonlinear response of the microbubbles can be modeled by a nonlinear system with memory by a Volterra series (Mleczko et al., 2009) when sub- and ultraharmonics are neglected.

$$y(t) = \sum_{i=1}^{\infty} h_i(\tau_1, \ldots, \tau_i)x(t - \tau_1)x(t - \tau_2) \cdot \ldots \cdot x(t - \tau_i). \qquad (11.27)$$

where the kernels h_i characterize the behavior of the nonlinear system for an input signal $x(t)$ and output signal $y(t)$. For a sinusoidal input signal of frequency f_0, the linear term with kernel h_1 generates only the original frequency f_0. The term with the quadratic kernel generates a constant output at frequency zero and a component at $2f_0$. The cubic term with kernel h_3 generates components at f_0 and $3f_0$. In general, the even kernels of order n generate a constant signal and all even multiples of f_0 up to nf_0. The odd order kernels of order n generate all odd multiples of f_0 up to nf_0. All odd order terms generate a component with the original transmit frequency that can be sensitively detected by the transducer.

To overcome the disadvantages of harmonic imaging by filtering the second harmonic, at the moment two different techniques are used, which send two or three pulses. The basic idea behind both schemes is that linear signal components cancel when the echoes of the pulses are added.

The first technique is Pulse Inversion (PI) imaging (Hope Simpson et al., 1999). Here, two pulses with opposite signs are transmitted in two transmit/receive cycles. When the received echoes are modeled according to Eq. (11.27), it can be seen that the addition of the two echo signals cancels all odd order components, including the linear term. The even order terms are still present in the sum signal, and the lowest frequency component is $2f_0$. This component will be the only one with a significant contribution to the received signal because of the bandpass character of the transducer and the lowpass characteristic of tissue attenuation. A disadvantage of this method is that higher odd order terms are cancelled, although they could contribute to signal energy around f_0 (Fig. 11.17).

Therefore, another pulsing scheme was proposed (Phillips, 2001) with three pulses (Contrast Pulse Sequencing, CPS), with the relative amplitudes $-1/2$, 1, $-1/2$ for the three pulses. Again, the echoes cancel the linear term for the three echoes according to Eq. (11.27). However, components with higher order still contribute to the sum signal, irrespective of even or odd order. Since the odd order components generate contributions at the fundamental frequency, the method gives higher amplitudes for the harmonic signal.

In addition, subharmonics and ultraharmonics can be used for better differentiation between tissue and microbubble nonlinearities because they are unique to microbubbles (Chomas et al., 2002).

11.3.2.3 Perfusion Imaging Techniques. To measure tissue perfusion, that is, the blood supply to capillary vessels in the tissue, different approaches exist.

Wei et al., (1998) introduced a technique known as *destruction–reperfusion* or replenishment, later successfully used for the assessment of myocardial perfusion (Tiemann et al., 1999). They proposed a constant venous infusion with contrast agent. Then, after an equilibrium concentration of the contrast agent in tissue is reached, a high MI burst pulse is used to destroy all microbubbles in the imaging plane. Subsequently, the amount of the inflow of new microbubbles is observed with low MI imaging pulses after varying delays. With this method, it has to be taken into account that the imaging pulse itself may also destroy microbubbles. Thus, for each delay, a new destruction–reperfusion experiment has to be performed. Therefore, this measurement technique is time consuming.

A less time-consuming alternative to the replenishment technique is the depletion method (Eyding et al., 2003), which uses the imaging pulses to destroy a certain percentage of contrast microbubbles. Again, at the beginning, a constant perfusion with contrast agent is realized by intravenous infusion. It can be shown that an exponential decay can be observed with a fast sequence of semidestructive

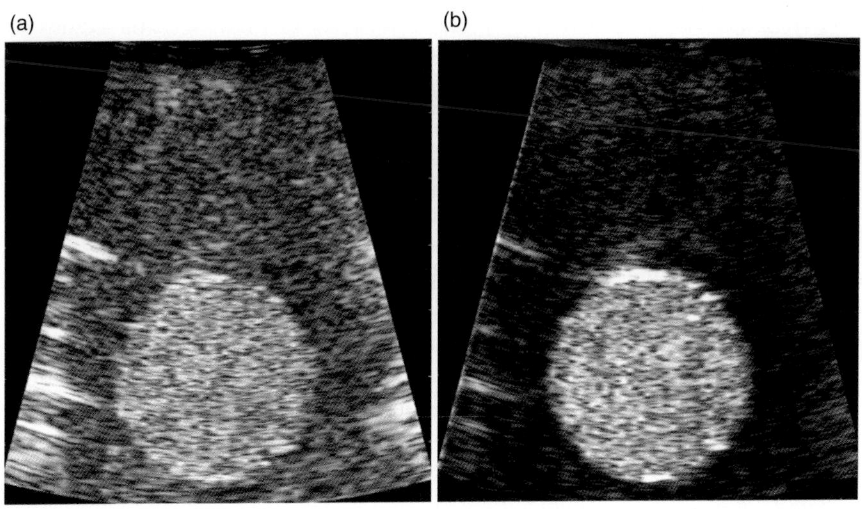

Figure 11.17. Pulse inversion contrast image (b) of a tissue mimicking phantom with a circular inclusion filled with contrast medium in water compared to the B-mode image without pulse inversion (a).

imaging pulses. Using mathematical models, perfusion can be calculated from the measurements by fitting of the model parameters.

The fastest way to find perfusion parameters is the bolus method (Eyding et al., 2002): one bolus of contrast microbubbles is administered and flows into the imaging plane with a time delay. Several parameters can be calculated from time–intensity curves in the imaging plane that are imaged by nondestructive pulses: peak intensity, time to peak, and peak width. Especially, time to peak has shown good correlation with perfusion quantification with Nuclear Magnetic Resonance (NMR) imaging (Meves et al., 2002, Chapter 5). Techniques for quantification of perfusion are still under development and have to be adapted to the specific application and contrast agent.

Another method to quantify contrast microbubbles in the capillaries is the detection of SAE or loss of correlation. Up to microbubble concentrations of 15,000 bubbles per milliliter, a linear relationship of the square root of the Doppler signal intensity could be demonstrated (Tiemann et al., 2000). At higher concentrations, the acoustic attenuation of microbubbles close to the transducer hinders the destruction of deeper ones, thus rendering quantitative measurements impossible. Therefore, Sensitive Particle Acoustic Quantification (SPAQ) has been proposed to quantify higher microbubble concentrations (Reinhardt et al., 2005). With this method, the volume of interest is slowly scanned by a lateral transducer movement in steps of 10–100 μm, so that only a few microbubbles have to be destroyed after one motion step. This technique allows quantification of higher concentrations (30,000 bubbles/mL), but has not been realized in real time so far.

11.3.2.4 Targeted Imaging. Advances in molecular biology drive the demand for imaging techniques that can show the presence or absence of molecules that are connected with certain disease states, especially in oncology and cardiovascular applications. For this application field, named molecular imaging, the sensitivity of the imaging method for small amounts of the target molecule is crucial for success. So far, nuclear imaging with Positron Emission Tomography (PET, Chapter 7) is the only modality that is clinically established for molecular imaging and has the highest sensitivity. However, for molecules expressed by vascular endothelial cells, ultrasound molecular imaging also shows promising results in preclinical studies (Bloch et al., 2004; Dayton and Ferrara, 2002; Lindner, 2004).

In principle, two different mechanisms are used to bind microbubbles to the target cells: in so-called passive targeting, either the chemical composition of the microbubble shell is responsible for binding or ligands binding to the targeted molecule are attached to the bubble surface. The main application field is better diagnosis of inflammation, thrombus, and angiogenesis.

Passive targeting of Albunex microbubbles was described by Wei et al., (2001) for myocardial inflammation. Activated leukocytes cling to albumin in the shell of the microbubbles and thus transport them to the inflammation. A similar effect was also used for imaging myocardial inflammation in dogs *in vivo* with passive targeting caused by phosphatidyl serine as part of the lipid composition of the microbubble shell (Christiansen et al., 2002), showing high sensitivity comparable to radionuclide imaging.

Active targeting has been demonstrated by, Weller et al., (2003) and Villanueva et al., (2007), with ICAM-1 (intracellular adhesion molecule) and selectins as target molecules expressed during inflammation. The study by Villanueva et al., (2007) showed the possibility of diagnosing a recent ischemia event by such methods.

Quantification in these applications is currently realized by the following imaging protocol: after bolus injection of the targeted contrast media, an image is taken after a delay to record the concentration of bound and unbound microbubbles in the tissue. Then, a destructive ultrasound pulse clears all microbubbles, and after a shorter delay, a second image records only unbound microbubbles. Subtraction of the intensity of both frames results in a quantitative measure of targeted microbubble concentration.

The second application field, thrombus imaging, has been addressed using microbubbles targeted to GPIIb/IIa, a glycoprotein overexpressed in thrombi. For example, with quantitative techniques, a significant increase in microbubble concentration in thrombi could be shown (Alonso et al., 2007).

Especially in the detection of cancer, markers of angiogenesis are of interest, such as $\alpha_v\beta_3$ (Ellegala et al., 2003), $\alpha_5\beta_1$ (Leong-Poi et al., 2005), or VEGFR2 (vascular endothelial growth factor receptor). Apart from cancer diagnosis, quantitative molecular imaging techniques for angiogenesis can be used to monitor the effect of antiangiogenic drugs in cancer therapy. The development of ultrasound molecular imaging techniques is currently a constantly growing application field.

11.4 APPLICATION EXAMPLES OF BIOMEDICAL SONOGRAPHY

11.4.1 B-Mode, M-Mode, and 3D Imaging

The standard imaging mode of ultrasound scanners is the B-scan or B-mode image relying on the pulse-echo imaging principle. In current systems, it is typically electronically scanned with transducer arrays and the beamforming techniques described earlier. Depending on the transducer, the resolution of these images is in the range from 0.1 to 3 mm. Figure 11.18 shows an example of B-mode imaging of a fetus with a convex array. The dots show a centimeter scale. Often, arrows on the depth scale mark the position of one or more transmit foci; in the image, one transmit focus at 5-cm depth was used. The frequency of the array was chosen in the range from 3 to 10 MHz because with the total image depth of 9 cm, maximum attenuation is still low enough to use this frequency range. This results in an axial resolution in the direction of the soundbeam below 1 mm and lateral resolution in the range of 1 mm at the focal depth of 5 cm. In the image, several artifacts of ultrasound imaging can be observed: surfaces give a stronger echo signal if the incidence is at 90°. This can be seen at the tip of the nose showing a bright spot in the position where it is insonified perpendicular to the

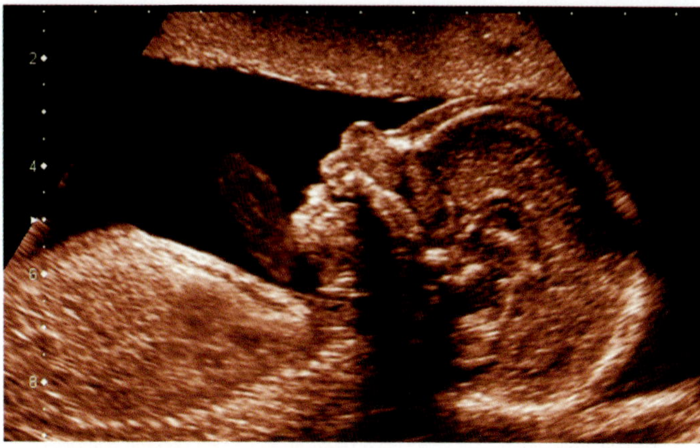

Figure 11.18. B-mode image of fetal profile showing minute details of brain and thorax. A convex array with a bandwidth from 3 to 10 MHz was used. The electronic transmit focus is at 5 cm depth, as indicated by the arrow on the left. In receive mode, dynamic focusing moves the focus continually to the depth of echo origin. Image courtesy of Toshiba Medical Systems.

surface. Furthermore, acoustic shadowing by the strong reflection and absorption of bone structures inside the head can be seen leading to missing echo signals at 4 cm behind the nose. However, imaging the brain through the skull bone is no problem in fetal imaging, because the fetal skull is still acoustically transparent.

By mechanically moving the array in a direction perpendicular to the electronic scan direction, 3D images can be acquired. This can also be achieved by electronic beamforming with a two-dimensional array as discussed earlier. If imaging is fast enough or synchronized with the Electrocardiogram (ECG) signal, volume images of the moving heart can be acquired.

However, the most popular three-dimensional images are fetal faces, as shown in Figure 11.19. This image is a snapshot of a movie that was taken with a fast mechanical scan of a one-dimensional array resulting in real-time images of the moving fetus. In both applications, cardiac imaging and fetal imaging, 3D rendering is easier than in other applications because the contrast between the low echo level from blood or amniotic fluid and the high echo level from tissue allows good surface detection.

For cardiac imaging, it is often of interest to study the motion of the valves or the myocardium over the heart cycle. To facilitate this, ultrasound scanners offer the M-mode (motion mode, sometimes also called TM-mode for time-motion mode). In this mode, one line along a fixed position is measured continuously and presented as in B-mode with brightness-coded intensity. The temporal changes of echo signals are shown by plotting one line next to the other in a moving window, similar to an ECG signal. This is shown in Figure 11.20 on the left. Therefore, the horizontal scale is a time scale. On the right side, a typical B-mode image of the heart can be seen. For cardiac imaging often phased arrays are used, which

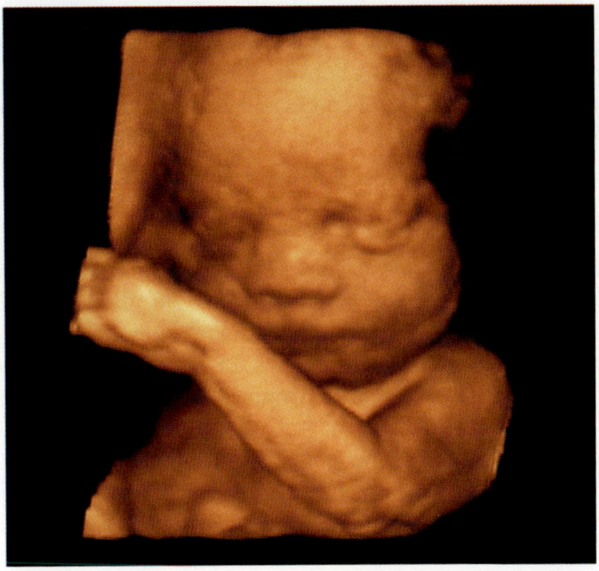

Figure 11.19. Three-dimensional rendering of fetal face and arm. The image is a snapshot of a movie sequence recorded with a mechanically scanned convex array with 2- to 7-MHz bandwidth. Image courtesy of Toshiba Medical Systems.

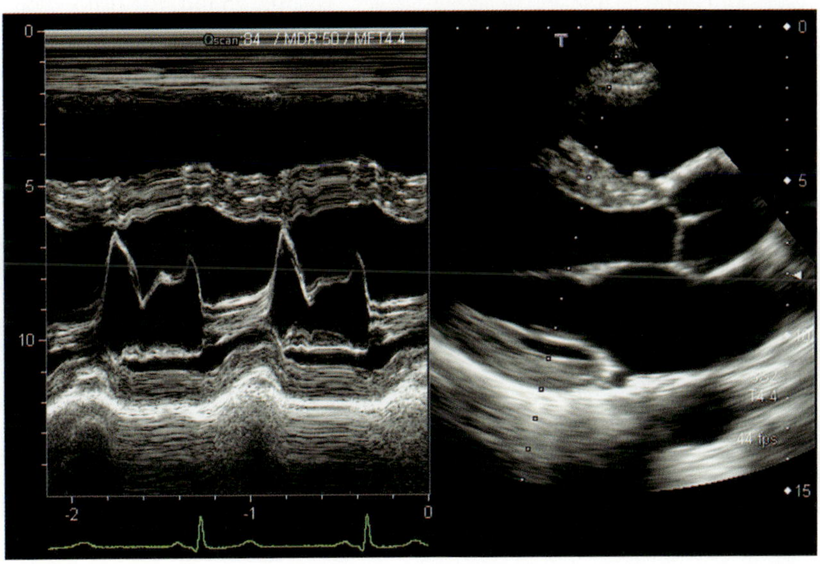

Figure 11.20. B-mode sector scan image of the adult heart (right), with the dotted line marking the measurement position for the M-mode image presented on the left. The vertical scale in the M-mode is in centimeters; the horizontal scale is in seconds. The continuously measured A-scan line cuts through the mitral valve. The strong movement of the valve over a period of 2 s can be observed clearly and can be related to the ECG signal shown in green at the bottom. Image courtesy of Toshiba Medical Systems.

scan the image only by steering the beam. This leads to a sector image with all scan lines originating at one point in the middle of a relatively small transducer. This is due to the small windows between the ribs that have to be used to get acoustic access to the heart. The B-mode image is used to determine the position of the M-mode measurements, indicated in the right image by the dotted line.

11.4.2 Flow and Perfusion Imaging

Functional imaging of flow and perfusion is a particular strength of ultrasound imaging. Examples have already been presented and discussed in the sections on Doppler and perfusion measurement techniques, and this section gives further examples for the most important applications. In vascular imaging, flow can either be assessed quantitatively with color Doppler imaging or just be detected, to demonstrate organ perfusion or patency of vessels. Figure 11.21 shows examples for both modes. In Figure 11.21a, color Doppler is used to image the carotid bifurcation with blood flow going from right to left. Owing to the bifurcation, turbulence is induced and leads to a backflow of blood, which is shown in red. A much lower blood flow speed is seen in the radial artery on the right side (Fig. 11.21b) and is detected with power Doppler imaging. In both images, the green parallelogram indicates the measurement area, which is restricted to speed up imaging and can be placed in the image by the user. The images also show the excellent resolution that can be achieved with today's ultrasound scanners. In both cases, the arteries are close to the skin surface and image depth is 3 and 2 cm, respectively. Therefore, high frequency arrays can be used. For the image in Figure 11.21a, 11.21a 6- to 11-MHz bandwidth transducer and that in Figure 11.21b, an 8- to 14-MHz transducer were used to image the radial artery of 3 mm diameter.

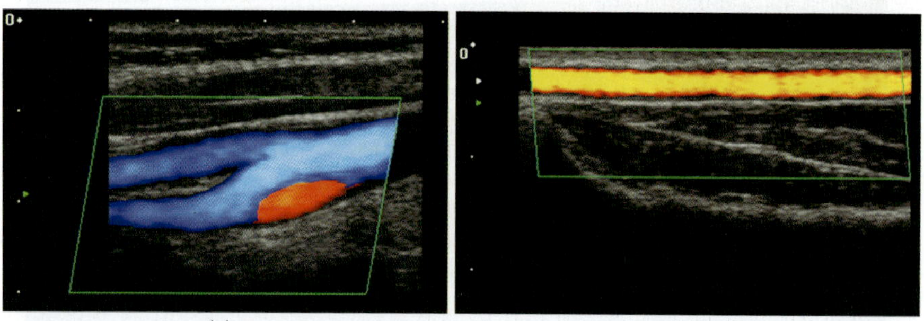

(a) (b)

Figure 11.21. (a) Color Doppler flow measurement of the carotid bifurcation. The blue color codes flow with a component away from the transducer (down to the left). A reverse flow due to turbulence is visible as a red signal. Image depth is 3 cm, and a linear array with 6- to 11-MHz bandwidth was used. (b) Power Doppler image of flow in the radial artery. Image depth is only 2 cm, and a high frequency transducer array with 8- to 14-MHz bandwidth was used. Image courtesy of Toshiba Medical Systems.

A main application of color Doppler imaging is blood flow measurement in the heart. For this, phased array transducers are used and center frequencies are chosen around 2–3 MHz to avoid aliasing in the Doppler signals: according to Eq. (11.20), the Doppler shift frequency is proportional to the center frequency of the pulse and to the blood flow speed. At the same time, the measurement depth has to reach up to 15 cm, as can be seen in Figure 11.22, which determines the maximum Pulse Repetition Frequency (PRF) ($1540\ \mathrm{ms}^{-1}/0.3\ \mathrm{m} = 5.1\ \mathrm{kHz}$). In Figure 11.22, an even lower PRF of 3 kHz was used, allowing a maximum Doppler shift frequency of 1.5 kHz to avoid aliasing. The center frequency chosen was 2.5 MHz. With Eq. (11.20), the maximum speed that can be measured can be calculated using the maximum Doppler shift:

$$v_{\max} = \frac{\Delta f_{\max} \cdot c}{2 \cdot f} = \frac{1500\ \mathrm{Hz} \cdot 1540\ \mathrm{m\,s}^{-1}}{2 \cdot 2.5\ \mathrm{MHz}} = 46.2\ \mathrm{cm\ s}^{-1} \tag{11.28}$$

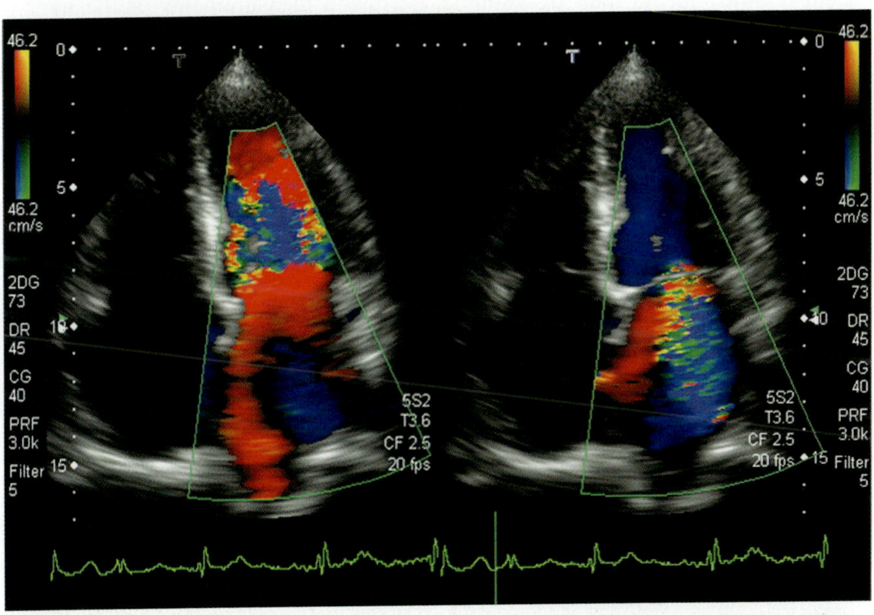

Figure 11.22. Color-coded blood flow in the heart. Flow to the transducer (to the top) is shown in red; flow in the downward direction is blue. In addition, turbulence is detected and color coded by a green/yellow overlay. Left: inflow of blood into the left ventricle through the open mitral valve (shown in red). Turbulent flow with downward components or aliasing occurs in the left ventricle. Right: the mitral valve is closed; however, a high speed leakage jet shown in blue, with turbulent components in green, can be seen and demonstrates malfunction of the valve. Blue color in the ventricle shows outflowing blood through the aortic valve. Images were recorded with a phased array with 2- to 5-MHz bandwidth and 2.5-MHz center frequency. Image courtesy of Toshiba Medical Systems.

This is also indicated by the velocity scale on the color bar at the side of Figure 11.22. The color Doppler processing relies on a certain number N of consecutive pulses with the PRF. The mean Doppler frequency is calculated according to Eq. (11.25). In addition, the variance of subsequent measurements can be analyzed and gives for large values an indication that flow may be turbulent. This is used in some systems to change the color scale if turbulent flow is assumed. This is also shown in Figure 11.22: an additional green-yellow color scale is used for turbulent flow, which is, for example, present in the high speed jet on the right side of the figure.

Low perfusion is better imaged with the use of contrast media as described earlier. In Figure 11.23, an example of a contrast study of thyroid perfusion is shown. In the normal thyroid, the perfusion is homogeneous, and the good contrast to tissue ratio of PI imaging at low MI can be seen on the left in comparison to the normal B-mode image on the right. The carotid artery clearly shows the strong contrast increase of blood relative to the B-mode image. The suppression of the linear signals from normal tissue is demonstrated by the low intensity of muscle tissue in front of the thyroid. Clinically, further applications for ultrasound contrast media are, for example, perfusion measurements of the liver to detect focal liver disease or brain perfusion imaging for stroke detection. Perfusion imaging techniques are under continuous development and can be expected to be extended by applications of targeted imaging in the future.

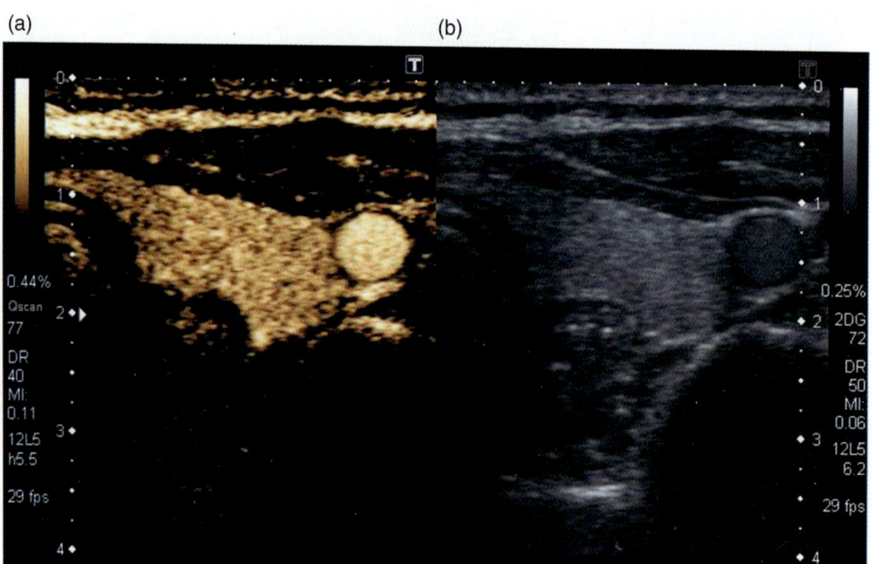

Figure 11.23. Simultaneous real-time display of normal thyroid in B-mode (b) and low MI pulse subtraction contrast harmonic imaging (a). Homogeneous uptake of microbubbles in the left lobe of the thyroid and microbubbles in the carotid artery can be seen. The MI of the imaging modes is 0.11 for the harmonic imaging mode and 0.06 for the normal B-mode image. Image courtesy of Toshiba Medical Systems.

REFERENCES

Albrecht T, Blomley M, Bolondi L, Claudon M, Correas J-M, Cosgrove D, Greiner L, Jäger K, de Jong N, Leen E, Lencioni R, Lindsell D, Martegani A, Solbiati L, Thorelius L, Tranquart F, Weskott H P, Whittingham T. Guidelines for the use of contrast agents in ultrasound. Ultraschall Med 2004;25:249–256.

Alonso A, Della Martina A, Stroick M, Fatar M, Griebe M, Pochon S, Schneider M, Hennerici M, Allemann E, Meairs S. Molecular imaging of human thrombus with novel abciximab immunobubbles and ultrasound. Stroke 2007;38(5):1508–1514.

Baker DW. Pulsed ultrasonic blood-flow sensing. IEEE Trans Son Ultrason 1970;SU-17:170–185.

Bamber JC. Ultrasonic properties of tissue. In: Duck FA, Baker AC, Starrit HC, editors. *Ultrasound in Medicine*. Bristol: Institute of Physics Publishing; 1998.

Bloch SH, Dayton PA, Ferrara KW. Targeted imaging using ultrasound contrast agents. IEEE Eng Med Biol Mag 2004;23:18–29.

Chomas JE, Dayton P, Allen J, Morgan K, Ferrara KW. Mechanisms of contrast agent destruction. IEEE Trans Ultrason Ferroelectr Freq Control 2001;48(1):232–248.

Chomas J, Dayton P, May D, Ferrara K. Nondestructive subharmonic imaging. IEEE Trans Ultrason Ferroelectr Freq Control 2002;49(7):883–892.

Christiansen JP, Leong-Poi H, Klibanov AL, Kaul S, Lindner JR. Non-invasive imaging of myocardial reperfusion injury using leukocyte-targeted contrast echocardiography. Circulation 2002;105:1764–1767.

Dayton PA, Ferrara KW. Targeted imaging using ultrasound. J Magn Reson Imaging 2002;16:362–377.

Doinikov AA, Dayton PA. Spatio-temporal dynamics of an encapsulated gas bubble in an ultrasound field. J Acoust Soc Am 2006;120(2):661–669.

Duck FA. *Physical Properties of Tissue*. New York: Academic Press; 1990.

Ellegala D, Leong-Poi H, Carpenter JE, Klibanov AL, Kaul S, Shaffrey ME, Sklenar J, Lindner JR. Imaging tumor angiogenesis with contrast ultrasound and microbubbles targeted to $\alpha_v\beta_3$. Circulation 2003;108:336–341.

Evans DH. In: Wells PNT, editor. *Advances in Ultrasound Techniques and Instrumentation*. New York: Churchill Livingstone; 1993. Chapter 8.

Eyding J, Wilkening WG, Postert T. Brain perfusion and ultrasonic imaging techniques. Eur J Ultrasound 2002;16:91–104.

Eyding J, Wilkening WG, Reckhardt M, Schmid G, Meves SH, Ermert H, Przuntek H, Postert T. Contrast burst depletion imaging (CODIM): a new imaging procedure and analysis method for semiquantitative ultrasonic perfusion imaging. Stroke 2003;34:77–83.

Gramiak R, Shah PM. Echocardiography of the aortic root. Invest Radiol 1968;3: 356–366.

Hickling R. Analysis of echoes from a solid elastic sphere in water. J Acoust Soc Am 1962;34:1582–1592.

Hope Simpson D, Chin CT, Burns PN. Pulse inversion Doppler: a new method for detecting nonlinear echoes from microbubble contrast agents. IEEE Trans Ultrason Ferroelectr Freq Control 1999;46(2):372–382.

Jensen JA. A model for the propagation and scattering of ultrasound in tissue. J Acoust Soc Am 1991;89(1):182–190.

Jensen JA. *Estimation of Blood Flow Velocities Using Ultrasound*. Cambridge: Cambridge University Press; 1996.

de Jong N. Acoustic properties of ultrasound contrast agents [PhD thesis]. Erasmus University Rotterdam: 1993.

de Jong N, Bouakaz A, Frinking P. Basic acoustic properties of microbubbles. Echocardiography 2002;19(3):229–240.

Kasai C, Namekawa K, Koyano A, Omoto R. Real-time two dimensional blood flow imaging using an autocorrelation technique. IEEE Trans Son Ultrason 1983;SU-32:458–464.

Leong-Poi H, Christiansen J, Heppner P, Lewis CW, Klibanov AL, Kaul S, Lindner JR. Assessment of endogenous and therapeutic arteriogenesis by contrast ultrasound molecular imaging of integrin expression. Circulation 2005;111(24):3248–3254.

Lindner JR. Microbubbles in medical imaging: current applications and future directions. Nat Rev: Drug Discov 2004;3:527–532.

Meves SH, Wilkening WG, Thies T, Eyding J, Finger THM, Schid G, Ermert H, Postert T. Comparison between echo contrast agent-specific imaging modes and perfusion weighted magnetic resonance imaging for the assessment of brain perfusion. Stroke 2002;33:2433–2437.

Miller DL, Quddus J. Diagnostic ultrasound activation of contrast agent gas bodies induces capillary rupture in mice. Proc Natl Acad Sci U S A 2000;97(18):10179–10184.

Mleczko M, Postema M, Schmitz G. Discussion of the Application of Finite Volterra Series for the Modeling of the Oscillation Behaviour of Ultrasound Contrast Agents. Applied Acoustics. 2009;70(10):1363–1369.

Morse PM, Ingard KU. *Theoretical Acoustics*. New York: McGraw-Hill; 1968.

Phillips P. Contrast pulse sequences (CPS): imaging nonlinear microbubbles. Proc IEEE Ultrason Symp 2001;2:1739–1745.

Postema M, van Wamel A, Lancée CT, de Jong N. Ultrasound-induced encapsulated microbubble phenomena. Ultrasound Med Biol 2004;30(6):827–840.

Reinhardt M, Hauff P, Briel A, Uhlendorf V, Linker RA, Mäurer M, Schirner M. Sensitive particle acoustic quantification (SPAQ): a new ultrasound-based approach for the quantification of ultrasound contrast media in high concentrations. Invest Radiol 2005;40(1):2–7.

Rubin JM, Bude RO, Carson PL, Bree RL, Adler RS. Power Doppler ultrasound: a potential useful alternative to mean-frequency-based color Doppler ultrasound. Radiology 1994;190:853–856.

Schmitz G. Ultrasound in medical diagnosis. In: Pike R, Sabatier P, editors. *Scattering, Scattering and Inverse Scattering in Pure and Applied Physics*. London: Academic Press; 2002. pp. 161–174.

Schrope BA, Newhouse VL. Second harmonic ultrasonic blood perfusion measurement. Ultrasound Med Biol 1993;19(7):567–579.

Shi WT, Forsberg F, Hall AL, Chiao RY, Liu J, Miller S, Thomenius KE, Wheatley MA, Goldberg BB. Subharmonic imaging with microbubble contrast agents: initial results. Ultrason Imaging 1999;21:79–94.

Shi WT, Forsberg F, Goldberg BB. Subharmonic imaging with contrast microbubbles. In: Goldberg BB, Raichlen JS, Forsberg F, editors. *Ultrasound Contrast Agents: Basic Principles and Clinical Applications*. London: Martin Dunitz Ltd; 2001. pp. 47–57.

Shung KK, Thieme GA. *Ultrasonic Scattering by Biological Tissues*. Boca Raton (FL): CRC Press; 1993.

Tiemann K, Lohmeier S, Kuntz S, Köster J, Pohl C, Burns PN, Porter TR, Nanda NC, Lüderitz B, Becher H. Real-time contrast echo assessment of myocardial perfusion at low emission power: first experimental and clinical results using power pulse inversion imaging. Echocardiogr J Cardiovasc Ultrasound Allied Tech 1999;16:799–809.

Tiemann K, Pohl C Schlosser T, Goenechea J, Bruce M, Veltmann C, Kuntz S, Bangard M, Becher H. Stimulated acoustic emission: pseudo-Doppler shifts seen during the destruction of nonmoving microbubbles. Ultrasound Med Biol 2000;26(7):1161.

Villanueva FS, Lu E, Bowry S, Kilic S, Tom E, Wang J, Gretton J, Pacella JJ, Wagner WR. Myocardial ischemic memory imaging with molecular echocardiography. Circulation 2007;115(3):345–352.

Wei K, Jayaweera AR, Firoozan S, Linka A, Skyba DM, Kaul S. Quantification of myocardial blood flow with ultrasound-induced destruction of microbubbles administered as a constant venous infusion. Circulation 1998;97:473–483.

Wei K, Ragosta M, Thorpe J, Coggins M, Moos S, Kaul S. Noninvasive quantification of coronary blood flow reserve in humans using myocardial contrast echocardiography. Circulation 2001;103(21):2560–2565.

Weller GER, Lu E, Csikari MM, Klibanov AL, Fischer D, Wagner WR, Villanueva FS. Ultrasound imaging of acute cardiac transplant rejection with microbubbles targeted to intercellular adhesion molecule-1. Circulation 2003;108(2):218–224.

Wells PNT. A range gated Doppler system. Med Biol Eng 1969;7:641–652.

Wild JJ. The use of ultrasound pulses for the measurement of biological tissues and the detection of tissue density changes. Surgery 1950;27:183–188.

12

ACOUSTIC MICROSCOPY FOR BIOMEDICAL APPLICATIONS

JÜRGEN BEREITER-HAHN
Institut für Zellbiologie und Neurowissenschaft, Johann-Wolfgang-Goethe-Universität, Frankfurt/M, Germany

12.1 SOUND WAVES AND BASICS OF ACOUSTIC MICROSCOPY

Similar to other microscopic procedures, acoustic microscopy provides images of specimens. However, in contrast to most light microscopic techniques, these images cannot be interpreted in a straightforward manner; instead, a detailed analysis is required to extract the information hidden within the images. The difference between light and acoustic microscopy corresponds to the difference between visual comprehension of our world and the information gained by feeling with fingers. Thus, the information gained is complementary.

Investigating mechanics on a microscopic scale seems strange in a biomedical world considering genomics, proteomics, and the interactions of signal transduction chains as the main clues for understanding how a cell or an organism functions. Indeed, all these molecular processes determine the function of a cell, which finally is a physical unit with a given shape and thus exerting mechanical forces, electrical currents, just physical properties. Comprehension of cells or organs on this level of organization is a holistic one, because mechanical forces as well as voltages and currents require a complete system of action and reaction where forces can be balanced or can produce movements in cases where they would not be in equilibrium. Major difficulty lies in bridging the description levels of biochemistry and biophysics.

Biomedical Imaging: Principles and Applications, First Edition. Edited by Reiner Salzer.

Acoustic microscopy provides unique information on the shape and mechanical properties of an object at a microscopic level. The biological material may even be placed on optically opaque materials such as ceramics or steel used for implantation purposes. The message has to be deciphered from the interaction of sound waves with the object and the image and the subsequent amplification and imaging procedure. As in sonography, x/y scans (= C-scan) or x/z scans (=B-scan) may be used for specimen characterization.

12.1.1 Propagation of Sound Waves

Sound waves are material waves propagated by fast compression–rarefactions cycles (longitudinal waves) and therefore probe the mechanical properties of the investigated specimen. The speed of phase movement (c) of an acoustic wave depends on the elasticity of the material (ε) and its density (ρ):

$$c = \sqrt{\frac{\varepsilon}{\rho}} \tag{12.1}$$

When sound waves impinge on a solid surface, part of the energy is reflected (Eq. 12.2). Reflectivity is a function of the impedance (Z_s and Z_F) differences at the boundary between the reflecting surface and the contacting material (e.g., water/solid or saline/tissue interface) and the angle of incidence (Θ). In the case of normal (i.e., vertical) incidence, reflectivity (R) is given by the following:

$$R^2 = \frac{I_r}{I_0} = \left(\frac{Z_s - Z_F}{Z_s + Z_F}\right)^2 \tag{12.2}$$

where I_r and I_0 denote the reflected intensities and Z_S and Z_F represent the impedances of sample and fluid layer.

Impedance Z of a material is defined by the product of its density (ρ) and the speed of sound wave propagation (c):

$$Z = \rho \bullet c \tag{12.3}$$

The unit of impedance is 1 rayl = 1 kg m^{-2} s^{-1}; practically often the megarayl (1 Mrayl = 10^6 rayl) is used.

The general equation describing reflection at an angle (Θ) is given by

$$R(\theta) = \frac{A_r}{A_0} = \frac{Z_F \cos^2 2\theta_S + Z_S \sin^2 2\theta_S - Z_F}{Z_F \cos^2 2\theta_S + Z_S \sin^2 2\theta_S + Z_F} \tag{12.4}$$

where A_0 and A_r are the amplitudes of the impinging and the reflected waves, respectively.

The nonreflected part penetrates the solid where it further propagates as a longitudinal wave. Excitation of the boundary surface causes it to move up and down, and this oscillation propagates as a transversal surface wave. At a specific angle of incidence (the Rayleigh angle), the whole impinging acoustic wave may move along the surface of a surface, being split into a longitudinal and a transversal surface wave, both propagating with the same phase velocity and finally leaking back to the lens. These waves are called *Rayleigh waves* or *leaky surface waves*. Interference of Rayleigh waves with waves reflected from the surface of a probe is the basis of $V(z)$ characteristics (Fig. 12.1).

In fluids or soft materials (as in biological tissues), no surface waves are induced, or they will be strongly attenuated.

Contrary to electromagnetic wave spectra, no transparency window exists for acoustic waves. They become monotonically attenuated, increasing with the square of frequency. Attenuation at a given frequency is defined by the decrease of amplitude of a wave depending on the distance (x) passed:

$$A = A_0 \exp(-\alpha_I x) \tag{12.5}$$

where α_I is the attenuation coefficient related to intensity decrease and is measured in Neper (Np) or in Bel. Normally, it is given as 1/10 of a Bel (dB)

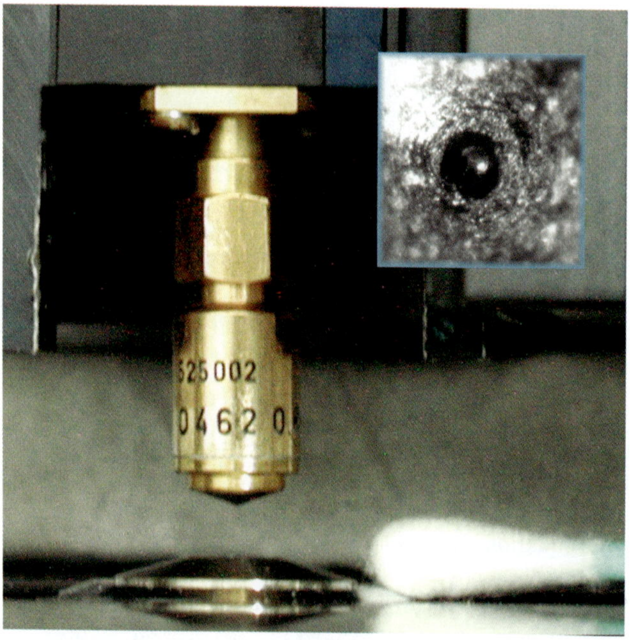

Figure 12.1. Acoustic broadband lens (gigahertz range) mounted on an ELSAM® microscope scanner and adjusted to a light microscope (lens is facing an objective lens of the light microscope). Inset: Top view of the acoustic lens with the spherical cavity in the middle. This cavity, with about 30 μm diameter, focuses the ultrasound. The broad surface around this cavity is roughened to decrease internal lens reflections. Photo by C. Blase.

corresponding to

$$\alpha_I x = 20 \log_{10}(I_0/I)\text{dB} \tag{12.6}$$

where I_0 and I are the sound intensities at the beginning and end of the distance, respectively.

12.1.2 Main Applications of Acoustic Microscopy

Because acoustic-wave-based images reveal mechanical parameters only, no staining is required to produce contrast in the case of tissue sections or isolated cells. This consideration was the motivation of Lemons and Quate (1974) for the development of a Scanning Acoustic Microscope (SAM) in the early 1970s. Whether this anticipation will hold true remains doubtful after the very slow increase in biomedical applications. Until now, most of the applications have been found in materials sciences, where, for example, delaminations of thin layers or microcracks can be detected with extreme sensitivity.

In the biomedical field, the main studies have been on tissue sections of the cardiovascular system, skin, and intestine, as well as investigations on the mechanical properties of bone and cartilage. In addition, cells in culture were the favourite specimens of the author and a few others. Many of the previous difficulties in image analysis have been overcome during the past years, and diagnostic as well as therapeutic sonography experienced a huge advancement.

A first comprehensive review on theory and applications was edited by Andrew Briggs in 1992 and continued in further issues in 1995. More recently, an updated view on theory and applications in material sciences as well as in biology and medicine has been edited by Kundu (2004).

12.1.3 Parameters to Be Determined and General Introduction into Microscopy with Ultrasound

The main parameters of biological tissues revealed by acoustic microscopy are geometry (thickness), mass, and elasticity, which taken together are related to the speed of the sound waves within the materials and structural organization represented by sound attenuation. Depending on the frequency used, the lateral resolution is in the range of a light microscope (around 1 μm at 1 GHz); under specific conditions (e.g., at liquid He temperatures), frequencies up to 8–10 GHz can be reached, corresponding to resolutions close to 100 nm (Foster and Rugar, 1983, 1985). A resolution of 10–20 nm in the vertical axis of an acoustic lens is easily achieved if interference phenomena are evaluated. Very high intensities within the focal spot can give rise to nonlinear phenomena by multiple phonon reactions and, by this, considerably increase resolution (Foster and Rugar, 1985). In general, a strict determination of lateral resolution is not possible; it strongly depends on the transfer characteristics of the acoustic lens, the contrast, and the wavelength. Experimentally it is best determined by calculating the spatial frequencies from the Fourier spectrum of a line scan of a specimen containing high spatial frequencies (Block et al., 1990). Commercial instruments are operated up to a maximum of 2 GHz. The lower frequency limit is more difficult to define; in most cases, it will be considered around 100 MHz. Sound waves of this frequency are strongly attenuated in air; therefore, the transducer has to be coupled to the specimen via a fluid layer. Attenuation of waves within this coupling fluid layer represents the main limit for using high frequencies; another limiting factor is lens design for high frequency imaging.

The idea of using ultrasound for microscopic imaging dates back to Sokolov (1949) who first viewed ultrasound waves projected via a lens on the surface of water. Most acoustic microscopes used are SAMs. One of the goals envisaged by investigators performing acoustic microscopy is a better understanding of the parameters controlling diagnostic sonography. Another source of interest is the increasing acceptance of mechanical forces as mediators in embryonic development (Beloussov, 1998; Beloussov et al., 1994), cell migration (i.e., in wound healing, invasiveness of cancer cells or embryonic foldings), cellular differentiation (e.g., Emerman and Pitelka, 1977; Kippenberger et al., 2000; Lyall and El Haj, 1994), and health impairments by pathological changes of tissue mechanical properties as in atherosclerosis (e.g., Saijo, 2004; Saijo et al., 2001) or osteoporosis (eg. Maia et al., 2002; Paschalis et al., 2004). Combined with specific contrast techniques (gold or nanobubble coupling of target molecules), acoustic microscopy will be extended to the molecular level (van Wamel et al., 2006). This, however, remains to be studied in future experiments. Therapeutic applications of ultrasound have not been performed on the microscopic level, although ultrasound in the lower megahertz region can be used for local membrane permeabilization (sonoporation) as required, for example, in cell transfection (Bao et al., 1997; Frenkel et al., 2002; van Wamel et al., 2006) and a variety of therapeutic approaches as in tumor treatment (Liu et al., 2005) and drug delivery (Bekeredjian et al., 2005). Tumor cell killing very much depends on the type of tumor and seems to be based on cellular membrane disruption, including plasma membrane as well as mitochondrial membranes, and therefore require quite high energy densities, that is, 3–4 W cm^{-2} for 60 s at 2.2 MHz (Wang et al., 2009). At even higher intensities reached by focusing ultrasound on the muscle of mice that were fully alive (800–300 W cm^{-2} at 1 MHz for 20 s four times with 2 weeks interval and spot size of 1.5 mm), expression of Cytomegalovirus (CMV)-promoted luciferase expression in transfected mouse muscle had been stimulated up to 6.5 fold (Hundt et al., 2009). Thus, the reaction of different tissues to ultrasound cannot be predicted at the moment.

12.2 TYPES OF ACOUSTIC MICROSCOPY

In principle, transmission and reflection techniques have been developed. For transmission systems, see, for instance, Ashman and Rho (1990), Kulik et al., (1992), and Maev and Levin (1997). From the very beginning, acoustic microscopes have been combined with other imaging techniques, that is, confocal laser scanning microscopy, fluorescence microscopy (Blase and Bereiter-Hahn, 2004; Kanngiesser and Anliker, 1991; Lüers et al., 1992; Lemor et al., 2004; Rabe et al., 2002) with microinterferometry (Bereiter-Hahn, 1987b) or with scanning force microscopy (Kopycinska-Müller et al., 2004). Scanning acoustic microscopy operated in the reflection mode became the most widely used principle since its introduction by Lemons and Quate (1974), because it was provided commercially, for example, by Olmypus, Leica (now SAM Tec), and Honda Electronics. Therefore, I will concentrate on this type of microscopes, the evaluation procedures, and some of the results achieved. In addition, the combination of a light microscope with an ultrasound transducer unit to observe ultrasound-induced oscillations of microbubbles (or cells in suspension), which was constructed by Postema at the Erasmus Medical Center in Rotterdam (Postema et al., 2004), will not be included.

12.2.1 Scanning Laser Acoustic Microscope (LSAM)

The general setup of this type of microscope was the first type of acoustic microscope brought to work (Korpel et al., 1971). The Laser Scanning Acoustic Microscope (LSAM; Kessler, 1976; Rudd et al., 1987) combines interaction of a specimen with plane ultrasound waves (typically 100 MHz) and a readout via scanning laser interferometry, revealing its shifts in phase and amplitude of the deformation of a thin gold layer, which acts as a receiver of the sound waves after passing the specimen. This principle has been used widely for the investigation of tissue sections (e.g., Agemura and O'Brien, 1990). Because this is a transmission-based microscopy and flat specimens are investigated, some of the interpretation problems that are due to varying slopes of reflecting surfaces are avoided, and therefore, attenuation and elasticity values are very well presented by this method.

12.2.2 Pulse-Echo Mode: Reflection-Based Acoustic Microscopy

These microscopes are all SAMs of the confocal type. Thus, the images are derived from point-by-point scanning of a specimen and represent data obtained for each pixel in a 2D matrix. The confocality and selection of a narrow time gate for the reflected pulse include the possibility of 3D imaging, which, however, was not very widely used in the past. Three-dimensional images have been calculated from thickness measurements (Fig. 12.11), but this is not real 3D imaging. More recently, real 3D images are reconstructed from time-resolved SAM.

In the very heart of such a microscope is the acoustic lens, which in the case of frequencies >100 MHz typically consists of a cylindrical sapphire with a plane side bearing the transducer element and a small spherical cavity on the opposite side directed toward the specimen (Figs 12.1 and 12.2). For gigahertz lenses, the cavity diameter is in the range of 30 μm within an area of about 5-mm diameter and has a roughened surface to reduce sound reflections within the lens. The velocity of sound is about 11.100 m s^{-1} in sapphire and 1500 m s^{-1} in

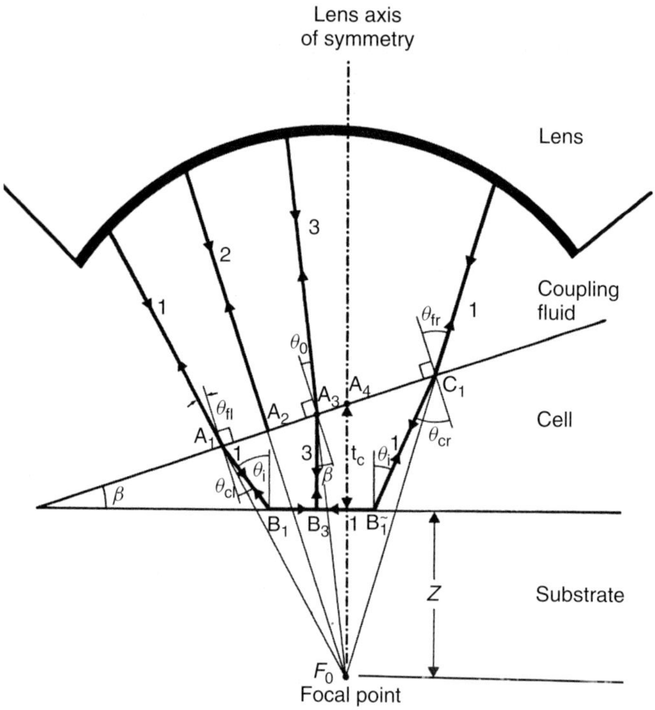

Figure 12.2. Scheme of an acoustic lens and course of sound waves interacting with a cell (oblique surface) on a solid substrate. The spherical cavity at the site where the lens is coupled to the object via a sound-propagating fluid renders the plane wave to converge in a focal spot. For ray 1, diffraction at the coupling fluid/cell interface (at A1) and then the formation of a Rayleigh wave from B1 to B1 is shown. With ray 2, sound reflection from the cell surface is exemplified, and ray 3 describes the reflection from the substrate. The focal spot in this case lies within the solid substrate. Angles θ mark the changes in the direction of sound propagation by diffraction. *Source:* From Kundu et al., 1991.

water (used as a coupling fluid); thus, the refractive index ratio amounts to 7.5 compared to 1.5 in light microscopy. Chromatic dispersion, therefore, is low, but losses at the lens/water interface due to reflections are a severe problem, which is overcome only in part by surface coatings. The influence of lens and electronic device on image generation has been discussed in detail by the group of Boseck (Block et al., 1990).

The transducer is a piezoelectronic actuator (a thin ZnO film), with its crystal axis perpendicular to the surface of the sapphire, which becomes activated by oscillating voltage and thus contracts and dilates periodically with the frequency of the oscillating voltage. By this, a plane wave is generated within the lens material, propagating along its length. The spherical cavity at the site where the lens is coupled to the object via a sound-propagating fluid renders the plane wave to converge in a focal spot (Fig. 12.2). Its size depends on the aperture of the acoustic lens, that is, the diameter of the cavity and focal length. As in every confocal method, the size of the focal spot determines the spatial resolution of the microscope. For 100 MHz, the resolution limit is about 15 μm, with a penetration depth of 4 mm; at 2 GHz, resolution is 0.75 μm (or better), but penetration depth decreases to 10 μm.

In the reflection mode, the same lens that sends the acoustic pulse (typically 4–25 ns long) acts as a receiver; however, two lenses may be used arranged in opposite positions, one sending the sound wave and the other focused to the same plane acting as a receiver. Most of the commercial instruments (Fig. 12.3) are operated in the reflection mode; therefore, only this type is discussed. In these cases, a fast circulator switches between the oscillating frequency inducing the ultrasound and the amplifier chain processing the signal produced by transforming the reflected sound wave into a voltage oscillation. This is superimposed on a carrier frequency, and after amplification within a heterodyne amplifier, it may be visualized on a screen or digitized and stored as a digital image. Considerable diversification of instrumental details occurred within 20 years of the introduction of commercial instruments.

Many of these modifications are laboratory prototypes and can be used only by personal collaboration; the development of commercial instruments was impaired by a relatively low number of instruments sold. The main advantage of the more recent developments is in the signal stored. The early high resolution instruments working in the gigahertz range, such as the ELSAM from Leica (Wetzlar) and the high frequency operated Evolution PII from PVA Tepla/KSI (Herborn and Westhausen, Germany), use the amplitude of the reflected sound signal received within a certain adjustable time window for image generation, which then might be digitized (32 bit in the case of the PII SAM). The "Evolution PII" instrument, for instance, sets time gates with a width down to 2 ns. In some recent brands working between 50 and 300 MHz (e.g., HMC by Honda Electronics, Toyohashi) or at about 900 MHz (SASAM from IBMT, St. Ingbert, Lemor et al., (2004)), the whole reflected signal along a series of meandering scanning lines (C-scan, including the B-scan for each pixel) is collected and may later on be processed to produce images either by using an amplitude overall image or by filtering certain time gates representing, for example, surface reflections only from a specimen or separating the reflections from a solid surface bearing the biological material from other reflections and thus allowing for the determination of attenuation. At gigahertz sound frequencies, full signal collection represents a high technical challenge.

The main features of instruments determining their practical use are as follows.

1. The frequency of the ultrasound is the main factor determining resolution. Production of lenses with reproducible high quality for the upper megahertz and gigahertz range is difficult. High aperture for high resolution images and low signal because of frequency-dependent attenuation force the reduction of working distance between the lens and the specimen (above 1 GHz typically 30 μm) and thus limits microscopy to very

(a)
(b)
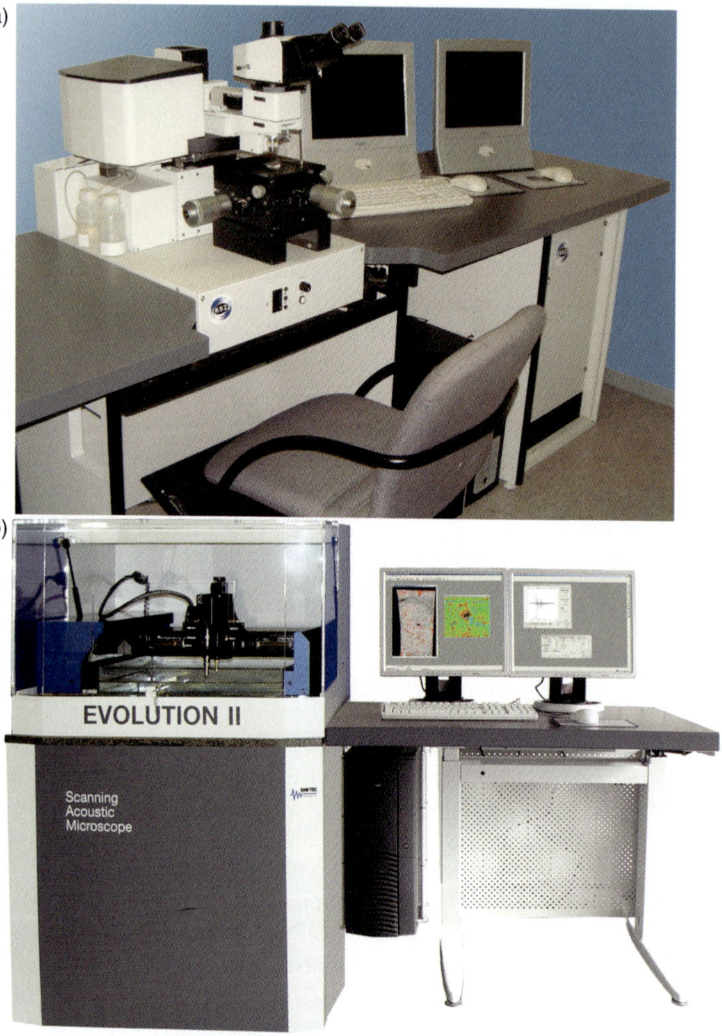

Figure 12.3. Two acoustic microscopes that are distributed by PVA Tepla (Westhausen, Germany). (a) High resolution instrument "Evolution PII" (f $\leq$ 2 GHz) with integrated light microscope. In this image, the head with the acoustic scanner is moved toward the left. (b) Instrument of the Evolution-series (Evolution II) in the frequency range between 3 and 400 MHz with large motorized scan width for samples up to 520 mm $\times$ 380 mm $\times$ 45 mm (w/l/h) and water tank for the specimen. (Images courtesy of PVA Tepla, Westhausen, Germany).

flat specimens. Frequencies up to 8 or 10 GHz are possible to transmit through superfluid helium only, and by this, the resolution barriers of light microscopy have been broken (Foster and Rugar, 1983). Larger focal lengths and deeper penetration instruments working at lower frequencies

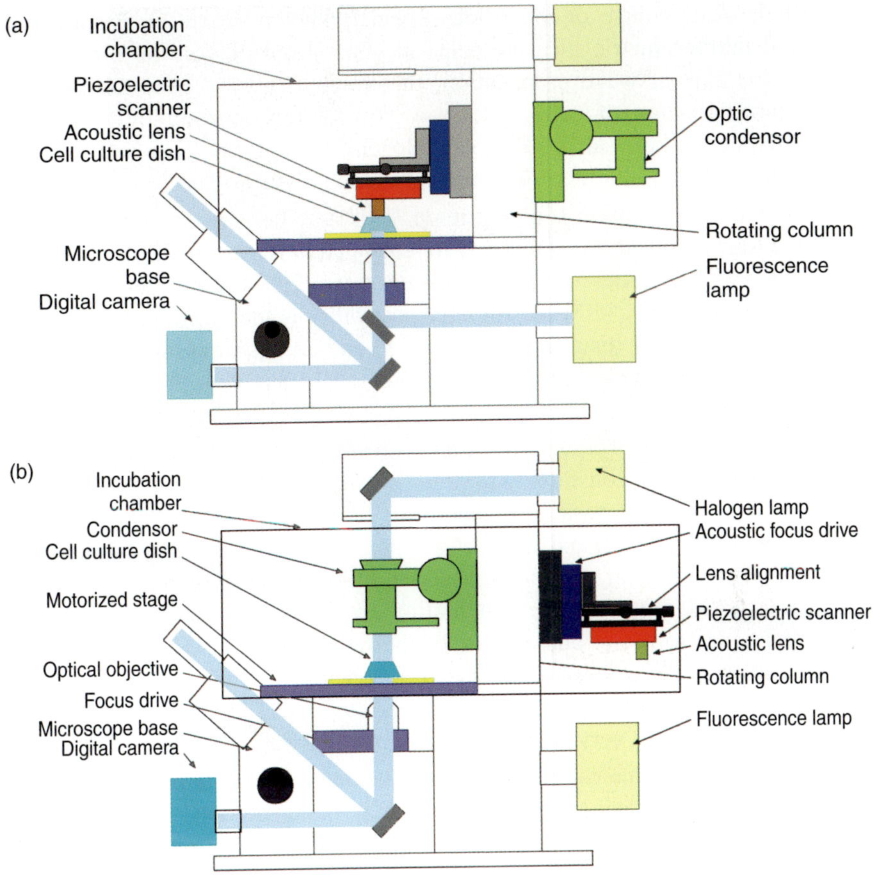

Figure 12.4. Schematic drawings of the SASAM system, an acoustic head integrated into an inverted fluorescence microscope, produced by the Institut für Biomedizinische Technik (St. Ingbert). (a) Acoustic head in active position (above the specimen). (b) Transmitting light condensor in active position, acoustic head turned to opposite side. Drawings courtesy of E.C. Weiss and R. Lemor.

(≤200 MHz) are superior for imaging structures that are not really flat. A good example for the application of SAM up to 200 MHz for *in vivo* studies has been given by Jörgensen and his group at the Centre of Experimental Medical Ultrasound at the Aarhus University Hospital. They imaged blood vessels in the thigh of a rat after removing the overlaying tissues.

2. Pulse length: pulses of 15–25 ns length contain 10–20 cycles for gigahertz sound, a coherence length sufficient for interference fringe generation resulting from interference between sound waves reflected at different interfaces (Figs 12.7 and 12.8). Very thin layers may also cause interferences within very short pulses (<5 ns); however, if pulse length allows only for one or two oscillations, the wavelength and frequency are no longer defined.

If the time course of the whole signal is known, it can be deconvolved and interferometric measurements in general are of very high resolution in the axis of wave propagation; therefore, they have been used for the characterization of cells and tissues by various quantitation procedures (Bereiter-Hahn et al., 1992, 1995; Hozumi et al., 2004; Karl and Bereiter-Hahn, 1998; Litniewski and Bereiter-Hahn, 1990; Zoller et al., 1997).

3. Acquisition of phase and amplitude. This may be performed by acquiring the fully resolved original signal for each pixel (as, for instance, realized for the instruments described by Hozumi et al., (2004), Lemor et al., (2004), and Raum et al., (2003a). Another possibility is the immediate generation of two different images, a phase image and an amplitude image as it was brought to action by Grill and his group (Hillmann et al., 1994; Grill et al., 1999; Pluta and Grill, 2002).
4. Time resolution. These systems take advantage of the relatively slow phase propagation of acoustic waves, thus allowing the determination of time of flight of a signal passing a specimen. Such a system was introduced by Briggs et al., (1993) and also underlies the instruments built by Lemor et al., (2004) (Fig. 12.4) and Hozumi et al., (2004). The Evolution instruments from SAM TEC/PVA Tepla operating up to 400 MHz automatically shift time gates to detect phase shifts of the reflected sound at the positive and negative peak positions. However, for very thin specimens, time resolution is insufficient for straightforward interpretations. These shortcomings may be overcome by very sophisticated signal analysis.
5. Scanning movements: In general, at least one scanning direction (x) is provided by the moving lens; the other may either be done by stepping the specimen or by shifting the lens. Step motors have been used for large-scale scanning (almost unlimited) with long acquisition times; the shortest acquisition times may be reached using fast scanning via piezoelements. Mechanical oscillators allow large-scale scanning (up to a few millimeters) as well as fast scanning in the micrometer range (e.g., 200 μm width), and because of its universal application this type has been used in the high resolution SAM constructed by Leica, which was improved (up to 60 scan lines per second) and purchased by SAM TEC (Fig. 12.3) and developed further as a 3D instrument by PVA Tepla (Westhausen, the company following SAM TEC). The type of scanner that is suited best depends on the requirements. One important factor is the strict correlation between the scanning position and the acoustic signal, thus the accuracy of the positioning. Fast scanning is related to smaller fields of viewing, but in addition, signal averaging may become a limiting factor at high sound frequencies that are subjected to strong attenuation. Then single signals may be accumulated for each point to improve signal to noise ratio, which finally results in an increase in image acquisition time.

12.2.2.1 Reflected Amplitude Measurements. Measuring sound reflected at the interface between coupling fluid and specimen (I_r/I_0) allows straightforward calculation of impedance (Z_S) and sound velocity (c_S) of a specimen using Eq. 12.2 or 12.4.

Sound velocity (c) in a body is a function of the appropriate elasticity modulus. In fluids, this is primarily the compression modulus (K):

$$c = \sqrt{\frac{K + \frac{4}{3} \cdot G}{\rho}} \tag{12.7}$$

where G is the shear modulus and ρ is the density of the liquid in grams per cubic centimeter. Commonly $G \ll K$; therefore, Eq. 12.8 is approximated to

$$c = \sqrt{\frac{K}{\rho}} \tag{12.8}$$

The relationship between the elastic modulus, E, and the compression modulus, K, is given by

$$K = \frac{E}{3 \cdot (1 - 2\mu)} \tag{12.9}$$

where μ is the Poisson ratio (e.g., for actin filaments about 0.4; Ziemann et al., 1994). The elastic modulus, E, is then 0.6 times the compression modulus, K.

Surface reflectivity has been widely used in a broad range of frequencies for the determination of elastic properties of biological hard tissues such as bone, dentin, or enamel (e.g., Maev et al., 2002; Meunier et al., 1988; Peck and Briggs, 1987; Raum et al., 2003a).

An example for measurements with this method is given: an "allmax" projection of a set of acoustic images taken from an isolated rat cardiomyocyte (Fig. 12.5). Adult cardiomyocytes are a good example for a specimen well suited for analysis by sound reflection measurements, but it also shows the limitations of this method. Because of cell thickness, reflections from the plastic material of low impedance supporting the cell do not interfere with the measurements. Separation of reflections from different surfaces can be improved by setting a narrow time gate for the reflected signal used to image a specimen. This is available for most of the commercially available instruments. From a single image, no distinction can be made between local differences in reflectivity caused by impedance differences or by the slope of the surface. This would require monitoring the phase of the reflected sound (which would shift with local thickness variations) or focus series. This was done by taking a series of images with a 0.5-μm increment in focal position; then, the brightest value for each pixel position (x_i, y_i) found in the whole set of about 20 images was written into a new image, thus showing only the brightest reflections at each point ("allmax image"). The focus

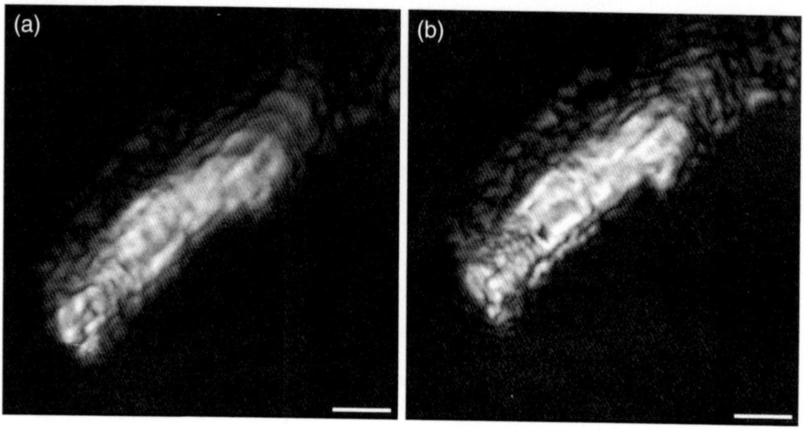

Figure 12.5. An “allmax” projection of a set of acoustic images taken from an isolated rat cardiomyocyte in relaxed (a) and contracted (b) state. Bar: 10 μm (courtesy of Dr M. Riehle).

increment has to be smaller than the focal depth of the acoustic lens to fulfill the Nyquist sampling theorem. In the case of 1 GHz, vertical resolution of the amplitude image is in the range of 3 μm; therefore, a recommended step size of 0.5 μm corresponds to sixfold oversampling. A detailed description of the physics of image reconstruction from such series has been provided by Raum et al., (2003a).

Additional limitations of this method are represented by the anisotropic structure of the probe. Only sections will allow for determination of acoustic anisotropy.

The simple relationship described by Eq. (12.2) is valid only for normal incidence. The assumption of normal incidence of ultrasound focused on a plane surface is justified in the focal plane because of the specific propagation pattern in the focal spot of an acoustic lens. If the focal plane of a lens is positioned several wavelengths above the surface to be imaged, only normally incident sound waves contribute to image formation. In many cases, the slope of the reflecting surface is not exactly known; therefore, the extended formula (including this obliqueness) cannot be applied, and thus only those parts of specimens that lie at approximately 90° to the incident sound beam can be studied. Examples of almost plane surfaces are tissue sections and very flat cells in culture (reflectivity does not change more than 5% if the slope of the reflecting surface of a cell is up to 15° (Weise et al., 1994)).

12.2.2.2 V(z) Imaging. A special case of reflection mode scanning is $V(z)$ scanning (voltage vs focus position). While focusing beyond the surface, because of interference between the acoustic waves reflected from the surface and the Rayleigh wave emitted back to the lens, periodic changes in reflected amplitude occur, which are characteristic for each material (Fig. 12.6). This method can

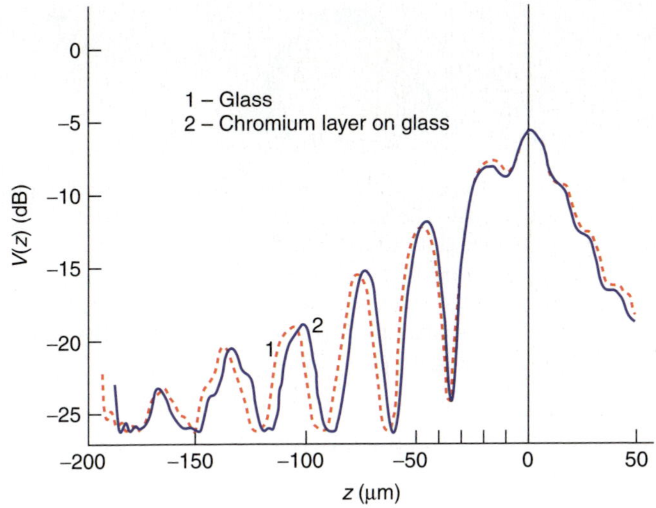

Figure 12.6. $V(z)$ curve for glass and glass covered with a 200-nm thick chromium layer (broken line) taken at 200 MHz (with an Olympus UH2 microscope). This curve has been obtained by plotting the reflected signal while focussing from the focus position on the glass surface (0—position) into the glass (negative focus positions) or above this surface (positive focus position). The thin chromium layer modulates the $V(z)$ signal. These modulations can be used to determine the acoustic properties of any superimposed layer with unknown properties. (From Block et al. 1990, with permission).

well be applied to biological hard materials (e.g., Block et al., 1990; Raum et al., 2006). The reflected voltage (V) in relation to focus position (z), as shown in Figure 12.6, is given by

$$V(z) = \int_0^{f \sin\alpha} U^2 2(r) P^2(r) R \frac{r}{f} \mathrm{e}^{-2jk_0 Z\sqrt{1-\left(\frac{r}{f}\right)^2}} r \, \mathrm{d}r \tag{12.10}$$

where U is the sound field produced by the transducer, P is the pupil function of the acoustic lens, R is the reflection function of the specimen, r is the radial position of the signal in the back focal plane of the lens, f is the focal length of the lens, r/f is the sinus of the aperture angle of the lens in combination with the coupling fluid, α is the half aperture angle of the lens, and k_0 is the wave number in the coupling fluid.

Although Rayleigh waves are missing within soft biological material, this material shifts the maxima and minima of the Rayleigh spectrum because sound velocity in the sample differs from that in the environment.

Modulations of hard material $V(z)$ curves by thin layers of soft material can also be used to calculate the acoustic properties of a thin layer of biological material. The theory of this model has been developed independently by several groups (Block et al., 1990; Chubachi et al., 1991; Kundu et al., 1991; Litniewski

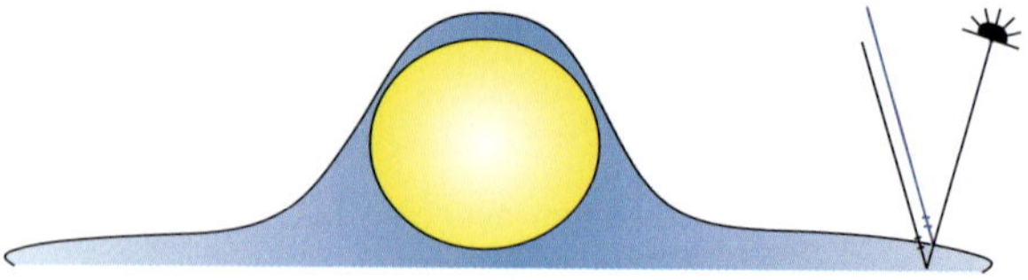

Figure 12.7. Schematic drawing of the cross section of a cell (blue, cytoplasm; yellow, nucleus) interacting with sound. The sound wave emitted from the acoustic lens (black ray) is partly reflected from the cell surface (blue line) and partly penetrates the cell to the solid substratum (e.g., plastic material or glass), where a fraction is reflected according to the acoustic impedance of the solid. Both these reflections interfere with each other, yielding a cell picture as exemplified for a group of HaCaT cells shown in Figure 12.8. (image width, 200 μm). (Courtesy of Dr. C. Blasé).

and Bereiter-Hahn, 1992; Yu and Boseck, 1992). Using a small part of $V(z)$ characteristics, allowed for the first time, mapping of elasticity (sound velocity) and attenuation over a cell with full resolution of the SAM (Bereiter-Hahn et al., 1992) (Fig. 12.13). More recently, Raum et al., (2003b) used the full Rayleigh spectrum obtained by large defocusing. Kundu et al., (1991) modeled cell properties from small defocusing only. The advantage of large defocus is the unambiguity of the calculations, which has to be introduced by setting limits in the calculations with the simplex approach used for small defocus images. The latter method was chosen because, for living cells, data acquisition time has to be as short as possible to avoid changes in cell parameters while the images are taken. Such active movements may be enhanced by fluid perturbation over the very small distance between the scanning lens and the cell surface: approaching the moving lens even more toward the cell increases the influence of fluid mechanics on the cell surface and supposedly evokes physiological reactions, thus obscuring the "real" situation. However, this influence has never been investigated systematically. For the investigation of tissue sections, large-range $V(z)$ analysis is a very elegant and reliable method.

The main advantages of this method are that it is a well developed theory, it is widely used in materials sciences, it offers high lateral resolution, and thin cytoplasmic layers can be analyzed. All the parameters can be calculated separately only in the microrange $V(z)$; bounds for the values are required to allow the simplex algorithm to converge to the correct set of values. A broad variety of substrata can be used to mount the specimen, and no interferences are required for the calculations.

The main disadvantages are the long acquisition time (several images are required) and the dependence on substrate properties, which must give distinct $V(z)$ curves.

12.2.2.3 V(f) Imaging. Variation of frequency has been used in light interference microscopy for the determination of two unknowns: thickness and refractive index (Bereiter-Hahn et al., 1979). A similar procedure can be applied in SAM (Kundu et al., 2000, 2006 and others). Using a phase- and amplitude-sensitive modulation of a SAM (Hillmann et al., 1994), longitudinal wave speed and attenuation in a cell or tissue section, as well as thickness profile are obtained from the voltage versus frequency or $V(f)$ curves. The challenge to determine at least four unknown parameters (speed of sound, attenuation, specimen thickness, and density) from acoustic images requires at least five images for reliable calculations. Grabbing a series of pictures in the range from 980 to 1100 MHz, with an increment of 20 MHz, allows the experimental generation of $V(f)$ curves for each pixel by simply changing the signal frequency while keeping the lens–specimen distance unchanged. Both amplitude and phase values of the $V(f)$ curves are used for obtaining cell properties and the cell thickness profile. Cell thickness, longitudinal wave speed, and attenuation can be estimated from the phase and amplitude for each pixel by the simplex inversion algorithm in a manner similar to $V(z)$ analysis. Theoretical analysis shows that the thin liquid layer, between the cell and the substrate, has a strong effect on the reflection coefficient and should not be ignored during the analysis (Kundu et al., 1991).

The main advantage of this method is that imaging can be done near the focal plane. Therefore, an optimal signal to noise ratio is achieved, no interference with Rayleigh waves occurs, and the method is independent from the properties of the solid substratum where the cells are growing on. This method allowed us to monitor by SAM the reaction of cells to mechanical stretch (Karl and Bereiter-Hahn, 1998). However, this method requires appropriate broadband lenses, which still cannot be produced reproducibly with the desired properties.

12.2.2.4 Interference-Fringe-Based Image Analysis. Thin layers of biological material on the supporting glass or plastic surfaces may give rise to interference of reflections from the surface of the sample with those from the supporting material. Prerequisites for such interferences are a sufficiently long sound pulse, small thickness of the sample ("small" relates to wavelength of sound, $<6-8\lambda$), and almost parallel reflecting surfaces (slope $<15-20^\circ$). Cells in culture exhibit an oblique surface relative to the supporting glass or plastic surface. Therefore, reflections from the substratum and from the surface of the biological sample cause a series of concentric interference fringes (Figs 12.8 and 12.9). These provide a useful signal for a fast and orienting analysis of shape, elasticity, and attenuation of the cells. The contrast of the interferences depends on the impedance of the solid material bearing the cells. Materials with high impedance, such as tungsten layers on glass or glass itself, give rise to very strong reflections that are only slightly modulated by the weak reflections from the surface of the cells; thus, the images are dominated by attenuation, while plastic materials have lower impedance and therefore interference fringes exhibit higher contrast. From the sum of adjacent bright and dark peak values, attenuation by the specimen can be calculated, while the difference of those values allows to calculate sound velocity (for detailed description of the method, see Litniewski and Bereiter-Hahn, 1990).

The approximate cell shape (topography) is immediately obvious from the pattern of interference fringes seen in SAM images. When applied to cells growing

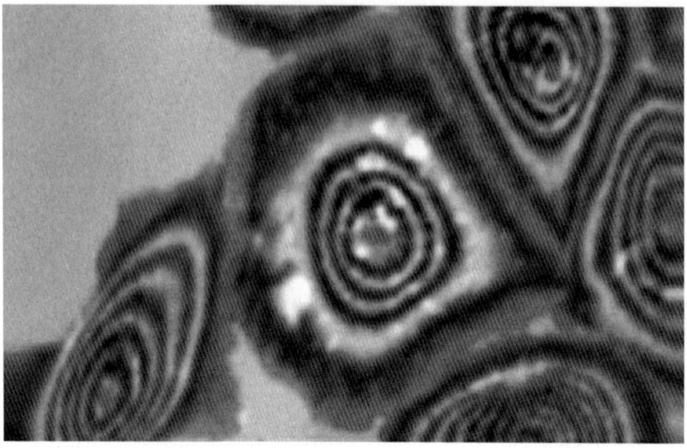

Figure 12.8. HaCaT cells on plastic as viewed by 1GHz acoustic microscopy (ELSAM). The course of the interference fringes indicates surface topography. Where the cells are not in contact with neighbors the develop a broad flat cytoplasmic layer (very broad interference fringes). The bright spots in the central cell indicate zones lacking contact to the plastic surface.

on a flat, solid substratum, these interference fringes delineate zones of equal acoustical path lengths between the reflecting boundaries, cell/culture medium and cell/substratum. Local variations in V_c would shift the position of an interference fringe; therefore, their pattern is only a first approximation to surface topography.

The big advantage of this method is its speed: a single amplitude image (scanning time <5 s) of a specimen is sufficient to calculate sound velocity, giving an estimation of elasticity. However, the method has several shortcomings: lateral resolution is limited to the distance between adjacent maxima and minima of interferences, and mechanical properties are assumed to be constant over this space. Reliable measurements require a solid substratum with relatively high impedance, that is, glass, and thus the overall contrast of these images is low, and the distance between lens and specimen is about 8λ apart to reach normal incidence, thus intensity is low. The procedure is limited to those areas showing interferences, and the order of interferences must be estimated properly. The density of the cytoplasm is assumed to be constant at an estimated level.

Therefore, this method was primarily used to follow dynamic events. The local dynamics of elasticity are easily visualized by Sobel filtering of the primary images taken at z-values a few wavelengths above the specimen. Sobel filtering reveals the steepness of gray level changes in between constructive and destructive interferences and thereby visualizes contrast (Fig. 12.9). Thus, as a first approximation, this filtering can be used to show elasticity distribution and is well suited for comparative observations of force distributions in migrating cells (Bereiter-Hahn and Lüers, 1998).

Contribution of substrate reflections can be avoided or at least strongly reduced by using substrates with an impedance close to that of the specimen under investigation or if the investigated specimen is thick, by sufficiently large defocusing.

(a)
(b)
(c)

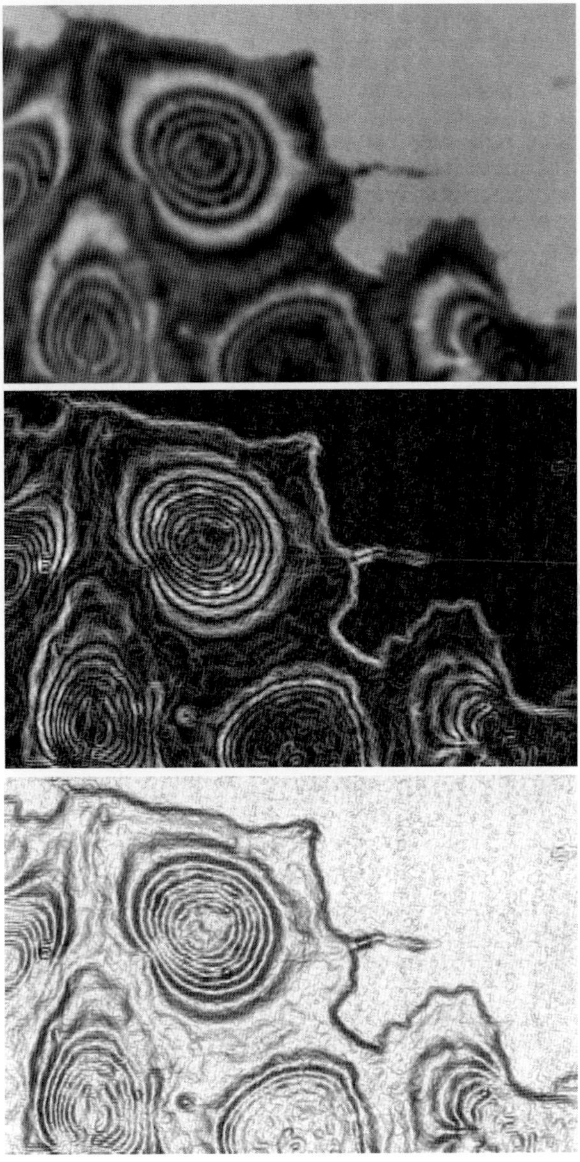

Figure 12.9. Example for visualization of the contrast function in an acoustic image by Sobel filtering. (a) The original SAM image of a group of HaCaT grown on a plastic culture dish, 1 GHz. (b) The first derivation of the original picture representing the intensity changes within the picture (Sobel filtering). To facilitate interpretation of this image, it will be inverted and thus results in (c). High contrast in the original is revealed by the black appearance, low contrast by brighter or gray areas. In addition, very fine structures become visible.

Materials almost matching cytoplasmic impedance are concentrated agar (>3%) or soft polyvinylchloride (Kanngiesser and Anliker, 1991).

12.2.2.5 Determination of Phase and the Complex Amplitude. Acoustic microscopy based on imaging phase and amplitude gives an easy access to all the data necessary for unequivocal evaluation of mechanical parameters of specimen in the reflected sound mode. For this purpose, an ELSAM has been equipped with an electronic circuit, allowing separation of the phase and the amplitude of the reflected signal (Fig. 12.10). The method has been presented in detail by Hillmann et al., (1994) and Grill et al., (1999). The probe-dependent phase shift of the signal can be achieved by comparing it with a reference derived from the sending oscillator. This multiplication is technically realized with a mixer followed by a lowpass filter. The complex amplitude has to be determined by splitting the reference and the probe wave path and extending the probe path by a quarter wavelength before it is mixed with the reference signal.

12.2.2.6 Combining V(f) with Reflected Amplitude and Phase Imaging. Speed was the main advantage of the interference-based method for cell mechanical properties (Litniewski and Bereiter-Hahn, 1990). However, it allowed only rough estimations of impedance (speed of sound, i.e., elasticity) and attenuation, all these at lateral resolution defined by the distance of constructive and destructive interferences. Shifting interference fringes using different frequencies can fill the gap of low spatial resolution. Frequency shifts can easily be programmed, and thus a few images can be sufficient to fill all the gaps between the maxima and minima of the interferences. In addition, combining phase and amplitude information provides an easy means to precisely calculate sound velocity and attenuation.

The acoustic path length is unequivocally determined at any maximum or minimum of an interference fringe: it represents a multiple of the wavelength λ. Because in the reflection mode sound passes twice through a specimen, destructive interferences (dark rings) occur at a multiple of $\lambda/4$, while constructive interferences represent multiples of $\lambda/2$. The multiple is given by the order (m) of the interference. Because λ results from c/f, and frequency f is known, λ can be replaced by the sound velocity c and frequency f:

$$d = mc_c/4f \tag{12.11}$$

in the case of destructive interferences, and

$$d = mc_c/2f \tag{12.12}$$

in the case of constructive interferences.

From the phase image, $\Delta\Phi$ (the phase difference between the sound waves reflected from an area devoid of specimen and the sound wave passing through a given volume of the specimen) can be defined by

$$\Delta\Phi = 4\pi df(1/c_f - 1/c_c) \tag{12.13}$$

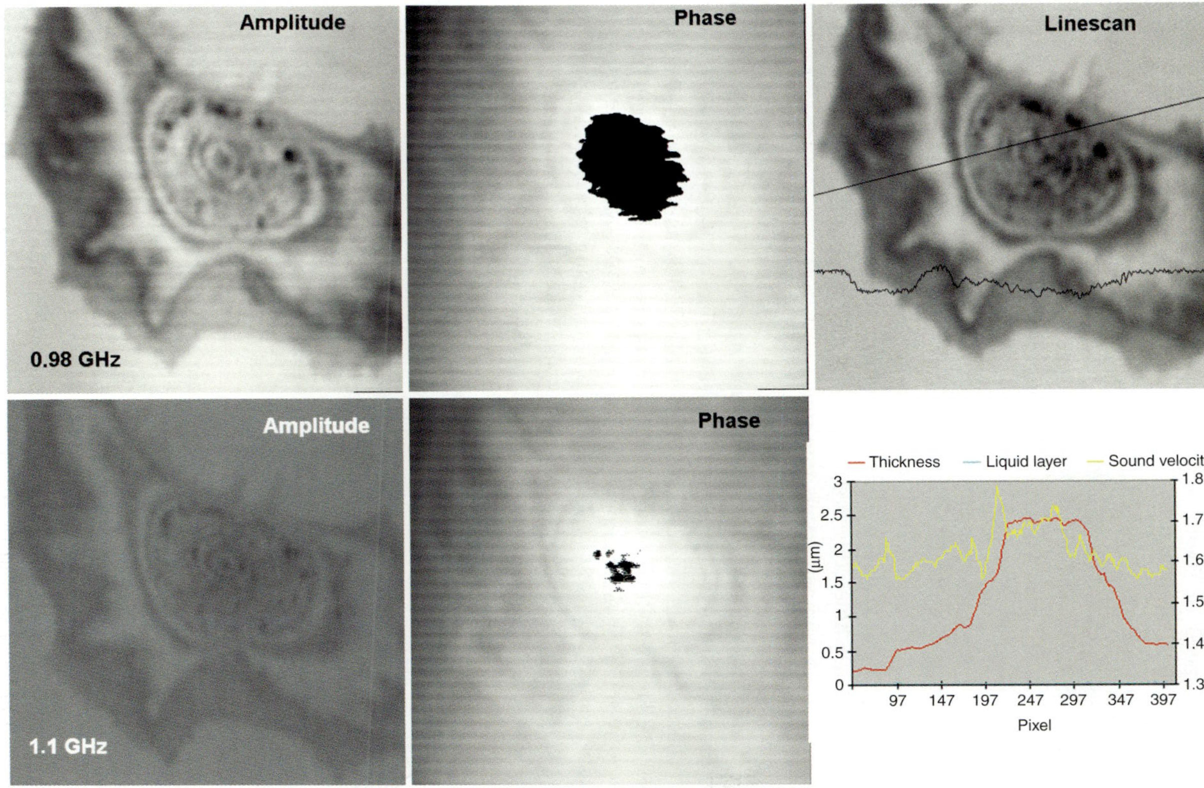

Figure 12.10. SAM images of an endothelial cell (XTH-2 cell) on plastic material taken at a series of different frequencies (here are shown 0.98 and 1.1 GHz). The phase change of the reflected sound and its intensity modulation by attenuation and interference phenomena are presented and then used to calculate the thickness and speed of sound along a chosen scan line, plotted in the graph. In this case, the presence of a thin layer of fluid between the cell and the solid substrate was assumed and incorporated into the calculations *Source:* From Kundu et al., 2000, with permission.

from which the following equation may be obtained:

$$c_c = c_f(1 + \Delta\Phi/\pi m) \tag{12.14}$$

where c_f is the speed of sound in the coupling medium and c_c is the speed of sound within the cytoplasm. Young's modulus may be calculated according to Eq. (12.9). Attenuation is calculated from the sum of adjacent maximal and minimal amplitudes according to Litniewski and Bereiter-Hahn (1990).

If this procedure is performed for a single frequency only, 5 s of image acquisition (512 × 512 pixel) is sufficient with the Leica ELSAM, but the values have to be integrated for the spaces in between the extrema of the interference fringes. If pictures were taken at several frequencies (Δf in the range of 20 MHz at a basic frequency close to 1 GHz), the shifts of the fringes fill in the gaps left by the first image and thus spatial resolution increases up to covering all areas of a cell with the desired density of measurement points. Figure 12.11 gives an example of such a whole-cell reconstruction using three different frequencies, corresponding to 15 s image acquisition time.

12.2.2.7 Time-Resolved SAM and Full Signal Analysis. Time-resolved microscopy has been constructed independently several times in the past and has been used for characterization of soft and hard biological tissues (for review, see Briggs, 1992). The short temporal extent of the impulse excitation allows separate echo pulses from the top and bottom of a thin specimen or from separate interfaces in a layered specimen to be identified in the received signal, and hence the vertical structure in specimens can be resolved. High reflectivity of the supporting surface combined with low reflectivity of the specimens and attenuation by the samples normally impede this type of imaging soft biological samples. Cells grown on a polyvinylchloride surface, which almost matches the acoustical impedance of the coupling fluid (reflectivity 18 dB lower than the reflection of the surface of a polystyrene petri dish), were viewed using ultrasound pulses in the nanosecond range. This method permitted acoustical sectioning and thus 3D imaging and x/z scans (B-scans) with a resolution of 1.24 μm in the axial direction (0.54 μm lateral resolution at 1.5 GHz) (Kanngiesser and Anliker, 1991).

Analysis of time-resolved measurements does not require any a priori assumptions about the acoustic properties of the specimen and works well with tissue sections of about 10 μm thickness. Data from very thin cytoplasmic layers of cells in culture require extensive processing by the appropriate deconvolution algorithms.

Recent developments allow for storage of the whole course of a pulsed signal reflected from a specimen for all scanning positions at varying frequencies. Such systems are realized, for instance, by Honda Electronics, for the frequency range up to 200 MHz, step size of scanning is 4 μm constructing images of 480 × 480 pixels, and beam width is 5 μm at 200 MHz (Hozumi et al., 2004). This instrument has been extensively used by the group of Saijo for the analysis of cardiovascular tissues. This group considerably improved the acoustic system

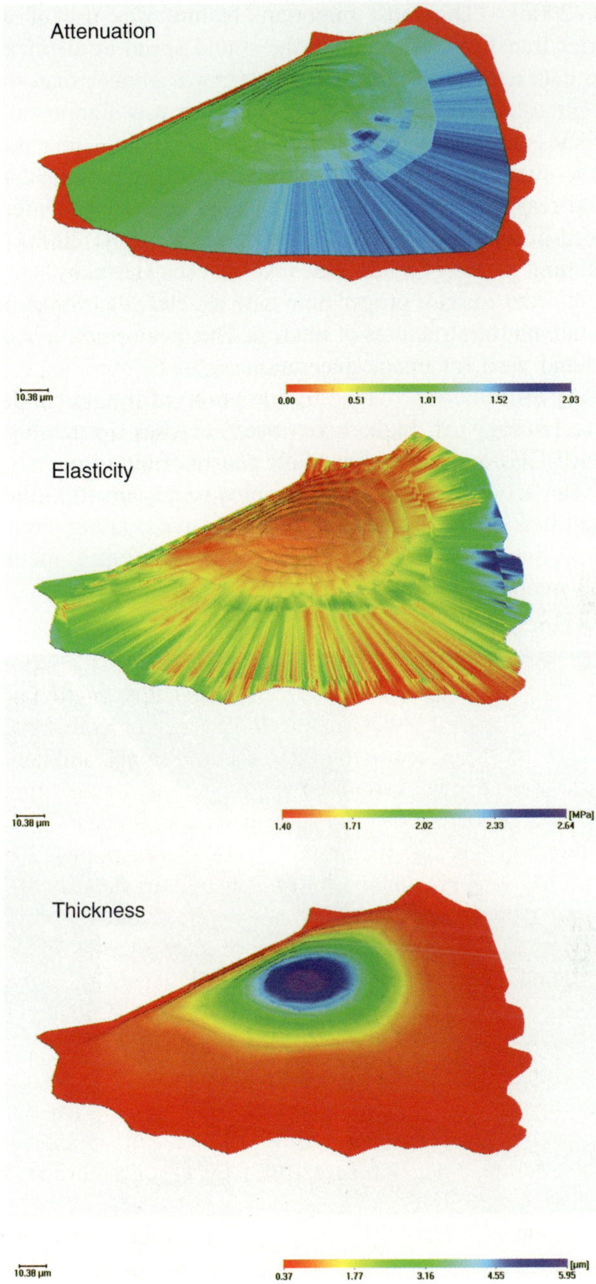

Figure 12.11. Reconstruction of the distribution of thickness, elasticity, and attenuation all over an endothelial cell (XTH-2 cell) in culture. This reconstruction is based on pictures taken at three different frequencies (from Hartmann, 2002).

(Saijo et al., 2006): "The most important feature was use of a single pulse and the Fourier transform to calculate the sound speed at all measuring points. Although the data acquisition time of a frame was greater than that in conventional SAM, the total time required for calculation was significantly shorter that can measure the speed of sound of thin slices of biological material." Deconvolution of the signal in the time domain enabled separation of the reflections from front and rear sides, and frequency domain analysis provided reliable data on sound speed in the range of 50–150 MHz (Saijo et al., 2006).

The "Evolution" series of SAM TEC (Westhausen Germany) shows the course of the signal in order to set a proper time gate to select the reflections from those distances containing the structures of interest. The mean amplitude of this selected part is stored and used for image generation.

The SASAM instrument provided by the group of. Lemor in the Institute for Biomedical Technology (St. Ingbert, Germany) reaches a much higher resolution by using about 1 GHz and saving the whole course of ultrasound signal for further calculations. The acoustic head can be coupled to any inverted light microscope (Fig. 12.4) and thus opens up the possibility of investigating simultaneously the very same area, for example, with fluorescence techniques, including confocal laser scanning microscopy and SAM (Fig. 12.12).

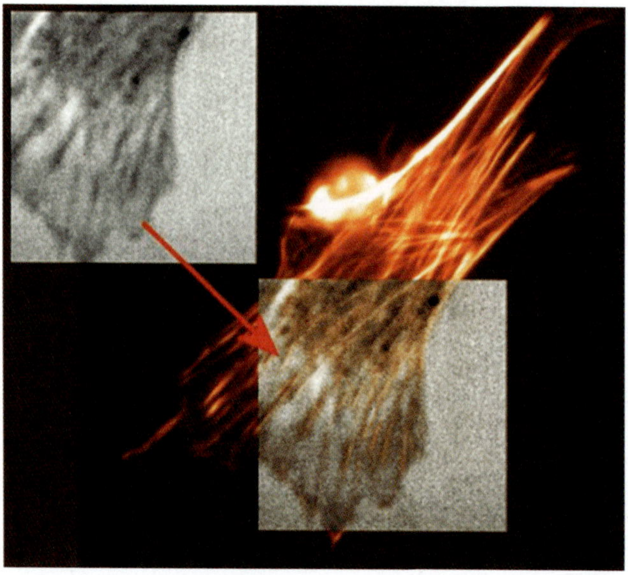

Figure 12.12. Coincidence of structures revealed by SAM imaging and fluorescence microscopy: embryonic chicken myoblasts were stained with Alexa-phalloidin (Molecular Probes: Eugene, Oregon) and the same positions were viewed with the SASAM and by fluorescence revealing F-actin. Focal contacts are represented as dark streaks in the acoustic image and can further be identified as the ends of stress fibers in the fluorescence image. The image size is 65 μm × 65 μm. (Courtesy of E. C. Weiss and R. Lemor, IBMT St. Ingbert).

12.3 BIOMEDICAL APPLICATIONS OF ACOUSTIC MICROSCOPY

12.3.1 Influence of Fixation on Acoustic Parameters of Cells and Tissues

Acoustic microscopy of biological samples does not depend on staining; fixation alone will be sufficient to reveal acoustic properties of cells and tissue sections (Hildebrand et al., 1981). Thus, the influence of freezing and thawing cycles—as required for freeze sectioning of organs—has been investigated qualitatively by Kessler, 1973; Parker, et al., 1984; and D'Astous and Foster, 1986; and quantitatively by van der Steen et al., (1991, 1992). This treatment does not significantly change acoustic parameters. Formalin fixation (4%, 1 week) of 5-mm liver cubes, on the other hand, has been found to leave speed of sound almost unaffected, while attenuation (at 5 MHz) increased it from 4.47 in fresh tissue to 4.96, paraffin embedding increased it to 11.62, and hematoxylin–eosin staining increased it to 16.01.

The first qualitative study on the influence of tissue fixation and processing on acoustic properties using 1.2 GHz transducer has been performed by van der Steen et al., (1992). They used 6-μm thick liver sections that were prepared in different ways: fixed either in ethanol or formalin; stained by hematoxylin–eosin, toluidin blue, or nonstained; cryostat sections or paraffin sections. Paraffin sections had to be deparaffinized to display any structure. Finer structures were displayed after ethanol fixation.

For cell cultures, fast air drying followed by rehydration in saline, Karnovsky fixation (mixture of glutaraldehyde and paraformaldehyde), and formalin fixation have been tested (Bereiter-Hahn et al., (1992)). Best preservation of morphology was reached by Karnovsky fixation; the acoustic parameters did not behave uniformly at 1–1.5 GHz showing many subcellular details. Least alterations were observed after air drying and rehydration. In general, attenuation was increased after fixation, in some cell areas up to fourfold as in the living state. Speed of sound decreased in the central cell areas and became more homogenous in the cell periphery. The interpretation was that local contractions no longer occur in dead cells. An example of fixation-related changes is given in Figure 12.13.

SAM investigations on soft tissue sections have been done on fixed or freeze-sectioned material. In paraffin sections, after deparaffinization, all the fat material of the tissue is removed, which is known to be of considerable influence on the acoustic properties of tissues (Brand et al., 2003; Sasaki et al., 2003). Thus, most researchers agree that freeze sectioning will influence acoustic parameters the least. Whether this represents elasticity in the organism remains an open question, because many tissues, for example, of the cardiovascular system, are under tension and this tension is released in the excised and sectioned material, thus the elasticity values measured are only elasticity values after full relaxation.

In hard tissues, the water content may be of more significant influence on the parameters to be measured than fixation (Currey et al., 1995). The influence of storage conditions on the elastic properties of dentin and enamel of human wisdom teeth has been investigated (Raum et al., 2006d), and it was revealed that artificial saliva was the fluid of choice for prolonged storage.

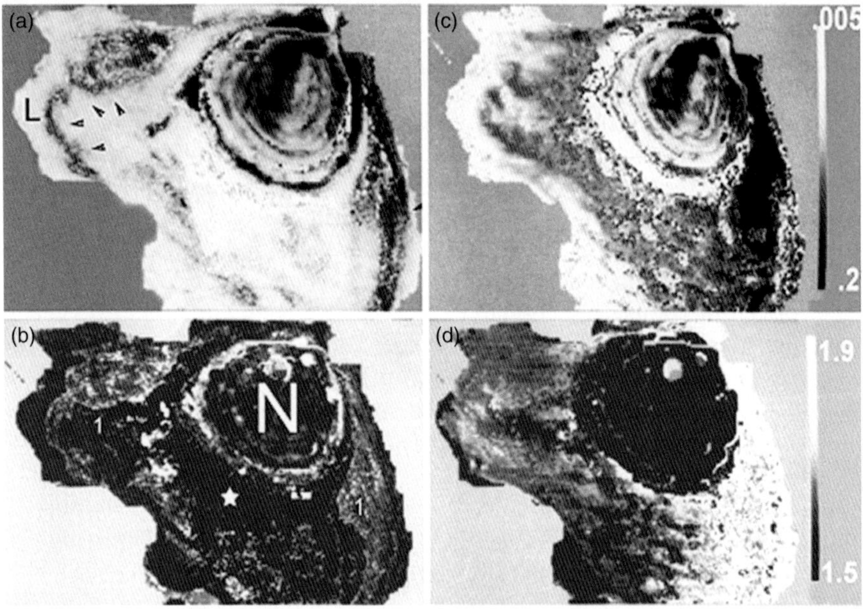

Figure 12.13. XTH-2 endothelial cell before (a, b) and after (c,d) fixation: Using a small part of $V(z)$ characteristics, for the first time allowed, mapping of elasticity (sound velocity: b,d) and attenuation (a,c) over a cell with full resolution of the SAM. Attenuation is increased after fixation and in the living cell represents areas with thick bundles of F-actin (arrowheads). Inverse behaviour of attenuation and sound velocity is seen in the two areas marked "1" in (b). The zone marked with the asterisk exhibits low attenuation and low elasticity as is typical for loose cytoskeletal networks often found in this area with the scanning electron microscope. 1 GHz, image width: 200 μm (from Bereiter-Hahn et al. (1992)).

Calculating acoustic parameters of tissue sections has to deal with thickness variations as an additional factor of uncertainty (Okawai et al., (1988)).

12.3.2 Acoustic Microscopy of Cells in Culture

For isolated cells and soft tissue, calculations of impedance differences from the acoustic signal seems a relatively simple method to determine elasticity because the contribution of surface waves and Rayleigh waves can be neglected. Problems arise because reflectivity for ultrasound is low and, in addition to the elasticity of the cytoplasm or tissue structures, sound reflection may be modulated by surface topography, which depends on overall cell shape and presence of microstructures on top of the cells and at their surfaces adhering to a solid substratum (e.g., glycocalix, ridges, microvilli, microstructures exposed by sectioning of tissues). Several unknowns determine a SAM image of a cell or tissue: cytoplasmic elasticity, density, and, probably, viscosity have to be calculated from the acoustic parameters, sound velocity and attenuation, which are derived from sound reflections. These may be supplemented by measurements of time of flight and phase of the acoustic signal from which cell or section thickness (topography) can be derived. In the case of cells in culture, a thin layer of fluid in between the cell and the supporting substrate has to be considered because this layer may considerably influence SAM images (Bereiter-Hahn et al., (1992); Kundu et al., 1991).

How to cope with these unknowns? A variety of methods has been developed to solve this problem and to calculate physiologically relevant parameters from SAM images. The principles of the different approaches have been summarized above. In general, $V(z)$ and $V(f)$ procedures ($V(z)$ and $V(f)$ curves) require frequency or focus variations and need several images to be taken before the calculations can be done. This limits temporal resolution. Methods based on the evaluation of interference fringes provide high temporal resolution combined with loss in spatial resolution, and they do not allow measurements of very thin cytoplasmic layers because the maxima and minima of interferences are difficult to localize. Procedures taking advantage of the information in time, phase, *and* amplitude of the acoustical signal are superior. If all these parameters are collected, they require long time for image acquisition, extensive calculations, and space for data storage. All high resolution imaging methods are very sensitive to external disturbances (temperature, scanning plane, vibrations), which may impose difficulties for practical work.

Almost all the possibilities and shortcomings, the imaging and interpretation problems of SAM, can be demonstrated with live cell imaging; therefore, this application is discussed in detail according to the application of various methods to cell cultures that have been used in the author's and others' laboratories.

12.3.3 Technical Requirements

12.3.3.1 Mechanical Stability. SAM imaging is very vibration sensitive; therefore, the instruments are posed on vibration-reducing tables by the manufacturers.

12.3.3.2 Frequency. With increasing sound frequency and thus resolution, attenuation of the coupling fluid increases and thus the signal to noise ratio becomes worse. Heating to 37°C reduces attenuation in relation to room temperature, and the required heating hood also stabilizes focus and thus is an indispensable tool for live cell investigation; also, in tissue section investigation, temperature must be kept stable.

12.3.3.3 Coupling Fluid. For biomedical investigations, saline is normally used as a coupling fluid. This gives optimal results because it has the least possible influence on the biological material, and the matching layer on the acoustic lens is optimized for sapphire/water interface. Sometimes methanol has been used as a coupling fluid, which also imbibes the probe. The advantage of using methanol is the lower sound velocity and thus smaller wavelength at a given frequency, which provides a chance for increasing spatial resolution; however, methanol itself changes the acoustic properties of the biological material and attenuates sound more than water, thus signal to noise ratio may become a limiting factor. This coupling fluid may be of help if frozen sections are going to be analyzed for morphological features without staining.

Protein-containing coupling fluids (cell culture media) may cause precipitations (probably of fibronectin) within the lens cavity and on the surface of cells, reducing the acoustic signal. Therefore, saline is preferable in all cases of investigation of tissues or cells.

12.3.3.4 ***Time of Image Acquisition.*** Scanning procedures produce sharp images even when the specimen is moving while the image is taken. So far, acquisition time does not seem to cause severe problems in SAM. However, mechanical properties of cells also underlie shape generation and motility, and these features can be studied only if the method of measurement (SAM) is fast in relation to the process to be analyzed (motility). Furthermore, all the analytic methods that require several images for calculation of the unknown cell parameters (e.g., $V(z)$- and $V(f)$-based SAM) have to start with the assumption that nothing changes during the time required for image acquisition, which was about 40 s for the $V(z)$ series and has now been reduced to 25 s for a $V(f)$ series. However, cells are dynamic as long as they are alive. As a consequence, fast moving cells (e.g., the speed of epidermal cells is up to 30 μm/min) cannot be analyzed at all by using $V(z)$- or $V(f)$-based evaluation methods. Cells that remain stationary on the scale of a few minutes might undergo shape changes. Therefore, we analyzed the overall cytoplasmic motility of nonlocomoting cells (i.e., keeping a constant position for at least several minutes) in culture. This is easily performed by subtraction of two subsequent images taken at a certain time interval (Fig. 12.14). By mathematical processing, the contrast of these different images can be improved. The differences were very small in most of the cultures; however, they led to the detection of clearly outlined domains of cytoplasmic motility (Vesely et al., 1994). These activities depended on cell density in those cultures that show contact-mediated control of locomotion and proliferation (Zoller et al., 1997). The motile activity measured by subtraction scanning acoustic microscopy (SubSAM) correlates well with the invasive potential of rat sarcoma cells and seems to be mediated by rac-activation (I. Karl and P. Vesely, personal communication).

Enhancement by selective receptor stimulation is in favor of the interpretation that these motility domains represent receptor fields (Fig. 12.15), probably membrane rafts. Because the motility domains become visible through the subtraction of interference images (sound waves reflected from the medium-facing surface interfere with those reflected from the substratum), surface topography changes down to about 15 nm are revealed and can be related to small local bulges also identified by light microscopic methods or by scanning electron microscopy.

12.3.4 What Is Revealed by SAM: Interpretation of SAM Images

The primary parameters that can be achieved from SAM images are sound velocity and attenuation and thickness of the sample. According to Eqs 12.7 and 12.8,

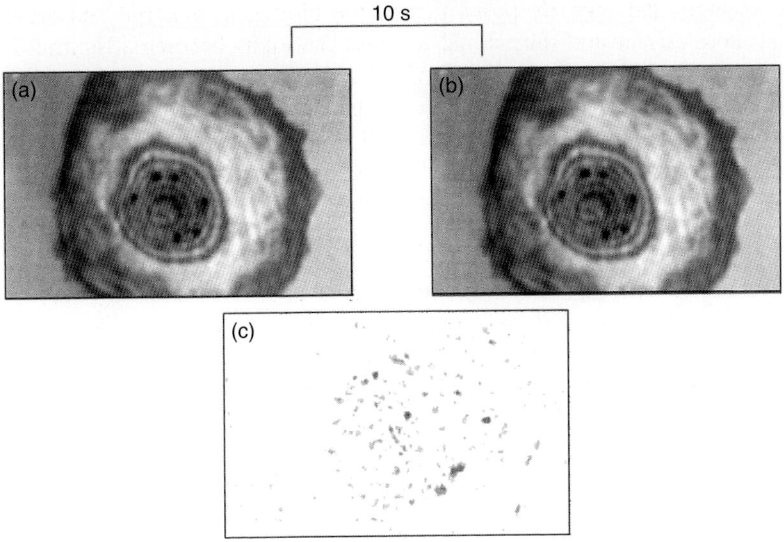

Figure 12.14. The method SubSAM is based on the subtraction of images gray level per pixel by gray level of the corresponding pixel in the second image. The absolute gray level differences were represented in the resulting subtraction image. The subtraction of images (a,b) taken from a living cell in a distinct time interval by scanning acoustic microscopy reveals domains, which represent the surface changes the cell undergoes in the meantime (c). Some of these domains represent ruffles (at the outermost cell margins); those in the more central parts of the cells just move up and down. The motility domains are related to receptor activations (compare Fig. 12.15), and cells differ in this behavior whether they are normal or tumor cells (from Karl and Bereiter-Hahn, (2001)).

sound velocity is a measure of elasticity including density, but which elasticity is revealed, the one of the whole cytoplasm along the focus line or only that of the surface structures, is not known. Which of the cellular structures is primarily responsible for the elastic properties of a cell or tissue? What does attenuation mean in physiological terms? These questions are discussed in the present section.

12.3.4.1 Sound Velocity, Elasticity, and the Cytoskeleton. Mechanical properties of cells cannot be considered to be constant throughout the cytoplasm, neither laterally, that is, in the periphery and the center of a cell, nor along the acoustical axis, because the cytoskeletal and membrane arrangements in cortical cytoplasm layers often considerably differ from those in the central parts. Sound velocity derived from impedance changes at an interface, as, for instance, revealed by measuring surface reflection only is a measure of surface elasticity, while sound velocity revealed in a transmission mode measures the mean speed of sound throughout a specimen. $V(z)$ and $V(f)$ methods provide those mean values, while amplitudes of sound reflected from the surface of cells or tissue sections reveal impedance differences and thus the product of density and speed of sound. The structure responsible for the mechanical properties of the cell surface in fact

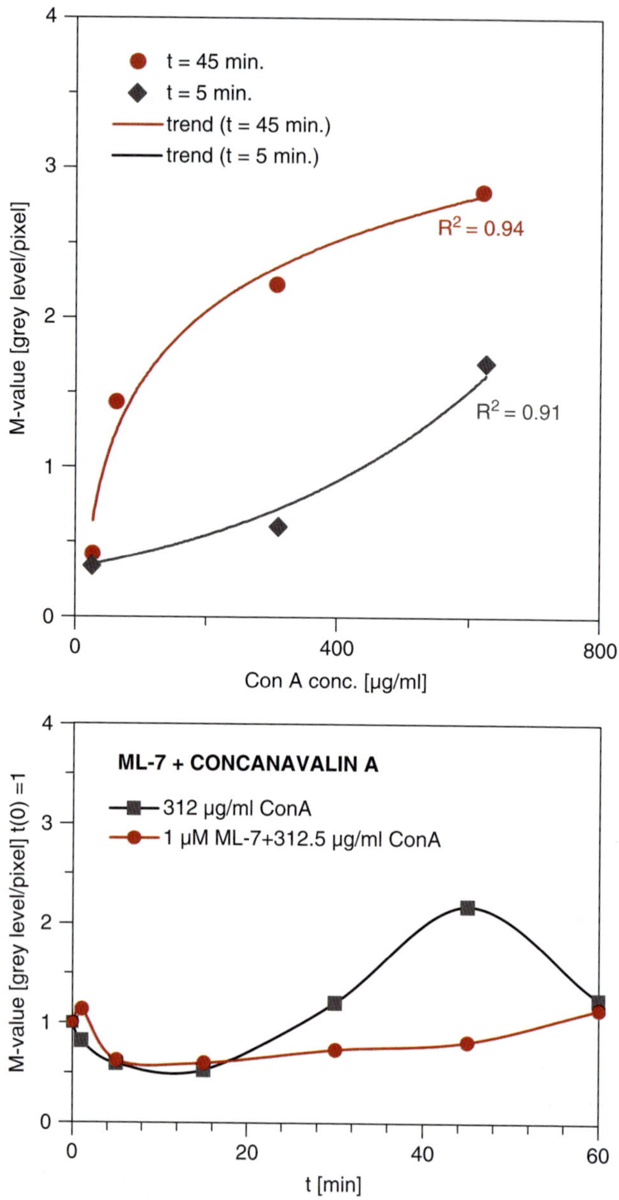

Figure 12.15. Quantitation of surface mobility as revealed by the procedure described in Figure 12.13. For reasons of comparability, an area-independent M-value was calculated on the basis of the gray level differences and the number of pixels in the SubSAM images. These M-values provide a measure of the surface mobility (Zoller et al., 1997). These curves give an example of stimulation of surface mobility by different concentrations of concanavalin A, its time dependence and its suppression by inhibition of myosin light chain kinase via ML-7 (lower panel). (From Karl and Bereiter-Hahn, 2001).

is the fibrillar cortex (Fig. 12.16), which forms a mechanical unit with the membrane: actin fibrils are anchored to intrinsic membrane proteins. Changes in cortex tension will affect the activity of ion channels and influence the distribution of signaling molecules (i.e., receptors, adhesion molecules). Therefore, the mechanical properties of the cortex are of great importance for the control of a variety of cell activities, including proliferation activity (e.g., Ingber et al., 1995).

The next question is about the depth of the interface layer responsible for reflection. According to knowledge from light microscopy (i.e., total internal reflection techniques) this depth is restricted to a very thin layer of a few nanometers, much less than the extension of the focal spot along the acoustical axis. Thus, amplitude measurements of reflected sound, compared with amplitudes reflected from interfaces with known impedance differences reveal the speed of sound in the reflecting medium. Density of cytoplasm will be close to 1.06, and variations between 1.04 and 1.1 will not have considerable influence on acoustic impedance, which thus measures sound velocity. This is done in all cases where surface reflections are clearly separated from any signals of underlying material. Equations 12.8 and 12.9 can be used to calculate elasticity, but this term needs further consideration.

Cellular elasticity depends highly on the strain rate; in slow deformation processes viscous creep may become prominent (e.g., Hiramoto, 1986). In SAM,

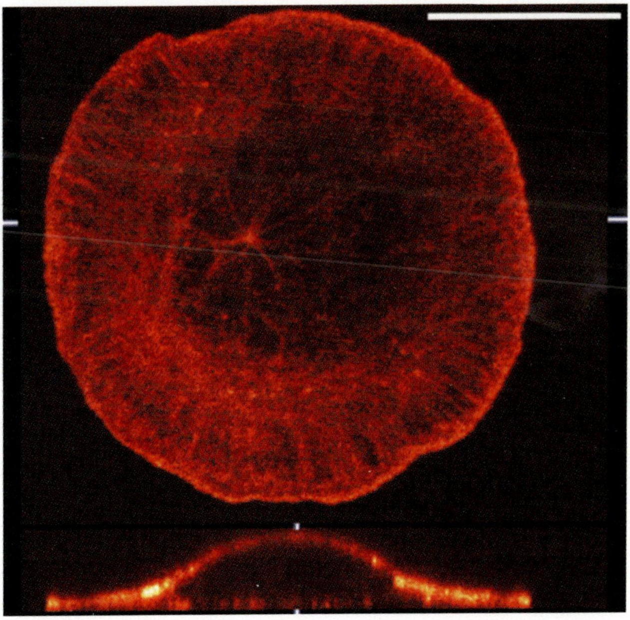

Figure 12.16. Optical section in x/y direction through a "fried-egg shaped" keratinocyte, and its cross section along the line indicated by the two marginal streaks in the x/y image. F-actin in this cell has been fluorochromed using TRITC–phalloidin. The cross section reveals the continuous F-actin layer beyond the cell membrane. Image by M. Voeth.

one can assume an extremely high strain rate (megahertz to gigahertz) together with an extremely small deformation (in the subnanometer range), thus viscosity does not influence the measurement that exclusively shows elasticity.

Further interpretation requires some basic assumptions on the physical state of cytoplasm, whether it is treated as a viscoelastic fluid (the widely accepted model) or a quasi solid, fibrous (or porous) matrix filled with fluid. This approach guides the interpretation whether bulk modulus or Young's modulus determines the longitudinal sound velocity according to:

$$c_c^2 = E/\rho \tag{12.15}$$

where c_c is the longitudinal sound velocity in the cytoplasm, E is the appropriate modulus of elasticity, and ρ is the density).

Physiological interpretation of data derived from SAM measurements requires some further considerations.

For calculation of these properties, which are independent of the volume fraction of the material involved, the basic sound speed in saline (c_s) has to be subtracted from the value determined for the whole cell (c) because it represents the compression modulus of the ubiquitous saline, while the speed exceeding this value must be due to constants other than water and ions, which then are responsible for a cell's mechanical properties. In the case of cells or tissues in an aqueous medium, the sound velocity derived for the sample includes the sound velocity of the aqueous medium and that of the proteinaceous content. The contribution of the aqueous phase can be considered to be a constant in most tissues and cells. The proteinaceous fraction is the one causing the variation in the mechanical properties. It can be evaluated only when an assumption is made on the volume fractions of the protein (p) and the fluid space (q) of a cell.

$$p + q = 1 \tag{12.16}$$

where p and q are a measure of the relative path a sound wave travels through a specimen.

The overall speed of sound determined for a cell (c) is presented by

$$c = pc_s + qc_p \tag{12.17}$$

Thus, the speed of sound of the protein fraction (c_p) amounts to

$$c_p = 1/q(c - pc_s) \tag{12.18}$$

and

$$c^2{}_p\rho_p = E_p \tag{12.19}$$

For living cells in culture, a relative dry mass of about 20% is reasonable according to interferometric determinations. The sound velocity of the fluid phase in a cell is about 1550 m s^{-1} (at 30°C); thus, in the case of a mean sound velocity of 1600 m s^{-1}, sound velocity of the protein fraction can be estimated to be 1800 m s^{-1}; in the rare cases when sound velocities of 1800 m s^{-1} have been measured, that of the protein fraction would be 2800 m s^{-1}. These values are in the range of polycarbonates.

The next question is, whether we are measuring bulk modulus (compressibility) or Young's modulus. In the case of a fluid, the situation is clear; fluids only have shear and bulk elasticity. Although the incident sound beam has a small diameter (in the range of 1–1.5 μm in water at 1 GHz), lateral displacements of the volume units exposed to sound are effectively attenuated; therefore, sound propagation is determined by compressibility only. The same can be assumed for highly hydrated proteins. This does not exclude, however, that Young's modulus of protein filaments under tension is the factor determining sound propagation. Mechanical properties of cells and tissues highly depend on the tension of fibers. In the case of tissues, these are primarily elastin and collagen; in the case of living cells, F-actin; thus the Poisson ratio determined for these fibrillar elements opens the possibility of relating compressibility to its modulus of elasticity (Young's modulus). Ziemann et al., (1994) determined the Poisson ratio (ν) for actin to be 0.33. In this case, the numerical value of the bulk modulus equals that of Youngs modulus (Eq. 12.9).

Tension caused by contractions of the actomyosin system thus will primarily contribute to the elastic modulus, as revealed by sound velocity. This can be shown experimentally by a short treatment with cytochalasin D, which releases tension from the actin fibrillar network almost immediately (30–60 s) (Bereiter-Hahn, 1987a), or on the other hand, by treatment with colcemid, which evokes strong contractions (Kolodney and Elson, 1995) resulting in extremely high sound speeds (Karl and Bereiter-Hahn, 1998). In both cases, mass does not change; only the arrangement and interactions of the fibrillar elements is altered. Another approach to clarify the cellular components and processes responsible for cytoplasmic elasticity as revealed by SAM was an experiment using the Ca^{2+}-selective ionophore ionomycin. Addition of this drug in the presence of Ca^{2+} ions (1–2 mM) causes calcium influx into the cytoplasm, thus activating actin–myosin interaction and causing disruption of microtubules. This contraction immediately raises sound velocity in a site-dependent manner, that is, different cell areas react to a different extent. Finally, the high internal calcium concentration leads to disassembly of all the cytoskeletal fibrils, and sound velocity decreases to a level below that of the untreated cell (Lüers et al., 1992). These interpretations are possible because the very same cells have been investigated by fluorescence microscopy after SAM images have been taken.

These experiments showed the significance of active processes, of contractions of the actomyosin system in particular. Because of the intimate interaction of the three cytoskeletal fiber types and their control by signaling pathways, the contribution of a single fiber type to the elastic properties has not been revealed unequivocally. Very short cytochalasin treatment is the most specific one, which causes an immediate reduction of sound reflectivity from the cell surface.

The contribution of active contraction processes to the elastic properties of cells implies that investigations of any dead—fixed—biological material does not reveal the real *in vivo* elastic properties. This is also valid for determining elasticity of tissues that are exposed to stresses in the body; all these stresses are missing after fixation and sectioning. This explains the big differences in sound velocity as determined in tissue sections and in living cells with intact cytoskeleton.

12.3.4.2 Attenuation. Attenuation is an important factor in ultrasound imaging because no window of transparency exists in materials for sound. Attenuation theoretically increases with the square of frequency; however, linear increase has been reported for several biological tissues. What does attenuation tell us? This is a difficult question to answer. Early findings on cirrhotic liver suggested that attenuation increases with the protein content (Okawai et al., 1988). First hints on the structural basis of ultrasound attenuation came from the ratio of dry mass and attenuation in the cell periphery and the cell center. In the periphery, a small increase in dry mass led to a much higher increase in attenuation than in the cell center (Bereiter-Hahn, 1987b). The attenuation coefficient can be regarded to represent viscosity and thermal relaxation. Experimental data with biogels show that the influence of viscosity on attenuation is small and does not correlate. Using an oscillatory rod rheometer we continuously measured viscosity increase, speed of sound, and attenuation of 1 GHz ultrasound during the polymerization of actin (Wagner et al., 1999, 2001). During the nucleation phase, attenuation slightly decreased when actin polymerization (this does not influence viscosity) started and increased considerably after polymerization was almost finished. After polymerization, entanglement and bundling of F-actin occurs, and only this process is reflected by attenuation increase. To prove the hypothesis that fibrillar cross-linking is the main determinant for attenuation, actin has been polymerized in the presence of the F-actin cross-linking protein α-actinin. In this case, attenuation increases much more, and in step with polymerization. Other cross-linking proteins evoke the same behavior, and the high attenuation of collagen bundles (e.g., Saijo et al., 1996) can thus be hypothesized to be based on the extensive cross-linking of the collagen fibers within the bundles. Contrary to these findings and interpretations, breaking intermolecular cross-links in collagen reduced the attenuation coefficient of articular cartilage at 100 MHz SLAM investigations (Agemura and O'Brien, 1990). Increase of attenuation by various chemical fixation procedures can also be attributed to extended cross-linking by the fixative itself and/or by freezing steady-state cross-linking. On the other hand, elastic fibers that have a chemical composition similar to that of collagen attenuate ultrasound less than the cellular components of tissues (Saijo et al., 1996). Thus, thermal relaxation can be considered the main determinant of the attenuation coefficient (α) corresponding to

$$\alpha = 2\pi^2\tau/c\nu^2 \tag{12.20}$$

where ν is the frequency of ultrasound; τ is thermal relaxation, that is, time required for a molecule to reach its ground position again after being displaced by a force, according to (1-1/e); and c is the velocity of sound.

This relaxation time finally is a measure of viscosity. However, the numerical value of viscosity strongly depends on the size of the probe, that is, in an entangled fibrillar net, all molecules that are small in relation to the pore size experience low resistance against movement, while large organelles may not move at all through such a net, and thus viscosity appears to be very high at this level of probe size.

12.3.4.3 Viewing Subcellular Structures. As pointed out earlier, lateral resolution of SAM operated in the 1- to 2-GHz range comes down to <1 μm. This feature will be revealed only for organelles or structures that differ in their acoustic impedance from that of their environment. In living cells, most organelles may not provide interfaces to be detected because their impedance matches that of the cytoplasm, and only in the case of cell death phase separation takes place. Figure 12.17 shows such an example.

These cells have been exposed to tetramethyl-rhodamin-labeled phalloidin (TRITC-phalloidin). TRITC-phalloidin does not penetrate living cells; impaired or dead cells become permeable, and in these cells, the phalloidin strongly binds to F-actin. The fluorescence image and the acoustic image (taken at 1.5 GHz) show exactly the same field. Small granular substructures are revealed by SAM in the TRITC-phalloidin permeable cells, while the cytoplasm of the uninjured cells appears homogenous. This shows that although SAM resolution would be sufficient to reveal subcellular structures, they are hidden because of matching acoustic impedance. At this point, we should become aware that ultrasound at high frequency provides a nondestructive interaction with the biological material; the intensities are too small, and the attenuation is too high to allow for cavitation phenomena or for any living cell destruction. This, however, does not exclude that by stimulating surface receptors; biological effects other than cell death are evoked. We have made several long-term (up to 10 h) observations of living cells with an acoustic microscope, As an example the full process of mitosis in cell culture is shown in Figure 12.18, produced by the group of Lemor.

12.3.5 Conclusions

Acoustic microscopy provides unique possibilities for probing elastic properties of cells and tissues (for detailed introduction and review see Bereiter-Hahn et al., 1995; Briggs, (1992), (1995)). SAM has reached a state of development that allows routine investigations of biological samples (isolated cells, tissue sections, and tissue blocks). Specimens with large surface topographic variations may be reconstructed from focus series or from deconvolution of the reflected signal pixel by pixel. The maximum reflectivity at any point can be used to calculate local impedance and, thus, elasticity values. Evaluation of $V(z)$ and $V(f)$ provides a convenient key to subcellular distribution of elasticity and fibrillar interactions.

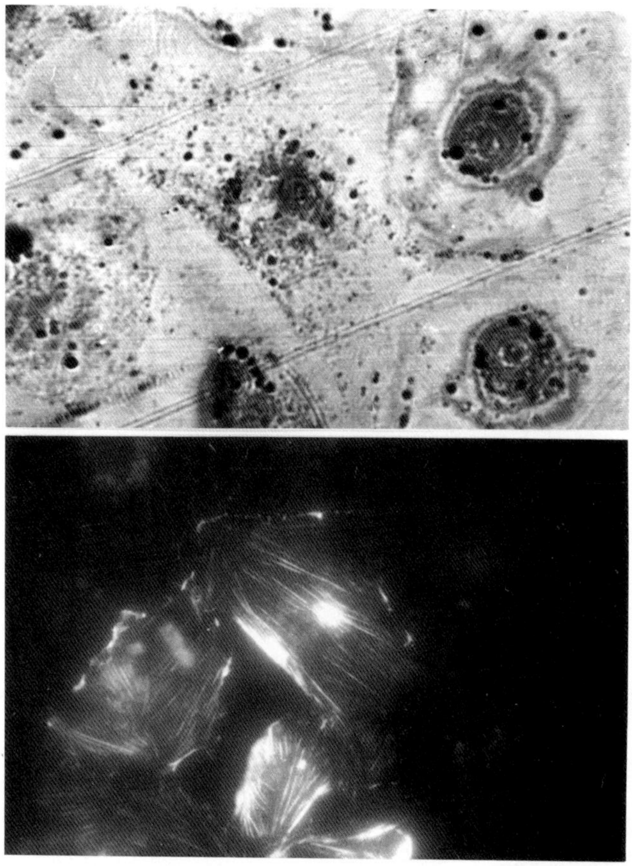

Figure 12.17. Culture of endothelial cells (XTH-2) exposed to TRITC-phalloidin, which does not penetrate living cells. Upper image: SAM, 1.5 GHz, cells on glass. Lower image: Fluorescence microscope image of the same area. In cells that show TRITC-phalloidin fluorescence, small "vesicular" structures are visible in the SAM image, while in the unstained, living cells, the cytoplasm is almost unstructured; only a few black granules show up because of impedance differences to the cytoplasm. Image width: 200 μm.

Cytoplasm and cellular organelles exhibit viscoelastic properties, that is, they are not adequately described as solid bodies or as fluids. In addition, cytoplasm and the organelles form microdomains that differ in their mechanical properties. A broad range of methods has been developed to determine viscosity (e.g., Hiramoto, (1986); Sackmann, (1997)); cytoplasmic elasticity, however, is more difficult to assess. Atomic force microscopy (e.g., Schoenenberger et al., (1997)) and the related poking methods are the most widely used principles to test cell elasticity. More recently, magnetic twisting cytometry added considerably to cytomechanical measurements and analysis of the physiological transduction of mechanical signals (Huang et al., 2005; Ingber et al., 1995).

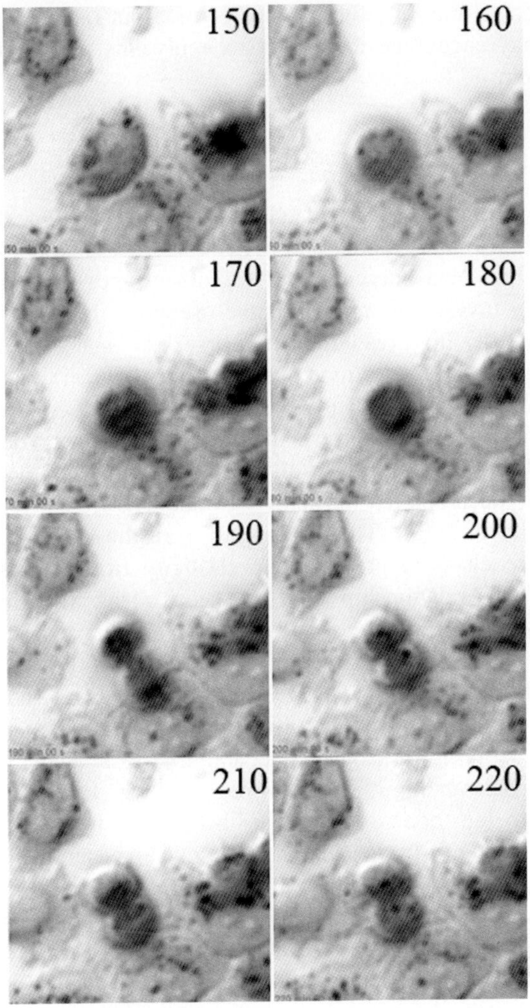

Figure 12.18. A group of HeLa cells was observed in the acoustic microscope SASAM. The numbers indicate the time of observation in minutes. At 150 min, the cell starts rounding and the nucleus is still visible; at 170 min, chromosomes are aligned in the equatorial plane and appear as a dark band; anaphase is going on at 180 min; at 190 min, the cleavage furrow is clearly visible; and cell spreading just starts at 220 min. At this time, the nucleus in the lower cell can be seen with its two nucleoli. Image size is 80 μm ×80 μm. This series has been taken by E.C. Weiss (St. Ingbert).

12.4 EXAMPLES OF TISSUE INVESTIGATIONS USING SAM

This section describes some results that have been achieved using ultrasound in the range above 100 MHz, thus of microscopy in a strict sense, with a lateral resolution approaching that of a light microscope. I do not intend to give a full overview on all the investigations performed but rather present a few basic findings that may encourage the reader to apply this technique to his/her own scientific problems.

12.4.1 Hard Tissues

Bone and cartilage are tissues with clear functions in biomechanics. They are a favorite object for sonographic and SAM investigations, because sonic investigation avoids the invasivity required for other types of biomechanical measurements. Early investigations on the microscope level were those of Meunier et al., (1988) and by high resolution by Hirsekorn et al., (1995). Turner et al., (1999) compared the Young's modulus of trabecular bone with that of cortical bone. The former was slightly higher than the transverse Young's modulus of cortical bone, but substantially lower than the longitudinal Young's modulus of cortical bone. More recently, the full range of frequencies between megahertz and 1 GHz have been applied for studying bone at different levels of resolution (Raum et al., 2003b, 2004). The challenge for all the applied experimental and mathematical models is to predict bone elasticity from structure, density, and mineralization. This relationship is by no means clear. Therefore, experimental data from SAM and other ultrasound-based studies have been compared with other types of mechanical and structural measurements, that is, microindentation (Bumrerraj and Katz, 2001), micro-CT (Chapter 4), and Raman spectroscopy (Chapter 9). In particular, probing cortical bone for porosity and mineralization, the comparison between the acoustic data and micro-CT on the very same sample enhanced the understanding of the CT images (Raum et al., 2005, 2006, 2008). A model for cancerous bone interacting with 1 MHz ultrasound accounts for spatial density distribution of trabeculae and includes measurement conditions such as pressure–time waveform of the probing ultrasound wave, the emitted field structure and transfer function of the instrument working in pulse-echo mode (Litniewski et al., 2009).

Interindividual and regional variations (i.e., osteons, interstitium; anisotropy) as well as genetically determined characteristics (Hofmann et al., 2006b) have been assessed. Interstitial tissue exhibited a higher elastic modulus than the osteonal tissue, an observation that coincided with nanoindentation studies (Raum et al., 2006); however, the absolute values obtained by SAM were higher. This may be due to the extremely high frequency of measurement with SAM and a slow one with nanoindentation, which gives the tissue a chance for viscous creep, thus reducing elasticity values. Bone can be considered to represent a highly anisotropic tissue; however, measurements of elastomechanical properties by Eckardt and Hein (2001) at different cutting angles referring to the axis of human femoral bones showed only weak variations, while. Hofmann et al., (2006a) found that acoustic impedance Z clearly reflects elastic anisotropy. Calibration of impedance versus the reflected sound was performed by correlating the square root of the integrated SAM signal of known materials (e.g., PMMA, Teflon, polypropylene, perspex, aluminum) with the reflection coefficients of the specimen (Bumrerraj and Katz, 2001; Laugier et al., 2005; Raum et al., 2004). As proved in an experimental model, fracture forces can be derived for healing callus tissue from acoustic impedance measurements (50 MHz) (Hube et al., 2006). Raum (2004, 2008) recently reviewed ultrasonic characterization of hard tissues.

Acoustic microscopy provides an excellent method to investigate mechanical properties of cartilage in a state as close to the *in vivo* situation as possible (Hagiwara et al., 2009), and 200 MHz are sufficient for detailed analysis of the local elasticity, shape, and spatial distribution of chondrocyte lacunae and their changes with age (Denisova et al., 2004).

12.4.2 Cardiovascular Tissues

The cardiovascular system is continuously mechanically stressed, and pathological alterations such as atherosclerosis or aneurisms cause severe health problems, which are also of great epidemiologic significance. Thus, several groups concentrated on the investigation of mechanical parameters of myocardium, veins, and arteries in the healthy state as well as in pathological situations. Final goals are, for example, early detection of infarcted tissue and beginning of rejection of transplants and risk assessment in dilated blood vessels. Thus, a few typical studies are mentioned here.

In a frequency range of 3–8 MHz, the dispersion of sound velocity in lamb myocardium proved to show anisotropy: 1.2 m s^{-1} perpendicular to the myofibrils versus 3.7 m s^{-1} in the direction of myofibril orientation (Marutyan et al., 2006). At 450 MHz, endocardial and myocardial elasticity were found to show a strong and different correlation to age, left atrial wall elasticity increased with advancing age (Masugata et al., 1999), and ultrasonic speed in canine myocardium arrested in systole was 1591 ± 11 m s^{-1} and 1575 ± 4.2 m s^{-1} in diastole (O'Brien et al., 1995a).

Comparison of normal, viable but stunned, and of infarcted myocardium in dogs on the 100-MHz level revealed a significantly lower speed of sound propagation in the infarcted area (decline from 1597 to 1575 m,s^{-1}), which, in addition, proved less homogenous, and attenuation was significantly higher in the normal myocardium (O'Brien et al., 1995b).

Arterial plaques have been intensively investigated by the group of Y. Saijo (2004, 2002, 2004, 2006). At 200 MHz, all the important tissue elements such as intima, calcified plaque, lipid deposition, and underlying fibrous cap can be distinguished and elasticity determined from sound velocity. The lower content of elastin in the arteries of patients with Marfan syndrome and disordered matrix organization in these patients makes them prone to aneurism development. These alterations are revealed by 50-MHz sonography (Recchia et al., 1995). Real microscopic studies (100–200 MHz) on aneurisms were performed by Saijo and his group (2004). They related increased attenuation to macrophage infiltration of the tissue and lower speed of sound to decreased elasticity of the intima in aneurysmal tissues.

12.4.3 Other Soft Tissues

Skin was among the first tissues to be investigated with high resolution SAM (Bamber et al., 1992a,b; Bereiter-Hahn and Buhles, 1987). Because of higher impedance, stratum corneum can easily be identified in the reflection mode, while unambiguous distinction between naevi and basiliomas has not been possible. However, tumor dimension, internal structure, and particularly the pattern of collagen and keratin could be assessed even at 20 MHz imaging (Bamber et al., 1992a, 1992b), and inflammatory infiltration zones showed reduced ultrasound reflectivity (Hoffmann et al., 1992). More recently, clear mechanical differences between ageing and photodamaged human skin have been reported (Miyasaka et al., 2005).

First microscale mechanical data of the small intestine were revealed by Jorgensen et al., (2001). Different layers were easily distinguishable on nonstained sections at 500 MHz, and the values (median values) of sound velocity ranged from 1550 to 1669 m s^{-1}, and impedance ranged from 2.10 to 2.60 MPa s m^{-1}. Elastic stiffness differed between all layers ranging from 3.25 to 4.27 GPa with the following sequence of magnitude: circular muscle > submucosa >mucosa >longitudinal muscle ($p < 0.001$).

The approach to investigate elastic properties of tissue while being compressed or stretched is very promising to evaluate the real mechanical behavior of tissues. Such an approach was successfully applied to porcine cornea by Hollman et al., (2002).

SAM made possible imaging of rat renal glomeruli (Hitomi et al., 2000). These authors were also able to demonstrate an increase in sound velocity under inflammatory conditions.

For clinical diagnostic purposes, discrimination of tumor tissue from normal tissue is of paramount importance. Therefore, several investigators focused on this topic. Renal tumors, for instance, show lower elasticity and attenuation than the surrounding tissue (Sasaki et al., 1996). This seems to be contradictory to the higher contrast of tumors in diagnostic sonography. High internal pressure within tumors (Hofmann et al., 2006) may explain these different measurements.

ACKNOWLEDGEMENTS

Funding by the Gesellschaft der Freunde und Förderer der Johann Wolfgang Goethe-Universitat is gratefully acknowledged. Our work has continuously been supported by the Deutsche Forschungsgemeinschaft under the scope of the "Schwerpunkt: Neue mikroskopische Techniken für Biologie und Medizin."

REFERENCES

Agemura DH, O'Brien WD Jr. Ultrasonic propagation properties of articular cartilage at 100 MHz. J Acoust Soc Am 1990;87(4):1786–1791.

Ashman RB, Rho JY. Use of a transmission ultrasonic technique for the in vitro evaluation of bone ingrowth. J Biomech 1990;23:941–943.

Bamber JC, Harland CC, Gusterson BA, Mortimer PS. Correlation between histology and high resolution echographic images of small skin tumours. Acoust Imaging 1992a;19:369–374.

Bamber JC, Crawford CD, Bell DA, Harland CC, Gusterson BA, Mortimer PS. Effects of speckle reduction processing on ultrasound B-mode images of skin tumours. Acoust Imaging 1992b;19:447–461.

Bao S, Thrall BD, Miller DL. Transfection of a reporter plasmid into cultured cells by sonoporation in vitro. Ultrasound Med Biol 1997;23:953–959.

Beloussov LV. *The Dynamic Architecture of a Developing Organism*. Dordrecht: Kluwer; 1998. p 238.

Beloussov LV, Saveliev SV, Naumidi II, Novoselov VV. Mechanical stresses in embryonic tissues: patterns, morphogenetic role, and involvement in regulatory feedback. Int Rev Cytol 1994;150:1–34.

Bekeredjian R, Grayburn PA, Shohet RV. Use of ultrasound contrast agents for gene or drug delivery in cardiovascular medicine. J Am Coll Cardiol 2005;45:329–335.

Bereiter-Hahn J. Scanning acoustic microscopy visualized cytomechanical responses to cytochalasin D. J Microsc 1987a;146:29–39.

Bereiter-Hahn J. Comparison of the appearance of cultured cells observed using scanning acoustomicroscopy with that obtained by interference and fluorescence microscopy. In: *Scanning Imaging Technology*. Berlin: Volume 809, SPIE; 1987b. p 162–165.

Bereiter-Hahn J, Buhles N, Wamsteker K, Jonas U, van der Veen G, van Waes PFGM Basic principles of interpretation of scanning acoustic images obtained from cell cultures and histological sections. In: Wamsteker K et al. editors. *Imaging and Visual Documentation in Medicine*. 2nd ed. New York: Elsevier Science Publishing Co., Inc; 1987. p 537–543.

Bereiter-Hahn J, Fox CH, Thorell B. Quantitative reflection contrast microscopy of living cells. J Cell Biol 1979;82:767–779.

Bereiter-Hahn J, Berghofer F, Kundu T, Penzkofer C, Hillmann K. Evaluation of mechanical properties of cells by scanning acoustic microscopy using V(z) characteristics. In: Gracewski SM, Kundu T editors. *Acousto-Optics and Acoustic Microscopy*. Am Soc Mech Engineers. Volume 140, 1992. p 71–80.

Bereiter-Hahn J, Karl I, Lüers H, Vöth M. Mechanical basis of cell shape: investigations with the scanning acoustic microscope. Biochem Cell Biol 1995;73:337–348.

Bereiter-Hahn J, Lüers H. Subcellular tension fields and mechanical resistance of the lamella front related to the direction of locomotion. Cell Biochem Biophys 1998;29:243–262.

Blase C, Bereiter-Hahn J. Correlative fluorescence and acoustic microscopy in the study of cell volume regulation. In: Arnold W, Hirsekorn S, editors. *Acoustical Imaging*. Volume 27, 2004. p 573–577.

Block H, Boseck S, Heygster G. Description of the defocus effects on an acoustic reflection scanning microscope (SAM). Optik 1990;86:27–37.

Brand S, Moerlein D, Rosner R, Wicke M, Jenderka KV. Estimation of intramuscular fat content in the longissimus dorsi of pigs by analysis of RF echo signals. Ultrasound Med Biol 2003;29:206–207.

Briggs GA. *Acoustic Microscopy*, Oxford Univ Press, New York; 1992. p 325.

Briggs GA, editor. *Advances in Acoustic Microscopy*. Volume 1, New York and London: Plenum Press; 1995. p 350.

Briggs GA, Wang J, Gundle R. Quantitative acoustic microscopy of individual living human cells. J Microsc 1993;172:3–12.

Bumrerraj S, Katz JL. Scanning acoustic microscopy study of human cortical and trabecular bone. Ann Biomed Eng 2001;29(12):1034–1042.

Chubachi N, Kanai H, Sannomiya T, Wakahara T. Acoustic microscope for measuring acoustic properties by micro-defocusing method. Acoust Imaging 1991;19:685–689.

Currey JD, Brear K, Zioupos P, Reilly GC. Effect of formaldehyde fixation on some mechanical properties of bovine bone. Biomaterials 1995;16:1267–1271.

D'Astous FT, Foster FS. Frequency dependence of ultrasound attenuation and backscatter in breast tissue. Ultrasound Med Biol. 1986;12:795–808.

Denisova LA, Denisov AF, Maev RG, Denisov-Nikolsky YI, Matveichuk IV, Maslennikova TV. Acoustic microscopy methods in morphological study of the articular cartilage and subchondrial bone. Acoust Imaging 2004;27:535–540.

Eckardt I, Hein HJ. Quantitative measurements of the mechanical properties of human bone tissues by scanning acoustic microscopy. Ann Biomed Eng 2001;29:1043–1047.

Emerman JT, Pitelka DR. Maintenance and induction of morphological differentiation in dissociated mammary epithelium on floating collagen. In Vitro 1977;13:316–328.

Foster JS, Rugar D. High resolution acoustic microscopy in superfluid helium. Appl Phys Lett 1983;42:869–871.

Foster JS, Rugar D. Low–temperature acoustic microscopy. IEEE Trans 1985;SU-32:139–151.

Frenkel PA, Chen S, Thai T, Shohet RV, Grayburn PA. DNA-loaded albumin microbubbles enhance ultrasound-mediated transfection in vitro. Ultrasound Med Biol 2002;28:817–822.

Grill W, Hillmann K, Kim TJ, Lenkeit O, Ndop J, Schubert M. Scanning acoustic microscopy with vector contrast. Physica B 1999;263:553–558.

Hagiwara Y, Ando A, Chimoto E, Sajo Y, Ohmori-Matsudea K, Itoi E. Changes of articular cartilage after immobilization in a rat knee contracture model. J Orthop Res 2009;27:236–242.

Hartmann S. Konzeption und evaluierung einer viskualiserungstechnik für mechanische eigenschaften von biologischen zellen. Diplomarbeit am Fachbereich Biologie und Informatik d. Johann Wolfgang Goethe Universität Frankfurt am Main; 2002.

Hildebrand JA, Rugar D, Johnston RN, Quate CF. Acoustic microscopy of living cells. Proc Natl Acad Sci USA 1981;78:1656–1660.

Hillmann K, Grill W, Bereiter-Hahn J. Determination of ultrasound attenuation in small samples of solid material by scanning acoustic microscopy with phase contrast. J Alloys Compd 1994;211/212:625–627.

Hiramoto Y, Bereiter-Hahn J, Anderson OR, Reif WE. Evaluation of cytomechanical properties. In: Bereiter-Hahn J et al. editors. *Cytomechanics*. New York, Wien: Springer Verlag; 1986. p 31–46.

Hirsekorn S, Pangraz S, Weides G, Arnold W. Measurement of elastic impedance with high spatial resolution using acoustic microscopy. Appl Phys Lett 1995;67:745–747.

Hitomi H, Kiyomoto H, Hashimoto M, Aki Y, Uchida K, Takahashi N, Fukunaga M, Mizushige K, Senda S, Sakamoto H, Matsuo H, Yuasa S. A new approach for glomerular lesions: evaluation of scanning acoustic microscopy (SAM) for experimental glomerular disease in rats. Ultrasound Med Biol 2000;26:571–577.

Hofmann M, Guschel M, Bernd A, Bereiter-Hahn J, Kaufmann R, Tandi C, Wiig H, Kippenberger S. Lowering of tumor interstitial fluid pressure reduces tumor cell proliferation in a xenograft tumor model. Neoplasia 2006;8(2):89–95.

Hofmann T, Heyroth F, Meinhard H, Fraenzel W, Raum K. Assessment of composition and anisotropic elastic properties of secondary osteon lamellae. J Biomech 2006a;39:2284–2294.

Hofmann T, Raum K, Leguerney I, Saied A, Peyrin F, Vico L, Laugier P Assessment of bone structure and acoustic impedance in C3H and BL6 mice using high resolution scanning acoustic microscopy. Ultrasonics 2006b. doi:10.1016j. ultras.2006.05032.

Hoffmann K, Schatz H, el Gamal S, Altmeyer P. B-scan-sonography in dermatological routine diagnostics. Acoust Imaging 1992;19:453–461.

Hollman KW, Emelianov SY, Neiss JH, Jotyan G, Spooner GJ, Juhasz T, Kurtz RM, O'Donnell M. Strain imaging of corneal tissue with an ultrasound elasticity microscope. Cornea 2002;21:68–73.

Hozumi N, Yamashita R, Lee CK, Nagao M, Kobayashi K, Saijo Y, Tanaka M, Tanaka N, Ohtsuki S. Time-frequency analysis for pulse driven ultrasonic microscopy for biological tissue characterization. Ultrasonics 2004;42:717–722.

Huang H, Kamm RD, Lee RT. Cell mechanics and mechanotransduction: pathways, probes, and physiology. Am J Cell Physiol 2005;287:C1–C11.

Hube R, Mayr H, Hein W, Raum K. Prediction of biomechanical stability after callus distraction by high resolution scanning acoustic microscopy. Ultrasound Med Biol 2006;32:1913–1921.

Hundt W, Steinbach S, Mayer D, Bednarski MD. Modulation of luciferase activity using high intensity focused ultrasound in combination with bioluminescence imaging, magnetic resonance imaging and histological analysis in muscle tissue. Ultasonics 2009;49:549–557.

Ingber DE, Prusty D, Sun ZQ, Betensky H, Wang N. Cell shape, cytoskeletal mechanics, and cell cycle control in angiogenesis. J Biomech 1995;28:1471–1484.

Jorgensen CS, Assentoft JE, Knauss D, Gregersen H, Briggs GA. Small intestine wall distribution of elastic stiffness measured with 500MHz scanning acoustic microscopy. Ann Biomed Eng 2001;29:1059–1063.

Kanngiesser H, Anliker M. Ultrasound microscopy of biological structures with weak reflecting properties. Acoust Imaging 1991;19:517–522.

Karl I, Bereiter-Hahn J. Cell contraction caused by microtubule disruption is accompanied by shape changes and an increased elasticity measured by scanning acoustic microscopy. Cell Biochem Biophys 1998;29:225–241.

Karl I, Bereiter-Hahn J. Scanning acoustic microscopy reveals distinct motility domains in living cells. In: Kundu T, editor. *Advanced Nondestructive Evaluation for Structural and Biological Health Monitoring*. Volume 4335, Proceedings of SPIE. 2001. p 254–269.

Kessler LW. VHF ultrasonic attenuation in mammalian tissue. J Acoust Soc Am 1973;53:1759–1760.

Kessler LW. Imaging with dynamic ripple diffraction. Acoust Imaging 1976;16:229–239.

Kippenberger S, Bernd A, Loitsch S, Guschel M, Müller J, Bereiter-Hahn J, Kaufmann R. Signaling of mechanical stretch in human keratinocytes via MAP kinases. J Invest Dermatol 2000;114:408–412.

Kolodney M, Elson E. Contraction due to microtubule disruption is associated with increased phosphorylation of myosin regulatory light chain. Proc Natl Acad Sci USA 1995;92:10252–10256.

Kopycinska-Müller M, Reinstädtler M, Rabe U, Caron A, Hirsekorn S, Arnold W. Ultrasonic modes in atomic force microscopy. In: Arnold W, Hirsekorn S, editors. *Acoustical Imaging*. Volume 27, 2004. p 699–706.

Korpel A, Kessler LW, Palermo PR. Acoustic microscope operating at 100 MHz. Nature 1970;232(5306): 110–111.

Kulik PR, Satish S, Gremaud G. Continuous wave transmission measuring scanning acoustic microscope. Acoust Microsc 1992;19:697–701.

Kundu B, Bereiter-Hahn J, Karl I. Cell property determination from the acoustic microscope generated voltage versus frequency curves. Biophys J 2000;78(5):2270–2279.

Kundu T. *Ultrasonic Nondestructive Evaluation: Engineering and Biological Material Characterization*. Boca Raton: CRC Press; 2004. p 872.

Kundu T, Bereiter-Hahn J, Hillmann K. Measuring elastic properties of cells by evaluation of scanning acoustic microscopy V(z) values using simplex algorithm. Biophys J 1991;59:1194–1207.

Kundu T, Lee J, Blasé C, Bereiter-Hahn J. Acoustic microscope lens modeling and its application in determining biological cell properties from single- and multi-layered cell models. J Acoust Soc Am 2006;120(3):1646–1654.

Laugier P, Padilla F, Peyrin F, Raum K, Saied A, Talmant M, Vico L. Apport des ultrasons dans l'exploration du tissue osseux. Current trends in the ultrasonic investigation of bone. ITBM-RBM 2005;26:299–311.

Lemons RA, Quate CF. Acoustic microscope-scanning version. Appl Phys Lett 1974;24:163–165.

Lemor RM, Pilarczyk G, Weiss EC, Westphal I. Combination of acoustic and optical microscopy for investigation of biological cell properties. In: Arnold W, Hirsekorn S,editors. *Acoustical Imaging*. Volume 27, 2004. p 563–572.

Litniewski J, Bereiter-Hahn J. Measurements of cells in culture by scanning acoustic microscopy. J Microsc 1990;158:95–107.

Litniewski J, Bereiter-Hahn J. Acoustic velocity determination in cytoplasm by V(z) shift. Acoust Imaging 1992;19:535–544.

Litniewski J, Nowicki A, Lewin PA. Semi-empirical bone model for determination of trabecular structure properties from backscattered ultrasound. Ultrasonics 2009;49:505–513.

Liu Y, Kon T, Li C, Zhong P. High intensity focused ultrasound-induced gene activation in sublethally injured tumor cells in vitro. J Acoust Soc Am 2005;118:3328–3336.

Lüers H, Hillmann K, Litniewski J, Bereiter-Hahn J. Acoustic microscopy of cultured cells: Distribution of forces and cytoskeletal elements. Cell Biophys 1992;18:279–293.

Lyall F, El Haj AJ. *Biomechanics and Cells*. Society for Experimental Biology Seminar Series 54. Cambridge, New York and Melbourne: Cambridge University Press; 1994. p 275.

Maev RG, Levin VM. Principles of local sound velocity and attenuation measurements using transmission acoustic microscope. IEEE Trans Ultrason Ferroelectr Freq Control 1997;44:1224–1231.

Maev RG, Denisova LA, Maeva EY, Denisov AA. New data on histology and physico-mechanical properties of human tooth obtained with acoustic microscopy. Ultrason Med Biol 2002;28:131–136.

Maia JM, Costa ET, Button VLSN, Neto JFM. An ultrasound system for the diagnosis of osteoporosis. Acoust Imaging 2002;26:77–83.

Marutyan KR, Yang M, Baldwin SL, Wallace KD, Holland MR, Miller JG. The frequency dependence of ultrasonic velocity and anisotropy of dispersion in both freshly excised and formalin-fixed myocardium. J Ultrasound Med Biol 2006;32:603–610.

Masugata H, Mizushige K, Senda S, Lu X, Kinoshita A, Sakamoto H, Nozaki S, Sakamoto S, Matsuo H. Evaluation of left atrial wall elasticity using acoustic microscopy. Angiology 1999;50(7):583–590.

Meunier A, Katz JL, Christel P, Sedel L. A reflection scanning acoustic microscope for bone and bone-biomaterials interface studies. J Orthop Res 1988;6:770–775.

Miyasaka M, Sakai S, Kusaka A, Endo Y, Kobayashi M, Kobayashi K, Hozumi N, Tanino R. Ultrasonic tissue characterization of photodamaged skin by scanning acoustic microscopy. Tokai J Exp Clin Med 2005;30:217–225.

O'Brien PD, O'Brien WD Jr., Rhyne TL, Warltier DC, Sagar KB. Relation of ultrasonic backscatter and acoustic propagation properties to myofibrillar length and myocardial thickness. Circulation 1995a;91:171–175.

O'Brien WD Jr, Sagar KB, Warltier DC, Rhyne TL. Acoustic propagation properties of normal, stunned, and infarcted myocardium. Circulation 1995b;91:154–160.

Okawai H, Tanaka M, Dunn F, Chubachi N, Honda K. Quantitative display of acoustic properties of the biological tissue elements. Acoust Imaging 1988;17:193–201.

Parker KJ, Lerner RM, Waag RC. Attentuation of ultrasound: magnitude and frequency dependence for tissue characterization. Radiology 1984; 153:785–788.

Paschalis EP, Shane E, Lyritis G, Skarantavos G, Mendelsohn R, Boskey AL. Bone fragility and collagen cross-links. J Bone Miner Res 2004;19:2000–2004.

Peck SD, Briggs GAD. The caries lesion under the scanning acoustic microscope. Adv Dent Res 1987;1 50–63.

Pluta M, Grill W. Phase sensitive acoustic microscopy image quality estimation by volume imaging in anisotropic media. Acoust Imaging 2002;26:213–221.

Postema M, van Wamel A, Lancée CT, de Jong N. Ultrasound-induced encapsulated microbubble phenomena. Ultrasound Med Biol 2004;30:827–840.

Rabe U, Kopycinska M, Hirsekorn S, Arnold W. Evaluation of the contact resonance frequencies in atomic force microscopy as a method for surface characterisation (invited). Ultrasonics 2002;40 49–54.

Raum K, Jenderka KV, Klemenz A, Brandt J. Multilayer analysis: quantitative scanning acoustic microscopy for tissue characterization at a microscopic scale. IEEE Trans Ultrason Ferroelectr Freq Control 2003a;50:507–516.

Raum K, Brandt J. Simultaneous determination of acoustic impedance, longitudinal and lateral wave velocities for the characterization of the elastic microstructure of cortical bone. Proc World Congress Ultrasound (Paris) 2003b;31:321–324.

Raum K, Reisshauer J, Brandt J. Frequency and resolution dependence of the anisotropic impedance estimation in cortical bone using time-resolved scanning acoustic microscopy. J Biomed Mater Res A 2004;71:430–438.

Raum K. Ultrasonic characterization of hard tissues. In: Kundu T, editor. *1994 Ultrasonic Nondestructive Evaluation: Engineering and Biological Material Characterization*. Boca Raton: CRC Press; 2004. p 761–782.

Raum K. Microeleastic imaging of bone. IEEE Trans Ultrason Ferroelectr Freq Control 2008;55:1417–1431.

Raum K, Leguerney I, Chandelier F, Bossy F, Talmant M, Saied A, Peyrin F, Laugier P. Bone microstructure and elastic tissue properties are reflected in AUS axial transmission measurements. Ultrasound Med Biol 2005;31:1225–1235.

Raum K, Leguerney I, Chandelier F, Talmant M, Saied A, Peyrin F, Laugier P. Site-matched assessment of structural and tissue properties of cortical bone using scanning acoustic microscopy and synchroton radiation μCT. Phys Med Biol 2006a;51:733–746.

Raum K, Cleveland RO, Peyrin F, Laugier P. Derivation of elastic stiffness from site-matched mineral density and acoustic impedance maps Phys Med Biol 2006b;51:747–758.

Raum K, Hofmann T, Leguerney I, Saied A, Peyrin F, Vico L, Laugier P. Variations of microstructure, mineral density and tissue elasticity in B6/C3H mice. Bone 2006c;44S: e1307–e1311.

Raum K, Kempf K, Hein HJ, Schubert J, Maurer P. Preservation of microelastic properties of dentin and tooth enamel in vitro—a scanning acoustic microscopy study. J Dental Mat 2006d. doi:10.1016/j.dental.2006.11.00F.

Recchia D, Sharkey AM, Bosner MS, Kouchoukos NT, Wickline SA. Sensitive Detection of abnormal aortic architecture in Marfan syndrome with high-frequency tissue characterization. Circulation 1995;91:1036–1043.

Rudd EP, Müller RK, Robbins WP, Skaar T, Soumekh B, Zhou ZQ. Scanning laser acoustic microscope with digital data acquisition. Rev Sci Instrum 1987;58(1):45–53.

Sackmann E. Viscoelasticity, rheology and molecular conformational dynamics of entangled and cross-linked actin networks. In: Isenberg G, editor. *Modern Optics, Electronics, and High Precision Techniques in Cell Biology*. New York: Springer Verlag Berlin; 1997. p 211–258.

Saijo Y. Ultrasonic measurement of micro-acoustic properties of the biological soft materials. In: Kundu T, editor. *Ultrasonic Nondestructive Evaluation: Engineering and Biological Material Characterization*. Boca Raton: CRC Press; 2004. p 783–827.

Saijo Y, Hozumi N, Lee C, Nagao M, Kobayashi K, Oakada N, Tanaka N, dos Santos Filho E, Sasaki H, Tanaka M, Yambe T. Ultrasonic speed microscopy for imaging coronary artery. Ultrasonics 2006;44(1 Suppl): e51–e55.

Saijo Y, Jorgensen C, Mondek P, Sefranek V, Paaske W. Acoustic inhomogeneity of carotid arterial plaques determined by GHz frequency range acoustic microscopy. Ultrasound Med Biol 2002;28: 933.

Saijo Y, Miyakawa T, Sasaki H, Tanaka M, Nitta SI. Acoustic properties of aortic aneurysm obtained with scanning acoustic microscopy. Ultrasonics 2004;42:695–698.

Saijo Y, Ohashi T, Sasaki H, Sato M, Jorgensen CS, Nitta SI. Application of scanning acoustic microscopy for assessing stress distribution in atherosclerotic plaque. Ann Biomed Eng 2001;29:1048–1053.

Saijo Y, Sasaki H, Okawi H, Tanaka M. Development of ultrasonic spectroscopy for biomedical use. Acoust Imaging 1996;22:335–340.

Sasaki H, Saijo Y, Okawai H, Terasawa Y, Nitta S-I, Tanaka M. Acoustic properties of renal cell carcinoma tissues. Acoust Imaging 1996;22:185–190.

Sasaki H, Saijo Y, Tanaka M, Nitta SI. Influence of tissue preparation on the acoustic properties of tissue sections at high frequencies. Ultrasound Med Biol 2003;29:1367–1372.

Schoenenberger CA, Müller DJ, Engel A. Atomic force microscopy provides molecular details of cell surfaces. In: Isenberg G editor. *Modern Optics, Electronics, and High Precision Techniques in Cell Biology*. New York: Springer Verlag Berlin; 1997. p 1–32.

Sokolov S. The ultrasonic microscope. Akad Nauk SSSR, Dokl 1949;64:333–345.

van der Steen AFW, Cuypers MHM, Thijssen JM, Ebben GPJ, de Wilde PCM. Preparation techniques in acoustical and optical microscopy of biological tissues, a study at 5MHz and at 1.2GHz. Acoust Imaging 1992;19:529–533.

van der Steen AFW, Cuypers MHM, Thijssen JM, de Wilde PCM. Influence of histochemical preparation on acoustic parameters of liver tissue, a 5MHz study. Ultrasound Med Biol 1991;17:879–891.

Turner CH, Rho J, Takano Y, Tsui TY, Pharr GM. The elastic properties of trabecular and cortical bone tissues are similar: results from two microscopic measurement techniques. J Biomech 1999;32:437–441.

Vesely P, Lüers H, Riehle M, Bereiter-Hahn J. Subtraction scanning acoustic microscopy reveals motility domains in cells in vitro. Cell Motil Cytoskelton 1994;29:231–240.

van Wamel A, Kooiman K, Harteveld M, Emmer M, ten Cate FJ, Verluis M, de Jong N. Vibrating microbubbles poking individual cells: drug transfer into cells via sonoporation. J Control Release 2006;112:149–155.

Wagner O, Schuler H, Hofmann P, Langer D, Dancker P, Bereiter-Hahn J. Sound attenuation of polymerizing actin reflects supramolecular structures: viscoelastic properties of actin gels modified by cytochalasin, profilin and alpha-actinin. Biochem J 2001;355:771–778.

Wagner O, Zinke J, Dancker P, Grill W, Bereiter-Hahn J. Viscoelastic properties of f-actin, microtubules, f-actin/a-actinin and f-actin/hexokinase determined in microliter volumes with a novel non-invasive method. Biophys J 1999;76(5):2784–2796.

Wang XB, Liu QH, Wang P, Wang ZZ, Tong WY, Zhu B, Wang Y, Li CD. Comparisons among sensitivities of different tumor cells to focused ultrasound in vitro. Ultrasonics 2009;49:558–564.

Weise W, Zinin P, Boseck S. Modelling of inclined and curved surfaces in the acoustic microscope. J Microsc 1994;176:245–253.

Yu Z, Boseck S. Inversion of V(z) data in the scanning acoustic microscope (SAM) to determine material properties of a layered solid. Acoust Imaging 1992;19:617–622.

Ziemann F, Radler J, Sackmann E. Local measurements of viscoelastic moduli of entangled actin networks using an oscillating magnetic bead micro-rheometer. Biophys J 1994;66:2210–2216.

Zoller J, Brändle K, Bereiter-Hahn J. Cellular motility in vitro as revealed by scanning acoustic microscopy depends on cell-cell contacts. Cell Tissue Res 1997;290:43–50.

INDEX

Biomedical Imaging: Principles and Applications, First Edition. Edited by Reiner Salzer.